COMPLEX CARBOHYDRATES IN FOODS

FOOD SCIENCE AND TECHNOLOGY

A Series of Monographs, Textbooks, and Reference Books

1. Flavor Research: Principles and Techniques, *R. Teranishi, I. Hornstein, P. Issenberg, and E. L. Wick*
2. Principles of Enzymology for the Food Sciences, *John R. Whitaker*
3. Low-Temperature Preservation of Foods and Living Matter, *Owen R. Fennema, William D. Powrie, and Elmer H. Marth*
4. Principles of Food Science
   Part I: Food Chemistry, *edited by Owen R. Fennema*
   Part II: Physical Methods of Food Preservation, *Marcus Karel, Owen R. Fennema, and Daryl B. Lund*
5. Food Emulsions, *edited by Stig E. Friberg*
6. Nutritional and Safety Aspects of Food Processing, *edited by Steven R. Tannenbaum*
7. Flavor Research: Recent Advances, *edited by R. Teranishi, Robert A. Flath, and Hiroshi Sugisawa*
8. Computer-Aided Techniques in Food Technology, *edited by Israel Saguy*
9. Handbook of Tropical Foods, *edited by Harvey T. Chan*
10. Antimicrobials in Foods, *edited by Alfred Larry Branen and P. Michael Davidson*
11. Food Constituents and Food Residues: Their Chromatographic Determination, *edited by James F. Lawrence*
12. Aspartame: Physiology and Biochemistry, *edited by Lewis D. Stegink and L. J. Filer, Jr.*
13. Handbook of Vitamins: Nutritional, Biochemical, and Clinical Aspects, *edited by Lawrence J. Machlin*
14. Starch Conversion Technology, *edited by G. M. A. van Beynum and J. A. Roels*
15. Food Chemistry: Second Edition, Revised and Expanded, *edited by Owen R. Fennema*

16. Sensory Evaluation of Food: Statistical Methods and Procedures, *Michael O'Mahony*
17. Alternative Sweetners, *edited by Lyn O'Brien Nabors and Robert C. Gelardi*
18. Citrus Fruits and Their Products: Analysis and Technology, *S. V. Ting and Russell L. Rouseff*
19. Engineering Properties of Foods, *edited by M. A. Rao and S. S. H. Rizvi*
20. Umami: A Basic Taste, *edited by Yojiro Kawamura and Morley R. Kare*
21. Food Biotechnology, *edited by Dietrich Knorr*
22. Food Texture: Instrumental and Sensory Measurement, *edited by Howard R. Moskowitz*
23. Seafoods and Fish Oils in Human Health and Disease, *John E. Kinsella*
24. Postharvest Physiology of Vegetables, *edited by J. Weichmann*
25. Handbook of Dietary Fiber: An Applied Approach, *Mark L. Dreher*
26. Food Toxicology, Parts A and B, *Jose M. Concon*
27. Modern Carbohydrate Chemistry, *Roger W. Binkley*
28. Trace Minerals in Foods, *edited by Kenneth T. Smith*
29. Protein Quality and the Effects of Processing, *edited by R. Dixon Phillips and John W. Finley*
30. Adulteration of Fruit Juice Beverages, *edited by Steven Nagy, John A. Attaway, and Martha E. Rhodes*
31. Foodborne Bacterial Pathogens, *edited by Michael P. Doyle*
32. Legumes: Chemistry, Technology, and Human Nutrition, *edited by Ruth H. Matthews*
33. Industrialization of Indigenous Fermented Foods, *edited by Keith H. Steinkraus*
34. International Food Regulation Handbook: Policy • Science • Law, *edited by Roger D. Middlekauff and Philippe Shubik*
35. Food Additives, *edited by A. Larry Branen, P. Michael Davidson, and Seppo Salminen*
36. Safety of Irradiated Foods, *J. F. Diehl*
37. Omega-3 Fatty Acids in Health and Disease, *edited by Robert S. Lees and Marcus Karel*
38. Food Emulsions: Second Edition, Revised and Expanded, *edited by Kåre Larsson and Stig E. Friberg*
39. Seafood: Effects of Technology on Nutrition, *George M. Pigott and Barbee W. Tucker*
40. Handbook of Vitamins: Second Edition, Revised and Expanded, *edited by Lawrence J. Machlin*
41. Handbook of Cereal Science and Technology, *Klaus J. Lorenz and Karel Kulp*
42. Food Processing Operations and Scale-Up, *Kenneth J. Valentas, Leon Levine, and J. Peter Clark*
43. Fish Quality Control by Computer Vision, *edited by L. F. Pau and R. Olafsson*

44. Volatile Compounds in Foods and Beverages, *edited by Henk Maarse*
45. Instrumental Methods for Quality Assurance in Foods, *edited by Daniel Y. C. Fung and Richard F. Matthews*
46. Listeria, Listeriosis, and Food Safety, *Elliot T. Ryser and Elmer H. Marth*
47. Acesulfame-K, *edited by D. G. Mayer and F. H. Kemper*
48. Alternative Sweeteners: Second Edition, Revised and Expanded, *edited by Lyn O'Brien Nabors and Robert C. Gelardi*
49. Food Extrusion Science and Technology, *edited by Jozef L. Kokini, Chi-Tang Ho, and Mukund V. Karwe*
50. Surimi Technology, *edited by Tyre C. Lanier and Chong M. Lee*
51. Handbook of Food Engineering, *edited by Dennis R. Heldman and Daryl B. Lund*
52. Food Analysis by HPLC, *edited by Leo M. L. Nollet*
53. Fatty Acids in Foods and Their Health Implications, *edited by Ching Kuang Chow*
54. *Clostridium botulinum*: Ecology and Control in Foods, *edited by Andreas H. W. Hauschild and Karen L. Dodds*
55. Cereals in Breadmaking: A Molecular Colloidal Approach, *Ann-Charlotte Eliasson and Kåre Larsson*
56. Low-Calorie Foods Handbook, *edited by Aaron M. Altschul*
57. Antimicrobials in Foods: Second Edition, Revised and Expanded, *edited by P. Michael Davidson and Alfred Larry Branen*
58. Lactic Acid Bacteria, *edited by Seppo Salminen and Atte von Wright*
59. Rice Science and Technology, *edited by Wayne E. Marshall and James I. Wadsworth*
60. Food Biosensor Analysis, *edited by Gabriele Wagner and George G. Guilbault*
61. Principles of Enzymology for the Food Sciences: Second Edition, *John R. Whitaker*
62. Carbohydrate Polyesters as Fat Substitutes, *edited by Casimir C. Akoh and Barry G. Swanson*
63. Engineering Properties of Foods: Second Edition, Revised and Expanded, *edited by M. A. Rao and S. S. H. Rizvi*
64. Handbook of Brewing, *edited by William A. Hardwick*
65. Analyzing Food for Nutrition Labeling and Hazardous Contaminants, *edited by Ike J. Jeon and William G. Ikins*
66. Ingredient Interactions: Effects on Food Quality, *edited by Anilkumar G. Gaonkar*
67. Food Polysaccharides and Their Applications, *edited by Alistair M. Stephen*
68. Safety of Irradiated Foods: Second Edition, Revised and Expanded, *J. F. Diehl*
69. Nutrition Labeling Handbook, *edited by Ralph Shapiro*
70. Handbook of Fruit Science and Technology: Production, Composition, Storage, and Processing, *edited by D. K. Salunkhe and S. S. Kadam*

71. Food Antioxidants: Technological, Toxicological, and Health Perspectives, *edited by D. L. Madhavi, S. S. Deshpande, and D. K. Salunkhe*
72. Freezing Effects on Food Quality, *edited by Lester E. Jeremiah*
73. Handbook of Indigenous Fermented Foods: Second Edition, Revised and Expanded, *edited by Keith H. Steinkraus*
74. Carbohydrates in Food, *edited by Ann-Charlotte Eliasson*
75. Baked Goods Freshness: Technology, Evaluation, and Inhibition of Staling, *edited by Ronald E. Hebeda and Henry F. Zobel*
76. Food Chemistry: Third Edition, *edited by Owen R. Fennema*
77. Handbook of Food Analysis: Volumes 1 and 2, *edited by Leo M. L. Nollet*
78. Computerized Control Systems in the Food Industry, *edited by Gauri S. Mittal*
79. Techniques for Analyzing Food Aroma, *edited by Ray Marsili*
80. Food Proteins and Their Applications, *edited by Srinivasan Damodaran and Alain Paraf*
81. Food Emulsions: Third Edition, Revised and Expanded, *edited by Stig E. Friberg and Kåre Larsson*
82. Nonthermal Preservation of Foods, *Gustavo V. Barbosa-Cánovas, Usha R. Pothakamury, Enrique Palou, and Barry G. Swanson*
83. Milk and Dairy Product Technology, *Edgar Spreer*
84. Applied Dairy Microbiology, *edited by Elmer H. Marth and James L. Steele*
85. Lactic Acid Bacteria: Microbiology and Functional Aspects: Second Edition, Revised and Expanded, *edited by Seppo Salminen and Atte von Wright*
86. Handbook of Vegetable Science and Technology: Production, Composition, Storage, and Processing, *edited by D. K. Salunkhe and S. S. Kadam*
87. Polysaccharide Association Structures in Food, *edited by Reginald H. Walter*
88. Food Lipids: Chemistry, Nutrition, and Biotechnology, *edited by Casimir C. Akoh and David B. Min*
89. Spice Science and Technology, *Kenji Hirasa and Mitsuo Takemasa*
90. Dairy Technology: Principles of Milk Properties and Processes, *P. Walstra, T. J. Geurts, A. Noomen, A. Jellema, and M. A. J. S. van Boekel*
91. Coloring of Food, Drugs, and Cosmetics, *Gisbert Otterstätter*
92. *Listeria*, Listeriosis, and Food Safety: Second Edition, Revised and Expanded, *edited by Elliot T. Ryser and Elmer H. Marth*
93. Complex Carbohydrates in Foods, *edited by Susan Sungsoo Cho, Leon Prosky, and Mark Dreher*
94. Handbook of Food Preservation, *edited by M. Shafiur Rahman*

Additional Volumes in Preparation

Food Safety: Science, International Regulation, and Control, *edited by C. A. van der Heijden, Sanford Miller, Maged Younes, and Lawrence Fishbein*

Fatty Acids and Their Health Implications: Second Edition, Revised and Expanded, *edited by Ching Kuang Chow*

COMPLEX CARBOHYDRATES IN FOODS

edited by

SUSAN SUNGSOO CHO
The Kellogg Company, Battle Creek, Michigan

LEON PROSKY
Prosky Associates, Rockville, Maryland

MARK DREHER
Nabisco, Inc., East Hanover, New Jersey

MARCEL DEKKER, INC. NEW YORK • BASEL

ISBN: 0-8247-0187-9

This book is printed on acid-free paper.

Headquarters
Marcel Dekker, Inc.
270 Madison Avenue, New York, NY 10016
tel: 212-696-9000; fax: 212-685-4540

Eastern Hemisphere Distribution
Marcel Dekker AG
Hutgasse 4, Postfach 812, CH-4001 Basel, Switzerland
tel: 44-61-261-8482; fax: 44-61-261-8896

World Wide Web
http://www.dekker.com

The publisher offers discounts on this book when ordered in bulk quantities. For more information, write to Special Sales/Professional Marketing at the headquarters address above.

Current printing (last digit):
10 9 8 7 6 5 4 3 2

PRINTED IN THE UNITED STATES OF AMERICA

Preface

To establish the effect that any nutrient has on human physiology takes years of research, punctuated by ongoing scientific debate. The task of determining what benefits can be derived from eating complex carbohydrates is no less rigorous. The term "complex carbohydrates" became popular in February of 1977, when the U.S. Senate Committee on Human Needs and Nutrition loosely indicated it as available starch. In their report, the committee encouraged liberal consumption of complex carbohydrates to achieve better health. In 1991 the U.S. Food and Drug Administration (FDA) proposed listing its quantities on food labels (as starches and any dextrins of 10 or more saccharide units). However, when the final regulations were issued in 1993, complex carbohydrates were not included in the labeling guidelines. During the 2-year interim, the FDA and U.S. Department of Agriculture (USDA) had concluded that although increased consumption of complex carbohydrates was desirable, neither a specific definition of nor a methodology for analyzing complex carbohydrates was clearly enough established to commence the labeling. The 1995 USDA dietary guidelines continued to recommend diets high in complex carbohydrates (defined as starch and dietary fiber). Yet the tool that would ultimately inform consumers about the levels of complex carbohydrates in their food (the nutrition label) still does not exist.

Because less conflict occurred in defining "dietary fiber," an analytical methodology was developed, validated, and has been now used in nutrition labeling since the 1980s. Labeling for complex carbohydrates, on the other hand, has not yet achieved its place in consumer nutrition education.

As with any scientific issue that results in debate and public policy, each idea and method about how to define and analyze complex carbohydrates has its supporters, detractors, and those whose opinions vacillate (sometimes frequently). Current efforts to educate the public about the health benefits of complex carbohydrates through publicity and food labeling continue to be offset, in part, by individuals and groups who want the term discontinued. Such arguments are similar to ones heard in the course of creating a methodology and labeling system for dietary fiber, although there was more universal agreement.

In 1990, after initially supporting the term ''dietary fiber,'' members of a task force from the British Nutrition Foundation decided that they wanted instead to make the term obsolete in scientific literature. They wanted to refer to just a portion of dietary fiber, the entity ''non-starch polysaccharides.'' However, their position was not accepted among international scientists and the term dietary fiber prevailed. Today, it is accepted and used even by members of the task force. Books and research continue to focus on dietary fiber and reinforce the importance of a liberal dietary fiber intake. One need only look at the number of workshops and symposia to realize that the term and its definition will continue to form the base of discussions for years to come.

Mirroring this earlier debate over dietary fiber, a small but vocal number of scientists want the term ''complex carbohydrates'' to be discontinued. These scientists are suggesting that because of unresolved differences of opinion on small details regarding the makeup of complex carbohydrates, we should throw out the term and ignore the important strides that have been made in understanding this important component of our diet. However, the majority of scientists working in the field support a continued effort in researching analytical methodologies and physiological effects even though the definition of complex carbohydrates remains loose. The term ''dietary fiber'' returned to routine use after years of debate. We predict that over the next few years the term ''complex carbohydrates'' will also return on food labels as consensus over its definition continues to be accepted.

As with any developing research, informed scientists must continue to speak out about their findings and pursue answers to questions of analytical methods and physiological impact. Unlike marketing or advertising careers where professionals must keep pace with fads, most scientists and nutritionists have the opportunity to stick with a subject until key issues are resolved and results show that their work will either benefit mankind or must be set aside because it has little or no value. The public understands how important complex carbohydrates are. Health recommendations made by government agencies as well as those of health and nutrition professionals have been pivotal in establishing this awareness.

The editors of this book seek to bring the issues that have been raised for adding complex carbohydrates to the nutrition label closer to a solution. They have also sought to bring health benefits and applications of complex carbohydrates to new food products development. This book includes international patent activities on the use of complex carbohydrates (starch gums and dietary fiber) in low fat and low calorie food products development as well as food content of dietary fiber and carbohydrates. In all, it is hoped that a valuable view of the current literature, practices, and prespectives is presented.

Susan Sungsoo Cho
Leon Prosky
Mark Dreher

Contents

Preface *iii*
Contributors *xi*

1. Introduction 1
   Susan Sungsoo Cho, Leon Prosky, and Jonathan W. Devries

Part I: Health Benefits and Definition of Complex Carbohydrates and Dietary Fiber **5**

2. Dietary Guidelines for Complex Carbohydrates/Dietary Fiber 7
   Joanne L. Slavin

3. Complex Carbohydrates and the Food Label: An FDA Perspective 15
   F. Edward Scarbrough

4. Dietary Fiber Properties and Health Benefits of Non-Digestible Oligosaccharides 25
   M. B. Roberfroid

5. Suggested Alternatives to the Term ''Complex Carbohydrates'' 35
   F. W. Scott, R. Mongeau, and P. Wood

6. Complex Carbohydrates: The Science and the Label 39
David R. Lineback, Mark Dreher, Jonathan W. Devries, Joanne L. Slavin, Alison Stephen, Dennis Gordon, Leon Prosky, F. Edward Scarbrough, Gary Henderson, Susan Sungsoo Cho, Beth Olson, and Fergus Clydesdale

7. The Role of Dietary Fiber in the Prevention of Lipid Metabolism Disorders 53
Elzbieta Bartnikowska

8. Health Benefits of Complex Carbohydrates 63
David Kritchevsky

9. Worldwide Dietary Fiber Intake: Recommendations and Actual Consumption Patterns 71
Susan Sungsoo Cho, K. O'Sullivan, and Sharon Rickard

Part II: Complex Carbohydrates—Chemistry and Analytical Methodology 113

10. The Chemistry of Complex Carbohydrates 115
David R. Lineback

11. Complex Carbohydrates: Definition and Analysis 131
Susan Sungsoo Cho and Leon Prosky

12. Determination of Complex Carbohydrate Fractions in Foods 145
Betty W. Li

Part III: Resistant Starch—Analysis 155

13. In Vivo Techniques to Quantify Resistant Starch 157
M. Champ, L. Martin, L. Noah, and M. Gratas

14. Analytical Methods for Resistant Starch 169
M. Champ, L. Martin, L. Noah, and M. Gratas

Part IV: Resistant Oligosaccharides—Analytical Methodology 189

15. A Sensitive and Reproducible Analytical Method to Measure Fructooligosaccharides in Food Products 191
F. Ouarne, A. Guibert, D. Brown, and F. Bornet

16. Inulin and Oligofructose as Dietary Fiber: Analytical, Nutritional and Legal Aspects 203
Paul Coussement

17. Determination of Inulin and Oligofructose in Food Products (Modified AOAC Dietary Fiber Method) 213
P. Dysseler, D. Hoffem, J. Fockedey, B. Quemener, J.-F. Thibault, and Paul Coussement

18. Polydextrose as Soluble Fiber and Complex Carbohydrate 229
S. A. S. Craig, J. F. Holden, J. P. Troup, M. H. Auerbach, and H. Frier

Part V: Dietary Fiber—Analytical Methodology 249

19. Progress in the Certification of Five New Food Reference Materials by AOAC, Englyst and Uppsala Methods of Dietary Fiber Analysis 251
Alan W. Pendlington

20. High Performance Anion Exchange Chromatography with Pulsed Amperometric Detection (HPAE-PAD): A Powerful Tool for the Analysis of Dietary Fiber and Complex Carbohydrates 267
Alan Henshall

21. NIR Analysis of Dietary Fiber 291
Sandra E. Kays, Franklin E. Barton II, and William R. Windham

22. Definition and Analysis of Dietary Fiber 305
R. Mongeau, F. W. Scott, and R. Brassard

23. Estimation of Psyllium Content in Ready-to-Eat Cereals 317
Susan Sungsoo Cho and Mike Bussey

24. Food Sources and Uses of Dietary Fiber 327
Mark Dreher

25. Chemical and Physical Modifications of Dietary Fiber 373
Mary Ellen Camire

26. Production of Resistant Starch 385
Pierre Würsch

27. Effect of Processing on Dietary Fiber in Foods 395
Eckhard Rabe

28. Application of Complex Carbohydrates to Food Product Fat Mimetics 411
Susan Sungsoo Cho and Leon Prosky

29. Patent Literature Review on Complex Carbohydrates as Fat Mimetics 431
Susan Sungsoo Cho

30. The Application of Complex Carbohydrates to Functional Food Development 593
Susan Sungsoo Cho and M. Jenab

Appendix I Perspectives on Dietary Fiber Definition 605
Appendix II Total Carbohydrates and Total Dietary Fiber Content in Grain-Based Foods 609
Index 661

Contributors

M. H. Auerbach H. I. Cultor Food Science, Groton, Connecticut

Elzbieta Bartnikowska Warsaw Agricultural University, Warsaw, Poland

Franklin E. Barton II Richard B. Russell Agricultural Research Center, Agricultural Research Service, U.S. Department of Agriculture, Athens, Georgia

F. Bornet Eridania Béghin-Say, Vilvoorde Research and Development Centre, Vilvoorde, Belgium

R. Brassard Food Directorate, Nutrition Research Division, Banting Research Centre, Ottawa, Ontario, Canada

D. Brown Golden Technologies Co., Johnstown, Colorado

Mike Bussey The Kellogg Company, Battle Creek, Michigan

Mary Ellen Camire University of Maine, Orono, Maine

M. Champ I.N.R.A., Laboratoire de Technologie Appliqué la Nutrition, Nantes, France

Susan Sungsoo Cho The Kellogg Company, Battle Creek, Michigan

Fergus Clydesdale University of Massachusetts, Amherst, Massachusetts

Paul Coussement ORAFTI, Tienen, Belgium

S. A. S. Craig H. I. Cultor Food Science, Groton, Connecticut

Jonathan W. Devries General Mills, Inc., Minneapolis, Minnesota

Mark Dreher Nabisco, Inc., East Hanover, New Jersey

P. Dysseler Institut Meurice, Brussels, Belgium

J. Fockedey Sucrerie de Warcoing, Pecq-Warcoing, Belgium

H. Frier H. I. Cultor Food Science, Groton, Connecticut

Dennis Gordon North Dakota State University, Fargo, North Dakota

M. Gratas I.N.R.A., Laboratoire de Technologie Appliqué la Nutrition, Nantes, France

A. Guibert Béghin-Say, INSA, Toulouse, France

Gary Henderson Kraft Foods, White Plains, New York

Alan Henshall Dionex Corporation, Sunnyvale, California

D. Hoffem Institut Meurice, Brussels, Belgium

J. F. Holden H. I. Cultor Food Science, Groton, Connecticut

M. Jenab University of Toronto, Toronto, Ontario, Canada

Sandra E. Kays Richard B. Russell Agricultural Research Center, Agricultural Research Service, U.S. Department of Agriculture, Athens, Georgia

David Kritchevsky The Wistar Institute, Philadelphia, Pennsylvania

Betty W. Li Food Composition Laboratory, Beltsville Human Nutrition Research Center, Agricultural Research Service, U.S. Department of Agriculture, Beltsville, Maryland

David R. Lineback College of Agriculture, University of Idaho, Moscow, Idaho

L. Martin I.N.R.A., Laboratoire de Technologie Appliqué la Nutrition, Nantes, France

R. Mongeau Food Directorate, Nutrition Research Division, Banting Research Centre, Ottawa, Ontario, Canada

L. Noah I.N.R.A., Laboratoire de Technologie Appliqué la Nutrition, Nantes, France

K. O'Sullivan The Kellogg Company, Arabic Areas

Beth Olson The Kellogg Company, Battle Creek, Michigan

F. Ouarne Béghin-Say, INSA, Toulouse, France

Alan W. Pendlington RHM Technology Ltd., High Wycombe, Bucks, England

Leon Prosky Prosky Associates, Rockville, Maryland

B. Quemener INRA, Nantes, France

Eckhard Rabe Federal Center for Cereal, Potato and Lipid Research, Detmold, Germany

Sharon Rickard University of Toronto, Toronto, Ontario, Canada

M. B. Roberfroid Département des Sciences Pharmaceutiques, Université Catholique de Louvain, Brussels, Belgium

F. Edward Scarbrough U.S. Food and Drug Administration, Washington, D.C.

F. W. Scott Food Directorate, Nutrition Research Division, Banting Research Centre, Ottawa, Ontario, Canada

Joanne L. Slavin University of Minnesota, St. Paul, Minnesota

Alison Stephen University of Saskatchewan, Saskatoon, Saskatchewan, Canada

J.-F. Thibault INRA, Nantes, France

J. P. Troup H. I. Cultor Food Science, Groton, Connecticut

William R. Windham Richard B. Russell Agricultural Research Center, Agricultural Research Service, U.S. Department of Agriculture, Athens, Georgia

P. Wood Centre for Food and Animal Research, Agriculture and Agri-Food Canada, Ottawa, Ontario, Canada

Pierre Würsch Nestlé Research Centre, Vers-chez-les-Blanc, Switzerland

1

Introduction

Susan Sungsoo Cho
The Kellogg Company, Battle Creek, Michigan
Leon Prosky
Prosky Associates, Rockville, Maryland
Jonathan W. DeVries
General Mills, Inc., Minneapolis, Minnesota

Over the past two decades consumers, health nutrition professionals, and the media have received extensive education about the importance of increasing complex carbohydrates in one's diet. Research linking the consumption of complex carbohydrates and the reduced risk of chronic disease (including cardiovascular diseases and cancers) has been passed on to consumers. Nevertheless, the government has yet to establish regulations that would quantify complex carbohydrates on food packaging labels and help consumers to make educated choices at the supermarket.

The lack of labeling results from an ongoing debate in the scientific community over the definition of complex carbohydrates. This debate has created a rift between the knowledge of nutrition scientists and the general population that they ordinarily serve. In January 1993 the U. S. Food and Drug Administration

(FDA) announced that in spite of general scientific evidence showing that complex carbohydrates were beneficial to human health it could not recommend that they be labeled on food product nutrition panels as part of the of the final Nutrition Labeling and Education Act (NLEA) regulations (1, 2). As its rationale the FDA cited the lack of consensus in the scientific community over the definition of complex carbohydrates. It reported that without a consensual definition no meaningful analysis of complex carbohydrates or labeling could occur.

Between 1990 and 1991 the FDA proposed a definition of complex carbohydrates as total carbohydrates minus sugar minus dietary fiber (3, 4). However, many professional and trade organizations, as well as many industries, reacted in opposition with another proposal that suggested expanding the definition to include dietary fiber or making the same calculation as total carbohydrates minus sugar (1).

Between 1991 and 1996 new steps were taken by this scientific community to expedite an agreement. The Food and Nutrition Methods Committee of the Association of Official Analytical Chemists (AOAC) International arranged three international surveys (one on complex carbohydrates and two on dietary fiber) (5-10). The surveys were conducted by referees (5, 6) who solicited the opinion on the definitions of dietary fiber and complex carbohydrates from professionals in the field.

The results showed that scientists generally defined complex carbohydrates as polysaccharides or starch plus dietary fiber and that they also supported expanding the definition of complex carbohydrates to include dietary fiber (5). The survey indicated interest in including resistant oligosaccharides, non-starch polysaccharides, resistant starches, and lignin in the term dietary fiber. However, more work was needed before agreement could be reached on augmenting the definition of complex carbohydrates with the components of resistant oligosaccharides and lignin.

In September 1995 the AOAC International held a workshop in Nashville, Tennessee. Fifty-seven participants attended from the United States and Europe (8). They represented industry, academia, and government and included the world's foremost authorities on complex carbohydrates. Their discussions focused on the recent international surveys by Lee and Prosky and a workshop that had also deliberated over complex carbohydrate labeling by the International Life Science Institute (ILSI) North American Workshop in Washington, D.C. (9).

During the panel discussion moderator L. Prosky and panelists J. Slavin, D. Gordon, M. Roberfroid, F. Scott, E. Bartnikowska, and R. Wood analyzed the appropriateness and advantages of labeling complex carbohydrates. The discussion centered around how the term "complex carbohydrates" is interpreted by lay persons, scientists, and politicians. In addition, the panel raised the point that certain components (resistant oligosaccharides) were not fully recovered in the dietary fiber fraction prepared by currently available AOAC methods. These resistant oligosaccharides (oligofructans, polydextrose) exert many of the physiological properties of dietary fiber. To improve the recovery of this fraction, they suggested that a new method for determining it be studied under the auspices of the AOAC.

Because of general agreement that dietary fiber should be included in the definition of complex carbohydrates and that resistant oligosaccharides are part of dietary fiber, the panel recommended that a vote be taken to establish a working definition of complex carbohydrates. Twenty-nine participants representing 85% of the 34 who gave definitions of complex carbohydrates agreed that the definition should be the sum of dietary fiber and starch (technically speaking, available or enzyme-available starch). They concurred that for use in labeling complex carbohydrates could be derived either from the sum of analytically measured starch and dietary fiber values or from the calculation of total carbohydrates minus sugar minus available oligosaccharides.

Among the 29 scientists agreeing that the complex carbohydrates definition should be the sum of starch and dietary fiber, 16 (55%) supported labeling analytically derived values (total dietary fiber and available starch) and 13 (45%) felt that values calculated by the difference method would also be acceptable. The panel recommended that the associate referee coordinate a study among different laboratories to validate a methodology. Only 2 participants of the workshop had supported the FDA's 1991 definition of complex carbohydrates as total carbohydrates minus dietary fiber minus simple sugars. Other definitions of complex carbohydrates considered by the workshop participants included the sum of starch and non-starch saccharides (3 votes). No one supported the definition as the sum of starch and non-starch polysaccharides (corresponding to polysaccharides) which received some support in the previous survey. Many showed a strong interest in developing analytical methods for resistant oligosaccharides, and they recommended establishing new associate refereeships in this area.

By the end of the workshop participants unanimously supported including resistant oligosaccharides in dietary fiber and complex carbohydrates definitions and expanding the complex carbohydrates definition to include dietary fiber and available starches. They agreed, too, that the new definition would not include the available oligosaccharides present in candy.

With this understanding complex carbohydrates could be derived as the sum of analytically measured starch and dietary fiber values or as the calculation of total carbohydrates minus sugar minus available oligosaccharides for most nutrition labeling. This complex carbohydrate definition would satisfy both the scientific community and government agencies. It would alleviate the FDA's concern about the possibility of candy producers claiming that their products are a source of complex carbohydrates simply because they contain a significant amount of maltotriose and maltotetrose. This problem might occur if complex carbohydrates values were derived by calculating total carbohydrates minus simple sugar.

Now that a group of scientists has reached a general consensus in defining complex carbohydrates we must collaborate to develop a method that analyzes and validates it. With these decisions made we can move ahead and reactivate research in the areas of nutrition and food technology. It is now possible to develop a common understanding of complex carbohydrates including resistant oligosaccharides, and to study the physiological effects of these nutrients. We want to emphasize that although the new complex carbohydrate definition will change the analytical methodology it will not affect the complex carbohydrate and dietary fiber values for most food products unless they are formulated with ingredients containing resistant oligosaccharides.

REFERENCES

1. Food and Drug Administration. (1993) Food Labeling, General Provisions: Nutrition Labeling: Label Format: Nutrient Content Claims: Ingredient Labeling: State and Local Requirements; and Exemptions: Final Rules. Fed. Register 58:2301–2964.
2. Department of Agriculture. (1993) Food Labeling; General Provisions: Nutrition Labeling: Label Format: Nutrient Content Claims: Ingredient Labeling: State and Local Requirements; and Exemptions: Final Rules. Fed. Register 58:631–691.
3. Department of Health and Human Services. (1990) Food Labeling. Fed. Register 55:29476–29486.
4. Department of Health and Human Services. (1991) Food Labeling; Proposed Rules. Fed. Register. 56:60366–61878.
5. Lee, S.C., and Prosky, L. (1994a) Summary of AOAC International Survey on Complex Carbohydrates. International Life Sciences Institute. North American Workshop on Complex Carbohydrates, Washington, D.C. November 2, 1994.
6. Lee, S.C., and Prosky, L. (1995) International Survey on Dietary Fiber Definition, Analysis, and Reference Materials. J. AOAC Int. 78:22–36.
7. Lee, S.C. and Prosky, L. (1994b) ''Perspectives on New Dietary Fiber Definition.'' Cereal Foods World 39:767–768.
8. Anonymous. (1995a) International Workshop on Complex Carbohydrates Definition. The Referee 19(10):15.
9. Anonymous. (1995b) Special Report: Complex Carbohydrates: The Science and the Label. Nutr. Rev. 53:186–193.
10. Lee, S.C., and Prosky, L. (1996) Perspectives on complex carbohydrates definition. Cereal Foods World, 41:88–89.

I

HEALTH BENEFITS AND DEFINITION OF COMPLEX CARBOHYDRATES AND DIETARY FIBER

2

Dietary Guidelines for Complex Carbohydrates/Dietary Fiber

JOANNE L. SLAVIN
University of Minnesota, St. Paul, Minnesota

INTRODUCTION

Nutrition educators agree consumers should increase intake of complex carbohydrates and dietary fiber, both for the beneficial health effects of these dietary ingredients and as a means to reduce dietary fat intake. Interest in dietary fiber has varied throughout the 20th century, but dietary guidance since the 1970s has consistently recommended increased dietary fiber in our diets. The USDA food pyramid recommends 6-11 servings from the grain group, 3-5 servings from the vegetable group, and 2-4 servings from the fruit group. Dietary Guidelines for Americans support increased intake of starch and dietary fiber in the form of bread, cereal, rice, pasta, and foods from the vegetable and fruit group. The National Research Council in 1989 recommended Americans eat every day five or more servings of a combination of vegetables and fruits, especially green and yellow vegetables and citrus fruits. They also recommend an increase in starches and other complex carbohydrates by eating six or more daily servings of a combination of breads, cereals, and legumes. Specifically, the 1987 FASEB report recommended Americans consume 10-13 grams of dietary fiber per 1,000 kilocalories consumed. Other dietary fiber recommendations have been published and are in the range of 20-35 grams/day.

Although there is general agreement that we should include more dietary fiber and complex carbohydrates in our diet, it is difficult to give specific recommendations for complex carbohydrates because of lack of agreement on definitions and methods. Nutrition labels listing dietary fiber have helped consumers assess their dietary fiber intake and select foods rich in fiber. Consumers are not able to estimate their complex carbohydrate intake and compare it to a nutrition standard.

In the United States, the term complex carbohydrates was used in the McGovern report and included digestible carbohydrates or starch. The British Nutrition Foundation Report included both starch and non-starch polysaccharides as complex carbohydrates. Consumers are familiar with the term complex carbohydrate and need more information on the complex carbohydrate content of foods to follow existing dietary guidance to increase complex carbohydrate intake.

DIETARY GUIDANCE

Since the 1940s scientific bodies have met to discuss nutrition recommendations. Recommended Dietary Allowances (RDAs) have been developed to provide nutrient allowances for the maintenance of good health. These guidelines are most useful to health professionals in planning and evaluating diets. For consumers, more general nutrition education tools have been developed. Food groups, meal plans, or exchange lists are examples of food guides available to help consumers plan and prepare more nutritious meals. These tools have evolved and generally try to meet the need for a simple nutrition education system that still provides the nutritional detail needed.

The U. S. Department of Agriculture (USDA) has published food guides to help Americans choose a healthful diet for almost 100 years (1). A food guide is a conceptual framework for selecting the kinds and amounts of foods of various types that together provide a nutritionally satisfactory diet. Food guides are not dietary standards (such as the Recommended Dietary Allowances or the Dietary Guidelines for Americans) but are translations of these recommendations on nutrient intake into quantities of food that people should eat on a daily basis.

The first food guide was issued in 1916, the Basic Seven in the 1940s, and the Basic Four in the 1950s. In the 1970s the focus of dietary recommendations shifted to concerns about dietary excesses. The release of the Dietary Goals by a U. S. Senate Select Committee on Nutrition and Human Needs in 1977 was a turning point in that quantitative limits were set for the dietary intake of certain food components that were linked to chronic diseases such as heart disease and cancer (2). The Dietary Goals were followed in 1980 by the first edition of Nutrition and Your Health: Dietary Guidelines for Americans, jointly released by USDA and the Department of Health and Human Services (DHHS) (3). The Dietary Guidelines are updated every five years and are currently being re-released (1995).

The USDA Food Guide Pyramid was developed to help people follow the Dietary Guidelines for Americans. The pyramid graphic is designed to emphasize the importance of increased consumption of vegetables, fruits, and grain products for a healthful diet and decreased consumption of fats, sugars, and alcohol.

As reviewed by Truswell (4) there is almost complete agreement on the following six dietary recommendations:

1. Eat a nutritionally adequate diet composed of a variety of foods.
2. Eat less fat, particularly saturated fat.
3. Adjust energy intake for weight control; exercise.
4. Eat more foods containing complex carbohydrates and fiber.
5. Reduce salt intake.
6. Drink alcohol in moderation, if at all.

Other recommendations on specific fats, sugars, cholesterol, and others vary among different dietary guidelines.

DIETARY GUIDANCE FOR CARBOHYDRATES

Dietary guidance for consumption of carbohydrates has resembled laboratory analysis of carbohydrates: take away the fat and protein and the remainder must to be carbohydrate. Nutritionists generally accept the fact that humans don't need more than 10-12% of kilocalories from protein, and less than 30% of kilocalories from fat. Subsequently, intake of carbohydrate should be 55% of kilocalories or more. Human diets historically have contained 40-80% of their energy as carbohydrate (5), although as income increases, so does the fat content of the diet while the carbohydrate content of the diet, especially the starch, decreases.

More specific recommendations for carbohydrate have become more likely in dietary guidance. In the 1980s the number of recommendations for carbohydrate intake increased and these recommendations became more specific. The recommendations generally divide carbohydrate intake into sugars and complex carbohydrates and starch. Sugar recommendations are often divided into naturally occurring sugars and refined sugars, despite the recognition that metabolically differences among sugars are not great. The Dietary Goals for the United States recommended Americans "increase the consumption of complex carbohydrates and naturally occurring sugars from about 28% of energy intake to 48% of energy intake." Such a recommendation would be difficult to follow with the limited information on the complex carbohydrate content of foods.

According to the RDA, 10th edition, of the carbohydrates in individual diets, an average of 41% comes from grain products and 23% comes from fruits and vegetables (6). About half of the total digestible carbohydrate intake is made up of monosaccharides and disaccharides. These are found naturally in fruits and milk and also enter the diet as sugars in soft drinks, candies, jams, and sweet desserts mainly composed of sucrose and high-fructose corn syrup. Complex carbohydrates, which constitute the other half of digestible carbohydrate intake, are starches found predominantly in cereal grains, potatoes, legumes, and a few other vegetables. In 1985 sugars and starches provided an average of 45.3% of the energy in the diet of adult men in the United States. This is less than the levels recommended for overall carbohydrate consumption and disproportionately high in simple sugars.

DIETARY GUIDANCE FOR DIETARY FIBER

Dietary guidance recommendations generally agree that Americans should increase their consumption of dietary fiber. For example, Dietary Guidelines for Americans recommends ". . . choose a diet with plenty of vegetables, fruits, and grain products." Recommended Dietary Allowances, 10th edition, suggests we ". . . achieve a desirable fiber intake by consumption of fruits, vegetables, legumes, and whole-grain cereals." Other general recommendations for increased dietary fiber intake are given in the Surgeon General's Report on Nutrition and Health (7) and Diet and Health, National Research Council, National Academy of Sciences(8).

Specific recommendations for dietary fiber intake are offered by some organizations. In Physiological Effects and Health Consequences of Dietary Fiber, Life Sciences Research Office, Federation of American Societies for Experimental Biology, the recommendation is to consume a wide variety of whole-grain products, fruits, and vegetables, leading to a dietary fiber intake range of 20 to 35 g/day (10-13 g/1000 kcal) for the healthy adult population (9). The American Dietetic Association (ADA) states that ". . . although a recommended dietary allowance for fiber has not been established, the current evidence suggests that high-carbohydrate, low-fat diets containing 20 to 35 grams dietary fiber per day from a variety of food sources may be beneficial for health promotion and disease risk reduction in the healthy adult population of the United States"(10). The ADA note that this recommendation is not appropriate for the pediatric or geriatric populations. Food, not dietary fiber supplements, provides the best means of increasing daily consumption of both soluble and insoluble fiber. The practice of taking fiber supplements to replace consumption of high-carbohydrate, nutrient-dense foods is not supported at this time by any health care authorities as a component of a balanced diet. In 1991 the United Kingdom issued recommendations for dietary fiber that state that ". . . diets should contain an average of 18 g/day (range of 12-24) non-starch polysaccharide (NSP) from a variety of foods whose constituents contain it as a naturally integrated component"(11).

Despite widespread acceptance that dietary fiber intakes are too low and need to be approximately doubled, little progress has been seen in increasing dietary fiber consumption in this country. Dietary fiber intake has been estimated at about 12 grams per day in the United States. A recent study found no increase in dietary fiber consumption despite widespread nutrition education efforts to increase dietary fiber consumption (12). A recent technical report on modeling nutrition intake by the USDA's Economic Research Service found that nutritional education strategies emphasizing general attitudinal messages such as five-a-day intake are likely to have greater effect in modifying dietary patterns than strategies emphasizing specialized knowledge about the nutrient content of foods. Higher intakes of dietary fiber consumption were also linked to years of formal education and consumption of a vegetarian diet.

DIETARY GUIDANCE FOR COMPLEX CARBOHYDRATES

In the U.S. the term complex carbohydrates was used in the McGovern report and included digestible carbohydrates or starch (2). The British Nutrition Foundation Report (13) included both starch and non-starch polysaccharides as complex carbohydrates. The British report defined polysaccharides as carbohydrates with 20 or more sugar residues. The British report stated that there are a variety of foods which are rich in complex carbohydrates and display great diversity in their physical and biological properties. Thus, it is difficult to make generalizations about properties of complex carbohydrates. They also noted that there is more overlap between the behavior and properties of the starches and non-starch polysaccharides than was previously thought.

Resistant starch is probably metabolized similar to some dietary fiber components in the gut. Thus, it appears that complex carbohydrate should contain both dietary fiber and starches and we must recognize that substances (such as phytate, phenolic compounds) and micronutrents (such as zinc and magnesium) are important nutritional components associated with complex carbohydrates. Dietary recommendations to increase intake of complex carbohydrate assume that the carbohydrates are not isolated, but come from intact foods.

Most dietary guidance is offered as a general endorsement of starches and complex carbohydrate to replace dietary fat. For example the U. S. Department of Agriculture food pyramid recommends 6-11 servings from the grain group, 3-5 servings from the vegetable group, and 2-4 servings from the fruit group (1). Such a diet would contain significantly more complex carbohydrate than the typical American diet. Dietary Guidelines for Americans also support increased intake of starch and dietary fiber in the form of bread, cereal, rice, pasta and foods from the vegetable and fruit group (3). The Surgeon General's Report on Nutrition and Health (7) recommends increased consumption of whole grain foods and cereal products, vegetables (including dried beans and peas), and fruits. In 1989 the National Research Council examined the relationship between diet and health and issued new recommendations (8). They recommend that Americans consume five or more servings of a combination of vegetables and fruits (especially green and yellow vegetables and citrus fruits) and increase starches and other complex carbohydrates by eating six or more daily servings of a combination of breads, cereals, and legumes daily.

There is growing acceptance that isolated carbohydrates provide different physiological responses than whole foods. Thus, it is difficult to study complex carbohydrates since they must be fed in their refined state. It is then difficult if not impossible to generalize the results to the unrefined complex carbohydrates fed in their native state. This is compounded further by the fact that many other nutritional ingredients cloud the physiological results of the experiment. If an exciting physiological response is seen with intake of a whole grain high in complex carbohydrate the question arises as to the true origin of the response: is it due to the carbohydrate, a specific component of the carbohydrate or an associated substance such as an antioxidant, phytoestrogen, trace mineral, and so on.

Another important consideration in devising nutrition guidance for carbohydrates is how they are metabolized. As discussed by Hirsch (14), more research is needed on the roles and benefits of carbohydrates in the diet. To determine how carbohydrates fit into dietary guidelines, he suggests we consider three issues:

1. The role of carbohydrate in the control of food intake in humans.
2. The effect of carbohydrate on energy metabolism as measured by long-term feeding experiments in small numbers of human subjects.
3. Whether a large carbohydrate intake leads to increased lipogenesis in humans.

Obviously, these are all important issues when considering the metabolic effects of carbohydrates. But such experiments are costly and dietary recommendations will have to be made before all experiments on these topics have been conducted.

Determining the appropriate metabolic tests to compare complex carbohydrates will also be difficult. Metabolic studies use human subjects and results tend to vary greatly among subjects. If we accept a physiological definition of dietary fiber as complex carbohydrate that escapes digestion in the small intestine, do we measure dietary fiber by gut fermentation? If we are convinced that slow digestion and absorption determines a complex carbohydrate from a simple carbohydrate, do we use glycemic index as the physiological determinant of a complex carbohydrate? As more research is available it may be easier to answer these questions, but meanwhile consumers need the best dietary guidance on complex carbohydrate intake.

Complex carbohydrates also need further definition. Should complex carbohydrates be only long chain (>10 DP) carbohydrates or should shorter carbohydrates that resist digestion in the smaller intestine be included in complex carbohydrates, especially if we accept a physiological definition for complex carbohydrates. If carbohydrates are isolated from non-traditional food sources or are manufactured in laboratory, can they qualify as complex carbohydrates if they act similarly to long chain carbohydrates in the gut? If we as an industry accept a chemical definition for complex carbohydrates it would be difficult to argue that we only accept complex carbohydrates that are in their native state and will not accept chemically altered or manufactured carbohydrates if they meet our chemical definition. If consumers are unwilling or unable to increase consumption of complex carbohydrate and dietary fiber with usual food sources, should we fortify the diet with isolated carbohydrates that have been shown to have the desired physiological effects? The questions are many but need answers if consumers are to be able to select high complex carbohydrate foods that are convenient or if they are to have access to useful data on complex carbohydrate content of foods to help in food selection.

CONCLUSION

Dietary recommendations for complex carbohydrates must be based on a synthesis of epidemiological, metabolic, animal, and mechanistic data (15) and by necessity will be non-specific. The British report notes that for most adults consuming nutritionally adequate diets and increased intake of complex carbohydrates it is unlikely to lead to deficiencies in micronutrents. Further, it appears sensible for adults to increase their intake of a variety of foods that are rich in complex carbohydrates. Obviously a wide range of carbohydrate intake is consistent with health (16) and dietary recommendations for carbohydrate intake will not be based on classical approaches for defining nutrient requirements since there is no clear-cut deficiency disease for carbohydrates.

In the past 25 years, dietary fiber has been defined, methods have been developed, and foods have been analyzed for dietary fiber. As a result, nutrition labels now contain information on the dietary fiber content of food. This information allows consumers to select foods high in dietary fiber and increase the dietary fiber content of their diet. Complex carbohydrates are universally recommended as the base of our diet, but scientific agreement is not available on a definition or a method to measure complex carbohydrate. Like dietary fiber, complex carbohydrate is not a single entity and many issues surround its definition and measurement. Should we accept a chemical or physiological definition, should isolated carbohydrate compounds be included, or should the term be discarded and something better found? Because of the industry's equity position in complex carbohydrates and the universal recommendation to increase consumption of complex carbohydrates, the term should be kept and further efforts exerted to see that it is better defined and measured to be included as part of the nutrition label.

REFERENCES

1. S Welsh, A Shaw, D Davis. Crit. Rev. Food Sci. Nutr. 34:441–451, 1994.
2. Dietary Goals for the United States, Select Committee on Nutrition and Human Needs, US Senate, 2nd ed.: US Government Printing Office, 1977.
3. Nutrition and Your Health: Dietary Guidelines for Americans. 3rd Ed., US Depts of Agriculture and Health and Human Services, Home and Garden Bulletin No. 232, Washington D.C., 1990.
4. AS Truswell. In: ME Shils, JA Olson, M Shike, eds. Modern Nutrition in Health and Disease. vol 2, , Philadelphia, PA: Lea and Febiger, 1994, pp. 1612–1625.
5. N Asp. Am. J. Clin. Nutr. 59S:679S-681S, 1994.
6. Recommended Dietary Allowances, National Academy Press, Washington, D.C., 1989.
7. US Department of Health and Human Services, The Surgeon General's Report on Nutrition and Health, Public Health Service. DHHS (PHS) Publication no. 88-50210, Washington, D.C., 1988.
8. National Research Council, Diet and Health Implication for Reducing Chronic Disease Risk, National Academy Press, Washington, D.C., 1989.
9. S Pilch. Physiological effects and health consequences of dietary fiber, Life Sciences Research Office, Federation of American Societies for Experimental Biology, Bethesda, MD, 1987.
10. Position of the American Dietetic Association: Health implications of dietary fiber, J. Am. Diet. Assoc. 93:1446–1447, 1993.
11. Department of Health: Dietary Reference Values for Food Energy and Nutrients for the United Kingdom. London, HMSO, pp. 61–71, 1991.
12. T Nicklas, R Farris, L Myers, GS Berenson. J. Am. Diet. Assoc. 95, 209–214, 1995.
13. The British Nutrition Foundation. Complex Carbohydrates in Foods, Chapman and Hall, London, 1990.
14. J Hirsch. Am. J. Clin. Nutr. 61S:996S-1000S, 1995.
15. WC Willett. Science 264:532–537, 1994.
16. BO Schneeman. J. Nutr. 124:1747S–1753S, 1994.

3

Complex Carbohydrates and the Food Label: An FDA Perspective

F. EDWARD SCARBROUGH
U.S. Food and Drug Administration, Washington, D.C.

INTRODUCTION

From their first issuance in 1980 the Dietary Guidelines have advised Americans to increase the amount of complex carbohydrates in their diets. Largely because of consumers' familiarity with the term "complex carbohydrate," certain segments of the food industry have sought for years to include quantitative amounts of this nutrient within nutrition labeling. However, current nutrition labeling regulations continue to prohibit listing of complex carbohydrate within the "Nutrition Facts" panel for at least four reasons. First, the mandatory inclusion of complex carbohydrate on the label may suggest that this food component has greater public health significance than has been established by existing diet and health studies. Second, dietary guidance documents have not specified a recommended level of intake for complex carbohydrates. Third, the term "complex carbohydrate" has not been clearly or consistently defined. And fourth, available analytical methods for carbohydrates in foods are not considered sufficiently specific for regulatory purposes. The Food and Drug Administration is working closely with health and science professional groups and the food industry to address these issues, particularly the questions of definition and analytical methodology.

THE FOOD LABEL AND DIETARY GUIDELINES

The Dietary Guidelines for Americans which is issued every five years jointly by the Departments of Health and Human Services and of Agriculture represent fundamental, federal government public health policy. The fourth edition of the Dietary Guidelines recognizes the food label, especially the new "Nutrition Facts" label, along with the Food Guide Pyramid as the educational tools American consumers should use to put the Dietary Guidelines into practice. Consumers are advised to: "use the Nutrition Facts Label to choose a healthful diet" (1, page 4). The same guidelines advise Americans to "choose a diet with plenty of grain products, vegetables, and fruits . . ." because they provide complex carbohydrates (1, page 22). However, for the nutrient "complex carbohydrates" the food label is not a very useful tool because "complex carbohydrates" do not appear in the Nutrition Facts panel.

This has been the case since the issuance of the first edition of the Dietary Guidelines in 1980. The first edition advised Americans to

> Eat foods with adequate starch and fiber . . . complex carbohydrate foods are better than simple carbohydrates . . . . Complex carbohydrate foods–such as beans, peas, nuts, seeds, fruits and vegetables, and whole grain breads, cereals and products–contain many essential nutrients in addition to calories (2, page 13).

The Guidelines advise that to eat more complex carbohydrates daily, substitute starches for fats and sugars and select foods that are good sources of fiber and starch (2, page 14). The second edition of the Dietary Guidelines in 1985 continued the advice to

> Eat foods with adequate starch and fiber . . . [S]imple carbohydrates, such as sugars, and complex carbohydrates, such as starches, have about the same caloric content. Most foods high in sugars . . . contain no vitamins or minerals. . . . Foods high in starch contain many of these essential nutrients. . . . Eating more foods containing complex carbohydrates can also help to add dietary fiber to your diet (3, page 17).

The third edition of the guidelines advised "choose a diet with plenty of vegetables, fruits, and grain products," with the explanation that "complex carbohydrates, such as starches are in breads, cereals, pasta, rice, dry beans and peas, and other vegetables such as potatoes and corn" (4, page 18).

PRE-NUTRITION LABELING AND EDUCATION ACT OF 1990

Even before the issuance of the first Dietary Guidelines for Americans in 1980, the FDA and the food industry had realized the problems created by there being no indication on the food label of the "complex carbohydrate" content of a food. At the same time dietary guidance almost universally advised consumers to increase their consumption of "complex carbohydrates". For example, in 1978, the Kellogg Company had submitted a petition to the FDA to voluntarily permit the declaration of (1) "grams per serving of starch and related carbohydrates", (2) "grams per serving of sucrose and other sugars", and (3) "grams per serving of total carbohydrates [the sum of (1) and (2)]". The Agency did not grant the Kellogg petition, but in the years from 1980 to 1993 many cereal companies listed either "complex carbohydrates" or "starches" and "related carbohydrates" on the labels of their products and the FDA took no regulatory actions.

In 1979 the FDA in cooperation with the United States Department of Agriculture (USDA) and the Federal Trade Commission (FTC) undertook a major food label reform initiative. The tentative positions of the three agencies were published in the Federal Register of December 29, 1979. However, the issue of complex carbohydrates did not surface as one of the major issues of the initiative. (5) Because of a number of factors, including a change in political administrations, little came of the 1979 food label reform initiative.

In the late 1980s the FDA again launched a food label reform effort. This effect was primarily based on the recognition that the food label continued to be out of step with the shifts in public health concerns from nutrient deficiencies to the health consequences of over-consumption. This label initiative was announced by Secretary of Health and Human Services, Dr. Louis Sullivan, in March 1989. On August 8, 1989, the FDA published an Advance Notice of Proposed RuleMaking (ANPRM) asking all interested parties to comment on a number of specific labeling issues. (6) The agency specifically asked, "How should the listing of components of carbohydrates be treated within the context of nutrition labeling (e.g., complex starches, total sugars)?" (6) Throughout the fall of 1989, the FDA conducted a series of Public Hearings and Consumer Exchange meetings on how the food label could be improved. The inclusion of complex carbohydrate content on the food label was often raised in these discussions.

In July 1990 the agency proposed to modify the nutrition label. (7) In that document, the FDA clearly set out the factors that it considered in deciding whether a nutrient or food component should be mandatory or voluntary in nutrition labeling.

> The agency has proposed to make the declaration of a nutrient or food component mandatory in nutrition labeling when quantitative intake rec-

> ommendations with respect to the nutrient or component are high-lighted in the reports cited above (e.g., "Reduce total fat intake to 30% or less of calories.". . .), and the nutrient or component is of particular public health significance as defined in several recent consensus documents. . . . On the other hand, for those nutrients or food components for which quantitative intake recommendations are not highlighted but that do have some public health significance (e.g., ". . . increase intakes of starches . . ."), or for which quantitative recommendations are available but that are not of pressing public health importance (e.g., the Recommended Dietary Allowances for several vitamins and minerals . . .), the agency is proposing to make declaration of the nutrient or component voluntary" (7, p 29493).

Following these principles, the FDA did not propose to require the mandatory declaration of complex carbohydrates in nutrition labeling. It should also be noted that the National Academy of Sciences, in their report, Nutrition Labeling, had recommended that the declaration of complex carbohydrates be voluntary. (8)

In response the FDA in July of 1990 proposed to make the declaration of complex carbohydrates voluntary with the following statement.

> The FDA is proposing in 101.9(c)(6)(i) to permit the voluntary declaration of the complex carbohydrate content because recent dietary reports have discussed the need to increase consumption of complex carbohydrates. (9, 10) Because recommendations to increase consumption of complex carbohydrates have not been quantified, however, the agency finds that a basis for requiring declaration of this food component in nutrition labeling has not been established (7, page 29497).

For labeling purposes the FDA defined complex carbohydrates in the proposal as the sum of dextrins and starches, or more specifically those carbohydrate components that contain 10 or more saccharide units exclusive of dietary fiber (7, p. 29497). The agency, however, expressed concern that the inclusion of dextrins (saccharide units of 10 or more) within the definition of complex carbohydrates may inappropriately classify the relatively low molecular weight carbohydrates in some nutritive sweeteners as complex carbohydrates.

This definition may result in some foods, such as coffee whiteners and ice cream, that contain large amounts of low conversion (low dextrose equivalent) corn sweeteners, being classified as sources of complex carbohydrates. These low molecular weight carbohydrates may have nutritional or metabolic effects different from those of commonly recognized complex carbohydrates. Thus, it may be misleading to consumers if these foods are labeled as containing complex carbohydrate.

Comments on this proposal indicated consumer interest in having complex carbohydrates as a mandatory part of nutrition labeling, based largely on the dietary guidance recommendations. Industry comments, however, generally supported a voluntary declaration of complex carbohydrates. There were four main reasons cited by comments advocating voluntary listing.

First, the mandatory inclusion of complex carbohydrate on the label may suggest that this food component has greater public health significance than has been established by existing diet and health studies. The identification of a specific health benefit for complex carbohydrates is confounded by the fact that diets high in complex carbohydrates are usually mixed diets that contain significant amounts of cereal grains, fruits, and vegetables which are high in vitamins, minerals, and fiber and low in fat. It is unclear the extent to which complex carbohydrates impart health benefits separate from these factors.

Second, dietary guidance documents have not specified a recommended level of intake for complex carbohydrates and thus the agency would be unable to establish a label reference value, such as a Daily Recommended Value (DRV), for labeling purposes. It was felt that DRVs would be helpful in planning overall diets and the extent to which the absence of a DRV for complex carbohydrates would be problematic or confusing to consumers was unknown.

Third, the term "complex carbohydrate" had not been clearly or consistently defined. For labeling purposes the agency needed a chemical definition that reflected the physiological effects and health benefits. For voluntary labeling purposes the agency had defined "complex carbohydrates" as the sum of dextrins and starches, or those carbohydrate components that contain 10 or more saccharide units, exclusive of dietary fiber. But FDA was concerned about the appropriateness of this rather arbitrary definition.

Fourth, and perhaps most important of all, available analytical methods for carbohydrates in foods were not considered sufficiently specific for regulatory purposes. For example, methods generally measured carbohydrates either as more than 4 saccharide units or as single saccharide units up to 4 units. Suitable analytical procedures were needed if complex carbohydrates were to be defined as those carbohydrates that contain a specified number of saccharide units.

POST–NUTRITION LABELING AND EDUCATION ACT OF 1990

When Congress passed the Nutrition Labeling and Education Act of 1990 (NLEA) one of the principal differences of that act compared to the FDA's 1990 proposal was the inclusion of "complex carbohydrates" as one of the components that was mandatory on the nutrition label (Section 403(q)(1)(D)) (11). In November 1991 the FDA published a revised proposal for mandatory nutrition labeling to conform agency regulations to the NLEA requirements. (12) Following the lead of Congress the agency proposed that complex carbohydrates be made mandatory on nutrition labels in that document. The definition (starches and dextrins with 10 or more saccharide units) remained as had been proposed in July 1990. However, the November 1991 re-proposal recognized that the NLEA gave the FDA some latitude in determining which nutrients should be listed on the nutrition label. Section 403(q)(2)(B) of the act allows the Secretary (and, by delegation, the FDA) to determine whether information relating to nutrients specified in section (q)(1)(D) inter alia is necessary to assist consumers in maintaining healthy dietary practices and, if not, to delete such nutrients from the required list of nutrients in nutrition labeling. The agency raised the four concerns cited above and requested specific comment.

Many comments on the revised proposal expressed opposition to the FDA's proposed definition of complex carbohydrate. The comments raised concerns about the feasibility of compliance and the economic burden of developing databases and analytical methods. Many comments recommended that the definition of "complex carbohydrate" be changed to be the difference between total carbohydrate and sugars because this difference could be readily calculated. Comments also noted that carbohydrates with saccharide units of 5 through 9 would not be accounted for in any of the labeled sub-components of carbohydrate, leading to possible consumer confusion. The cut-off of 10 saccharide units was criticized as being arbitrary because there are no known nutritional or physiological differences to justify a distinction between polysaccharides at this dividing line. Several comments suggested that the commonly accepted usage of "complex carbohydrate" includes all carbohydrates larger than disaccharides. Other comments suggested that complex carbohydrate should be defined as all digestible polysaccharides (e.g., dextrins, starch, and glycogen) rather than on the basis of the number of saccharide units, but no information was provided on reliable methods for determining carbohydrate digestibility or for distinguishing energy derived from intestinal digestion from that derived from colonic fermentation. Comments emphasized that while there was not a consensus on a precise definition for "complex carbohydrate," the agency's proposed definition was not commonly recognized, nor was it consistent with the use of the term in the IOM report. (8) One comment from a state government recommended that to avert undue emphasis on complex carbohydrate substances added to foods and to avoid the potential for misleading claims about complex carbohydrates, the term "other carbohydrate" should be used rather than "complex carbohydrate."

In the final regulations implementing the NLEA, published in the Federal Register on January 6, 1993, the FDA concluded that the comments indicated that there was not sufficient consensus on the meaning of the term "complex carbohydrate" to justify adopting a definition and requiring mandatory inclusion in the nutrition label. (13) Further, because there was no apparent consensus on the health benefits or physiological effects of "complex carbohydrates" per se, the agency determined that the term "other carbohydrates" should be used voluntarily on the label. "Other carbohydrate" is calculated as the amount of carbohydrate remaining after subtraction of dietary fiber, sugars, and sugar alcohols from total carbohydrate. The agency recognized that this new definition will include many substances added to processed foods for technical purposes, such as for texture modification or as bulking agents. The FDA stated the belief that to declare these substances as complex carbohydrates would be misleading. The intent of dietary recommendations to increase the consumption of complex carbohydrates and dietary fiber is to select diets with plenty of fruits, vegetables, and grain products, not foods that have complex carbohydrates as added texturizers or bulking agents.

Because "other carbohydrate" is calculated as that amount of carbohydrate remaining after subtraction of the amount of dietary fiber, sugars, and sugar alcohols (when declared) from total carbohydrate, it was logical to rearrange the subcomponents of total carbohydrate to place "other carbohydrate" at the bottom of the list. This reordering was intended help to reduce any potential confusion over the meaning of the term "other carbohydrate."

When "other carbohydrate" is omitted from the label, the declared subcomponents of total carbohydrate (i.e., dietary fiber and sugars) will not add up to the value for total carbohydrate in most foods. The agency recommended that consumer education programs should inform interested persons that other forms of carbohydrate beyond those declared on the label are in the food product. This situation is analogous to the fat category where the sum of saturated, polyunsaturated, and monounsaturated fatty acids often do not add up to 100 percent of the value for total fat because trans fatty acids are not included in the definition of the fatty acids but are included in the value for total fat.

CONCLUSION

The issue of "complex carbohydrates" clearly has not been settled. Many in academia, professional societies, and the food industry continue to express interest in including "complex carbohydrate" on the food label. In November 1994 the International Life Sciences Institute (ILSI) sponsored a workshop to evaluate the scientific issues associated with complex carbohydrates and, in light of these issues, address the rationale for adding complex carbohydrates to the nutrition label. (14) This workshop concluded that "it is clear that this is not a simple task. Classifications cannot be made simply for chemical or analytical expediency if they do not express physiological significance." As a follow-up to the ILSI Conference the AOAC (Association of Official Analytical Chemists) International sponsored a Workshop in September 1995 with a goal of reaching a consensus on the definition of complex carbohydrates to support food labeling and dietary guidelines, to discuss state-of-the-art techniques in analytical methods, and to set the direction for future improvement in analytical methods. (15) Growing out of this workshop, the AOAC International has launched a collaborative study of a promising analytical methodology and in which the FDA is participating as a collaborator.

Building on the firm scientific basis that will be provided by these above efforts, the FDA will then be able to move to a regulatory position that will allow complex carbohydrate content to be declared on the nutrition label, thus bringing about greater correspondence between the nutrition label and dietary guidance.

REFERENCES

1. Nutrition and Your Health: Dietary Guidelines for Americans. Fourth Edition. (1995) Department of Agriculture and Department of Health and Human Services, Home and Garden Bulletin No. 232.
2. Nutrition and Your Health: Dietary Guidelines for Americans. (1980) Department of Agriculture and Department of Health and Human Services, Home and Garden Bulletin No. 232.
3. Nutrition and Your Health: Dietary Guidelines for Americans. Second Edition. (1985) Department of Agriculture and Department of Health and Human Services, Home and Garden Bulletin No. 232.
4. Nutrition and Your Health: Dietary Guidelines for Americans. Third Edition. (1990) Department of Agriculture and Department of Health and Human Services, Home and Garden Bulletin No. 232.
5. U. S. Department of Health Education, and Welfare, U. S. Department of Agriculture, and Federal Trade Commission. (1979) Advance Notice of Rulemaking, Tentative Positions of the Agencies, Federal Register 44:75990-76020, U. S. Government Printing Office, Washington, D.C., December 21, 1979.
6. Food and Drug Administration. (1989) Food Labeling; Advance Notice of Proposed Rulemaking, Federal Register 54:32610-32615, U. S. Government Printing Office, Washington, D.C., August 8, 1989.
7. Food and Drug Administration. (1990) Food Labeling; Reference Daily Intakes and Daily Reference Values; Mandatory Status of Nutrition Labeling and Nutrient Content Revision; Serving Size, Proposed Rules, Federal Register 55:29475-29533, U. S. Government Printing Office, Washington, D.C., July 19, 1990.
8. Committee on the Nutrition Components of Food Labeling, Food and Nutrition Board, Institute of Medicine, National Academy of Sciences. (1990) Nutrition Labeling: Issues and Directions for the 1990's (Porter, D.V. and Earl, R.O. editors), National Academy Press, Washington, D.C.
9. U. S. Department of Health and Human Services, Public Health Service. (1988) The Surgeon General's Report on Nutrition and Health, DHHS(PHS) Publication No. 88-50210, U. S. Government Printing Office, Washington, D.C.
10. Committee on Diet and Health, Food and Nutrition Board, Commission on Life Sciences, National Research Council, Diet and Health (1989): Implications for Reducing Chronic Disease Risk, National Academy Press, Washington, D.C.

11. Nutrition Labeling and Education Act of 1990, Public Law 101-535, 104 Stat. 2353, 1990.
12. Food and Drug Administration. (1991) Food Labeling; Proposed Rules, Federal Register 56:60366–60878, U. S. Government Printing Office, Washington, D.C., November 21, 1991.
13. Food and Drug Administration, Food Labeling; Final Rules, Federal Register 58: 2066-2941, U. S. Government Printing Office, Washington, D.C., January 6, 1993.
14. Lineback, D. et al. (1995) Complex Carbohydrates: The Science and the Label, Nutrition Reviews 53(7):186–193, July 1995.
15. AOAC Workshop on Definition and Analysis of Complex Carbohydrate / Dietary Fiber. (1995) Annual Meeting, September 15–16, 1995, Nashville, Tennessee.

4

Dietary Fiber Properties and Health Benefits of Non-Digestible Oligosaccharides

M. B. Roberfroid
Département des Sciences Pharmaceutiques, Université Catholique de Louvain, Brussels, Belgium

INTRODUCTION

Non-digestible oligosaccharides (NDOs, recently referred to as "resistant oligosaccharides") are complex carbohydrates which are resistant to hydrolysis by acid and enzymes in the human digestive tract due to the configuration of their osidic bonds. Most dietary oligo-/polysaccharides are quantitatively hydrolyzed in the upper part of the gastrointestinal tract. The resulting monosaccharides are transported via the portal blood to the liver and, subsequently, to the systemic circulation. Such carbohydrates are essential for health as they serve both as substrates and regulators of major metabolic pathways. They also trigger hormone secretion. But some of the dietary oligo-/polysaccharides do resist, more or less quantitatively, the digestive process. Consequently, such carbohydrates reach the caecocolon as they have been eaten and so do not provide the body with monosaccharides (1).

Once they have reached the caeco-colon, most (but not necessarily all) of the non-digestible oligosaccharides are hydrolyzed to small oligomers and monomers that are further metabolized by one, a few, or most of the anaerobic bacteria. Such a metabolic process, known as fermentation, not only serves the bacteria by providing energy for proliferation, but also produces gases (H_2, CO_2, CH_4) which are metabolically useless to the host. Small organic acids such as acetate, propionate, butyrate, and L-lactate, which are named short chain carboxylic acid (SCCA) are additional products. By a mechanism which is still a matter of some debate (2, 3) the SCCA are largely (90–95%) absorbed through the intestinal wall, in the caecum and the ascending part of colon. Except for butyrate (which is a major energy substrate for colonocytes) the other SCCA reach the portal circulation and enter the liver, the main site of their metabolism. However, part of acetate (25–50%) escapes hepatic metabolism and, via the systemic circulation, reaches the peripheral tissues, mainly the muscle (4, 5). Even though they do not provide the body with monosaccharides, the non-digestible oligo-/polysaccharides are, thus, indirect energy substrates and metabolic regulators. Thanks to the symbiosis between the caeco-colon and a myriad of colonizing bacteria, they are transformed to SCCA, which essentially via the same route as monosaccharides (portal blood), feed the liver and other important tissues with energy. Acetate, propionate, butyrate, lactate, and so on are indeed important substrates and/or intermediates in cell metabolism. Moreover, it has recently been demonstrated that, at least some of these molecules may also serve as modulators of key metabolic pathways.

The most important class of dietary non-digestible saccharides is that composed of short (up to 10 monomers) and medium (up to 50–60 units) chain-length homopolymers (Table 1). Some NDOs, like inulin and its hydrolysis product oligofructose, which belong to the group of fructans, are common natural food ingredients (6) while others like galactooligosaccharides or Neosugar are synthetic products resulting from the enzymatic and/or chemical modification of natural disaccharides like saccharose, lactose, and so on.

Among these NDOs the chicory fructooligosaccharides (inulin and its product of partial enzymatic hydrolysis, oligofructose) are authorized as food ingredients in most European countries. Others like trans-galactooligosaccharides (TOS or GOS), isomaltooligosaccahrides (IMO), soybean oligosaccharides (SOS) and xylooligosaccharides (XOS) are recognized as functional foods by Japanese authorities.

The aim of the present chapter is to review the nutritional and physiological properties of chicory fructooligosaccharides that are, so far, the most studied NDOs. Similar evidence exists, however, for the other NDOs. The objective is to give scientific support to the classification of chicory fructooligosaccharides as dietary fiber (7).

TABLE 1 Non-Digestible Oligosaccharides

Name (abbreviation)	Chemical structure	Osidic bond	Origin	Trade name
Fructooligosaccharides (FOS)				
Inulin	Glucosyl (fructosyl)$_n$ fructose (n = 2 → 20) Glucosyl (fructosyl)$_n$	β1 → 2	Plant	Raftiline® Fibrulin®
Oligofructose	Fructose (fructosyl)$_m$ fructose (n = 1 → 6, m = 2 → 7)	β1 → 2	Plant and enzymatic hydrolysis of inulin	Raftilose®
Neosugar	Glucosyl (fructosyl)$_n$ fructose (n = 1 → 3)	β1 → 2	Enzymatic synthesis from sucrose	Neosugar® Actilight®
Galactooligosaccharides (GOS or TOS)	Glucosyl (galactosyl)$_n$ galactose (n = 1 → 3)	β1 → 6	Enzymatic synthesis from lactose	Oligomate®
Transgalacto-oligosaccharides	(Galactosyl)$_n$ galactose (n = 2)	α1 → 6	Enzymatic synthesis from lactose	Cup-oligo®
Isomaltooligosaccharides (IMO)	(Glucosyl)$_n$ glucose (n = 2 → 7)	α1 → 4	Enzymatic rearrangement of maltose	Isomalto®
Palatinose Condensates (PC)				
Polydextrose	Randomly branched + citric acid (n = 2 → 100?)		Glucose pyrolysis-citric acid	Polydextrose®
Pyrodextrins	Complex mixture		Pyrolysis of corn or potato starch	
Sololigosaccharides (SOS)	Rafficose + stachyose (n = 3 → 4)		Enzymatic synthesis + pyrolysis	Soya-Oligo®
Xylooligosaccharides (XOS)	(Xylosyl)$_n$ xylose (n = 2 → 4)	β1 → 4		Xylooligo®

BEHAVIOR AND EFFECTS OF CHICORY FRUCTOOLIGOSACCHARIDES IN THE GASTRO-INTESTINAL TRACT

Non-Digestibility

The evidence that fructooligosaccharides are resistant to hydrolysis and are not absorbed in the upper part of the gastrointestinal tract comes from in vivo human studies, essentially performed in ileostomy subjects. More than 90–95% of ingested fructooligosaccharides are indeed recovered in the ileostomy effluent (8, 9). A study in rats fed 14C-labeled Neosugar® provided similar evidence (10).

Fermentation by Anaerobic Colonic Bacteria

In an extensive study using the model of mixed fecal culture, Wang and Gibson (11) have reported that the utilization of chicory fructooligosaccharides was much more specific than that of other substrates (like polydextrose, pectin, or fructose for example). Indeed, a marked proliferation of bifidus occurred, while populations of bacteroides, lactobacilli, clostridia, coliforms and gram positive cocci were maintained at a relatively low level or even reduced. Such a high specificity of chicory fructooligosaccharides for bifidobacteria is mainly due to the secretion by these bacteria of a β-fructosidase, as demonstrated in pure cultures (12). The accepted mechanism by which bifidobacteria inhibit the growth of other bacteria involves a decrease in pH as a consequence of the intense production of SCCA. However, the acidity is not the only mechanism of inhibition of growth of *E. coli* and *C. perfringens* as shown in fermentation systems in which pH is maintained constant (11,13).

Other authors have also shown that bifidobacteria are able to produce substances that would be bactericidal to others including some members of the genus *Clostridium* (14). The fermentability and the bifidogenic effect of chicory fructooligosaccharides, demonstrated in vitro were also confirmed in vivo. A marked increase in bifidobacteria and consequently a profound modification of the fecal flora have been demonstrated in vivo in human healthy volunteers fed 3 x 5 g a day of oligofructose or inulin for two weeks (15) or 8 g/day for up to 5 weeks (N. Guggenbuhl et al., personal communication).

Bulking Effect

An increase in fecal dry weight excretion observed in oligofructose-fed rats is also a parameter related to the increased number of bacteria resulting from its extensive fermentation. Calculations have indicated that about 40% of the carbon atoms ingested as oligofructose are incorporated into newly synthesized bacteria (16).

A bulking effect has also been observed in the human volunteers in the study performed by Gibson et al. (15). Such an effect expressed as grams of increase of fresh fecal weight by grams of chicory fructooligosaccharides eaten (bulking index) compares well, both in rats and in humans, with that obtained after eating soluble or mixed dietary fibers like pectin, oat bran, wheat bran or guar gum (Table 2).

Chicory Fructooligosaccharides as Prebiotics

It can thus be hypothesized that feeding chicory fructooligosaccharide has a major impact on gut microflora, by favoring the proliferation of beneficial bacteria like bifidobacteria and by reducing the number of potentially harmful anaerobes. It is thus likely to be beneficial for the host, but the exact role of gut microflora on health, as well as the definition of a healthy flora, still remains open questions (23).

By analogy, living bacteria that are added to food (e.g., in yogurt) which cross the upper gastrointestinal tract to colonize the caeco-colon have been called probiotics. We propose to call them prebiotics with NDO used as food ingredients to modify the composition of endogenous gut microflora (24).

TABLE 2 Bulking Effect of Chicory Fructooligosaccharides as Compared to Dietary Fiber

Species	Carbohydrates	Bulking index*	Reference
Rats	Oligofructose (10%)	+ 1	16
	Inulin (10%)		
	Pectin (10%)	+ 1	17
	Oat Bran (14%)	+ 0.7	18
	Wheat Bran (13%)	+ 1.3–2.0	17, 18
Humans	Oligofructose (15g)	+ 1.2	15
	Inulin (15g)	+2.1	
	Pectin	+ 1–2	19, 20
	Guar Gum	+ 1–2	19, 20
	Wheat Bran (15g)	+ 2.5–5	18–21

*Bulking index = g of increase in fresh fecal weight / g of carbohydrates eaten
( ) Indicates either % added to rat diet or g eaten per day

SYSTEMIC EFFECTS OF CHICORY FRUCTOOLIGOSACCHARIDES

Effects on Lipid Metabolism

The main systemic effect of NDOs so far studied is the effect on lipid metabolism. A few Japanese studies have suggested that feeding rats with fructans leads to modification of blood lipid concentration. Even if controversial studies are reported fructans administration often leads to a decrease in cholesterol and/or triglycerides concentration. By using chicory fructooligosaccharide as model substances we have analyzed the influence of feeding rats a diet containing these NDOs on lipidemia in protocols differing in the basal diet, the dose of NDOs, and the duration of the treatment. In all these protocols, the constant effect was a decrease in triglyceride concentration.

Our recent data have further shown that the hypotriglyceridemic effect of chicory fructooligosaccharides, given at 10% in the standard diet of rats for 3 months, was accompanied by a decrease in serum cholesterol and phospholipids. That decrease was most exclusively due to a change in the very low density lipoprotein (VLDL) fraction (25).

We hypothesize that such changes in lipid parameters are the consequence of a metabolic adaptation of the liver that might be induced by SCCA. Indeed, hepatocytes isolated from oligofructose fed rats have a reduced capacity to synthesize triglycerides from free fatty acids and acetate and a decreased fatty acyl synthase activity (26). Such an effect on triglyceridemia has been demonstrated in rats and compares rather well with similar effects reported for guar gum or sugar beet fiber (Table 3) and has to be confirmed in humans, in particular in hyperlipidemic patients.

Caloric Value

As a consequence of their fermentation and of the resorption of fermentation products the next nutritional property of chicory fructooligosaccharides to be

TABLE 3 Hypolipidemic Effects of Chicory Fructooligosaccharides as Compared to Dietary Fiber

		% change / g of dietary supplement		
Species	Carbohydrates	TC	LDL-C	TG
Rats	Oligofructose (10%)	− 10	0	− 20
	Guar Gum (10%)	− 5	–	− 5
	Sugar Beet Fiber (10%)	− 4	–	− 4

discussed concerns their caloric value. Indeed, being exclusive substrates for colonic fermentation, oligofructose and inulin have also much lower caloric value than equivalent but digested carbohydrates. Moreover, they are (at least) partly used as direct and indirect substrates for bacterial proliferation, a process that further reduces their bioavailability to the host. Based on experimental evidence as well as on basic biochemical knowledge a theoretical approach has been proposed to compare the metabolic efficiency (in term of ATP production) and thus the effective caloric value of a fructosyl moiety in chicory fructooligosaccharide and sucrose (as a typically digested substrate). As compared to sucrose chicory fructooligosaccharide has a relative caloric value of 25 to 35%, or 1 to 1.5 kcal/g or 4 to 6 kJ/g (16).

Mineral Bioavailability

As chicory fructooligosaccharides modify intestine and colon physiology, it should be asked whether they might influence the nutritional balance of several macro- or micronutrients.

Our recent studies (27) have shown that feeding rats with oligofructose or inulin at the dose of 10% leads to an increased fecal excretion of N, resulting most probably from an increase in fecal bacteria and leading to a decreased urinary excretion of urea and decreased uremia. Such results are in accordance with those obtained with other dietary fibers.

The possible interference of dietary fibers with ion absorption relative to their physiological effects on the small intestine and the colon has regularly been questioned. In a recent experiment in rats fed a diet supplemented with 10% FOS or inulin, we have demonstrated that the balance for Ca, Mg, and Fe is improved (27). This beneficial effect, quite surprising as compared to the effect of dietary fiber, may result from an increased intestinal absorption of the minerals. This effect has also been observed by Levrat et al. (28) in rats fed a diet containing 10% inulin, and by Ohta et al. (29). All showed that in rats fed a diet enriched in synthetic fructans the absorption of Ca^{++}, Mg^{++} and P was significantly higher than in rats fed a diet supplemented with lactose. They also showed that galactooligosaccharides had no effect. Neither Zn or Cu bioavailability nor lipid soluble vitamins (A and E) homeostasis was modified by chicory fructooligosaccharides.

DISCUSSION: NON-DIGESTIBLE OLIGOSACCHARIDES AS DIETARY FIBER

Within the vast group of dietary carbohydrates (Table 1) the non-digestible oligosaccharides belong to the class of compounds which resist digestion. The chicory fructooligosaccharides are extensively fermented in the colon, have prebiotic properties, and are likely to modulate systemic physiological function (24).

"Dietary fiber" must be defined more as a concept rather than as a chemical (or an analytical) entity (30). Such a concept must include "resistance to digestion" as a key factor together with the saccharidic nature and the plant origin of the material. The term dietary fiber must therefore cover any plant's oligo-/polysaccharides that resist hydrolysis in the human digestive tract and reach the colon where they can eventually be fermented. They belong to the group of colonic foods and, if selectively fermented by one or a limited number of colonic bacteria, become classified as prebiotics (24).

The non-digestible oligosaccharides in general, and the chicory fructooligosaccharides in particular, resist digestion, behave as colonic foods, are selectively fermented (e.g. by bifidobacteria) and exert systemic effects. As a consequence of these properties they have bulking effects and they might positively modulate lipid metabolism without interfering with mineral absorption. Indeed, they tended to enhance and improve said absorption.

From a conceptual perspective non-digestible oligosaccharides in general and chicory fructooligosaccharides in particular have to be classified as dietary fiber and they have to appear as such on nutrition labeling. From a nutritional perspective, chicory fructooligosaccharides have to be viewed as prebiotics: due to their selective fermentation by bifidobacteria they improve the composition of the colonic microbiota.

Finally, via their systemic effects, they might also positively modulate lipid metabolism. Within the recently promoted functional foods (defined as any food constituent which affects the functions of the body in a targeted way so as to have positive effect which may justify functional or health claims) the chicory fructoligosaccharides (the most developed non-digestible oligosaccharides) are likely to occupy a key position (31). In the frame of a stepwise strategy for research and development (32) they are eligible for a functional claim like "bifidogenic factor", but further studies in human volunteers might justify more of such claims. By allowing to quantitatively modify the composition of the colonic microbiota in favor of bifidobacteria, these food ingredients are a useful tool to study the positive effects on health (if any) of such a modification (23).

REFERENCES

1. Lee, S.C., and Prosky, L. (1995) J. Assoc. Org. Anal. Chem. 78, 22–36.
2. Ruppin, H., Bar Meir, S., Soergel, K.H., Wood, C.M., and Schmitt, M.G. (1980) Gastroenterology, 78, 1500–1507.
3. Yeo, S. (1991) Ph.D. Thesis, University of California, Berkeley, UNI-Dissertation information service, 174 p.
4. Rémésy, C., and Demigné, C. (1993) Ann. Nutrition. Metabol., 27, 57–70.

5. Schummann, W.C., Magnusson, I., Clandromouli, V., Rumaran, K., Wahren, J., and Landan, B. R. (1991) J. Biol. Chem., 266, 6985–6990.
6. Van Loo, J., Coussement, P., De Leenheer, L., Hoebregs, H., and Smits, G. (1995) C.R.C. Crit. Rev. Food Sci. Nutr. 35, 525–552.
7. Coussement, P. (1995) See chapter 20 in this book.
8. Knudsen, K.E.B., and Prosky, L. (1995) J. Assoc. Anal. Org. Chem. 78, 22–36.
9. Ellegärd, L., Andersson, H., and Hessou, I. (1995) Br. J. Nutr., 74, 101–113.
10. Tokunaga, T., Oku, T., and Hosoya, N. (1989) J. Nutr., 119, 553–559.
11. Wang, X., and Gibson, G.R. (1993) J. Appl. Bateriol., 75, 373–380.
12. McKellar, R.C., and Modler, H.W. (1989) Appl. Microbiol. Biotechnol. 31, 537–541.
13. Wang X. (1993) Ph.D. thesis, MRC Dunn Clinical Nutrition Center, University of Cambridge, England.
14. Meghrous, J., Euloge, A.M., Junelles, J., Ballongue, J., and Petitdemange, H. (1990) Biotechnol. Lett. 12, 575–580.
15. Gibson, G.R., Beatty, E.B., Wang, X. and Cummings, J.H. (1995) Gastroenterology, 108, 975–982.
16. Roberfroid, M., Gibson, G.R., and Delzenne, N. (1993) Nutr. Rev. 51, 137–146.
17. Armstrong, E.F., Eastwood, M. A., and Brydon, W.G. (1993) J. Nutr. 69, 913–920.
18. Hansen, I., Bach Knudsen, K.E., and Eggum, B. O. (1992) Br. J. Nutr. 68, 451–462.
19. Cummings, J.H. (1984) Postgrad Med. J., 60, 811–819.
20. Splliler, G.A. (1986) Handbook of Dietary Fiber in Human Nutrition, CRC Press Inc., Boca Raton, Florida, USA.
21. Spoiler, G.A., Story, J.A., Wong., L.G., Nooses, J.D., Alton, M., Petro, M.S., Furumoto, E.J., Whittman, J.H., and Scala, J. (1986) J. Nutr. 116, 778–785.
22. Tomlin, J. and Read, N. W. (1988) Eur. J. Clin. Nutr. 42, 857–861.
23. Roberfroid, M.B., Bornet, F., Bouley C., and Cummings J.H. (1995) Nutr. Rev. 53, 127–130.
24. Gibson, G.R., and Roberfroid, M.B. (1995) J. Nutr. 125, 1401–1412.
25. Fiordaliso, M.F., Kok, N., Desager, J.P., Goethals, F., Deboyser, D., Roberfroid, M., and Delzenne, N. (1995) Lipids 30, 163–167.
26. Kok, N., Roberfroid, M., and Delzenne, N. (1995) Arch. Biochem. Physiol. 103, B19.
27. Delzenne, N., Aertsens, J., Verplaetse, H., Roccaro, M., and Roberfroid, M. (1995) Life Sci. 57, 1579–1587.
28. Levrat, M.A., Rémésy C., and Demigné C (1991) J. Nutr. 121, 1730–1737.
29. Ohta A., Ohtuki M., Takizawa T., Inaba H., Adachi T. and Kumura S. (1994) J. Vit. Nutr. Res. 64, 316–323.
30. Roberfroid, M. (1993) C.R.C. Crit. Rev. Food Sci. Nutr. 33, 103–148.
31. Roberfroid, M.B. (1995) World Ingredients March-April, 42–44.
32. Roberfroid, M.B. (1996) Nutr. Rev. 54, 538–542.

5

Suggested Alternatives to the Term "Complex Carbohydrates"

F. W. Scott and R. Mongeau
Food Directorate, Nutrition Research Division, Banting Research Centre, Ottawa, Ontario, Canada

P. Wood
Centre for Food and Animal Research, Agriculture and Agri-Food Canada, Ottawa, Ontario, Canada

INTRODUCTION

The Canadian Nutrition Recommendations published in 1990 by Health Canada refer to the benefits of diets high in complex carbohydrates, defined essentially as starches. For the purposes of food labeling claims in Canada the term "complex carbohydrates" is permitted and has been taken to mean only starch which is the term used on the nutrition label itself. In other jurisdictions, the term "complex carbohydrates" has been taken to mean either starches or starches plus dietary fiber. Thus, the term is a source of confusion, is difficult to define in a manner that can be verified analytically and has little scientific meaning for many scientists and lay people alike (1, 2). There is a need to simplify and more clearly define in chemical terms what is meant by the advice to consume foods high in complex carbohydrates. It is time to re-think the use of this chemically undefined term and we suggest that "complex carbohydrate" be replaced by the terms starch and dietary fiber.

MEASUREMENT AND IDENTIFICATION OF CARBOHYDRATES

As the physiological effects of different polysaccharides become better understood it is appropriate to bring improved definition and precision to the area of food carbohydrates. This message is important when one considers that as recently as 1992 carbohydrate was still measured "by difference" in USDA Handbook 8, a practice subject to error because it includes minor non-carbohydrate components and is subject to cumulative analytical error derived from the analyses for protein, fat, moisture and ash. The FDA does not permit the term complex carbohydrate but requires the term "other carbohydrate" which is defined as the amount of carbohydrates remaining after subtraction of dietary fiber, sugars and sugar alcohols from total carbohydrates (3). This introduces another ill-defined and confusing term and continues to avoid mentioning by name the chemically well-defined term starch.

STARCH

We feel that a more useful and practical solution at present is to use the terms starch and dietary fiber separately. An appropriate definition of starch follows: "Starch is a large polymer of glucose consisting of glucose units formed into unbranched amylose chains composed of alpha-1,4 linked glucose residues and highly branched amylopectin with alpha-1,4 and alpha-1,6 bonds." There are several methods to measure starch (4–9). There are commercially available kits to measure starch based on converting it to soluble fragments with minimal production of glucose followed by quantitative hydrolysis by amyloglucosidase (4). (This kit can also provide an estimation of enzyme-"resistant" starch). In the method for total starch, starch is solubilized with DMSO or the sample is cooked in buffer with a thermostable alpha-amylase. Complete breakdown to dextrins is carried out by subsequent treatment with the de-branching enzyme pullulanase in combination with alpha-amylase to minimize the amount of free glucose formed by continued action of alpha-amylase. Quantitative hydrolysis of the resulting maltotrioses and maltoses, (which are not substrates for the bacterial alpha-amylase) to glucose is carried out with amyloglucosidase and glucose is measured using a standard enzyme/color reaction with samples read in a spectrophotometer. Unlike the term "complex carbohydrates", starch is a more defined chemical entity and can be measured by several methods.

DIETARY FIBER

Dietary fiber is essentially dietary non-starch polysaccharides and cell wall-associated components such as lignin. The report of the Canadian Expert Committee (10) strongly emphasized that dietary fiber excludes polymers formed during food processing or preparation and that the labeling of dietary fiber content in a food has value only because certain physiological benefits are expected of fiber.

To consider dietary fiber as complex carbohydrates also ignores the fact that the non-carbohydrate components participate in maintaining the botanical (plant cell wall) structure of dietary fiber and the structure of the food. The botanical structure and particle size may account for a significant proportion of the beneficial effects of dietary fiber on postprandial blood glucose response and intestinal function (11).

PHYSIOLOGICAL EFFECTS AND LABELING

The approach we suggest here focuses on two groups of components that can be analyzed using available methods.

The ingestion of starches can have a variety of effects depending on the plant source, cooking conditions and the individual's digestive tract. These variations result from interactions in both the upper gastrointestinal tract and in the colon and are not necessarily a consequence of chemical differences that are easily identified. Evidence that small amounts of "resistant starch" may have effects on gastrointestinal function and metabolism is important but this is just one aspect of a spectrum of effects originating from the same chemical entity. Information on these effects is not yet sufficient to include recommendations with respect to different starches and should not be of concern for the purpose of food labeling at this time.

Because high carbohydrate diets containing foods high in starches and dietary fiber can have beneficial health effects, the most useful and practical position at present for the purposes of labeling is to identify starches and dietary fiber separately. This approach to simplifying the definitions, analytical and labeling issues would facilitate healthy food choices by the consumer.

Products enriched in non-native or novel fiber sources also have a place in the market and may have benefit for particular segments of the population. Thus, the only justification for enriching foods in these materials should be the clear demonstration of beneficial physiological effects and not simply the artificial inflation of total carbohydrate and dietary fiber values.

REFERENCES

1. Asp, N.-G. (1994) Nutritional classification and analysis of food carbohydrates. Am J. Clin. Nutr. 59 (Suppl), 679S–681S.

2. Johnson, I. T., and Southgate, D.A.T. (1994) Dietary fibre and related substances. in Dietary fibre and related substances. Chapman and Hall, London. 132 pp.
3. Anonymous (1993) Discussion on other carbohydrates. Federal Register 58, 2177.
4. Total starch procedure TSA 9/92 (1993) Megazyme Australia, 2/11 Ponderosa Parade, Warriewood, (Sydney), NSW 2102, Australia (Fax: 612-979-8272).
5. Moreels, E. (1987) Measurement of the starch content of commercial starches. Starch 39, 414–416.
6. Mitchell, G. A. (1990) Methods of starch analysis. Starch 42, 131–134.
7. Henry, R. J., Balkeney, A. B., and Lance, R.C.M. (1990) Enzymatic determination of starch in samples with high sugar content. Starch 42, 468–470.
8. Batey, I.L. (1982) Starch analysis using thermostable alpha-amylases. Starch 34, 125–128.
9. Baur, M.C., and Alexander, R. J. (1979) Enzymatic procedure for determination of starch in cereal products. Cereal Chem. 56, 364–366.
10. Health and Welfare Canada (1985) Report of the Expert Advisory Committee on Dietary Fibre, National Health and Welfare Canada, Ottawa, Ontario.
11. Mongeau, R., Scott, F. W., and Brassard, R. (1997) Definition and analysis of dietary fiber. In Complex carbohydrates: Definition, analysis, and applications. Marcel Dekker, New York.

6

Complex Carbohydrates: The Science and the Label

David R. Lineback
University of Idaho, Moscow, Idaho
Mark Dreher
Nabisco, Inc., East Hanover, New Jersey
Jonathan W. DeVries
General Mills, Inc., Minneapolis, Minnesota
Joanne L. Slavin
University of Minnesota, St. Paul, Minnesota
Alison Stephen
University of Saskatchewan, Saskatoon, Saskatchewan, Canada
Dennis Gordon
North Dakota State University, Fargo, North Dakota
Leon Prosky
Prosky Associates, Rockville, Maryland
F. Edward Scarbrough
U. S. Food and Drug Administration, Washington, D.C.
Gary Henderson
Kraft Foods, White Plains, New York
Susan Sungsoo Cho and Beth Olson
The Kellogg Company, Battle Creek, Michigan
Fergus Clydesdale
University of Massachusetts, Amherst, Massachusetts

On November 2, 1994, the International Life Science's Institute (ILSI) North America Project Committee on Fiber/Complex Carbohydrates (now known as the Technical Committee on Carbohydrates) sponsored a workshop titled Complex Carbohydrates: The Science and the Label. This workshop evaluated the scientific issues associated with complex carbohydrates and, in light of these issues, addressed the rationale for adding complex carbohydrates to the nutrition label. Nutrition Reviews is pleased to publish the summary of this workshop.

PREFACE AND OVERVIEW*

The objectives for the workshop were: 1) To evaluate complex carbohydrates from the perspectives of definition and methodology, nutrition and health, and dietary guidelines and public health; 2) To evaluate critically the scientific issues associated with the possible addition of complex carbohydrates to the nutrition label; and 3) To explore issues associated with developing a rational public policy for the labeling of complex carbohydrates.

Since the 1970s, complex carbohydrates have been an important component of various dietary guidelines. However, the term has been used without much attention given to definition, analytic methodology, or physiologic effects. These issues must be resolved before complex carbohydrates can meet the criteria for use in food labeling.

The current opportunities to educate consumers utilizing clearly defined food labels have never been greater. Using the synergy between the Nutrition Labeling and Education Act (NLEA) and the revised Food Guide Pyramid has facilitated great strides toward a better understanding on the part of the public regarding the constituents of a healthy diet. Just as it has learned the terms "saturated fat", "soluble fiber," and "dietary cholesterol", the public is capable of understanding the term "complex carbohydrate" if the scientific issues are clarified. The primary questions are

1. What are the components included in the term "complex carbohydrate"?
2. Can analytic methodology be developed that reflects all of the components encountered in the broad definition of complex carbohydrates?
3. Is there a clear understanding of the physiologic benefits of complex carbohydrates?

This workshop was an initial step toward resolving these questions.

---

* David Lineback and Mark Dreher

INTRODUCTION*

On November 27, 1991, the term complex carbohydrates was proposed as a mandatory listing in the Nutrition Facts segment of the nutrition label. The calculation of complex carbohydrates was to be the sum of digestible polysaccharides with a degree of polymerization greater than nine. The final regulations of January 6, 1993, do not allow use of the term complex carbohydrates on the nutrition label because of lack of a clear definition and commensurate methodology. This is problematic because the term complex carbohydrate has become very familiar (even colloquial) to consumers by way of media reinforcement for the past 18 years. Although consumers are aware of the recommendations to increase their consumption of complex carbohydrates, they are unable to find this information readily on the food label.

Complex carbohydrates, with or without other concurrent nutrients, have been a significant topic of scientific research and public interest. This interest has spanned the three decades since the initial observations that populations that consumed diets high in complex carbohydrates and their sub-components suffered from a decreased prevalence of certain conditions such as coronary heart disease, diabetes, etc.

Public education about complex carbohydrates began in the United States in 1977, with Dietary Goals for the United States, a report from the United States Senate Select Committee on Nutrition and Human Needs (McGovern Commission) (1). Nutrition and Your Health: Dietary Guidelines for Americans, first issued in 1980, continues to recommend that consumers increase their intake of foods containing complex carbohydrates (2). In 1988 The Surgeon Generals Report on Nutrition and Health also recommended an increased consumption of complex carbohydrates and fiber, with an emphasis on diets high in whole-grain cereal products, vegetables, and fruits (3). The 10th edition of Recommended Dietary Allowances and Diet and Health: Implications for Reducing Chronic Disease Risk echoed the call for increased complex carbohydrate consumption (digestible complex carbohydrates and dietary fiber) (4,5). Finally, the 1992 Food Guide Pyramid reemphasized the need to increase consumption of complex carbohydrates relative to other foods (i.e., three times as many vegetables, fruits, and grain products) (6). Thus, consumers, health and nutrition professionals, and the media have been extensively educated about the need to increase complex carbohydrates in the diet. Consumers are aware of the need for increased consumption of complex carbohydrates, but the data are not readily available as part of the food label's nutrition facts.

The Association of Official Analytical Chemists (AOAC) International has responded to the Food and Drug Administration's (FDA) proposed regulations

---

* Jonathan W. Devries

about the labeling of complex carbohydrates by committing itself to pursuing and validating appropriate methodology if these new labeling regulations are adopted. AOAC International has initiated work to establish a single clear definition and to provide commensurate official methodology. Complex carbohydrates should include both dietary fiber and the digestible complex carbohydrate fractions of food. Analytic methods have been developed and proposed for collaborative validation. The definition and methods encompass both the physiologic and chemical bases for complex carbohydrates. Enzyme systems used for analysis mimic the human digestive system, thus providing a physiologic basis. Complexity of the carbohydrate is chemically established by the insolubility of the fraction in four parts alcohol and one part water, which has long been considered the standard basis for separating the simple from the more complex compounds in food matrices.

A potential scheme for listing carbohydrate information on labels and in nutrition data table might be:

Total carbohydrates
Complex carbohydrates
Dietary fiber
Digestible complex carbohydrates
Sugars
Sugar alcohols (optional)
Other carbohydrates

AOAC International is committed to validating appropriate methodology, and progress is being made. Nutrition knowledge will continue to increase and so will the validated methods, because inclusion of complex carbohydrate data on the nutrition label would be beneficial to consumers.

DIETARY GUIDANCE ISSUES*

Nutritionists generally accept that humans do not need more than 10–12% of their total energy from protein and that fat should provide no more than 30%. By mathematical difference, carbohydrate intake should be approximately 55–60% of total daily calories. Human diets have historically contained 40-80% of their energy as carbohydrate. However, as income has increased, fat content has increased as well, while the carbohydrate content, especially starch, has decreased.

In the 1980s the number of recommendations for increasing carbohydrate intake grew and became more specific. Generally, the recommendations divided

* Joanne Slavin

the carbohydrate intake into two groups: 1) sugars and 2) complex carbohydrates and starch. However, issues associated with definitions and methods of isolating complex carbohydrates need to be resolved before complex carbohydrates can be added to the nutrition label.

In the United States, the term "complex carbohydrates" was first used in the Senate Select Committee Report and included digestible carbohydrates or starch (1). The British Nutrition Foundation report included both starch and non-starch polysaccharides as complex carbohydrates and stated that because foods rich in complex carbohydrates have greatly diverse physical and biological properties, it is difficult to generalize about these properties (7). The report also noted that there is more overlap between the behavior and properties of the starches and non-starch polysaccharides than was previously thought. Resistant starch is probably metabolized similarly to some dietary fiber components in the gut. Thus, it appears that complex carbohydrates should contain both dietary fiber and starches and that certain substances (e.g., phytate and phenolic compounds) and micronutrients (e.g., zinc and magnesium) are important components associated with complex carbohydrates.

Classification of complex carbohydrates should not specify the minimum chain length of saccharides. Dietary recommendations to increase intake of complex carbohydrates are based on the assumption that the carbohydrates are not isolated, but rather are derived from intact foods. Most dietary guidance is offered as a general endorsement of starches and complex carbohydrates to replace dietary fat. There is growing acceptance that isolated carbohydrates provide different physiologic responses than do whole foods.

Dietary recommendations for complex carbohydrates must be based on a synthesis of epidemiological, metabolic, and mechanistic data and by necessity will be nonspecific. The British Nutrition Foundation report noted that for most adults consuming nutritionally adequate diets, an increased intake of complex carbohydrates is unlikely to lead to deficiencies in micronutrients (7). Further, it appears sensible for adults to increase their intake of a variety of foods that are rich in complex carbohydrates. A wide range of carbohydrate intake is consistent with health, but recommendations for carbohydrate intake cannot be based on classical approaches for defining nutrient requirements because there is no clear-cut deficiency disease related to carbohydrates.

THE PHYSIOLOGIC EFFECTS*

Complex carbohydrates are important sources of dietary energy, and those that resist digestion are now emerging as important components of the diet. Some of

---

* Alison Stephen

these carbohydrates are fermented like soluble dietary fiber. Others resist fermentation and are excreted in the same manner as insoluble dietary fiber.

The soluble fiber component of non-starch polysaccharides resists digestion within the small intestine and undergoes extensive fermentation to short-chain fatty acids within the large intestine. Production of acetic, propionic, and butyric acids from non-digestible non-starch polysaccharides by the microflora of the colon has been shown to benefit colonic health. Resistant starch could be considered to act like a non-starch polysaccharide within the complex carbohydrate umbrella now recognized to resist digestion and to undergo extensive colonic fermentation to butyric acid.

Numerous factors determine the proportion of dietary starch that becomes resistant starch. The extent of resistant starch fermentation is controlled by physical factors such as source, granular structure, degree of processing (cooking and/or cooling), and relative ratio to protein, fat, plant silica, lignin, and phytate. Physiologic factors such as extent of chewing, rate of passage through the small intestine, and activity of intestinal amylases also determine the amount of ingested starch available for colonic fermentation.

A growing body of evidence suggests that the preferential fermentation of resistant starch to butyric acid not only improves colonic health but also may protect against the development of colon cancer. Inhibition of uncontrolled cancer cell growth by butyric acid has been attributed to its ability to promote acetylation of histones, its direct interaction with genetic material, its effect on cell methylation, and its promotion of programmed cell death. The factors responsible for the inhibition of cancer cell growth by butyric acid are less well defined. Butyric acid is thought to affect cell growth by regulating the production of epidermal growth factor, estrogen receptors, or polyamines.

Epidemiological analysis of individual dietary intake has shown a significant inverse relationship between starch consumption and colon cancer mortality. This may be due in part to increased availability of resistant starch for colon fermentation.

DEFINING SIMPLE AND COMPLEX CARBOHYDRATES*

Carbohydrate-rich foods contain mixtures of sugars, starches, and fibers. Different criteria are used to define the analytic and physiologic distinctiveness of these components. Because the impact of carbohydrates on human nutrition is more rigorous than inherent in simplified definitions, integrated analytic and nutrition terminologies are necessary to convey the importance of carbohydrates in human health.

* Dennis Gordon

Although there is an established analytic nomenclature for carbohydrates, appropriate descriptors are required to indicate their collective physiologic attributes and roles. The term "complex carbohydrates" was adopted to simplify the dietary contributions of a broad and chemically diverse group of carbohydrates. For instance, variable inclusion or exclusion of total dietary fiber is one of the recognized incongruities related to the common use of the term.

The lack of accepted measurements for defining the components of complex carbohydrates resulted in the exclusion of information about complex carbohydrates from the recently implemented NLEA. Although the term complex carbohydrates is used in most education materials, human physiologic response to dietary carbohydrates is more complicated than that implied by the labels "simple" and "complex." Use of the terms "total carbohydrates" and "other carbohydrates" in nutrition labeling is without precedence; no quantitative measure of carbohydrates is represented by the calculated values.

The proposed classification of simple and complex carbohydrates requires establishment of an accepted system for determining solubility and requires reliable methods for the recovery of all non-digestible carbohydrates and commercially available bulking agents used in some foods. Establishment of an accepted system would require agreement to define the average degree of polymerization separating soluble and insoluble oligosaccharides or dextrins.

Under the proposed FDA definition complex carbohydrates would include starches and dietary fiber. Starches would include amylose, amylopectin, modified starches, resistant starches, and insoluble and digestible or non-digestible oligosaccharides and dextrins. Dietary fiber would include insoluble dietary fiber, soluble dietary fiber, soluble or insoluble non-digestible oligosaccharides and polysaccharides, non-digestible and non-absorbable disaccharides, non-absorbable monosaccharides, and sugar alcohols. Inclusion of resistant starches with dietary fiber is consistent with the proposed definitions. It may be more beneficial to list sugar alcohols as a separate category. Simple carbohydrates would include any soluble, digestible, and absorbable sugars and any soluble and digestible oligosaccharides and polysaccharides.

METHODOLOGY DEVELOPMENT*

The McGovern commission recommended that FDA establish a definition of complex carbohydrates. The FDA methodology for measuring complex carbohydrates is determined by summing the total dietary fiber and available starch measured in the sample. Using 80% aqueous ethanol simple carbohydrates (sugars

* Leon Prosky and Susan Sungsoo Cho

and low-molecular-weight dextrins) are removed from the food to be analyzed. Fat is extracted if the food contains more than 10% fat.

Duplicate samples of the de-sugared, sugar- and fat-extracted food are treated with a heat-stable amylase to degrade its starch. Each sample is then digested with a protease and an amyloglucosidase mixture to remove protein and starch. Incubation is performed under conditions specified in the AOAC International current method for dietary fiber in food and food products. After the addition of four volumes of ethanol, each sample is filtered. The filtrate is collected and set aside for analysis of available starch content. The residue collected on the filter is washed with ethanol and acetone to remove any remaining low-molecular-weight materials, dried, and weighed.

Total dietary fiber is calculated after correction for the protein and ash contents of the collected residue. The available starch content of the original food is calculated from the glucose content of the filtrate set aside after the addition of four volumes of ethanol. The collected filtrate is evaporated before various spectrophotometric or chromatographic procedures determine its glucose content. Spectrophotometric procedures include either an ultraviolet-enzymatic or a visible-colorimetric method. Chromatographic methods use high-pressure liquid chromatography (HPLC) with either a bonded-amine column, which is preferred, or an ion-exchange column.

In a recent survey conducted by the AOAC International Food and Nutrition Committee the FDA methodology appears to meet the definition criteria most frequently cited as appropriate by scientists working in the area of complex carbohydrates. However, a number of methodology issues still require resolution. Two basic issues concern completeness of starch digestion by the alpha-amylase-protease-amyloglucosidase mixture, and elimination of the long and tedious step of filtrate evaporation through implementation of newer, more sensitive HPLC detectors. Complex carbohydrate methodology must address quantification of oligosaccharides resistant to digestion in the human alimentary system. Finally, methodology implemented for determining complex carbohydrates requires multi-laboratory validation of its ruggedness, accuracy, and precision no matter how it is defined.

PERSPECTIVES ON LABELING*

Perspectives from both the U. S. government and the food industry about complex carbohydrates were presented.

FDA permits the term "other carbohydrate" (calculated as the amount of carbohydrate remaining after subtraction of dietary fiber, sugars, and sugar alco-

---

* F. Edward Scarbrough and Gary Henderson

hols from total carbohydrate) on the nutrition label rather than the term "complex carbohydrate". The reasons for this decision were: 1) The inclusion of complex carbohydrate on the label might have suggested greater public health significance than that established by diet and health studies; 2) The term "complex carbohydrate" had not been clearly defined; and 3) The analytic methodologies for complex carbohydrate were not sufficiently developed. Also, FDA was unable to establish a daily recommended value (DRV) for label reference purposes. FDA concluded from submitted comments that there was not sufficient consensus related to the meaning of the term "complex carbohydrate" and was persuaded to change the name to "other carbohydrate". The FDA has acknowledged that academia, professional societies, and the food industry continue to express interest in including complex carbohydrate on the label and hoped that this conference would give the agency some guidance about how to proceed.

From the perspective of the U. S. food industry, consumers do not understand the term "other carbohydrate". A study was conducted to compare consumer understanding of the terms "complex carbohydrate" and "other carbohydrate" in the cereal category 6 months before and 6 months after NLEA labels appeared in the marketplace. Results indicated that there is a fair amount of confusion among consumers regarding the term "other carbohydrate." The reason for this confusion is the equity in the term "complex carbohydrate" that has been building since 1977 through references in dietary guidelines, programs by health professionals and industry, and use in pre-NLEA labeling. The return to the term "complex carbohydrate" would reduce consumer confusion. Factors that should be considered in reinstatement are: 1) Opportunities for the use of complex carbohydrate as a marker nutrient; 2) Provision of quantitative information if the lack of consensus on daily value is seen as a barrier; and 3) Consideration of the physiologic effect in developing a definition.

SUMMARY OF AOAC SURVEY ON COMPLEX CARBOHYDRATES*

In 1992 the AOAC International Task Force on Nutrients Labeling Analysis and its Subcommittee on Carbohydrates Methodology concluded that more work was necessary to develop an analytic methodology for complex carbohydrates. In 1993 AOAC International subsequently established refereeship in the area of complex carbohydrates to accommodate the analytic needs. As the first step in establishing analytic methodology an international survey on complex carbohydrate definition and analysis under the auspices of AOAC International was initiated.

---

* Susan Sungsoo Cho and Leon Prosky

The survey was designed to determine if a consensus could be reached on the definition of complex carbohydrates and associated methodologies. Approximately 200 survey questionnaires were distributed to professionals in the area of carbohydrates and 114 replies were received. The survey results indicated that complex carbohydrates should include available starch and total dietary fiber. In the previous two international surveys on dietary fiber definition and analysis respondents generally supported including lignin (a non-carbohydrate substance closely associated structurally with other dietary fiber components) and resistant oligosaccharides in the definition, in addition to non-starch polysaccharides and resistant starches. Considering the results from these three international surveys and the traditional labeling of dietary fiber that has included lignins, it is logical to conclude that complex carbohydrates can be described for labeling purposes as the sum of available starches and dietary fiber including resistant oligosaccharides and lignin. The current AOAC International position is that analytic methodology can be developed to meet this proposed definition for complex carbohydrates.

PANEL DISCUSSION*

1. *What are the important scientific reasons for including complex carbohydrates on the label?*

The panel emphasized the need to increase the physiologic database supporting the overall benefits of a diet high in complex carbohydrates to support and substantiate the current dietary recommendations and reach a consensus on the definition and methodology to reduce the research fragmentation that currently exists. The panel suggested practical reasons for putting the term complex carbohydrate on the label:

1. Complex carbohydrates are a marker of foods people should be consuming.
2. Use of the term is a normal progression of knowledge about the health benefits of carbohydrates; complex carbohydrates and even types of complex carbohydrates (such as resistant starch) are an important component of the diet. It was noted that this is similar to the progression of knowledge on the importance of fiber and on specific types of fiber (for example, soluble and insoluble fiber).

---

* Moderator: Beth Olson. Panelists: Jonathan W. Devries; David Kritchevsky, Wistar Institute, Philadelphia, PA; Elaine Lanza, National Cancer Institute, Bethesda, MD; Betty W. Li, U.S. Department of Agriculture, Washington, DC; Linda Van Horn, Northwestern University Medical School, Chicago, IL; Thomas Wolever, University of Toronto, Ontario, Canada; John Vanderveen, U.S. Food and Drug Administration, Washington, DC.

3. There is a history to the use of the term and consumer recognition that they should look for it in foods.

There was consensus that use of the term "complex carbohydrate" will help the progress of science in the area.

2. *Given the current methodology, what should the definition of complex carbohydrates be for purposes of nutrition labeling?*

The panel suggested the following definitions: starch and dietary fiber, starch and non-starch polysaccharides, and carbohydrates with degree of polymerization greater than or equal to 10.

3. *If methodology could be developed, what would the ideal definition be for purposes of nutrition labeling?*

Future definitions would ideally be physiologically based. As more knowledge is gained about the health benefit of particular carbohydrates and how to measure them, they should be included on the label. Examples of future possibilities given for labeling purposes were lignin and resistant starch.

4. *What definition would best serve the purposes of current scientific recommendations to increase complex carbohydrates consumption (e.g., Dietary Guidelines for Americans, The Surgeon General's Report on Nutrition and Health)?*

The panel felt that to determine the best definition, analytic starch values would need to be available to researchers working on the health benefits of carbohydrate. Also, more knowledge is needed about healthful diets and what these diets comprise.

5. *What are the gaps in our scientific knowledge of complex carbohydrates?*

The gaps are in the three areas of the analytic, physiologic, and health benefits of complex carbohydrates. Some health benefits are known, but less is known about the physiologic effects behind these health benefits. The panel members agree that there needs to be more starch analysis done, particularly by the government. The analytic data must be available for researchers working in the area of carbohydrates so that they can find the components in food and then investigate health benefits.

6. *Is there sufficient scientific rationale to put the term complex carbohydrates on the nutrition label?*

Several members of the panel agreed that additional scientific evidence is required to provide the foundation for the labeling of complex carbohydrates. They emphasized the need to advance the definition, methodology, and physiologic data to support such labeling efforts. Members also indicated that the term could have a practical labeling purpose.

It was stated that the term "other carbohydrate" is not meaningful and that "complex carbohydrate" is preferable because of the history of its use. Some members felt that the best compromise for the definition should be: "starch plus dietary fiber or non-starch polysaccharides". This is because there is evidence that these components are important in the diet. In addition, these compounds are markers of a good diet, and people therefore should find that the term "complex carbohydrate" provides useful information on the Nutrition Facts label. It was felt that the term should be reconsidered for labeling after the standardization of definition and methodology.

SUMMARY AND CONCLUSION*

This conference resulted in a foundation upon which consensus will be built in the future. Further, it provided a forum for the articulation of the critical need for carbohydrates in human nutrition. We have come a long way in the past 25 years in the food and nutrition sciences and this conference well illustrated that point. At the White House Conference on Nutrition in 1969, macronutrients were never even mentioned as being necessary to nutrition; only micronutrients were emphasized. In 1977 the term "complex carbohydrate" was used without definition in the Dietary Goals for the United States (1). This conference encapsulated the tremendous strides that have been made concerning the chemical, nutritional, biologic, and physiologic importance of carbohydrates in health and disease.

It is fascinating to review the recommendations concerning complex carbohydrate from 1977 on. The list includes recommendations made by the Senate Select Committee in 1977, the Dietary Guidelines of 1980, 1985, and 1990, the Surgeon General's reports of 1979 and 1988, the 10th edition of Recommended Dietary Allowances, the 1989 National Academy of Sciences Diet and Health: Implications for Reducing Chronic Disease Risk, the 1991 FDA proposal for labeling, and the 1992 Food Guide Pyramid (1-6,8). Indeed, as Joanne Slavin pointed out, ". . . there is a wide range of consensus that increased complex carbohydrate is consistent with good health . . . " and certainly as Gary Henderson said, ". . . the term complex carbohydrate has equity with consumers."

With this level of apparent clarity it is difficult at first to identify a problem for the food label. After all, if consumer health would benefit why not simply do it? However, a problem does exist in that carbohydrates may be classified chemically in groups that are difficult to analyze and to define as to their physiologic function in the body. Indeed, complex carbohydrates defined by chain length may have molecular structures less complex than those of smaller units and may vary in solubility and digestibility. A continuum does exist in each of the chemical, analytical, and physiologic characteristics of carbohydrates. Scien-

---

* Fergus Clydesdale

tists do not like a continuum and regulators probably like it even less, but such a continuum holds great promise for future consensus. This continuum provided the thoughtful alternatives presented above by Jonathan Devries, Dennis Gordon, and Alison Stephen. Devries suggested a scheme of complex carbohydrates, sugars, and sugar alcohols, while Gordon suggested complex carbohydrates, dietary fiber, and simple carbohydrates, and Stephen suggested starch, sugar, and non-starch polysaccharides. Surely, we can develop a meaningful technique for labeling from these recommendations, which illustrate the continuum.

Further complicating the complicated scientific questions are the questions raised by consumer understanding and education. The label is not only a statement of truth for package content but is a tool for creating better-educated and better-fed consumers. Scarbrough pointed out that FDA was concerned because a DRV does not exist for complex carbohydrates and because health benefits should not be exaggerated. Both of these are legitimate concerns. We are currently recommending that carbohydrate be the major macronutrient in the diet, which seems to lessen the concern for a DRV and exaggerated claims to eat more.

Consumers will conceivably derive many benefits from the labeling of what we consider complex carbohydrate. We must obtain more data from consumers on what and how they understand some of the proposals put forth today. If we do this correctly we can certainly do a better job of educating consumers. By labeling carbohydrates rationally and tracking our scientific knowledge, we will be able to reduce the good food / bad food syndrome that is all too prevalent in much of our nutrition education system. We could also eliminate the term "other carbohydrate" which can only cause confusion and concern. Lastly, and perhaps most importantly, we will have the potential to increase the consumption of foods that are high in carbohydrates.

Aside from consumer education other benefits would be derived from including complex carbohydrates on the food label. Incentives would be created for the support of more research to better define the relationship between carbohydrates and health as well as more research into the development of new food products that are consistent with national dietary goals.

It is clear that this is not a simple task. Classifications cannot be made simply for chemical or analytic expediency if they do not adequately express physiologic significance. However, we are all committed to achieving a means to satisfy this continuum, and I have no doubt that in the future we will have labels presenting what we all think of as complex carbohydrate.

This summary has been reviewed and approved by each of the speakers and panel members from the workshop on Complex Carbohydrates: the Science and the Label. The views expressed herein are those of the individual authors and/or their organizations, and do not necessarily reflect the views of ILSI North America.

REFERENCES

1. U. S. Congress, Senate (1977) Dietary Goals for the United States, Stock no. 052-070-03913-2. U.S. Government Printing Office, Washington, D. C.
2. U. S. Department of Agriculture/U. S. Department of Health and Human Services (1985) Nutrition and Your Health: Dietary Guidelines for Americans, 2nd ed., Home and Garden Bulletin no. 232, U.S. Government Printing Office, Washington, D. C.
3. U. S. Department of Health and Human Services (1988) The Surgeon General's Report on Nutrition and Health, DHHS (PHS) Publ. no. 88-50210, U. S. Government Printing Office, Washington, D. C.
4. National Research Council (1989) Recommended Dietary Allowances, 10th ed., National Academy Press, Washington, D. C.
5. National Research Council (1989) Diet and Health: Implications for Reducing Chronic Disease Risk, National Academy Press, Washington, D. C.
6. U. S. Department of Agriculture and U. S. Department of Health and Human Services (1992) The Food Guide Pyramid, Home and Garden no. 252, U. S. Government Printing Office, Washington, D.C.
7. British Nutrition Foundation (1994) Starchy foods in the diet. British Nutrition Foundation, London, UK.
8. U. S. Department of Health, Education and Welfare (1979) Healthy people: the Surgeon General's report on health promotion and disease prevention, DHEW (PHS) Publ. no. 79-55071, U. S. Government Printing Office, Washington, D. C.

7

The Role of Dietary Fiber in the Prevention of Lipid Metabolism Disorders

ELZBIETA BARTNIKOWSKA
Warsaw Agricultural University, Warsaw, Poland

INTRODUCTION

The earlier assumptions regarding the importance of dietary fiber relate to the controversy on the differences of white and brown bread in terms of health and better nutrition. Popular taste has tended to prefer white flour. Therefore white bread with its higher cost and greater aesthetic appeal had social esteem, which generally persisted until today.

The first researchers to pay attention to the health contribution of whole cereal foods were S. Graham and J. H. Kellogg. History was not on their side at that time, and the components of dietary fiber have largely been neglected as they were considered to have no nutritive value. In the last three decades, however, attention has been focused on the fiber content in the diet. Interest in fiber arose from epidemiological studies indicating the low prevalence of coronary heart disease, diabetes, gallstones, obesity, appendicitis, diverticulosis, varicose veins and hemorrhoids in underdeveloped countries, but common in Western countries, may be due to the consumption of greater amounts of plant foods rich in fiber.

Epidemiological evidence linking the intake of dietary fiber and serum lipid levels indicates that the concentration of low-density lipoprotein (LDL) and total cholesterol and triglycerides in blood serum are significantly lower in populations habitually consuming high-fiber diets. Detailed experimental animal studies indicate the water soluble components of dietary fiber reduce serum total cholesterol and atherosclerotic changes in the aorta wall. The hypocholesterolemic effects of water soluble fibers were more visible when experimental diets were supplemented with cholesterol and/or saturated fats. Similar results were obtained in clinical studies in humans. The most effective dietary fiber components are pectins present in fruits and vegetables, guar gum in beans, and soluble beta-glucans in cereal grains, particularly in oat and barley. The hypocholesterolemic effect of the soluble components of dietary fiber depends on its form and amount of fiber intake, and was more pronounced in patients with hyperlipidemia than in persons without lipid metabolism disorders.

It should be stressed that it is very important to distinguish between the effects of food rich in fiber and diets containing fiber as an added ingredient. Foods rich in fiber are usually rich in complex carbohydrates, microelements, and vitamins with antioxidative properties like vitamin C, tocopherols, tocotrienols and carotenoids. Interactions between these dietary components may be responsible not only for the prevention of lipid metabolism disorders, but also for coronary heart disease (CHD).

INFLUENCE OF DIETARY FIBER ON LIPID METABOLISM

Epidemiologic Studies

Epidemiologic studies performed by Burkitt, Trowell, and Walker indicate there are great differences in intakes of dietary fiber depending on geographical location, and simultaneously significant negative correlation between the consumption of dietary fiber and the prevalence of CHD (1, 2). Nutritional studies in which diet composition of people living in rural areas in Africa and in urban areas in Europe were compared indicate that diets rich in fiber and complex carbohydrates may prevent lipid metabolism disorders and atherosclerosis (3, 4). This hypothesis was further confirmed by the observation that Africans who adopt European lifestyles and diets based on refined products showed a significant increase in the prevalence of hyperlipidemias and CHD.

It is well established that LDL and total cholesterol levels are correlated according to the exponential curve with the risk of CHD. Simultaneously, there is a negative correlation between high-density lipoprotein (HDL) cholesterol and the risk of CHD. Hence, there arises great need to perform indirect studies on the influence of dietary components on blood lipids and lipoprotein levels in experimental animals, as well as the comparison of obtained results with the results from histopathological studies. These findings also create the possibility of studying the influence of different dietary components on blood lipid metabolism indices and the risk of atherosclerosis in humans.

Studies performed by Sacks et al. (5) and other investigators (6) demonstrate that total, very low-density lipoprotein (VLDL) and LDL cholesterol levels are significantly higher in nonvegetarians than in matched vegetarian controls. Although the HDL-cholesterol levels also are higher in nonvegetarians, the ratio of HDL cholesterol to total cholesterol is significantly lower compared to vegetarians. Additionally, blood triglyceride levels in nonvegetarians are significantly higher than in vegetarians. Simultaneously, the prevalence of CHD in nonvegetarians is higher than in vegetarians (7).

The epidemiologic data linking the intake of dietary fiber and risk of CHD is less consistent than the data on blood lipid levels. Liu et al. (8) found the rate of CHD in 20 developed countries varied inversely with fiber intake. Morris et al. (9), for example, reported that fiber from cereals protect against CHD.

Animal Studies

The influence of dietary components on blood lipids and atherogenesis depends on the animal model, some of which are more susceptible than others to atherosclerotic lesions induced via the alimentary tract. Hence, this may account for difference in data obtained from animal studies. It should be also stressed that there are multidirectional interactions of dietary fiber and other diet components, which may be responsible for the observed effects.

As it appears from the summary of studies performed on rats by Anderson and Chen (10), water soluble components of fiber (pectin, guar gum) significantly lower the concentration of total cholesterol in blood, whereas the hypocholesterolemic effect of water insoluble components (cellulose) is less pronounced. From the detailed studies performed by Newman et al. (11), with the use of the enzyme beta-glucanase, beta-glucan has significant hypocholesterolemic properties.

It is generally accepted that dietary cholesterol, saturated fats, and animal protein increase the concentration of total cholesterol in blood and raise the risk of atherosclerosis. Results of experimental studies showed that fiber counteracts the hypercholesterolemic and atherogenic action of dietary cholesterol, saturated fats, and animal proteins (12).

Similar to the effects on blood cholesterol levels, separate components of dietary fiber differently influence liver cholesterol levels in laboratory animals. Supplementation of a rat diet with insoluble fibers such as cellulose raised liver cholesterol above that of the control group of rats. Contrary to this, in rats receiving soluble components such as pectin or carboxyl methylcellulose, less cholesterol was accumulated in the liver than in the control group (13).

Clinical and Metabolic Studies

Results of animal experiments as well as epidemiological observations encouraged many research workers to perform clinical studies on humans. It appears the influence of dietary fiber components added to the diet is different. A summary of studies with wheat bran and cellulose by Anderson and Chen (10) indicates the influence of these fiber sources may depend on the dose of fiber. However, in the majority of studies with wheat bran, the content of fiber was not specified. Due to production technology wheat bran may consist of 16% to 45% dietary fiber. Due to the lack of detailed characteristics of the wheat bran used most results are difficult to interpret. However, in humans and experimental animals wheat bran (as opposed to oat bran) has no hypocholesterolemic effect.

It should be mentioned that Hillman et al. (14) demonstrated the consumption of diet supplemented with lignin by persons with hypercholesterolemia is associated with a decrease of total cholesterol concentration in the blood. However, in persons without disorders of lipid metabolism lignin has no such effect. Studies performed in vitro demonstrate that lignin binds bile acids (15). The hypocholesterolemic action of lignin may be the result of binding bile acids in the intestinal lumen. This mechanism is similar to cholestyramine or plant sterols that have a marked hypocholesterolemic effect in persons with hypercholesterolemia (16). Although different doses of fiber were used in these separate studies it appears from these summaries that the water insoluble components of dietary fiber are relatively ineffective in lowering the total cholesterol concentration in blood in humans, while the water soluble components are moderately effective.

It should be stressed that it is very important to distinguish between the effects of food rich in fiber and diets containing dietary fiber components as an added ingredient. Guar gum and pectin are fiber sources that were commonly added to the diet as purified preparations of dietary fiber. It was found that the hypocholesterolemic effect of such preparations depends on the dose of fiber and the forms in which they were administered (biscuits, gelatin capsules and water gel form). The most effective are fibers (pectin) in water gel form without sugar. Additionally, the hypocholesterolemic effect of fiber (pectin and beta-glucans) was more pronounced in patients with hypercholesterolemia than in persons without lipid metabolism disorders.

Palmer and Dixon (17) reported that a dose of pectin below 10 grams per day is ineffective in lowering cholesterol levels. In turn, enlarging the dose of pectin to 40–50 grams per day did not multiply its hypocholesterolemic activity. In addition, a 40–50 gram per day dose caused unfavorable side effects, particularly flatulence, and sometimes diarrhea and vomiting (18). The most often-used dose of pectin was 15 g/day. Some authors suggest that such a dose of pectin included in the diet is optimal (19). Ershoff and Wells (20) demonstrated that pectin derivatives, such as pectic acid, galacturonic acid or polygalacturonic acid, at levels of 5% of diet did not affect serum and liver cholesterol concentrations in cholesterol fed rats. Likewise, methylated polygalacturonic acid had no hypocholesterolemic activity. Thus it would appear that only intact pectin has hypocholesterolemic activity, which is partially determined by its methoxyl content.

TABLE 1 Influence of Oat Products on Lipoprotein Cholesterol Level in Humans

References	Fiber source	Dose of fiber (g/day)	Percent of control Cholesterol HDL	Percent of control Cholesterol LDL
Kirby et al., 1981 (23)	Oat bran	27	0	−1.4
Kestin et al., 1990 (24)	Oat bran	95	−2.8	−6.8
Anderson et al., 1991 (25)	Oat bran	110	+10.4	−12.1
Leadbetter et al., 1991 (26)	Oat bran	30	−5.1	−2.5
	Oat bran	60	−4.5	1.7
	Oat bran	90	−8.9	−4.0
Lepre et al., 1992 (27)	Oat bran	60	+2.3	−3.0
Uusitupa et al., 1992 (28)	Oat bran	29.8	−1.3	−4.8
Whyte et al., 1992 (29)	Oat bran	123	+4.9	−5.6
Kashtan et al., 1992 (30)	Oat bran	100	−9.8	−12.4
Poulter et al., 1993 (31)	Oat bran	50	+3.4	−8.1
He et al., 1995 (32)	Oat bran	<25	0	−3.8
	Oat bran	25–90	+2.5	−16.8
	Oat bran	>90	−7.7	−4.9

Our results demonstrated that in patients with hyperlipidemia, high methoxylated pectin exerts significantly higher hypocholesterolemic activity than low methoxylated pectin. In persons with hyperlipidemia, the degree of hypocholesterolemic activity of pectin depends on the blood total cholesterol levels. Pectin exerts higher hypocholesterolemic activity in patients with hypercholesterolemia than in persons without disorders of lipid metabolism (2).

Similar results were obtained with oat preparations (meal, bran) rich in beta-glucans. Inclusion of oat preparation to the diet of persons with hypercholesterolemia caused significant reduction of blood total cholesterol, whereas in persons without disorders of lipid metabolism, the hypocholesterolemic effect of oat preparations was low (21). Similarly, the hypocholesterolemic effect of oat depends also on the dose of oat fiber, but exceeding such a dose does not give an appropriate hypocholesterolemic response.

In order to evaluate if oat products decrease total cholesterol concentration in blood, Ripsin et al. (22) performed a meta-analysis of the results of clinical studies with oat. This analysis provided strong support for the hypothesis that approximately 3 g per day of soluble fiber from oat products can lower total cholesterol level by 0.13 to 0.16 mmol/l, and that the reduction is greater in persons with initially higher blood cholesterol levels. From the summary of results of clinical studies with oat bran (23–32), it appears soluble beta-glucans decrease LDL cholesterol without marked influence on HDL cholesterol. As a result, the ratios of HDL cholesterol to LDL cholesterol as well as the ratio of HDL cholesterol to total cholesterol were increased.

MECHANISMS OF ACTION

The mechanism of lowering blood cholesterol by dietary fiber is not fully understood. Since dietary fiber is not absorbed, it may be expected that its effect would be exerted in the gastrointestinal tract. Dietary fiber binds cholesterol and bile acids in the intestinal lumen and increases their excretion (10). This may partly explain the observation that the hypocholesterolemic action of water soluble components of dietary fiber is more visible in cases of diets supplemented with cholesterol.

The results of a detailed study performed by Thomas et al. (33) demonstrated that fiber from black gram increases hydroxy-methyl-glutaryl CoA (HMG CoA) reductase activity in liver. Increased activity of HMG CoA reductase (the main enzyme controlling cholesterol biosynthesis) may reflect increased cholesterogenesis in response to increased losses of cholesterol and bile acids in faces after high fiber meals.

Studies performed by Marlett et al. (34) with the use of stable isotope labeled bile acids demonstrated that oat bran not only reduced bile acid absorption and increased bile acid synthesis, but also changed the proportion of separate bile acids in the total bile acid pool. The pool size of cholic acid was decreased, whereas the pool size of its secondary bile acid (chenodesoxycholic acid) doubled. Decreased absorption of bile acids leads to switching of cholesterol to synthesis of bile acids, resulting in less cholesterol is available for synthesis of lipoprotein in liver.

Dietary fiber alters transit time as well as the morphology of the intestinal mucosa in a manner that could influence lipid digestion and absorption (10). Gallaher et al. (35) in studies with radiolabeled cholesterol and triglycerides demonstrated that cellulose changed the site at which lipids are absorbed from the intestine. The incorporation of fiber into diets is associated with slowing digestion and promoting more absorption from ileum, which in turn alters the lipid and protein pattern in lymph. Altered size and composition of chylomicrons influence their subsequent metabolism (10).

The other experimental studies performed on rats adapted short or long term to a high fiber diet with canulated mesenteric lymph system demonstrated that after a test meal, transport of cholesterol to the lymph is decreased (36). The results of our experiment performed on canulated pigs not adapted to a high fiber diet demonstrated that supplementation of test meal with pectin delayed transport of cholesterol to the lymph (37).

Similarly, in animals fed diets supplemented with water soluble fiber components for a long time secretion of chylomicrons to the lymph after a test meal was slowed down (36). The delayed secretion of chylomicrons to the lymph by water soluble components of fiber may be the result of transit time elongation by slowing gastric emptying (35), changes in peristaltic movements, modifications of pancreas enzymes activity (38), inhibition of lipid diffusion to the intestinal wall or their defusion though an unstirred water layer (35). Sustained supplementation with fiber alters intestinal surface morphology, the membrane function involved in the transmural transport of nutrients, and biosynthetic events in mucosal cells (36). Farness and Schneeman (39) reported that the ingestion of pectin increases the length of the small intestine and mucosal weight in rats relative to a fiber free diet.

Water soluble components of fiber, unlike insoluble components, are fermented almost completely by colonic bacteria to short chain fatty acids, acetate, propionate and butyrate. The concentration of these fatty acids in hepatic portal venous blood of rats fed pectin were higher than those fed cellulose. It has been shown that in isolated rat hepatocytes, acetate and propionate suppress de novo cholesterol synthesis. However, these inhibitory effects of short chain fatty acids are influenced by their higher concentration than those produced during fermentation of soluble fiber in large intestine (40, 41). Short chain fatty acids might additionally help to reduce blood cholesterol concentration.

Mechanisms of hypocholesterolemic effect of fiber may also include the influence of fiber on increased catabolism of LDL and possibly on increased peripheral LDL receptors and LDL clearance (42).

DIETARY FIBER AND ANTIOXIDANTS

Recently, considerable attention has been focused on the role of dietary antioxidants (particularly vitamin E, carotenoids and vitamin C) in counteracting the formation of lipid peroxides and oxidative modifications of LDLs, which play an important role in the progression of atherosclerosis. Dietary fiber binds bile acids and increases formation of micelles in the intestinal lumen. It may lead to decreased absorption of fat-soluble vitamins. In experiments on the influence of dietary fiber components on absorption of vitamin A and β-carotene in animals, conflicting results were obtained (43, 44). It should be mentioned, however, that diets rich in plant foods and high in fiber are also rich in antioxidants such as vitamin C, tocopherols and tocotrienols, carotenoids and other phenolic compounds such as tannins with high antioxidative properties. If dietary fibers were to suppress the absorption of dietary antioxidants, such action of fiber would be compensated by a simultaneous rise in dietary antioxidant intake.

Hostmark et al. (45) observed that in nonvegetarians who consumed a typical vegetarian diet for three weeks, apart from a reduction of total cholesterol, the concentration of lipid peroxides in blood decreased significantly. This observation suggests that the antioxidant status in humans is influenced by dietary habits, and may explain why many epidemiological studies show an inverse relationship between intake of fresh fruits and vegetables, rich in fiber and antioxidants, and mortality from CHD.

ACKNOWLEDGMENT

This work was partly supported by grant No. 5830701006 from the State Committee for Scientific Research in Poland.

REFERENCES

1. Anderson J.W., Deakins D. A., Bridges S. R. (1990) in Dietary Fiber Chemistry, Physiology, and Health Effects. D. Kritchevsky, C. Bonfield, & J.W. Anderson (Eds), Plenum Press, New York, pp.339–363.
2. Bartnikowska E., & Michajlik A. (1980) Kardiol. Pol. 23, 131–138.
3. Burkitt D.P., Walker A.R.P., Painter N.S. (1974) J. Am. Med. Assoc. 229, 1068–1074.
4. Burkitt D.P. (1973) Br. Med. J. 1, 274–278.

5. Sacks F.M, Castelli W.P., Donner A., Kass E. (1975) N. Engl. J. Med. 292, 1148–1151.
6. Resnicow K., Barone J., Engle A., Miller S., Haley N.J., Fleming D., & Wynder E. (1991) J. Am. Diet. Assoc. 91, 447–453.
7. Burr M.L., & Sweetman P.M. (1982) Am. J. Clin. Nutr. 36, 873–877.
8. Liu K., Stamler J., Trevison M., Moss D. (1982) Arteriosclerosis 2, 221–227.
9. Morris J.N., Marr J.W., Clayton D.G. (1977) Br. Med. J. 2, 1307–1314.
10. Anderson J.W., & Chen W.J.L. (1979) Am. J. Clin. Nutr. 32, 346–363.
11. Newman R.K., Klopfstein C.F., Newman C.W., Guritno N., Hofer P.J. (1992) Cereal Chem. 69, 240–244.
12. Kritchevsky D., Tepper S.A. (1968) J. Atheroscl. Res. 8, 357–369.
13. Chen W.L., Anderson J.W., Jennings D. (1984) Proc. Soc. Exp. Biol. Med. 175, 215–218.
14. Hillman L.C., Peters S.G., Fisher C.A. (1985) Am. J. Clin. Nutr. 42, 207–213.
15. Story J.A. (1982) in: Dietary Fiber in Health and Disease. G.V. Vahouny and D. Kritchevsky (Eds), Plenum Press, New York, pp. 253–264.
16. Von Bergman K. (1990) Current Opinion in Lipidology 1, 48–50.
17. Palmer G.H., Dixon D. G. (1966) Am. J. Clin. Nutr. 18, 437–442.
18. Miettinen T. A., Tarpila S. (1977) Clin. Chim. Acta 79, 471–477.
19. Kay R.M. (1976) Lancet II, 799–800.
20. Ershoff B.H., Wells A. F. (1963) Exp. Med. Surgery 21, 108–112.
21. Lund E.K., Farleigh C.A., Johnson I. T. (1990) in Dietary Fibre: Chemical and Biological Aspects. D.A.T. Southgate, K. Waldron, I. T. Johnson R. Fenwick (Eds), The Royal Society of Chemistry, pp.296–299.
22. Ripsin C. M., Keenan J.M., Jacobs D. R., Elmer P.J., Welch R.R., Van Horn L., Kiang L., Turnbull W.H., Thye F. W., Kestin M., Hegsted M., Davidson M.H., Dugan L.D., Demark-Wahnefried W., Beling S. (1992) J.A.M.A. 267, 3317–3325.
23. Kirby R.W., Anderson J.W., Sieling B., Rees E.D., Chen W.L., Miller R.E., Kay R.M. (1981) Am. J. Clin. Nutr. 34, 824–829.
24. Kestin M., Moss R., Clifton P.M., Nestel P.J. (1990) Am. J. Clin. Nutr. 52, 661–666.
25. Anderson J.W., Gilinsky N. H., Deakins D.A., Smith S.F., Spencer O'Neil D., Dillon D.W., Oeltgen P.R. (1991) Am. J. Clin Nutr. 54, 678–683
26. Leadbetter J., Ball M.J., Mann J.I. (1991) Am. J. Clin. Nutr. 54, 841–845.
27. Kromhout D., de Lezenne Coulander C. (1984) Am. J. Epidemiol. 119, 733–741.
28. Uusitupa M.I.J., Ruuskanen E., Makinen E., Laitinen J., Toskala E., Kervinen K., Kesaniemi Y.A. (1992) J. Am. Coll. Nutr. 11, 651–659.
29. Whyte J.L., McArthur R., Topping D., Nestel P. (1992) J. Am. Diet. Assoc. 92, 446–449.
30. Kashtan H., Stern H.S., Jenkins D.J.A., Jenkins A.L., Hay K., Marcon N., Minkin S., Bruce W.R.(1992) Am. J. Clin. Nutr. 55, 976–980.
31. Poulter N., Chang C.L., Cuff A., Poulter C., Sever P., Thom S. (1993) Am. J. Clin. Nutr. 58, 66–69.
32. He J., Klag M.J., Whelton P.K., Mo J.P., Chen J.Y., Qian M.C., Mo P.S., He G.Q. (1995) Am. J. Clin. Nutr. 61, 366–372.
33. Thomas M., Leelamma S., Kurup P.A. (1983) J. Nutr. 113, 1104–1108.

34. Marlett J.A., Hosig K.B., Vollendorf N.W., Shinnick F.L., Haack V.S., Story J. A. (1994) Hepatology 20, 1450–1457.
35. Gallaher D., Schneeman B. O. (1985) Am. J. Physiol. 249, G184-G191.
36. Vahouny G.V., Cassidy M.M. (1986) in Dietary Fiber: Basic and Clinical Aspects. G.V. Vahouny D. Kritchevsky (Eds), Plenum Press, New York & London, pp.181–209.
37. Bartnikowska, E., Zabielski, R. (1990) J. Anim. Physiol., Anim. Nutr. 64, 174–176.
38. Ikegami S., Tsuchihashi F., Harada H., Tsuchihashi N., Nishide E., Innami S. (1990) J. Nutr. 120, 353–360.
39. Farness, P.L., Schneeman, B.O. (1982) J. Nutr. 112, 1315–1319.
40. Kritchevsky D., Beynen A.C. (1986) in Nutritional Effects on Cholesterol Metabolism. A. C. Beynen (Ed), Transmondial Voorthuiizen pp. 19–28.
41. Imaizumi K., Sugano M. (1986) in Dietary Fiber. Basic and Clinical Aspects. G.V. Vahouny, D. Kritchevsky (Eds), Plenum Press, New York and London, pp. 287–308.
42. Kay R.M., Sabry Z.I., Csima A. (1980) Am. J. Clin. Nutr. 33, 2566–2572.
43. Erdman J.W., Fahey G.C., White C.B. (1986) J. Nutr. 116, 2415–2423.
44. Khaw K.T., Barret-Connor E. (1987) Am. J. Epidemiol. 126, 1093–1102.
45. Hostmark A.T., Lystad E., Vellar O. D., Hovi K., Berg J.E. (1993) Plant Food Human Nutr. 43, 55–61.

8

Health Benefits of Complex Carbohydrates

David Kritchevsky
The Wistar Institute, Philadelphia, Pennsylvania

The modern fiber era was launched with a paper by Cleave (1) that attributed many of the diseases of developed countries to consumption of refined sugar and refined flour. Burkitt, Trowell and Walker, all of whom worked in Africa, noticed the low incidence of large bowel cancer, ischemic heart disease, diabetes, and gallstones in rural areas.

Burkitt and Trowell expanded these observations and brought them to the attention of the nutrition and medical communities (2–6). Hipsley (7) coined the term ''dietary fiber.'' Dietary fiber may be defined as plant material that resists digestion by human alimentary enzymes. It includes substances of unique chemical structure, distinct physical properties, and individual physiological effects. Except for lignin, all are carbohydrate in nature. They are degraded by enzymes of gastrointestinal bacteria to give by fermentation hydrogen, methane, carbon dioxide and short chain fatty acids (8). The chemical structure of fiber offers no clues to physiological effects but can be grouped into soluble (viscous, easily fermentable) and insoluble (non-viscous, slowly fermentable) fibers. These general types of fiber exhibit different physiological effects; the former may be useful in the treatment of diabetes and hyperlipidemia and the latter in the treatment of gastrointestinal problems such as constipation, diverticulitis and may even be protective against bowel cancer. The fiber era in the United States began with a paper by Burkitt, Walker and Painter (9) which summarized the view that a high fiber diet prevented or protected against the disease conditions most prevalent in this country.

There are many data relating to the beneficial effects of fiber but we lack an intellectually satisfying structure/function relationship and while dietary fiber is ingested in the form and structure native to individual plant foods much of our data are derived from experiments using a purified form of a specific fiber whose only relationship to its native state lies in similarity of structure.

For more than two decades evidence has been accumulating regarding the hypoglycemic action of soluble fiber. Jenkins et al. (10) reported that the addition of soluble fiber to a test meal lowered blood glucose and insulin response. Kiehm et al. (11) make a similar observation—soluble fibers such as guar or pectin were effective (12) but insoluble fibers such as cellulose or wheat bran were not (13). The soluble fibers increased viscosity of the food bolus and it was thought that this reduced the rate of gastric emptying (14). Wolever (15) has reviewed the role of dietary fiber in the management of diabetes: fasting serum glucose is reduced, on average, by 16% and plasma cholesterol and triglycerides by 18% and 10% respectively.

Dietary soluble fiber also tends to reduce serum or plasma lipid levels. In what may be regarded as the "Medieval Age" of fiber, Ershoff and Wells (16, 17) found that feeding several fibers could lower slightly the serum cholesterol and lower markedly the liver cholesterol compared to levels in rats fed 1% cholesterol in a fiber-free diet. Pectin, guar, or locust bean gum, and carrageenan were effective in this regard but cellulose and alginic acid were not. It has been demonstrated that certain types of fiber can reduce the severity of atherosclerosis in rabbits fed a semi-purified, cholesterol-free diet (18–20). Pectin will reduce the severity of atherosclerosis in cholesterol-fed chickens (21).

The possible influence of dietary fiber on heart disease in man cannot be studied directly but there have been numerous studies of fiber effects on hypercholesterolemia, which is one of the major risk factors for development of cardiovascular disease. A review by Truswell and Beynen (22) tabulated data on a number of different fibers that are effective in this regard. In most of the studies the fiber was used in a pharmacological sense as a lipid lowering agent. An earlier review (23) found that wheat bran was almost totally ineffective in lowering cholesterol levels. Cellulose is also without effect (24). Pectin, guar gum, and oat fiber are generally effective cholesterol lowering agents and Truswell and Beynen (22) cite single studies which showed that other soluble fibers namely gum arabic, xanthan gum, gum acacia, karaya gum, and locust bean gum were hypocholesterolemic. Psyllium has also been shown to lower cholesterol (25–

27). In general the active fibers will lower total and LDL-cholesterol but do not influence HDL-cholesterol (28). Epidemiological data have recently become available relating to the effects of high fiber diets on coronary disease mortality and these have been reviewed by Humble (29). Khaw et al. (30) studied a group of 356 men and 503 women aged 50–79 years over a 12 year period: they observed reduced mortality from coronary disease with increasing fiber intake. Humble et al. (31) studied 1801 men aged 45–59 years over a 9 year period and Rimm et al. (32) reported data from 43,757 men aged 40–75 years obtained over a 6 year period. In both cases a higher fiber diet led to significant reduction in death from coronary disease. Dietary fiber intake was judged to be more significant indicator of risk than fat intake.

Heaton (33) has pointed out that dietary fiber exerts its effects throughout the length of the gastrointestinal tract. In the mouth it stimulates salivary flow and in the stomach it dilutes the contents and prolongs storage. In the small intestine fiber is a diluent of the contents and delays absorption and in the large intestine it acts as a diluent, bacterial substrate and traps water. Finally, dietary fiber softens and enlarges the stool. To expand on some of the above, constipation is relieved by the addition of fiber to the diet, the most effective fiber being wheat bran (34). Fiber may also restore normal bowel function in individuals who have become laxative-dependent (35). Paradoxically, fiber may also reduce diarrhea (36). Patients with irritable bowel syndrome also respond to a high fiber diet (37) as do subjects with diverticular disease (38). Heaton (39) has also reviewed the role of dietary fiber in the prevention and treatment of gastrointestinal disorders. In addition to the conditions discussed above, he marshals data which suggest that dietary fiber can reduce risk of gallstones and possibly appendicitis.

The findings regarding the role of fiber in treatment, or possibly prevention, of obesity are moot (40). Probably the greatest emphasis on a particular health aspect of dietary fiber has been on its possible protective role against colon or colorectal cancer. The data are not unanimous but there is enough encouragement to stimulate interest in continuing trials. A thorough review, which covered the literature through 1986 (41), reported that among 22 ecological (population) studies there were 15 negative correlations, one positive correlation, and 6 in which no effect was seen. Among 22 case control studies, there were 8 negative correlations, 6 six positive correlations, and 8 in which there was no effect. Subsequently published reviews show a similar scatter of results (42–44). Meta-analysis of 13 studies leads to a conclusion that fiber is protective (45). Two Australian studies yielded opposite results. Potter and McMichael (46) in Adelaide found increasing risk with increasing fiber intake whereas Kune et al. (47) in Melbourne found risk to be reduced dramatically with increasing fiber intake. This dichotomy illustrates the importance of other factors, physiologic and dietary.

Jensen et al. (48) compared diet and incidence of large bowel cancer in Finland and Denmark. Total fiber intake, in men aged 50–59 years, was higher in the Finnish population. After analyzing 39 variables only two, alcohol intake and concentration of fecal bile acids, were correlated positively with risk. There were significant negative correlations with saturated fatty acids, carbohydrate, starch, protein, cereals and total dietary fiber. Hill et al. (49) found the average fecal bile acid concentration in three countries with low incidence of colon cancer (Uganda, Japan, India) to be 0.61 ± 0.13 mg/g feces, whereas for England, Scotland and the United States the average concentration was 6.15 ± 0.66 mg/g feces. Finns and Americans excrete about the same amount of bile acid daily (275 mg) but the concentration is 4.6 mg/g feces in the Finns and 12.3 mg/g feces in Americans (50).

Walker et al. (51) compared fiber intake with colon cancer risk in five groups of South Africans. These were rural and urban blacks (very low risk), Indians (low risk) and white (very high risk). Fiber intake was similar in the five groups, however one striking difference was in fecal pH which ranged from 6.12 in rural blacks to 6.88 in whites. This finding suggests a difference in colonic acidity which could be due, in part, to the short chain fatty acids produced by fermentation of dietary fiber by the colonic flora. Since the total fiber intake of the various groups was similar the differences may be due to different types of dietary fiber or different strains of resident microorganisms. The principal short chain fatty acids formed by fermentation in the colon are acetic, propionic, and butyric. Butyric acid has been shown to suppress cellular proliferation (52) and to alter properties of human colorectal cells grown in vitro (53).

Interaction between dietary fiber and bile acids may underlie its modes of action in reducing hyperlipidemic and cancer risk. Portman and Murphy (54) showed that substitution of a semi-purified diet for commercial ration increased bile acid turnover in rats. It has been demonstrated amply that bile acids and bile salts are bound to the fiber (52–58) or to fiber containing foods (59, 60). The degree of binding is a function of both the fiber and the bile acid or salt. Alberts et al. (61) have shown that a diet high in wheat bran and calcium carbonate leads to significant reduction in bile acid concentrations and excretion rates in subjects with resected colon adenomas. Two studies relating to the mechanisms by which psyllium or oat bran lower cholesterol have also shown effects on bile acid composition, pool size, and turnover (62,63).

The fiber hypothesis rests on data derived from observations of populations eating a diet high in fiber. Most chemical and physiological studies, however, are conducted using single substances. Fiber in the diet can be obtained from four sources (64), namely:

1. Whole food high in fiber
2. A high fiber fraction (such as wheat bran) which can be produced without affecting the structure or composition of the material as present in food

3. Concentrated fiber such as cellulose or pectin which has been altered in the course of extraction and purification
4. Fiber-enriched foods

There is no evidence to show that purified pectin, for instance, is biologically equivalent to a pectin-rich food.

Fiber-rich foods may also be sources of carotenoids, antioxidant vitamins (C and E), selenium, dithiolthiones, indoles and glucosinolates, flavonoids, coumarins, isothiocyanates and thiocyanates, saponins, phenols (such as ferulic or ellagic acid), sterols, inositol hexaphosphate, and allium compounds, all of which have demonstrated biological activity. Most of these compounds have inhibited tumor growth to some extent and some also have hypolipidemic properties. Proper understanding of the mode of action of fiber will involve elucidation of the individual roles played by all the plant components and their interactions.

Recommendations for daily intake of fiber are all in the range of 20–40 g or 13–25 g per 1000 kilocalories. This range represents a level of intake that poses no risk.

ACKNOWLEDGMENT

Supported, in part, by a Research Career Award (HL00734) from the National Institutes of Health.

REFERENCES

1. Cleave, T.L. (1956) J. Roy. Nav. Med. Serv. 42, 55–82.
2. Burkitt, D.P. (1969) Lancet 2, 1229–1231.
3. Burkitt, D.P. (1971) Cancer 28, 3–13.
4. Burkitt, D.P. (1973) Proc. Nutr. Soc. 32, 145–149.
5. Trowell, H. (1974) Plant Foods for Man 1, 91–97.
6. Trowell, H. (1978) Am. J. Clin. Nutr. 31, S3-S11.
7. Hipsley, E.H. (1953) Br. Med. J. 2, 20.
8. Kritchevsky, D. (1988) Ann. Rev. Nutr. 8, 301–328.
9. Burkitt, D.P., Walker, A.R.P. & Painter, N.S. (1974) JAMA 229, 1068–1074.
10. Jenkins, D.J.A., Leeds, A.R., Gassull, M.A., Cochet, B. & Alberti, K.G.M.M. (1977) Ann. Int. Med. 86, 20–23.
11. Kiehm, T.G., Anderson, J.W. & Ward, K. (1976) Am. J. Clin. Nutr. 29, 895–899.
12. Jenkins, D.J.A., Wolever, T.M.S., Ninehan, R., Taylor, R.H., Metz, G. L., Bacon, S. & Hockaday, T.D.R. (1978) Br. Med. J. 2, 1744–1746.
13. Eastwood, M.A. (1969) Lancet 2, 1222–1225.
14. Leeds, A.R., Ralphs, D.N.L., Ebied, F., Metz, G.L. & Dilwairi, J. (1981) Lancet 1, 1075–1078.
15. Wolever, T.M.S. (1990) in Dietary Fiber: Chemistry, Physiology, and Health Ef-

fects, D. Kritchevsky, C.Bonfield & J.W. Anderson (Eds), Plenum Press, New York, NY, pp. 287–300.
16. Wells, A.F. & Ershoff, B.H. (1961) J. Nutr. 74, 87–92.
17. Ershoff, B.H & Wells, A.F. (1962) Proc. Soc. Exp. Biol. Med. 11, 580–582.
18. Kritchevsky, D. & Tepper, S.A. (1965) Life Sci. 4, 1467–1471.
19. Moore, J.H. (1967) Br. J. Nutr. 21, 207–215.
20. Cookson, F.B., Altschul, R. & Federoff, S. (1967) J. Atheroscler. Res. 7, 69–81.
21. Fisher, H., Soller, W.G. & Grimminger, P. (1966) J. Atheroscler. Res. 6, 292–298.
22. Truswell, A. S. & Beynen, A.C. (1992) in Dietary Fiber—A Component of Food, T.F. Schweizer & C.A. Edwards (Eds), Springer-Verlag, London, pp. 295–332.
23. Kay, R.M. & Truswell, A.S. (1980) in Medical Aspects of Dietary Fiber, G.A. Spiller & R.M. Kay (Eds), Plenum Press, New York, NY, pp. 153–173.
24. Behall, K.M., Lee, K.H. & Moses, P.B. (1984) Am. J. Clin. Nutr. 39, 209–214.
25. Abraham, Z.D. & Mehta, T. (1988) Am. J. Clin. Nutr. 47, 67–74.
26. Anderson, J.W., Zettwoch, N., Feldman, T., Tretyen-Clark, J., Oeltgen, P. & Bishop, C.W. (1988) Arch. Int. Med. 148, 292–296.
27. Bell, L.P., Hectorne, K.J., Reynolds, H. & Hunninghake, D.B. (199) Am. J. Clin. Nutr. 52, 1020–1026.
28. Schneeman, B.O. & Lefevre, M. (1986) in Dietary Fiber: Basic and Clinical Aspects, G.V. Vahouny & D. Kritchevsky (Eds), Plenum Press, New York, NY, pp. 309–321.
29. Humble, C. (1996) Nutr. Disease Update 1, 9–13.
30. Khaw, K.T. & Barrett-Connor, E. (1987) Am. J. Epidemol. 126, 1093–1102.
31. Humble, C.G., Malarcher, A.M. & Tyroler, H.A. (1993) J. Prev. Med. 9, 197–202.
32. Rimm, E.B., Ascherio, A, Giovannucci, E., Spiegelman, D., Stampfer, M.J. & Willett, W.C. (1996) JAMA 275, 447–451.
33. Heaton, K.W. (1980) Human Nutr.: Clin. Nutr. 37C, 151–170
34. Graham, D.Y., Moser, S.E. & Estes, M.K. (1982) Am. J. Gastroenterol. 77, 599–603
35. Sandman, P.O., Adolfsson, R., Hallmans, G., Nygren, C., Nystrom, L. & Windblad, B. (1983) J. Am. Gereatric Soc. 31, 289–293
36. Zimmaro, D.M., Rolandelli, R.H., Korunda, M.J., Settle, R.G., Stein, T.P. & Rombfan, J.L. (1989) J. Parenteral Enteral. Nutr. 13, 117–123
37. Manning, A.P., Heaton, K.W., Harvey, R.F. & Uglow, P. (1977) Lancet 2, 417–418.
38. Painter, N.S. (1985) in Dietary Fibre, Fibre-Depleted Foods and Disease, H. Trowell, D. Burkitt & K. Heaton (Eds), Academic Press, New York, NY, pp. 145–160.
39. Heaton, K.W. (1992) in Dietary Fibre–A Component of Food, T.F. Schweizer & C.A. Edwards (Eds) Springer-Verlag, London, pp. 249–263.
40. Rššsner, S. (1992) in Dietary Fibre—A Component of Food, T.F. Schweizer & C.A. Edwards (Eds) Springer-Verlag, London, pp. 265–277.
41. Pilch, S.M. (Ed). (1987) Review of Physiological Effects and Health Consequences of Dietary Fiber, FASEB, Bethesda, MD.
42. Rogers, A.E. & Longnecker, M.P. (1988) Lab. Invest. 59, 729–759.
43. Byers, T. (1995) in Dietary Fiber in Health and Disease, D. Kritchevsky & C. Bonfield (Eds), Eagan Press, St. Paul, MN, pp. 183–190.

44. Potter, J.D. & Steinmetz, K. (1995) in Dietary Fiber in Health and Disease, D. Kritchevsky & C. Bonfield (Eds), Eagan Press, St. Paul, MN, pp. 191–218.
45. Howe, G.R., Benito, E., Castelleto, R., Cornee, J., Esteve, J. Gallagher, R. P., et al. (1992) J. Nat. Cancer Inst. 84, 1887–1896.
46. Potter, J.D. & McMichael, A.J. (1986) J. Nat. Cancer Inst. 76, 557–569.
47. Kune, S., Kune, G.A. & Watson, L.F. (1987) Nutr. Cancer 9, 21–42.
48. Jensen, O.M., MacLennon, R. & Wahrendorf, J. (1982) Nutr. Cancer 4, 5–19.
49. Hill, M.J., Drasae, B.S., Aries, V.C., Crowther, J.S., Hawksworth, G. & Williams, R.E.O. (1971) Lancet 1, 95–100.
50. Reddy, B.S., Hedges, A.R., Laakso, K. & Wynder, E. L. (1978) Cancer 42, 2832–2838.
51. Walker, A.R.P., Walker, B.F. & Walker, A.J. (1986) Br. J. Cancer 53, 489–495.
52. Hagopian, H.K., Riggs, M.G., Swartz, L.A. & Ingram, V.M. (1977) Cell 12, 855–860.
53. Kim, Y. S., Tsao, D., Morita, A. & Bella, A. (1982) in Colon Carcinogenesis, R.A. Malt & R.C.N. Williamson (Eds), MTP Press, Lancaster, UK, pp. 317–323.
54. Portman, O.W. & Murphy, P. (1958) Arch. Biochem. Biophys. 76, 367–376.
55. Eastwood, M.A. & Hamilton, D. (1968) Biochim. Biophys. Acta 152, 165–173.
56. Balmer, J. & Zilversmit, D.B. (1974) J. Nutr. 104, 1319–1328.
57. Kritchevsky, D. & Story, J.A. (1974) J. Nutr. 104, 458–460.
58. Story, J. A. & Kritchevsky, D. (1976) J. Nutr. 106, 1292–1294.
59. Birkner, N.J. & Kern, F., Jr. (1974) Gastroenterology 67, 237–244.
60. Story, J. A. & Kritchevsky, D. (1975) Nutr. Rep. Int. 11, 161–163.
61. Alberts, D.S., Ritenbaugh, C., Story, J.A., Aickin, M., Rees-McGee, S., Buller, M.K., Atwood, J., Phelps, J., Ramanujam, P.S., Bellapravula, S., Patel, J., Bettinger, L. & Clark, L. (1996) J. Nat. Cancer Inst. 88, 81–92.
62. Everson, G.T., Daggy, B.P., McKinley, C. & Story, J. A. (192) J. Lipid Res. 33, 1183–1192.
63. Marlett, J.A., Hosig, K.B., Vollendorf, N. W., Shinnick, F.L., Haack, V.S. & Story, J.A. (1994) Hepatology 20, 1450–1457.
64. Spiller, G.A. & Jenkins, D.J.A. (1986) in Proceedings of XIII International Congress of Nutrition 1985, T. G. Taylor & N.K. Jenkins (Eds), John Libbey, London, pp. 184–187.

9

Worldwide Dietary Fiber Intake: Recommendations and Actual Consumption Patterns

Susan Sungsoo Cho
The Kellogg Company, Battle Creek, Michigan
K. O'Sullivan
The Kellogg Company, Arabic Areas
Sharon Rickard
University of Toronto, Toronto, Ontario, Canada

INTRODUCTION

The role of dietary fiber (DF) in the prevention and treatment of constipation has been recognized for a century, but dietary fiber is now considered as an important nutrient in reducing the risk of Western diseases such as cancer, cardiovascular disease, and diabetes. Data exists to relate dietary fiber intake to certain diseases. However, lack of agreement on what dietary fiber is and how it should be measured often makes data interpretation difficult. In 1972–1976, dietary fiber was defined as the remnants of plant components that are resistant to hydrolysis by human alimentary enzymes. Most dietary fiber intake databases have been developed based on analytical values to meet this definition. Recently, the scientific community has supported the expansion of the definition to include resistant oligosaccharides and resistant starch in addition to non-starch polysaccharides and lignin. Except for special products, this new definition would not affect dietary fiber values in most food tables in the next decade. Typical recommendations in various countries are set at 20–30 grams of dietary fiber daily. Despite the enormous amount of scientific literature on the benefits of dietary fiber and dietary guidelines, dietary fiber intakes of the general public are well below the recommended levels. For example, the recommended DF intake in the United States is 20–30 g/day while actual consumption ranges from 11–13 g daily. In Arabic countries, dietary fiber intake levels have decreased significantly over the past decades as whole grains are replaced with refined grain flours. Special nutrition education may be required to improve public health related to optimum consumption of fiber-rich foods. Whole grain or bran-enriched food products should be promoted in such nutritional education programs.

Based on studies done in rural Africa, Burkitt and Trowell (1) proposed that the consumption of diets deficient in fiber is associated with increased incidence of diseases common to Western industrialized countries. In the past 25 years, evidence of the beneficial effects of dietary fiber (DF) in diabetes, heart disease, colon cancer and other chronic diseases of the gastrointestinal tract has accumulated (2). Studies on the relationship of DF to health and disease are dependent on accurate DF values for foods. However, the existing methodologies for the measurement of dietary fiber for a particular food give widely ranging values (3). This variability and inconsistency is then reflected in the variety of food composition tables utilized by epidemiologists and other research scientists to estimate DF intake.

Despite these difficulties, government agencies around the world have been able to set recommended levels of DF intake based on existing data. Unfortunately, the actual intake has been far below these recommended levels. Education on the benefits of consuming higher levels of fiber need to be implemented. In this review, the recommendations and intake levels in North America, Europe, Latin America, and the Asia-Pacific region will be discussed. However, before these issues are addressed, DF will be defined and the various methodologies for its measurement will be reviewed.

WHAT IS DIETARY FIBER?

Burkitt and Trowell's definition of DF, the sum of polysaccharides and lignin that are not hydrolyzed by human alimentary enzymes, has gained a wide acceptance (4,5). This physiological definition allows the inclusion of other compounds that may differ in chemical structure but have fiber-like characteristics. On the other hand, analytical chemists prefer the definition proposed by Southgate in

1982 (6) where DF is the sum of lignin and non-starch polysaccharides (NSP). The NSP consist of cellulose, hemicelluloses, β-glucans, pectin, gums, and mucilages. Lignin, the noncarbohydrate constituent of DF, is a complex three dimensional polymer of phenyl propane units. Resistant starches, formed by retrogradation of amylose that escapes digestion in the small intestine (7,8), are also included in the definition of DF because they behave like NSP in the gut.

Two international surveys were conducted by the AOAC International in order to fulfill two objectives: 1) to determine if a consensus could be reached on the definition of DF and associated methodologies; and 2) to consider appropriate classification of oligosaccharides that are not hydrolyzed by human alimentary enzymes (9). Results of the survey should help international harmonization of acceptable definitions of DF and its components. The survey results will also provide insight for chemists seeking to modify analytical methods and develop reference materials to meet the accepted definition.

The first survey was initiated in December 1992 and 144 professionals participated (9). A large majority of participants (70%) supported that the DF definition should reflect both chemical and physiological perspectives. The survey results indicated that 65% of people supported the current DF definition as polysaccharides and lignin that are not hydrolyzed by human alimentary enzymes. However, 59% supported the future expansion of DF definition to include oligosaccharides that are not hydrolyzed by human alimentary enzymes.

In December 1993, a follow-up survey was sent out, specifically addressing the issue of a new definition that may include oligosaccharides that are not hydrolyzed by human alimentary enzymes, along with the results from the first survey for confirmation (9). The second time, 65% of the participants supported the inclusion of these oligosaccharides. Eighty (80) % supported the inclusion of resistant starches and lignin in the DF definition beyond NSP. It is noteworthy that only 6% believe DF includes only NSP or plant cell wall components, suggesting a general agreement that the chemical entity of DF is not limited to these components.

Based on these survey results, Cho (formerly Lee) and Prosky (9) have proposed the expansion of the definition of DF to include resistant oligosaccharides, in addition to the currently included NSP, resistant starch, and lignin. Resistant oligosaccharides, defined as oligosaccharides that are resistant to hydrolysis by human alimentary enzymes, can be used synonymously with the term ''unavailable oligosaccharides.'' This proposal was adopted at the AOAC Workshop on Complex Carbohydrates held in Nashville, TN, USA in October, 1995.

The addition of resistant oligosaccharides to the DF definition may open up new avenues in the nutritional, analytical, and food technology research areas. Along this line, a common understanding on resistant oligosaccharides should be developed. Certain types of oligosaccharides may be claimed for DF in the future if the unavailability in the human upper gastrointestinal tract and the resulting physiological actions similar to other DF components are fully proven. It should be emphasized that most of the foods in today's market do not contain resistant oligosaccharides, except a few formulations using resistant oligosaccharides as ingredients. Thus this new definition would not affect the DF values of most food products. Nevertheless, the inclusion of resistant oligosaccharides would allow new product development efforts as well as nutrition research to more actively evolve. Subsequently, analytical methodology should be fine tuned to fully recover these resistant oligosaccharides as well as resistant starch in the DF analysis. Until a reliable methodology is developed to meet this new definition, current DF methods should continue to be used for DF labeling and dietary assessment studies (5).

ANALYTICAL METHODS FOR DIETARY FIBER

Dietary fiber analysis can be subdivided into gravimetric and component analysis procedures. Gravimetric methods are simpler and faster than component analysis methods but are limited to estimates of total dietary fiber (TDF) or soluble (SDF) and insoluble (IDF) components. Conversely, component analysis allows for the determination of individual sugars, both neutral and acidic (i.e. uronic acids), as well as a separate estimation for lignin in some cases. The TDF content can then be calculated as the sum of these components. A drawback of component analysis is that the procedures are longer and more complex, rendering them less suitable for routine dietary analysis. Table 1 summarizes the methods that have been collaboratively studied and used in the development of fiber tables.

Gravimetric Procedures

Crude Fiber Determination

The crude fiber (CF) method received official final action by AOAC in 1936 and was officially approved for flour (AOAC method 920.86) and animal feed (AOAC method 962.09) in 1920 and 1962, respectively (10). The technique involves digestion of the food sample with boiling, dilute acid and alkali with corrections for residual ash content. Under these harsh conditions, all of the soluble fiber is lost with variable amounts of insoluble fiber leaving mainly lignin and cellulose. Lignin and cellulose values are usually 10–40% and 50–90%, respectively, of their original levels (3). Thus, the CF estimate underestimates DF and does not give a constant value for any fiber component. Nevertheless, CF determination is still used for nutritional labeling purposes in some countries where Western diseases are not a major health concern.

TABLE 1 The Status of Methods Collaboratively Studied and Used in the Construction of Fiber Tables

Method	Status	Reference
AOAC 985.29 (Prosky enz.-gravimetric)	TDF	15, 80
AOAC method 991.42 (Prosky enz.-gravimetric)	IDF	80
AOAC method 993.19 (Prosky enz.-gravimetric)	SDF	80
AOAC method 991.43 (Lee, enz.-gravimetric)	TDF (measured and calculated), SDF/IDF	16, 80
AOAC method 994.24 (Uppsalla GLC method)	TDF, NSP Glucose, fructose, xylose, arabinose and uronic acids	18, 80
Englyst NSP method	Total, soluble, and insoluble NSP GLC and colorimetric	21–23

Detergent Methods of Fiber Analysis

The neutral detergent fiber (NDF) method was developed in 1967 by Van Soest and Wine (11). Food samples are boiled with a detergent solution (sodium lauryl sulfate) at neutral pH and the residue, consisting of cellulose, lignin, and some hemicelluloses, is collected by filtration. The acid detergent fiber (ADF) method includes dilute acid to solubilize the hemicelluloses leaving cellulose and lignin in the residue (12). Thus, by difference of the NDF and ADF, the amount of hemicellulose can be determined. Further treatment of the ADF with strong acid dissolves the cellulose, allowing quantification of all IDF components. The NDF detergent does not solubilize starch efficiently, leading to erroneously high fiber values for starchy foods like flours or potatoes (3). Schaller's modification of the NDF procedure, which was adopted by the American Association of Cereal Chemists as their official fiber method in 1977, employed α-amylase treatment of the sample after filtration to reduce starch interference (13).

Hellendoorn Method

Hellendoorn and colleagues (14) believed that quantification of undigestible carbohydrates required digestion with mammalian enzymes. However, although the method employs pepsin and pancreatin to digest protein and starch, respectively, some protein and starch residue still remains.

Total Dietary Fiber (TDF) Method

Growing awareness of the physiological importance of soluble fiber led to the development of the present official AOAC method (methods 985.29 and 991.42)

known as the TDF method (15). Food samples undergo sequential enzymatic digestion with a heat-stable α-amylase, protease, and amyloglucosidase to remove starch and protein. Precipitation of soluble fiber with 95% ethanol followed by filtration yields a residue containing cellulose, hemicelluloses, lignin, and pectin and corrections are made for residual protein and ash. Estimates of the insoluble and soluble fiber components can be determined by (a) filtering the fiber digest before the addition of ethanol to isolate the IDF and (b) ethanol precipitation followed by filtration to isolate the SDF in the filtrate. A minor modification of these methods (AOAC method 991.43) includes the addition of morpholinoethane sulfonic acid (MES) to the buffer solution used which minimizes the coprecipitation of buffer reagents in the ethanol. In addition, this buffer is not sensitive to changes in ethanol concentration nor to the final pH of the enzyme digestate, making the DF determination more rigorous (16). The AOAC TDF methods are the most ideal among all current techniques regarding their accuracy, precision, simplicity, cost-effectiveness, and suitability for routine use. They may require more fine tuning for more complete recovery of resistant starch and resistant oligosaccharides.

Component Analysis Procedures

Unavailable Carbohydrate Method

Southgate (17) had developed an analytical procedure to fractionate DF into its various components. Hot water digestion removes the soluble starches and pectins, the enzyme takadiastase dissolves the insoluble starch, dilute acid breaks down the hemicelluloses, and finally strong acid hydrolyzes the cellulose. The residue remaining is lignin. The insoluble starch and hemicelluloses can be quantified either colorimetrically or by liquid chromatography. The method has been criticized for both the incomplete removal of starch and the nonspecific colorimetric methods used for quantification of sugar components (3).

Uppsalla Gas-Liquid Chromatography (GLC) Method

The Uppsalla method (18) (AOAC method 994.24) involves gelatinization followed by treatment with Termamyl, an α-amylase, and amyloglucosidase to remove starches. After precipitation of the soluble fiber with 80% ethanol, the dried residues are subjected to acid hydrolysis for liberation of neutral sugars and uronic acids. Neutral sugars are determined as alditol acetate derivatives by GLC, and uronic acids are determined by either decarboxylation or colorimetric methods. The acid-insoluble fraction, called Klason lignin, can be determined gravimetrically. An important point to note is that this method does not use any protein digestion step (18). Marlett (19) has established fiber tables using the Uppsalla GLC method in the U.S. Although the AOAC enzymatic-gravimetric method and the Uppsalla GLC method will give comparable TDF values in most cases, the GLC method tends to be lower.

The DNS Reduction Method for Soluble and Insoluble NSP

The NSP method, developed by Englyst and colleagues (20), has gone through several modifications since its inception for evaluation of NSP alone, NSP plus resistant starch, resistant starch alone and/or lignin determination (21–23). Like the Uppsalla method, neutral sugars are quantified by GLC after derivitization with alditol acetate. Colorimetric techniques are also used. The soluble NSP content is calculated as the difference between TDF and IDF to avoid the problems of incomplete precipitation of SDF (23). The NSP method has been chosen to replace the unavailable (CHO) carbohydrate method for fiber labeling purposes in the United Kingdom based on the superior precision in comparison to other component analysis procedures. Although NSP are major components of dietary fiber, the values do not represent all the DF values. For high starch foods, grains, and cereals, NSP values are significantly lower than TDF values obtained by AOAC methods. Differentiating NSP from resistant starch does not sufficiently address the issue of the physiological effects of these fractions. The physiological function of DF as a quantified entity is more acceptable. Major improvements are required to measure TDF, resistant starch and lignin if separate labeling is the goal with the Englyst methods. The employment of dimethylsulfoxide (DMSO) in this method to solubilize starch makes the soluble and insoluble NSP value interpretation complicated since DMSO is a known solvent for hemicelluloses (24,25).

RECOMMENDATIONS FOR DIETARY FIBER INTAKE LEVELS

Before making DF recommendations, the physiological effects of its different components must be known. The two main types of DF, water-soluble (SDF) and water-insoluble (IDF), have some different mechanisms of action in vivo. The SDF such as soluble β-glucans, pectins, gums, mucilages, and some hemicelluloses delay transit time in the gut, delay gastric emptying, impede the absorption of certain nutrients like glucose, and decrease serum cholesterol levels (26). Insoluble DF like cellulose, lignin, and other hemicelluloses increase intestinal transit time and fecal weight, slow starch hydrolysis, and delay glucose absorption (26). Appropriate amounts of both types of fiber are important for overall health.

The health beneficial effects of a dietary recommendation should also outweigh potential deleterious consequences. Using the estimation that 35% of all cancer cases are attributable to diet, 315,000 new cancer cases or 166,000 cancer deaths would result in the United States if dietary goals for cancer prevention such as increasing DF intake levels are not achieved (27). This could cost as much as $25 billion a year. Based on international correlation statistics, an inverse relationship has been found between fiber and fiber-containing foods and colon cancer risk (28, 29). After examination of all fiber sources, the Life Science Research Office (LSRO) (30) determined that the IDF-rich wheat bran most consistently reduced colon tumor incidence in animal models. Recurrence of precancerous polyp lesions in the rectum has also been shown to be lower with wheat bran in humans (31). Both IDF and SDF may reduce breast cancer risk by binding estrogen, a potent promoter, and thus preventing enterohepatic reabsorption and lowering circulating levels (32). Although increased DF intake seems to be beneficial in terms of cancer, there are concerns about impaired mineral availability. Examination of populations that consume much higher levels of DF (e.g. vegetarians vs. omnivores) showed that mineral levels in various biological samples were comparable to those with lower DF intakes (30). In addition, bone mineral mass was observed to be higher or at least the same. Thus, bioavailability of minerals with higher DF intakes does not appear to be an issue as long as intakes are adequate.

Other issues that are considered in making a recommendation are the intended audience, the current intake levels of DF, and how the DF will be consumed (i.e. in foods vs. supplements) (30). Recommendations are generally based on a healthy, adult population and are not applicable to special populations like young children and the elderly. In reviewing existing data on current DF intakes of a population, the methods used for dietary assessment and chemical analysis of the DF content of a food are determined since they both influence the estimated intake level. Finally, recommendations are for DF in foods and not supplements. The use of DF supplements may affect the balance of nutrients in an otherwise healthy diet. Limited data exist on the effects of isolated DF which may differ from the DF naturally present in a food (30).

Worldwide Dietary Fiber Intake Recommendations

Recommendations for DF intake by the World Health Organization (WHO) are 16–24 g/d of NSP or 27–40 g/d of TDF (Table 2). The Food and Agriculture Organization (FAO) of the United Nations (1995) recommends that individuals should eat a variety of foods in order to obtain all the necessary nutrients for proper health (Table 3). Carbohydrates was one of seven food groups mentioned, with cereals listed as a choice. In contrast, the WHO Study group (33) advocated that complex carbohydrates should be a major portion of the diet at 50–70% of the total energy consumed. Suggested sources of NSP included fruits and vegetables (no less than 400 g/d) and pulses, nuts, and seeds (no less than 30 g/d but

TABLE 2 Dietary Fiber Daily Intake Recommendations

Country	Recommended intake	Basis	Source of recommendation
WHO	16–24 g 27–40 g	NSP TDF	Report: Diet, nutrition and the prevention of chronic diseases
Australia	30 g	DF	Australian Government Department of Community Services and Health
Belgium	26–38 g (male) 19–28 g (female)	DF	National Council for Nutrition (unofficial)
Canada	25–35 g	DF	Expert Panel in 1985 (unofficial)
Central America	18–24 g	DF	Institute of Nutrition of Central America and Panama (INCAP)
Columbia	15–20 g	NSP	Health Ministry (1992)
Denmark	25–30 g	TDF	National Food Agency/Nutrition Council
Finland	25–30 g	DF	National Food Agency/Nutrition Council
France	25–30 g	DF	French gastroenterologist–unpublished
Germany	30 g	DF	German Society of Nutrition
India	40 g	DF	Indian Council of Medical Research, National Institute of Nutrition
Ireland	25–35 g	DF	The Food Advisory Committee of the Department of Health (1987)
Italy	19 g	TDF	National Nutrition Institute
Japan	20–25 g	TDF	Ministry of Health and Welfare
Mexico	25–30 g	DF	National Nutrition Institute
Netherlands	3 g/MJ/day (24–30 g)	DF	Dutch Nutritional Values 1989: Nutritional Council
Norway	25 g	DF	National Food Agency/Nutrition Council
Puerto Rico	25 g/2000 kcal	DF	Food and Drug Administration (FDA)
South Africa	30–40 g	TDF	Heart Foundation, Cancer Association, Association of Dietetics, Department of Health (unofficial)
Spain	30 g	TDF	General literature references, no official figures
Sweden	25–30 g	DF	National Food Agency/Nutrition Council

Table 2 Continued

Country	Recommended intake	Basis	Source of recommendation
United Kingdom	18 g	NSP	Department of Health Committee on Aspects of Food Policy, Department of Health Dietary Reference Values Report
United States	25 g/2000 kcal (adult)	DF	Food and Drug Administration (FDA)
United States	''Age + 5'' to ''Age + 10'' g (3–20 years of age)	DF	American Health Foundation
United States	0.5 g/kg BW up to 25 g/day (adolescents)	DF	American Academy of Pediatrics
Venezuela	8–10 g/1000 kcal	DF	National Nutrition Institute (1993)

part of the 400 g recommendation for fruit and vegetables). The WHO further specified that free sugars should be no more than 10% of energy (33).

Dietary Fiber Intake Recommendations in North America

Final food labeling regulations by the U.S. Food and Drug Administration (FDA) and U.S. Department of Agriculture (USDA) were disseminated through the January 6, 1993 issue of the Federal Register (34, 35). Both the FDA and USDA recognize the AOAC methods 985.29 (TDF) (15) and 991.43 (TDF, SDF/IDF)

Table 3 Dietary Recommendations Around the World—References to ''Grain-Based'' Foods*

Country	Name/Source of recommendation	Reference to ''grain-based'' foods
Worldwide	Food and Agriculture Organization (FAO) of the United Nations. ''Get the best from your food'' (1995)	Recommend eating a variety of foods; 7 groups of foods listed. One is ''foods rich in carbohydrate'' which are ''. . . rice, maize, wheat and other cereals . . .''

*Source: L. O'Rourke and S. Cho, Kellogg Company, USA

(16) as suitable methodologies for the analysis of DF for nutrition labeling purposes. Professionals in the DF research field, however, strongly support the enzymatic-gravimetric technique as the most appropriate approach for nutrition labeling and quality control purposes (9). Thus, recommendations for DF intake in both the United States and Canada are generally based on the AOAC methods. Recommendations for DF intake in North America range from 25 to 35 g/d. The U.S. FDA recommends that DF goals be based on a caloric basis (Table 2). General dietary recommendations by organizations in the U.S. and Canada are to increase intakes of grain products, fruits and vegetables which will increase overall DF intake if followed (Table 4). Recent U.S. recommendations for intakes of grain-based foods are at least 6 servings per day. In Canada, recommended intake levels of breads, cereals and other grain products have increased from 3–5 servings/d to 5–12 servings/d (Table 4).

Even though pediatric guidelines for intakes in the U.S. have been set for the consumption of other macronutrients such as protein, fat and carbohydrates, no specific recommendations on DF levels have been made until recently. In 1993, the American Academy of Pediatrics (AAP) Committee on Nutrition made the recommendation that DF intake in children over age 2 should be 0.5 g/kg body weight (36) (Table 2). To avoid the potential hazards of excessive consumption, especially for overweight children, the AAP suggest a cap at 35 g/d. However, intakes up to 25 g/d should not be deleterious even with suboptimal mineral intake (36). The American Health Foundation (AHF) recommends that a range of DF intake, between ''Age + 5'' and ''Age + 10'' g/d may represent a safe and tolerable level for most children over the age of 2 years (37) (Table 2). Consistent with guidelines for adult DF intake, the AHF recommendation gradually increases the fiber intakes to the minimal adult DF level by age 20. Consumption of recommended levels of DF by children may help reduce the risk of developing chronic diseases such as cancer and cardiovascular disease later on in life (37).

Dietary Fiber Intake Recommendations in Europe

In the U.K., the recommendation for DF intake is based on NSP because it is the major fraction of DF regardless of the DF definition used and is chemically identifiable and measurable with reasonable precision. In the early 1970s, fiber tables in the U.K. had been constructed with Southgate's unavailable CHO method (17) which overestimates DF values of high-starch foods due to incomplete starch removal during the procedure (3). The NSP methods of analysis developed by Englyst and colleagues (21–23), classifying NSP into soluble and insoluble fractions, are now used for labeling purposes in the U.K. The U.K. Department of Health recommends an average NSP intake of 18 g/d to be consumed from a variety of foods and not supplements (Table 2). Confusion in data

TABLE 4 Dietary recommendations in the U.S. and Canada

Country	Name/Source of recommendation	References to "grain-based" and complex CHO/DF
U.S.	American Cancer Society (ACS), "Guidelines on Diet, Nutrition, and Cancer Prevention" (1996)	Eat 5 or more servings of fruits and vegetables each day. Eat other foods from plant sources, such as breads, cereals, grain products, rice, pasta, or beans several times each day. Choose whole grains over processed grains.
U.S.	U.S. Department of Health and Human Services (USDHHS), *Action Guide for Healthy Eating* (1996)	Eat lots of fruits and vegetables, grains, and beans.
U.S.	U.S. Department of Agriculture, *Report of the Dietary Guidelines, Advisory Committee on the Dietary Guidelines for Americans* (1995)	Choose a diet with plenty of grain products, vegetables, and fruits. Adults should eat at least 3 servings of vegetables, 2 servings of fruits, and 6 servings of grain products each day.
U.S.	U.S. Department of Agriculture and USDHHS, "Nutrition and Your Health: Dietary Guidelines for Americans," 4th edition (1995)	Choose a diet with plenty of grain products, vegetables, and fruits.
U.S.	American Cancer Society, *Nutrition and Cancer: Cause and Prevention* (1993)	Eat more high fiber foods. Fiber is found in fruits and vegetables, whole grains, and dried beans.
U.S.	American Cancer Society, *Eating Smart* (1993)	(indirect) Eat more high-fiber foods; eat a varied diet including fruits and vegetables.
U.S.	American Dietetic Association (ADA), *Position of the American Dietetic Association: Health Implications of Dietary Fiber* (1993)	The consensus drawn from numerous health authorities is that Americans should consume at least 5 servings of fruits/vegetables and 6 servings of breads/cereals/legumes per day.
U.S.	USDA Food Guide Pyramid (1992)	"At the base of the Food Guide Pyramid are the breads, cereals, rice and pasta–all foods from grains. You need the most servings of these each day (6–11)." Breakfast cereals mentioned in text as an option.
U.S.	USDHHS, *Eating to Lower Your High Blood Cholesterol* (1992)	(indirect) Choose foods high in complex carbohydrates (starch and fiber).

TABLE 4 Continued

Country	Name/Source of recommendation	References to "grain-based" and complex CHO/DF
U.S.	ACS, *Nutrition and Cancer: American Cancer Society Guidelines, Programs, and Initiative* (1990)	Include a variety of fruits and vegetables in the daily diet. Eat more high-fiber foods, such as whole grain cereals, vegetables, and fruits. "Whole grain cereals" recommended; i.e. breakfast cereals.
U.S.	American Heart Association (AHA) Report: *The Healthy American Diet* (1990)	(indirect) Increase consumption of complex carbohydrates and fiber.
U.S.	California Department of Health and Human Services, *The California Daily Food Guide: Dietary Guidance for Californians* (1990)	Adults in California should eat 4 servings of whole grain breads every day (plus addit'l servings of other grains to a total 6 servings per day). Eat 5 servings or more of fruits and vegetables every day.
U.S.	USDHHS, *Report of the Expert Panel on Population Strategies for Blood Cholesterol Reduction* (1990)	Eat a greater quantity and variety of fruits, vegetables, breads, cereals, and legumes. Carbohydrates should be increased to 50–60% of total calories.
U.S.	National Research Council, National Academy of Sciences *Diet and Health–Implications for Reducing Chronic Disease Risk* (1989)	"Every day eat 5 or more servings of fruits and vegetables and increase intake of starches and other complex carbohydrates by eating 6 or more daily servings of a combination of breads, cereals, and legumes." "Whole grain cereals" referred to in text as a good cereal choice; "cereals" is understood to include breakfast cereals.
U.S.	AHA, *Position Statement–Dietary Guidelines for Healthy American Adults, A Statement for Physicians and Health Professionals by the Nutrition Committee* (1988)	(indirect) Carbohydrate intake should constitute 50% or more of calories, with emphasis on complex carbohydrates.
U.S.	USDHHS, *The Surgeon General's Report on Nutrition and Health* (1988)	Increase consumption of whole grain foods and cereal products, vegetables, and fruits.

Table 4 Continued

Country	Name/Source of recommendation	References to ''grain-based'' and complex CHO/DF
U.S.	AHA, *Position Statement–Dietary Guidelines for Healthy American Adults, A Statement for Physicians and Health Professionals by the Nutrition Committee* (1988)	(indirect) Carbohydrate intake should constitute 50% or more of calories, with emphasis on complex carbohydrates.
U.S.	ACS, *Taking Control—10 Steps to a Healthier Life and Reduced Cancer Risk* (1987)	Add more high-fiber foods to the diet. Fiber occurs in whole grains (such as wheat and bran cereals), fruits, and vegetables. ''Bran cereals'' noted as a good fiber source.
U.S.	United States Senate, *Dietary Goals for the United States* (1977)	(indirect) Increase the consumption of complex carbohydrates.
Canada	Health and Welfare Canada, *Canada's Food Guide to Healthy Eating* (1992)	''Enjoy a variety of foods from each group every day.'' Groups include ''Grain Products''–''choose whole grain and enriched products more often (5–12 servings per day)''; ''Vegetables and Fruit''–''choose dark green and orange vegetables and orange fruit more often (5–10 servings per day).'' ''. . . Choose whole grain and enriched products more often.''
Canada	Health and Welfare Canada, *Summary of Report of the Scientific Review Committee and the Communications/Implementation Committee*	Emphasize cereals, breads, other grain products, vegetables, and fruits. ''Preferably whole grain'' products recommended.
Canada	Canada's Guidelines for Healthy Eating (1989)	''Preferably whole grain'' products recommended.
Canada	Canada Cancer Society, *Healthy Food Choices May Reduce Your Cancer Risk* (1988)	(indirect) Eat more fiber-containing foods. Eat several servings of fruits and vegetables daily.
Canada	*Canadian Consensus Conference on Cholesterol: Final Report* (1988)	(indirect) Thirty-five to 40 percent of energy should come from carbohydrates, with emphasis on polysaccharides from a variety of foods containing dietary fiber.

TABLE 4 Continued

Country	Name/Source of recommendation	References to "grain-based" and complex CHO/DF
Canada	Canadian Cancer Society, *Fact on Cancer and Diet–Your Food Choices May Help You Reduce Your Cancer Risk* (1986)	(indirect) Eat more fiber-containing foods. Have several servings of vegetables and fruits daily.
Canada	Health and Welfare Canada, *Canada's Food Guide Handbook* (1985)	Eat 3–5 servings of breads and cereals, "Preferably whole grain" products recommended. Eat 4–5 servings of fruits and vegetables.

interpretation had resulted in the previous recommendation of 30 g/d, based on the unavailable CHO method, by the British National Advisory Committee on Nutrition Education in 1983 (38).

The present NSP recommendation is based on its importance for overall colonic health and regularity. At NSP intakes of less than 12 g/d, stool weights are less than 100 g/d which is associated with an increased risk of bowel disease (39). However, a recent study showed that NSP plus resistant starch, and not NSP alone, correlated with colon cancer incidence (28). Carbohydrate metabolism, insulin metabolism, or blood lipid profiles were not considered in the recommendation due to the lack of evidence that NSP plays any significant role (39). There does not appear to be any significant reduction in mineral bioavailability with populations which habitually consume high levels of NSP. Because this may be a factor in those with marginal mineral intakes like the elderly, the recommendation is only applicable to healthy adults (39).

In Continental Europe, DF tables are generally based on the AOAC TDF method 985.29 (15). Since NSP represent most, but not all DF fractions, the NSP values used in the U.K. tend to be lower than TDF values, especially for grain-based foods (3). Using the TDF method as a basis, most countries in Europe recommend a daily DF intake of 20–35 g (Table 2). General recommendations are to increase consumption of fruits, vegetables, and cereals and cereal products, replacing energy intakes from fatty or sugary foods (Table 5).

Dietary Fiber Recommendations in the Asia-Pacific Region

Generally, DF tables in the Asia-Pacific region are based on the AOAC TDF method 985.29 and 991.43, sometimes with modifications for foods unique to the country (e.g. Japan). Korea, India, and Australia use "food pyramids" as in

TABLE 5 Dietary Recommendations in Europe

Country	Name/Source of recommendation	References to ''grain-based'' and complex CHO/DF
Europe	Health Directorate General of the European Commission. ''Europe vs. Cancer''	Increase intake of fresh fruits and vegetables. Eat high-fiber cereals more often. Recommend ''high fiber'' cereals.
Europe	European Atherosclerosis Society, *Strategies for the Prevention of Coronary Heart Disease: A Policy Statement of the European Atherosclerosis Society* (1987)	Increase intake of fruit, vegetables, and cereal fiber, with emphasis on legumes. ''Increase intake of . . . cereal fiber.''
France	French Health Education Committee	One of the recommended food groups is ''cereals and their derivatives, potatoes, and dried vegetables.'' Breakfast cereals are mentioned as a choice which offers several positive nutrition characteristic (''rich in carbohydrate, essentially starch and in fiber–for whole grain cereals. Also provide protein and minerals. Some are enriched in iron and vitamins.'')
France	National Center for Coordination of Research on Nutrition and Diet (edits RDA's from French population) (1992)	Refer to the food groups defined by the French Health Education Committee, one of which is ''. . . cereals and their derivatives'' (see above) In a section on fiber, indicate that it is ''. . . important to consume vegetables, cereals, legumes, wholemeal bread''
France	National Food Council. Campaign to reduce risk of cardiovascular disease and overweight (1989)	''One should eat every day . . . at least one food from each of the food groups–this includes the group 'bread, cereals, and pasta' . . .''
Germany	German Society for Nutrition	Recommendations for carbohydrates and fiber include grain-based foods.

TABLE 5 Continued

Country	Name/Source of recommendation	References to "grain-based" and complex CHO/DF
U.K.	Health Education Council, *A Discussion Paper on Proposals for Nutritional Guidelines for Health Education in Britain* (1983)	Fiber intake should increase on average to 30 g per day, the increase to come mainly from the increased consumption of whole grain cereals. An increase in vegetable and fruit should also be warranted. Specifies "whole brain cereals."
U.K.	Department of Health, Eat Well–An action plan from the Nutritional Task Force to achieve the Health of the Nation targets on diet and nutrition (1994)	(indirect) Any reduction in fat consumption will need to be balanced by an increased consumption of the basic staple foodstuffs–starchy, fiber-rich foods such as breads, potatoes, pasta and rice, and vegetables and fruit.
U.K.	Health Education Authority, The Balance of Good Health (1994)	(indirect) Eat plenty of foods rich in starch and fiber.
U.K.	U.K. Department of Health, *The Nutrition of Elderly People. Report of the Working Group on the Nutrition of Elderly People of the Committee on Medical Aspects of Food Policy* (1992)	Elderly people, in common with those of all ages, should be advised to eat more fresh vegetables, fruit, and whole grain cereals. "Whole grain cereals" recommended.
U.K.	The Health of the Nation. A Consultative Document for Health in England (1991)	. . . to replace fatty and sugary foods by cereal and starchy foods
U.K.	Ad Hoc Working Group on Coronary Prevention, *Prevention of Coronary Heart Disease in the United Kingdom* (1982)	(indirect) Reduce fat contribution to energy requirements by eating foods rich in complex carbohydrates, particularly breads, vegetables, potatoes, and fruits; this would also increase dietary fiber intake.
U.K.	Europe Against Cancer. Cancer Education Coordinating Group (HEA, Health Education Board for Scotland, Health Promotion Wales, and Health Promotion Agency for Northern Ireland)	For another source of fiber, choose foods made with whole grains and whole grain flours of all kinds.

Table 5 Continued

Country	Name/Source of recommendation	References to ''grain-based'' and complex CHO/DF
Ireland	Health Promotion Unit (Dublin), A Guide to Daily Healthy Choices. Food Pyramid (1995)	Eat plenty of foods rich in starch and fiber–choose whole grain products more often.
Ireland	Nutrition Advisory Group Recommendations for a Food Nutrition Policy for Ireland (1995)	Starchy foods such as bread (preferably wholemeal), cereals, pasta and rice, as well as fruit and vegetables, should be eaten daily.
Italy	National Institute of Nutrition, Dietary Guidelines	Reduce fat and increase use of fiber; eat grain-based food (pasta, rice, potatoes, bread, high fiber content cereals, and polenta). Recommend ''high fibre content cereals.''
Italy	Italian Association Against Cancer, 10 Recommendations	Reduce fat and increase use of fiber; eat grain-based food (pasta, rice, potatoes, bread, high fiber content cereals, and polenta). Specifies ''high fibre content cereals''. Suggests eating ready-to-eat cereals every day for breakfast.
Scandinavian Countries	Keys, A. *Official Collective Recommendation on Diet in the Scandinavian Countries* (1968)	The consumption of vegetables, fruits, potatoes, skimmed milk, fish, lean meat, and cereal products should be increased.
Norway	National Nutrition Council of Norway	Eat more bread and grain based foods.
Finland	National Public Health Institute, Finland	It is good to eat bread and porridge regularly, preferably whole grain products.
Sweden	Swedish National Food Administration	Eat foods with complex carbohydrates and fiber. Bread, cereals, grains, pasta, fruit, vegetables, potatoes, and root-crops.

the U.S. to demonstrate relative proportions in which different food groups should be consumed (Table 6). Recommendations are to emphasize grain-based foods like rice, breads, and cereals.

Recommendations for DF intake are lower in Japan (20–25 g/d) than in Australia (30 g/d) (Table 2). Australians have dietary habits similar to that of Americans. However, officials in Japan believe that the American RDA for DF is probably too high for the Japanese considering the lower energy consumption, lower fat intake, and insufficient calcium intakes which may be exacerbated by high DF levels (40). Another point for consideration was the recent fad in Japan to consume drinks containing 5 g/bottle or more of soluble oligosaccharides and the unknown health impact if DF recommendations were set at a higher level. In determining appropriate DF intakes for Japanese, Nishimune and colleagues estimated the TDF intakes in 1935, 1955, and 1990 using a database with values derived from the AOAC enzymatic-gravimetric method and, using the same method, measured the TDF of model duplicate meals and composites for the average Japanese in 1985 (40). Using the average Japanese energy intakes of 2,088 kcal in 1985, suggested daily DF intake levels are 10–12 g/1,000 kcal (about 20–25 g/d). The lower limit is based on the DF required for a daily fecal output of 140–150 g since this is associated with bowel disease risk (41). Factors considered in establishing the upper limit are mineral sufficiency, fat consumption, ratio of IDF to SDF intake, the decreasing trend in Japanese TDF intake, and the increase in mortality rates of diabetes mellitus, ischemic heart disease, and diverticulosis.

Dietary Fiber Recommendations in Latin America

The recommendations in Latin America, generally based on the AOAC TDF method 985.29 and 991.43, are similar to other countries around the world (Table 2). In the late 70s and early 80s, the NDF method was the basis for Latin American food labeling. Latin American government agencies advocate increasing complex CHO intake by increasing consumption of fruits, vegetables, legumes, and grain products (Table 7). Mexico, Chile, and Puerto Rico (which follows U.S. recommendations) give guidelines for relative consumption of DF from different food sources. Brazil and Argentina have no official guidelines in place (Table 7).

Dietary Fiber Recommendations in South Africa

The Department of Health Services and Welfare in South Africa and (HMAC) Subcommittee on Nutrition Services have published booklets containing recommendations to satisfy the normal requirements of healthy South Africans. They endorse the consumption of fiber-rich foods such as whole grain products, fruits, vegetables, and dry legumes. In concern for the unknown effects of consuming

Table 6 Dietary Recommendations in the Asia-Pacific Region

Country	Name/Source of recommendation	References to "grain-based" and complex CHO/DF
Taiwan	No official guideline	Eat cereals for three meals (?)
Korea	Korean Nutrition Society Food Pagoda	Eat more grain and starch of foods (pictoral demonstration)
India	Indian Dietetic Association, Food Pyramid	Recommends consumption of cereals. Ready-to-eat cereals are specified as a choice.
China	Chinese Nutrition Society, Recommended Dietary Allowances (1989)	Encourage consumption of more grain based foods–should contribute about 70% of calories
Japan	Ministry of Health and Welfare, Dietary Guideline for Japanese	Recommends variety . . . each "menu" should include a "staple" food which is defined as rice, bread, or other grain-based food
Singapore, Indonesia, Philippines	No official guideline	
Australia	Australian Nutrition Foundation, Healthy Eating Pyramid	"Bread, Cereal" group is at base of pyramid along with "vegetables, dried peas, beans, lentils, and fruits" group. States ". . . including whole grain cereals".
Australia	Anti Cancer Foundation (CSIRO) (1991)	"Breads and Cereals" groups are at the base of the Food Pyramid. Five or more servings per day are recommended. Ready-to-eat cereal is pictured as one option in the "bread and cereal" group.
Australia	National Health and Medical Research Council, Dietary Guidelines for Australia	". . . Eat plenty of breads and cereals (preferably whole grain) . . ." Breakfast cereals noted as an option in the "Cereal" group; recommend preferably whole grain cereals.
Australia	Department of Community Services and Health (Australia), *Towards Better Nutrition for Australians*, 1987	Eat more breads and cereals (preferably whole grains) and vegetables and fruits. Emphasis on "whole grain" cereal choices.

TABLE 7 Dietary recommendations in Latin America

Country	Name/Source of recommendation	References to "grain-based" foods and complex CHO/DF
Mexico	National Institute of Nutrition (Mexico), Food Pyramid	Grains and their products: eat in sufficient amounts . . . preferably their whole grain versions. ". . . Complex carbohydrates should make up 70% of total energy . . . grains are one of the best sources . . ." (Note: fruits and vegetables are at the base of the Mexican food pyramid.) All Bran is pictured as a grain-based food option.
Chile	Institute of Nutrition and Food Technology (INTA). Food guidelines (still in draft form) (1996)	First level of pyramid is cereals, potatoes, legumes, and peas
Central America	Nutrition Institute of Central America and Panama (INCAP). WHO affiliate (based in Guatemala), Dietary Recommendation.	Complex carbohydrates should be the main energy source. These can only be found in plant foods, particularly in cereals, legumes, roots, and tubers.
Venezuela	National Institute of Nutrition/ Cavendes Foundation	"Include in your daily diet grains, fruits, vegetables, or cereals to guarantee your organism the necessary fiber." ". . . to obtain more of your money's worth, buy foods that in addition to energy provide other nutrients, such as cereals and grains."
Puerto Rico	(Follows U.S. guidelines)	
Brazil and Argentina	No official guidelines	
Colombia	Colombian Institute of Well-being for Families, Food Composition Tables (1978)	One of the 3 food groups is ". . . energy supplying foods: this includes 'cereals and their products' . . ."

isolated DF products, they also state that it is preferable to consume foods naturally high in fiber than to add bran to low fiber foods. Increasing fiber intake by consuming unrefined cereal products like brown and whole wheat bread and high-fiber breakfast cereals is advocated. The recommended DF intake is 30-40 g TDF/d (Table 2).

PROBLEMS IN ASSESSING DIETARY FIBER INTAKES

One of the difficulties encountered in making specific recommendations for DF intake is in assessing the current intake levels. Variability in estimated DF intakes can be attributed in part to the type of dietary assessment and method of fiber analysis utilized.

There are three main methods for obtaining dietary data: (1) food balance (e.g. per capita disappearance) statistics; (2) household food surveys; and (3) studies of individuals (42). Dietary data obtained from food balance statistics tend to overestimate actual consumption by individuals (42, 43). Household food survey data need to be corrected for food waste, consumption of meals outside the home, locally grown produce, and household size and composition (42). Studies on individuals, which are probably more representative than the other two techniques, use a variety of methods to assess intake: 24-h recall, food frequency questionnaires, and food records for varying periods which may or may not include weighing of food consumed. Assessments through single 24-h recall tend to underestimate and detailed food records tend to overestimate intake levels (44). The coefficient of variation in day-to-day intake in individuals, which cannot be assessed by 24-h recall, is much greater than intake variability observed season-to-season (44). In comparing a food frequency questionnaire with 7-d weighed records, Saba et al. (45) found that TDF estimates were higher with the questionnaire for all categories of high DF foods. Weighed food records strongly correlate with chemical analysis methods of food composites and independent markers of food intake (i.e. urinary and fecal nitrogen excretion) (46). Thus, the most objective method available is the weighing and recording of all food eaten, but even the act of doing so can disturb a person's normal eating pattern (44).

Most of the fiber databases established in the 1970s were based on CF values. Subsequently, much of the fiber intake data in the 70s and early 80s are derived from the CF method. Bright-See and McKeown-Eyssen reported an estimation of CF and DF (as unavailable CHO) supply in different countries around the world (Table 8) (43). CF estimates drastically underestimate DF values. It should be noted that the DF values reported in this study are much higher than many of the studies cited below because the Southgate method generally reports the highest DF values for high-starch foods and per capita disappearance overestimates nutrient intakes. Marlett and Bokram (47) have tried to establish a relationship between CF and DF which has been used by subsequent studies

TABLE 8 Estimate of DF Intake in Various Countries Using Unavailable Carbohydrate (CHO) and CF Methods*

Region	Country	CF (g/d)	Unavailable CHO
North America	U.S.	5.9	27.4
	Canada	5.4	24.6
Latin America	Costa Rica	8.2	48.3
	Cuba	9.1	42.2
	Chile	12.8	55.9
	Mexico	13.2	93.6
	Uruguay	9.3	42.3
Asia-Pacific Region	Japan	6.0	31.9
	China (Hong Kong)	6.8	35.0
	Singapore	7.9	36.6
	Australia	4.5	22.8
	New Zealand	5.0	24.0
Europe	U.K.	5.0	23.5
	Ireland	5.0	26.0
	France	5.4	25.3
	Italy	7.0	36.1
	Portugal	14.7	71.4
	Spain	12.5	51.3
	Yugoslavia	7.3	45.6
	Romania	16	88.1
	Hungary	12.3	51.6
	Poland	7.5	37.2
	Germany	5.6	28.0
	Austria	8.9	39.6
	Belgium & Luxembourg	5.4	25.9
	Bulgaria	16.1	68.1
	Czechoslovakia	10.6	45.4
	Greece	14.9	62.4
	Sweden	4.4	22.1
	Switzerland	4.8	23.7
	Denmark	5.0	32.5
	Finland	4.5	23.1
	Netherlands	4.5	22.1
	Iceland	5.5	24.2
	Norway	8.2	35.3

*Data from ref. #43 based on FAO food disappearance data, 1972–1974

as a conversion factor (48–50). Since the CF level can vary from 10–50% of the TDF value depending on the nature of the food, dietary intake data employing the CF method should be interpreted with caution. Tables of DF levels in foods have been improved by employing AOAC TDF 985.29/991.43, NSP, or unavailable CHO methodology, but limited intake data are available using these new databases.

DIETARY FIBER INTAKE LEVELS AROUND THE WORLD

Dietary fiber intake levels in North America, the Asia-Pacific Region, and most industrialized nations in Europe are far below the recommended levels (Tables 9–11). In North America, usual intake levels of TDF are between 10 and 15 g/d (Table 9). Estimates of DF intakes in Europe, mostly based on Southgate's unavailable CHO method, are in the range of 18–25 g/d (Table 10). Two European studies, one in Italy (51) and one in the Netherlands (52), obtained much higher estimates of about 32 g/d. In the U.K. and Scandinavia, NSP intakes range from 13–18 g/d. Studies in Australia and New Zealand have found DF intake levels in the range of 18–20 g/d (unavailable CHO) whereas countries like Japan and Korea are even lower at 10–17 g TDF/d. However, South Asians who have immigrated to the U.K. were found to have much higher intake levels than the native British in one study (53). Dietary fiber consumption in Latin America are closer to recommended levels (20–23 g/d) but still fall below official guidelines (Table 9).

As mentioned previously, some of the variability in estimated DF intake levels is due to the fiber analysis method used in the assessment. Studies comparing values derived from the Southgate unavailable CHO method with the NSP (54, 55), TDF (56), or a combination of methods (57) always found Southgate estimates to be higher. In a Japanese study by Nakaji et al. (56), Southgate estimates were only slightly higher than the TDF estimates by the AOAC TDF method. However, the proportion of DF from different food sources differed greatly between the two methods, especially for grains and vegetables (Table 12).

The major source of DF varies from region to region. Kasper et al. (48) found that most of the DF in Germany was from cereals (44–52%) and then potatoes and vegetables (25-32%). Studies in Japan, the U.K., and Italy have found more of the DF intake to come from vegetables (51, 53, 58, 59). In Asia, rice constitutes the greatest proportion of grain products consumed at approximately 12% (58, 60). Decreasing trends in bread and cereal consumption have resulted in a concomitant rise in fruit consumption in the Netherlands (52, 61). Unfortunately, decreased consumption of cereals and cereal products can have a serious impact on DF intakes. Emmett and colleagues found that increasing

TABLE 9 Dietary Fiber Intake Levels in North America and Latin America

Investigator	Country/ Region	Data source/Subject	Fiber analysis method	DF intake (g/day)
Mueller et al., 1997 (74)	U.S.	USDA's Continuing Survey of Food Intakes by Individuals (1989–1991); children and adolescents (to age 20)	AOAC TDF (985.29, Prosky; and 991.43, Lee) USDA Handbook No. 8	Age 3: 9 Age 9: 14 Age 20: 15.6
Lytle et al., 1996 (75)	U.S.	Child and Adolescent Trial for Cardiovascular Health (CATCH), 24-h recall	AOAC TDF (985.29 Prosky; and 991.43, Lee) USDA Handbook No. 8	Caucasian; 15.1 ± 7.4 African-American: 15.1 ± 8.5 Hispanic: 14.8 ± 7.6 Other: 12.1 ± 3.6
Slesinski et al., 1996 (71)	U.S.	Food frequency questionnaire, 1992 National Health Interview Survey Epidemiology Supplement; adults stratified by supplement use (n = 11,643)	AOAC TDF (985.29, Prosky; and 991.43, Lee) USDA Handbook No. 8	Daily M: 14.6 ± 0.2 F: 11.9 ± 0.1 Occasionally M: 14.1 ± 0.3 F: 11.8 ± 0.3 Seldom M: 13.5 ± 0.1 F: 10.5 ± 0.8
Ballew and Sugerman, 1995 (68)	U.S.	24-h recall; low income Mexican women in Chicago, IL, USA (n = 186)	AOAC TDF (985.29 and 991.43) USDA Handbook No. 8	16.9
Marlett and Bokram, 1981 (47)	U.S.	2-d records; males (n = 57), females (n = 143), college students	Unavailable CHO (Southgate)	M = 19.91 ± 9.97 F = 13.41 ± 6.02

TABLE 9 Continued

Investigator	Country/ Region	Data source/Subject	Fiber analysis method	DF intake (g/day)
Hallfrisch et al., 1988 (49)	U.S.	Data from the Baltimore Longitudinal Study (1959–1975), 7-d diet records males (n = 843) aged 20–103	CF (originally) extrapolated to DF based Uppsalla method	15
Block and Lanza, 1987 (67)	U.S.	Data from the Second National Health and Nutrition Examination Survey (NHANES II, 1976–1980); males and females (both white and black), n = 11,658, aged 19–74 years	NDF (Van Soest), NDF plus water-soluble fraction, unavailable CHO, TDF (USDA Handbook No. 8), NSP (Englyst)	*Age: 20–29.5* WM 13.8 WF 9.2 BM 11.2 BF 8.1 *Age: 30–54* WM 13.0 WF 9.4 BM 10.9 BF 7.4 *Age: 55–74* WM 12.6 WF 10.4 BM 7.4 BF 9.1

Ahrens and Boucher, 1978 (81)	U.S.	Per capita use in 1965–1966, from USDA 1965 Household Food Consumption Survey	Unavailable CHO (Southgate)	19.1
Lanza et al., 1987 (57)	U.S.	Data from the Second National Health and Nutrition Examination Survey (NHANES II, 1976–1980), >19 years of age	TDF, NDF, NSP, unavailable CHO	*Southgate* Males, 15.7 Females, 11.1 *Combination* Males, 12.9 Females 9.4
Gibson and Scythes, 1982 (82)	Canada	3-d records; 100 females, 30 ± 6 years of age	Unavailable CHO (Southgate)	19.4 ± 6.6
Anderson et al., 1981 (72)	Canada	56 females, Seventh Day Adventists, 53 ± 15 years of age	Unavailable CHO (Southgate)	30.9 ± 11.0
Kay et al., 1980 (83)	Canada	24-h recall; 200 males, 50–59 years of age	Unavailable CHO (Southgate)	17.8 ± 9.4
Arauz, et al., 1991 (84)	Costa Rica	1-d weighed records; 51 families, urban	AOAC TDF (Prosky, 985.29)	20.3
Acevedo and Bressani, 1989 (64)	Central America and Panama	Per capita consumption, 1969 and 1986, preschool children	CF (USDA Handbook No. 8)	El Salvador 12.5 Costa Rica 5.4
Rosado et al., 1995 (50)	Mexico	Per capita consumption in 1979 and 1989, 219 rural communities	CF (USDA Handbook No. 8) recalculated as TDF (Prosky, 985.29)	1979: 19.8–4.0 (27.2 ± 3.3) 1989: 17.5–27.1 (22.5 ± 2.2)

Abbreviations: M = male; F = female; WM = white male; WF = white female; BM = black male; BF = black female

TABLE 10 Actual Dietary Fiber Intake Levels in Europe

Investigator	Country/ Region	Data source/Subject	Fiber analysis method	DF intake (g/day)
Emmett et al., 1993 (54)	Great Britain	Food frequency questionnaire; males (n = 739, aged 40–69), females (n = 976, aged 25–69)	NSP (Englyst), unavailable CHO (Southgate)	NSP M: 15.5–16.4 F = 14.3–5.1 Unavailable CHO: M = 23.2–25.3 F = 21.6–23.3
Lewis and Buss, 1988 (55)	Great Britain	Per capita consumption from National Food Survey in 1986	Unavailable CHO (Southgate); NSP (Englyst)	Unavailable CHO: 21.8 NSP: 12.9
O'Neill and Fehily, 1991 (85)	U.K.	7-d weighed records; comparison of survey taken in 1980–83 (n = 665) and in 1990 (n = 98)	Unavailable CHO (Southgate)	1980–1983: 19 ± 7 1990: 21 ± 9
McKeigue et al., 1989 (70)	U.K.	7-d record, food-frequency questionnaires; 299 households, South Asian vegetarian and non-vegetarian and British	Unavailable CHO (Southgate)	South Asian, nonvegetarian: 26.4 South Asian, vegetarian: 32.2 British: 17.9
Davies et al., 1986 (59)	U.K.	7-d weighed records; males (n= 41) and females (n = 53)	Unavailable CHO (Southgate)	preretirement 17.6 ± 6.5 postretirement 18.4 ± 6.1
Bingham et al., 1979 (86)	U.K.	7-d weighed records; M and F (n = 63), aged 20–80	Unavailable CHO (Southgate)	19.9 ± 5.3
Thomson et al., 1985 (87)	Scotland	7-d weighed records; 164 men, aged 45–54	Unavailable CHO (Southgate)	19.8

Thomson et al., 1982 (88)	Scotland	7-d weighed records; males (n = 97), age 49	Unavailable CHO (Southgate)	17.5 ± 0.6
Eastwood et al., 1982 (89)	Scotland	7-d diet history, 23 couples, aged 35–82	Unavailable CHO (Southgate)	M = 15.9 ± 6.1 F = 12.7 ± 4.6
Bull et al., 1982 (90)	Scotland	Food diary for 1 month; M (n = 16) and F (n = 27), aged 21–69	Unavailable CHO (Southgate)	M = 16.5 F = 15.0
Fielding and Melvin, 1979 (91)	Ireland	Retrospective 7-d diet history; M (n = 9) and F (n = 16)	Unavailable CHO (Southgate)	M = 22.6 ± 4.1 F = 22.7 ± 4.3
Bagheri and Debry, 1990 (92)	France	Per capita consumption	NSP (Englyst), Unavailable CHO (Southgate)	16.53
Le Quintrec and Gendre, 1986 (93)	France	Per capita consumption, EUROSTAT 1970–80	Unavailable CHO (Southgate)	17.85–24.6
Macquart-Moulin et al., 1983 (94)	France	Food frequency questionnaire; M (n = 122) and F (n = 129)	Unavailable CHO (Southgate)	M = 11.6 ± 6.4 F = 6.6 ± 4.0
Myer and Le Quintrec, 1981 (95)	France	24-h recall; 22 females, with or without constipation	Unavailable CHO (Southgate)	With/Without constipation: 12.4/12.7
Frexinos and Allegret, 1980 (96)	France	Retrospective 7-d diet history; males (n = 27) and females (n = 50), seasonal variations (May and October)	Unavailable CHO (Southgate)	(May) M: 10.61 ± 0.70 F: 11.81 ± 1.88 (October) M: 8.34 ± 1.08 F: 8.64 ± 0.70
Turrini et al., 1995 (51)	Italy	Food-frequency questionnaire twice a year, 24-h recall every 2 yr for 10 year period	Unavailable CHO (Southgate), AOAC TDF (Prosky, 985.29)	32.4
Bingham and Cummings, 1980 (97)	Yugoslavia	Records of duplicate food collections, males (n = 49)	Unavailable CHO (Southgate)	25.5 ± 7.5

TABLE 10 Continued

Investigator	Country/ Region	Data source/Subject	Fiber analysis method	DF intake (g/day)
Samuelson et al., 1996 (76)	Sweden	7-d weighed records, food frequency questionnaire; boys (n = 193) and girls (n = 218) age 15	Unavailable CHO (Southgate)	(Uppsala) Boys: 18 ± 6 Girls: 16 ± 5 (Trollhattan): Boys: 18 ± 6 Girls: 14 ± 4
Kasper et al., 1980 (48)	Germany	Food diaries for October to December; 150 Manual, Students, Teachers, Admin. (M, S, T, A respectively)	CF (USDA Handbook No. 8), unavailable CHO (Southgate)	*Unavail. CHO* M: 22.0 ± 5.5 S: 24.8 ± 8.4 T: 21.7 ± 5.5 A: 17.6 ± 7.7 *Crude fiber* M: 6.2 ± 1.8 S: 6.3 ± 2.0 T: 5.0 ± 1.4 A: 4.6 ± 2.4
Asp et al., 1979 (99)	Sweden	1-d duplicate; 35 men and women	NDF (Englyst), unavailable CHO (Southgate)	NDF: M = 17.8 ± 6.9 F = 11.1 ± 3.5 Unavailable CHO: M = 27.5 ± 5.9 F = 21.1 ± 4.8

Rottka, 1980 (98)	Germany	Food diary; 135,000 males and females	CF values (USDA Handbook No. 8) converted to unavail. CHO (Southgate)	M = 25.1 F = 22.3
Beer-Borst, et al., 1994 (65)	Switzerland	24-h recall, n = 3653	Unavailable CHO (Southgate)	M = 33 W = 30
Englyst et al., 1982 (69)	Scandinavia	4-d weighed records, males (n = 30), 50–59 years of age, rural and urban communities	NSP (Englyst)	rural Finland M18.4 ± 7.8 rural Denmark M18.0 ± 6.4 urban Finland F14.5 ± 5.4 urban Denmark F 13.2 ± 4.8
Kromhout et al., 1990 (52)	Netherlands	Data from Zutphen Study dietary surveys in 1960 (n = 1049) and 1985 (n = 51), retrospective dietary history	Unavailable CHO (Southgate)	1960: 33.2 1985: 31.5
Van Staveren et al., 1982 (61)	Netherlands	7-d food record; males (n = 44) and females (n = 56), aged 25–65	Unavail. CHO (Southgate), IDF (Hellendoorn)	M: 27.5 ± 7.8 F: 21.3 ± 4.7
Van Dokkum et al., 1982 (100)	Netherlands	Diet composites every 2 mo. for a 2 year period; M & F, aged 16–18	IDF (Hellendoorn)	17.7
Frost Andersen et al., 1995 (53)	Norway	Food frequency questionnaire; boys (n-710) and girls (n = 854), age 18	?–Unavailable CHO (Southgate)–?	Boy = 25 Girls = 19

the NSP contribution from cereals greatly increases the overall NSP intake (62). Unfortunately, negative trends in DF consumption have been observed in some countries. Dietary fiber intakes in Japan have been declining consistently since the 1950s (40, 63). Similar drops are being observed in certain rural and urban areas of Latin America (50, 64). So although some positive dietary patterns have been observed in certain regions (52, 65), especially in Italy where significant positive trends in DF intake have been observed (66), dietary intake levels of DF are still falling short of the recommended levels.

Dietary fiber intake levels can also vary according to sex, ethnicity, and lifestyle. Women usually have lower intakes than men. In some cases, this is due to lower energy intakes. Some investigators have found that although women's overall intake of DF was lower, they chose more fiber-dense diets (57) consisting of foods such as brown breads, cereals, raw fruit, and salads (54). However, men and younger people tended to consume more DF from potatoes cooked in fat and pulses in one study (54). In the U.S., Block and Lanza found trends in DF intakes also differ between the sexes. Dietary fiber intakes in women increased with age whereas the opposite occurred in men (67). In the same study, ethnic differences in DF intakes existed with Blacks tending to consume less than Whites in both sexes across all age groups (67). However, Ballew and Sugerman found that DF intakes in Mexican women living in Chicago were different than those living in Texas, suggesting that within an ethnic group there are also temporal and regional variations in dietary intake patterns (68). Greater DF intakes in rural vs. urban areas is not uncommon (69). Lifestyle plays a large role in the level of DF consumed. In general, those with healthier lifestyles or concerned about getting adequate nutrient intakes had higher intakes of DF (53, 70–73).

As in the adult population, DF intakes in children are lower than recommended levels, but their dietary patterns are also undesirable. In the U.S., DF intakes of children are not increasing with age according to the AHF ''Age + 5'' guideline (74). Mueller and colleagues found that as children age, their consumption of fruits, vegetables, and cereals decline (74). Dietary fiber intake levels are lowest in Japanese under the age of 19 (40). In the Child and Adolescent Trial for Cardiovascular Health (CATCH) study (Table 10), dietary intervention to reduce total fat in school children did indicate a shift in energy from fat to CHO while keeping energy level from protein stable. However, the relative proportions of energy from simple sugars and complex CHO remained the same (75). Norwegian adolescents consume too much fat and sugar and not enough DF (70). In Sweden, young people may have adopted advice about consuming less fat, but instead of increasing their fiber intake, consumption of sweets and soft drinks is considerable (76). Thus, it is important to educate the youth about the importance of consuming adequate amounts of dietary fiber as part of a healthy diet.

Adequate intakes of DF are necessary to prevent the onset of constipation

TABLE 11 Actual Dietary Fiber Intake Levels in the Asia-Pacific Region

Investigator	Country/Region	Data source/Subject	Fiber analysis method	DF intake (g/day)
Nakaji et al., 1993 (56)	Japan	Per capita consumption, Aomori Nutrition Survey	Modified AOAC TDF (Prosky, 985.29), unavailable CHO (Southgate)	Unavailable CHO: 23.7 ± 8.4 TDF: 22.2 ± 8.5
Bingham, 1985 (44)	European Economic Community (EEC), 11 regions	Monthly weighed food records over 3-year period (data from Cresta et al., 1969[101]); 30 families, 1963–65	Unavailable CHO (Southgate)	Holland: 22.6 Belgium: 26.8 to 28.9 Luxembourg: 29.1 Germany: 27.3 France: 23.8 to 29.6 Italy: 23.8 to 26.9
Nishimune et al., 1993 (40)	Japan	Menu-based questionnaire in 1990, duplicate analysis of food composites	Modified AOAC TDF (Prosky, 985.29)	≤19 years: 11.5 20–29 years: 13.5
Morita, 1987 (63)	Japan	3-day duplicate food collections; males (n = 6) and females (n = 6), aged 30–50	NDF and ADF (Van Soest)	M = 8.5 ± 0.9 to 16.5 ± 2.8 F = 6.6 ± 0.6 to 10.3 ± 1.5
Minowa et al., 1983 (102)	Japan	Per capita consumption in 1979, National Nutrition Survey	Unavailable CHO (Southgate)	19.4
Hwang et al., 1996 (60)	Korea	3-day food records, M college students (n = 80)	AOAC TDF (Prosky, 985.29)	20.54 ± 5.82
Lee et al., 1994 (58)	Korea	Per capita consumption in 1989, Nat'l Nutrition Survey	AOAC TDF (Prosky, 985.29)	10–15
Zhi-Ping and Su-Fang, 1986 (103)	China	Dietary survey in 1979, various parts of China	CF (USDA Handbook No. 8?)	6.6 to 11.3
Prior et al., 1981 (104)	Polynesia	7-d weighed records, 24 h recall; M (n = 95) and F (n = 161) on island of Tokelau	Unavailable CHO (Southgate), (105)	M = 16.5 F = 14.9

TABLE 12 Dietary Fiber Intake and Food Sources in Aomori, Japan Calculated Using Southgate and Prosky Methods*

	Southgate	Prosky
Total	23.7 ± 8.4 g/day	22.2 ± 8.5 g/day
Dietary fiber source		
Grains	32.3%	19.0%
Vegetables	22.7%	31.3%
Beans	15.6%	18.0%
Fruits	7.8%	11.6%

*Data from ref. #56.

which is more prevalent in the elderly. People over the aged 65+ have lower overall intakes of fiber because of reduced energy consumption. Because of this, it is difficult to increase intakes in the elderly to the general recommended levels of 25–30 g without resorting to supplements and this may have serious consequences in terms of mineral availability (59). However, there is still some indication that dietary fat intakes are still high in this population (77). Interestingly, Davies and colleagues found that despite increased awareness of DF and availability of high fiber foods, DF intake levels remained the same after retirement. This particular post-retirement study population believed that constipation was a problem for the ''elderly'' (59).

Thus, diet-related and health-related beliefs play an important role in one's ability to make changes in their dietary patterns such as increasing DF consumption. In a study on American rural energy workers, a worker's efficacy expectation, i.e. their perceived ability to perform a behavior, was an important variable in raising their DF intake level (78). Smith and Owen found that both diet and health related beliefs were independently associated with higher fiber density (79). Perceptions of external influences on food choices, not related to social status, were also positively associated. Thus, beliefs and perceptions related to diet and health should be addressed for interventions to be successful in raising DF intakes.

SUMMARY

It is important that regulatory agencies, researchers in nutrition and analytical areas, industry representatives, consumers, and health professionals have a common understanding of the definition of DF. International surveys like those conducted by the AOAC are a necessary step in keeping abreast of perceptions about the definition of DF. Chemical methodology for DF analysis needs to keep up with changing or expanding definitions of DF for proper food labeling for the consumer and for assessment in epidemiological studies. Although AOAC TDF methods appear to be the most ideal, improvements must be made for better recoveries of resistant starch and resistant oligosaccharides that are part of the new and expanded DF definition. Dietary recommendations for fiber must take into account several factors: (1) physiological effects of various fiber components; (2) long-term effects of fiber on health and disease; (3) potential adverse effects of mineral availability in more susceptible populations; (4) the intended population for the recommendation; (5) current intake levels to assess feasibility of the recommended level; and (6) whether DF will be consumed in foods or supplements. Although analysis and characterization of DF is one of the more popular areas of research according to the European Management Committee of COST 92 (42), research into DF epidemiology and intakes is severely lacking. Despite official recommendations and increased awareness around the world to increase DF consumption by increasing intakes of grain products, fruits, and vegetables, this advice is not being adhered to by the general public. Children and adolescents are an important group to reach since the early development of good dietary habits will most likely be carried throughout adulthood, affording protection against the development of chronic diseases associated with low fiber intakes. A necessary step is increased education about the importance of DF to change the existing perceptions about foods choices. Diet and health-related beliefs are crucial factors in changing dietary patterns.

REFERENCES

1. Burkitt DP, Trowell HC. (1975) Refined Carbohydrate Foods and Disease: Implications of Dietary Fiber. Academic Press, London, England.
2. Gray DS. (1995) The clinical uses of dietary fiber. Am. Family Phys. 51:419–26.
3. Lanza E, Butrum RR. (1986) A critical review of food fiber analysis and data. J. Am. Diet. Assoc. 86:732–43.
4. Cho, SS, Prosky, L. (1998) Definition and analysis of complex carbohydrates. In: Cho, SS, Prosky, L, Dreher, M, eds. Complex Carbohydrates. Marcel Dekker, pp. 131–143. New York, NY.
5. Lee SC, Prosky L. (1992) Dietary fiber analysis for nutrition labeling. Cereal Foods World 37:765–71.
6. Southgate DAT. (1982) Definitions and terminology of dietary fiber. In: Vahouny, GV, Kritchevsky, D, eds Dietary Fiber in Health and Disease. Plenum Press, 1982: 1–7. New York, NY.
7. Englyst HN, Cummings JH. (1987) Digestion of polysaccharides of potato in the small intestine of man. Am. J. Clin. Nutr. 45:423–31.
8. Berry CS. (1986) Resistant starch: formation and measurement of starch that survives exhaustive digestion with amolytic enzymes during the determination of dietary fibre. J. Cereal Sci. 4:301–14.

9. Lee SC, Prosky L. (1995) International survey on dietary fiber: definition, analysis, and reference materials. J. AOAC Int. 78:22–36.
10. AOAC. (1990) Official Methods of Analysis of the Association of Official Analytical Chemists, 15th ed. Arlington, VA.
11. Van Soest PJ, Wine RH. (1967) Use of detergents in analysis of fibrous feeds. IV. Determination of plant cell-wall constituents. J. Assoc. Off. Anal. Chem. 50:50–5.
12. Goering HK, Van Soest PJ. (1970) USDA Agriculture Handbook No. 379.
13. Schaller D. (1977) Analysis of dietary fiber. Food Prod. Devel. 11:70.
14. Hellendoorn EW, Noordhoff MG, Slagman J. (1976) Enzymatic determination of the indigestible residue content of human food. J. Sci. Food Agric. 26:1461–8.
15. Prosky L, Asp N-G, Schweizer TF, DeVries JW, Furda I. (1988) Determination of insoluble, soluble and total dietary fiber in foods and food products: interlaboratory study. J. Assoc. Off. Anal. Chem. 71:1017–23.
16. Lee SC, Prosky L, DeVries JW. (1992) Determination of total, soluble, and insoluble dietary fiber in foods- enzymatic-gravimetric method, MES-TRIS buffer: collaborative study. J. AOAC Int. 75:395.
17. Southgate DAT. (1969) Determination of carbohydrates in foods. II. Unavailable carbohydrates. J. Sci. Food Agric. 20:331–5.
18. Theander O, Aman P, Westerlund E, Graham H. (1994) Enzymatic/chemical analysis of dietary fiber. J. AOAC Int. 77:703–9.
19. Marlett JA. (1992) Content and composition of dietary fiber in 117 frequently consumed foods. J. Am. Diet. Assoc. 92:175–86.
20. Englyst HN, Wiggins HS, Cummings JR. (1982) Determination of the non-starch polysaccharides in plant foods by gas-liquid chromatography of constituent sugars as alditol acetates. Analyst 107:307–18.
21. Cummings JH, Englyst HN, Wood R. (1985) Determination of dietary fibre in cereals and cereal products–collaborative trials. Part I: Initial trial. J. Assoc. Off. Anal. Chem. 23:1–35.
22. Englyst HN, Cummings JH, Wood R. (1987) Determination of dietary fibre in cereals and cereal products–collaborative trials. Part II: Studies of the modified Englyst procedure. J. Assoc. Publ. Analysts 25:59–71.
23. Englyst HN, Cummings JH, Wood R. (1987) Determination of dietary fibre in cereals and cereal products. Part III: Study of further simplified procedures. J. Assoc. Publ. Analysts 1987;25:73–110.
24. Hagglund E, Lindberg B, McPherson J. (1956) Dimethylsulphoxide, a solvent for hemicellulose. Acta. Chem. Scand. 10:1160.
25. Woolard GR, Rathbone EB, Novellie. (1977) DMSO–soluble hemicelluloses from the husk of sorghum grain. Phytochem. 16:961.
26. Orman M. (1993) Position of the American Dietetic Association: health implications of dietary fiber. J. Am. Diet. Assoc. 93:1446–7.
27. Bal DG, Foerster SB. (1993) Dietary strategies for cancer prevention. Cancer 72: 1005–10.
28. Cassidy A, Bingham SA, Cummings JH. (1994) Starch intake and colorectal cancer risk: an international comparison. Br. J. Cancer 69:937–42.
29. Kritchevsky, D. (1991) Evaluation of publicly available scientific evidence regard-

ing certain nutrient-disease relationships: Dietary fiber and cardiovascular disease. Prepared by LSRO/FASEB for Center for Food Safety and Applied Nutrition, FDA, DHHS, under FDA Contract No. 223-88-2124, Task Order #9.
30. Pilch S.M (ed.). (1987) Physiological effects and health consequences of dietary fiber. Life Sciences Research Office, Federation of American Societies for Experimental Biology, Bethesda, MD.
31. DeCosse JJ, Miller HH, Lesser ML. (1989) Effect of wheat fiber and vitamins C and E on rectal polyps in patients with familial adenomatous polyposis. J. Natl. Cancer Inst. 81:1290–7.
32. Rose DP. (1990) Dietary fiber and breast cancer. Nutr. Cancer 13:1–8.
33. WHO. (1990) Diet, nutrition, and the prevention of chronic diseases. World Health Organization. Geneva, Switzerland.
34. Food and Drug Administration (FDA). (1993) Food labeling; general provisions; nutrition labeling; label format; nutrient claims; ingredient labeling; state and local requirements; and exemptions: final rules. Fed. Register. 58:2302–2906.
35. Department of Agriculture (USDA). (1993) Food labeling; general provisions; nutrition labeling; label format; nutrient claims; ingredient labeling; state and local requirements; and exemptions: final rules. Fed. Register. 58:631–691.
36. Committee on Nutrition, American Association of Pediatrics. (1993) Carbohydrate and dietary fiber. In: Barness, LA, ed. Pediatric Nutrition Handbook, 3rd ed. American Academy of Pediatrics, Elk Grove Village, IL.
37. Williams, CL, Bollella, M, Wynder, EL. (1995) A new recommendation for dietary fiber in childhood. Pediatrics. 96:985–8.
38. Horwath CC. (1989) Dietary intake studies in elderly people. World Rev. Nutr. Diet. 59:1–70.
39. Department of Health, UK. (1991) Dietary reference values for food energy and nutrients for the United Kingdom. Department of Health Report on Health and Social Subjects. 41:61–71.
40. Nishimune T, Sumimoto T, Konishi Y, Yakushiji T, Komachi Y, Mitsuhashi Y, Nakayama I, Okazaki K, Tsuda T, Ichihashi A, Nakahara S, Oda S. (1993) Dietary fiber intake of Japanese younger generations and the recommended daily allowance. J. Nutr. Sci. Vitaminol. 39:263–78.
41. Spiller GA, Chernoff MC, Shipley FA, Beigler MA, Briggs GM. (1977) Can fecal weight be used to establish a recommended intake of dietary fiber? Am. J. Clin. Nutr. 30:659–60.
42. Cummings JH. (1995) Dietary fibre intakes in Europe: overview and summary of European research activities, conducted by members of the Management Committee of COST 92. Eur. J. Clin. Nutr. 49:S5–S9.
43. Bright-See E, McKeown-Eyssen GE. (1984) Estimation of per capita crude and dietary fiber supply in 38 countries. Am. J. Clin Nutr. 39:821–9.
44. Bingham S. Dietary fibre intakes: intake studies, problems, methods and results. In: Trowell HC, Burkitt DP, Heaton K, eds. Dietary Fibre, Fibre-Depleted Foods and Disease. London, England: Academic Press, 1985:77–104.
45. Saba A, D'Amicis A, Turrini A. (1995) Evaluation of a fibre intake questionnaire using weighed records. Eur. J. Clin. Nutr. 49:S135–S8.
46. Bingham S, Wiggins HS, Englyst H, Seppanen R, Helms P, Strand R, Burton R,

Jorgensen IM, Poulsen L, Paerregaard A, Bjerrum L, James WP. (1982) Methods and validity of dietary assessments in four Scandinavian populations. Nutr. Cancer. 4:23–33.
47. Marlett JA, Bokram RL. (1981) Relationship between calculated dietary and crude fiber intakes of 200 college students. Am. J. Clin. Nutr. 34:335–42.
48. Kasper H, Rabast U, Ehl M. Studies on the extent of dietary fiber intake in West Germany. Nutr. Metab. 24:102–9.
49. Hallfrisch J, Tobin JD, Muller DC, Andres R. (1988) Fiber intake, age, and other coronary risk factors in men of the Baltimore Longitudinal Study (1959–1975). J. Gerontol. 43:M64–M8.
50. Rosado JL, Lopez P, Lopez G, Madrigal H, Huerta Z. (1995) Consumption of dietary fiber in rural Mexico. Ecol. Food Nutr. 34:129–36.
51. Turrini A, Saba A, D'Amicis A, Cialfa E, Lintas C. (1995) A study to investigate the relationship between dietary fibre intake and gastrointestinal diseases. Eur. J. Clin. Nutr. 49:S139–S44.
52. Kromhout D, de Lezenne Coulander C, Obermann-de Boer GL, van Kampen-Donker M, Goddijn E, Bloemberg BP. (1990) Changes in food and nutrient intake in middle-aged men from 1960 to 1985 (the Zutphen Study). Am. J. Clin. Nutr. 51:123–9.
53. Frost Andersen L, Nes M, Sandstad B, Bjorneboe G-EA, Drevon CA. (1995) Dietary intake among Norwegian adolescents. Eur. J. Clin. Nutr. 49:555–64.
54. Emmett PM, Symes CL, Heaton KW. (1993) Dietary intake and sources of non-starch polysaccharide in English men and women. Eur. J. Clin. Nutr. 47:20–30.
55. Lewis J, Buss DH. (1988) Trace nutrients: minerals and vitamins in the British household food supply. Br. J. Nutr. 60:413–24.
56. Nakaji S, Sakamoto J, Sugawara K, Iwane S, Ohta M, Mori B. (1993) Dietary fiber intake and intake patterns among the general population in Aomori, calculated using modified Southgate and Prosky methods. Nippon Eiseigaku Zasshi. 48:628–37.
57. Lanza E, Jones DY, Block G, Kessler L. (1987) Dietary fiber intake in the US population. Am. J. Clin. Nutr. 46:790–7.
58. Lee K-H, Park M-A, Kim E-S, Moon H-K. (1994) A study on dietary fiber intakes of Korean. J. Korean Soc. Food Nutr. 23:767–73.
59. Davies L, Holdsworth MD, Macfarlane D. (1986) Dietary fibre intakes in the United Kingdom before and after retirement from work. Hum. Nutr. Appl. Nutr. 10:431–9.
60. Hwang S-H, Kim J-I, Sung C-J. (1996) Assessment of dietary fiber intake in Korean college students. J. Korean Soc. Food Nutr. 25:205–13.
61. Van Staveren WA, Hautvast JGAJ, Katan MB, van Montfort MAJ, van-Oosten-van der Goes HGC. (1982) Dietary fiber consumption in an adult Dutch population. J. Am. Diet. Assoc. 80:324–30.
62. Emmett PM, Symos CL, Heaton KW. (1993) The contribution of breakfast cereals to non-starch polysaccharide intakes in English men and women. J. Hum. Nutr. Diet. 6:217–22.
63. Morita K. (1987) The relation of dietary fiber intake to large bowel cancer mortality in Japan. Eisei Kagaku. 33:185–90.

64. Acevedo E, Bressani R. (1989) Intake of dietary fiber in the Central American isthmus: nutritional implications. Arch. Latinoam. Nutr. 39:392–404.
65. Beer-Borst S, Wellauer-Weber B, Amado R. (1994) Dietary fiber intake of a collective Swiss population interested in nutrition. Z. Ernahrungswiss. 33:68–78.
66. Turrini A, Rosolini G, Cialfa E, Lintas C. (1995) Dietary fibre intake: trends in Italy. Eur. J. Clin. Nutr. 49:S219–S21.
67. Block G, Lanza E. (1987) Dietary fiber sources in the US by demographic group. J. Natl. Cancer Inst 79:83–91.
68. Ballew C, Sugerman SB. (1995) High-risk nutrient intakes among low-income Mexican women in Chicago, Illinois. J. Am. Diet. Assoc. 95:1409–13.
69. Englyst HN, Bingham S, Wiggins, HS, Southgate DAT, Sepparen R, Helms P, Anderson V, Day KC, Choolun R, Collinson E, Cummings JH. (1982) Analysis of and consumption of non-starch polysaccharides in four Scandinavian populations. Nutr. Cancer. 4:50–60.
70. McKeigue PM, Adelstein AM, Marmot MG, Henly PJ, Owen RW, Hill MJ, Thompson MH. (1989) Diet and fecal steroid profile in a South Asian population with a low colon-cancer rate. Am. J. Clin. Nutr. 50:151–4.
71. Slesinski MJ, Subar AF, Kahle LL. (1996) Dietary fat, fiber and other nutrients is related to the use of vitamin and mineral supplements in the United States: the 1992 National Health Interview Survey. J. Nutr. 126:3001–8.
72. Anderson BM, Gibson RS, Sabry JH. (1981) The iron and zinc status of long-term vegetarian women. Am. J. Clin. Nutr. 34:1042–8.
73. Potter J, Record SJ, Baghurst KI. (1986) Fiber consumption in Australian populations. In: Spiller GA, ed. CRC Handbook of Dietary Fiber in Human Nutrition. CRC Press, Inc., Boca Raton, FL. 415–22.
74. Mueller S, Keast DR, Olson BH. (1997) Intakes and food sources of dietary fiber in children. FASEB J. 11:A187 (abstr.).
75. Lytle LA, Stone EJ, Nichaman MZ, Perry CL, Montgomery DH, Nicklas TA, Zive MM, Mitchell P, Dwyer JY, Ebzery M, Evans MA, Galati TP. (1996) Changes in nutrient intakes of elementary school children following a school-based intervention: results from the CATCH study. Prev. Med. 25:465–7.
76. Samuelson G, Bratteby L-E, Enghardt H, Hedgren M. (1995) Food habits and energy and nutrient intake in Swedish adolescents approaching the year 2000. Acta. Paediatr. Suppl. 415:1–20.
77. Horwath CC. (1989) Dietary survey of a large random sample of elderly people: energy and nutrient intakes. Nutr. Res. 9:479–92.
78. Kuppens R, Eriksen MP, Adriaanse HP, Nijuis FJN, Aaron JC. (1996) Determinants of fat and fiber consumption in American rural energy workers. Prev. Med. 25: 212–7.
79. Smith AM, Owen N. (1992) Associations of social status and health-related beliefs with dietary fat and fiber densities. Prev. Med. 21:735–45.
80. AOAC. (1995) Official Methods of Analysis of the Association of Official Analytical Chemists, 16th ed. AOAC. Arlington, VA.
81. Ahrens EH Jr., Boucher CA. (1978) The composition of a simulated American diet. Comparison of chemical analyses and estimates from food composition tables. J. Am. Diet. Assoc. 73:613–20.

82. Gibson RS, Scythes CA. (1982) Trace element intakes of women. Br. J. Nutr. 48: 241–8.
83. Kay RM, Sabry ZI, Csima A. (1980) Multivariate analysis of diet and serum lipids in normal men. Am. J. Clin. Nutr. 33:2566–72.
84. Arauz AG, Monge RA, Munoz L, Rojas MT. (1991) Diet as a risk factor for cardiovascular disease in residents of the metropolitan area, San Jose, Costa Rica. Arch. Latinoam. Nutr. 41:350–62.
85. O'Neill O, Fehily AM. (1991) Nutrient intakes of men in South Wales: a comparison of surveys taken in 1980-1983 and 1990. J. Hum. Nutr. Diet. 4:413–9.
86. Bingham S, Cummings JH, McNeil NI. (1979) Intakes and sources of dietary fiber in the British population. Am. J. Clin. Nutr. 32:1313–9.
87. Thomson M, Fulton M, Wood DA, Brown S, Elton RA, Birtwhistle A, Oliver MF. (1985) A comparison of nutrient intake of some Scotsmen with dietary recommendations. Hum. Nutr. Appl. Nutr. 39:443–55.
88. Thomson M, Logan RL, Sharman M, Lockerbie L, Riemersma RA, Oliver MF. (1982) Dietary survey in 49 year old Edinburgh men. Hum. Nutr. Appl. Nutr. 36A: 272–80.
89. Eastwood MA, Brydon WG, Smith DM, Smith JH. (1982) A study of diet, serum lipids, and fecal constituents in spouses. Am. J. Clin. Nutr. 36:290–3.
90. Bull NL, Smart GA, Judson H. (1982) Food and nutrient intakes on the Westray in the Orkney Islands. Ecol. Food Nutr. 12:97–101.
91. Fielding JF, Melvin K. (1979) Dietary fibre and the irritable bowel syndrome. J. Hum. Nutr. 33:243–7.
92. Bagheri SM, Debry G. (1990) Estimation of daily dietary fiber intake in France. Ann. Nutr. Metab. 34:69–75.
93. Le Quintrec Y, Gendre JP. (1986) Consumption of dietary fiber in France. In: Spiller GA, ed. CRC Handbook of Dietary Fiber in Human Nutrition. CRC Press Inc., Boca Raton, FL. 425–32.
94. Macquart-Moulin G, Durbec JP, Corvee J, Berthezene P, Southgate DAT. (1983) Alimentation et cancer recto-colique. Gastroenterol. Clin. Biol. 7:277–86.
95. Meyer F, Le Quintrec Y. (1981) Relationship between dietary fibers and constipation. Nouv. Presse. Med. 10:2479–81.
96. Frexinos J, Allegret M. (1980) Evaluation de la ration en fibres alimentaires dans la region Midi-Pyrenees et en Nouvelle Caledonie. Gastroenterol. Clin. Biol. 4: 729–30.
97. Bingham S, Cummings JH. (1980) Sources and intake of dietary fiber in man. In: Spiller GA, Kay RM, eds. Medical Aspects of Dietary Fiber. Raven Press, New York, NY. 261–84.
98. Rottka, H. (1980) Pflanzenfasern–Ballastoffe in der menschlichen Ernahrung. Thieme, Stuttgart.
99. Asp N-G, Carlstedt L, Dahlqvist A, Johansson CG, Paulsson M. (1979) Dietary fiber. Scand. J. Gastroenterol. 14 (52 Suppl.):128–37.
100. Van Dokkum W, De Vos RH, Cloughley FA, Hulshof KFAM, Dukel F, Wijsman JA. (1982) Food additives and food components in total diets in the Netherlands. Br. J. Nutr. 48:223–31.
101. Cresta M, Ledermann S, Gardiner A, Lombardo E, Lacourly G. (1969) A dietary

survey of 11 areas of the EEC in order to determine levels of radioactive contamination. EUR. 4218F, Euratom, Leiden.
102. Minowa M, Bingham S, Cummings JH. (1983) Dietary fibre intake in Japan. Hum. Nutr. Appl. Nutr. 37:113–9.
103. Zhi-Ping S, Su-Fang Z. (1986) Consumption of dietary fiber-rich foods in China. In: Spiller GA, ed. CRC Handbook of Dietary Fiber in Human Nutrition. Boca Raton, FL: CRC Press Inc., Boca Raton, FL. 423–4.
104. Prior IA, Davidson F, Salmond CE, Czochanska Z. (1981) Cholesterol, coconuts, and diet on Polynesian atolls: a natural experiment: the Pukapuka and Tokelau island studies. Am. J. Clin. Nutr. 34:1552–61.
105. Holloway WD, Tasman-Jones C, Maher D. (1977) Towards an accurate measurement of dietary fibre. NZ Med. J. 85:420–3.
106. Margarey A, Nichols J, Boulton J. (1987) Food intake at age 8. I. Energy, macro- and micronutrients. Aust. Paediatr. J. 23:173–8.
107. Flint DM, Wahlqvist ML, Parish AE, Smith TJ. (1983) Dietary fiber intakes of elderly Australians. In: Wallace G, Bell L, eds. Fiber in Human and Animal Nutrition. Wellington, NZ: Royal Society of New Zealand. 33 (abstr.).
108. Pomare EW, Stace NH, Peters SG, Fisher A. (1983) Dietary intakes, stool characteristics and biliary bile acid composition in four South Pacific populations. In: Wallace G, Bell L, eds. Fiber in Human and Animal Nutrition. Wellington, NZ: Royal Society of New Zealand. 35 (abstr.).
109. Hillman LC, Stace NJ, Fisher A, Pomare EW. (1982) Dietary intakes and stool characteristics of patients with the irritable bowel syndrome. Am. J. Clin. Nutr. 36: 626–9.

II

COMPLEX CARBOHYDRATES—CHEMISTRY AND ANALYTICAL METHODOLOGY

10

The Chemistry of Complex Carbohydrates

DAVID R. LINEBACK
University of Idaho, Moscow, Idaho

INTRODUCTION

The term "complex carbohydrates" has been used in dietary recommendations for the past two decades in the United States. There is a lack of a clear definition of what is included in complex carbohydrates. Beginning with the second edition of the Dietary Goals in 1977 (1), the emphasis has been on complex carbohydrates as "starches," i.e. digestible (available) polysaccharides, primarily starch and dextrins. The 1979 Surgeon General's Report on Health Promotion and Disease Prevention (2) referred to complex carbohydrates in terms of whole grains, cereals, fruits and vegetables, a usage that appears to include starch and non-starch polysaccharides (dietary fiber). A task force of the British Nutrition Foundation proposed elimination of the term dietary fiber and that complex carbohydrates be defined as starches plus non-starch polysaccharides (3). However, it does not appear that these recommendations will be accepted. In its July 1990 proposal for food labeling, the Food and Drug Administration proposed that, for regulatory purposes, complex carbohydrates be defined as the sum of dextrins and starches including those carbohydrate components that contain 10 or more saccharide units, excluding dietary fiber (4). This was not allowed in the final regulations when the term ''other carbohydrates'' was adopted rather than complex carbohydrates because of the lack of an accepted definition and analytical methodology for the latter (5).

Recently, AOAC International conducted surveys to determine whether a consensus could be reached, among professionals in the carbohydrate area, on the definition of complex carbohydrates and dietary fiber. Results indicated that complex carbohydrates should include available starch and dietary fiber or its polysaccharides (6). There was also general support that the definition of dietary fiber should be expanded to include resistant oligosaccharides in addition to non-starch polysaccharides, resistant starches, and lignin. At an AOAC International Workshop on Definition and Analysis of Complex Carbohydrates/Dietary Fiber in November 1995, there was general agreement among the participants that dietary fiber should be included in the definition of complex carbohydrates and that resistant oligosaccharides are part of dietary fiber.

Thus, while the lack of an accepted definition and analytical methodology has limited the use and understanding of the term ''complex carbohydrates,'' there appears to be an increasing consensus that complex carbohydrates should be defined as available starch plus dietary fiber (non-starch polysaccharides plus lignin) with resistant oligosaccharides and resistant starch included in the definition of dietary fiber. This is the definition that will be used in this brief review concerning the chemistry of complex carbohydrates. Since lignin is not a polysaccharide, being a complex cross-linked polymer based on oxygenated phenylpropane units, it will not be discussed further.

The emphasis on increasing the consumption of complex carbohydrates probably had its origin in the desire to decrease the fat content of diets while increasing the amount of dietary fiber without increasing the consumption of simple sugars. This was partially based on long held understanding that complex carbohydrates are more slowly digested and absorbed than simple sugars, resulting in a decreased insulin and blood glucose response. It was believed that all complex carbohydrates had similar effects on these responses. Studies have indicated that this assumption is not universally true and that different types of complex carbohydrates produce significantly different responses (7).

The increased consumption of complex carbohydrates continues to be advocated in dietary recommendations. Since information on complex carbohydrates is not listed on labels, consumers lack a readily identified means of determining the complex carbohydrate content of foods and what foods are good sources of complex carbohydrates. This is an important driving force in arriving at an accepted definition of complex carbohydrates and the analytical methodologies needed to determine their content in foods.

The complex carbohydrates commonly encountered in foods include starch (available), resistant starch, cellulose, hemicelluloses, pectic substances, hydrocolloids (gums, mucilages), modified starches, and resistant oligosaccharides. There is much yet to be learned about this area and the components involved, e.g. isolation, structures, properties, physiological responses, definitive analytical procedures. It is made difficult by the fact that complex carbohydrates cannot be clearly defined on the basis of structure, analytical methodology, or physiological response. The components of complex carbohydrates/dietary fiber have traditionally been defined on the basis of the solvent extraction procedures used for their isolation. This does not result in clearly definitive separations of the components, nor in definition when a structural basis is used.

STARCH

Starch is the most important reserve polysaccharide of many higher plants where it occurs as discrete granules in the leaf, stem (pith), root (tuber), seed, fruit and pollen. The size, shape and gelatinization temperature of the granules depend on the botanical source of the starch. Common food starches are derived from seed (wheat, maize, rice, barley) and root (potato, cassava/tapioca) sources.

Starch consists of a mixture of two polymers, amylose and amylopectin, that are composed entirely of glucose units, i.e. homopolysaccharides. The glucopyranosyl units in amylose are linked through alpha-D-(1 $\rightarrow$ 4)-glucosidic linkages. Amylose has traditionally been considered to be a linear polymer with an average chain length and degree of polymerization of approximately 1000 or less. However, it is now known that it contains a limited amount of branching involving alpha-D-(1 $\rightarrow$ 6)-glucosidic linkages at the branch points. Amyloses, as isolated, are often a mixture of linear and branched molecules (Figure 1). The behavior of amylose is dominated by two major properties:

(a) Its ability to form inclusion complexes with iodine, aliphatic primary alcohols, lipids and surfactants. Amylose produces a deep blue inclusion complex with iodine, used in the detection of starch, in which the amylose chain forms a helix around the iodine molecule with six glucosyl units per turn of the helix.

(b) Its ability to form strong intermolecular interactions, hydrogen bonding, leading to precipitation or gel formation when a solution of amylose is cooled.

Amylopectin is a high molecular weight, highly branched polymer containing about 5–6% alpha-D-(1 $\rightarrow$ 6)-glucosidic linkages. It has an average chain length of 20 to 25, an average degree of polymerization in the thousands, and molecular weights in the millions. The structure of amylopectin contains clusters in which about 20–25 chains containing 12–16 glucose units are involved (8) (Figure 1). These clusters, in which many of the chains exist as double helices, are responsible for the crystalline regions of starch granules.

While the manner in which amylose and amylopectin are organized to form the granule is not clearly understood, the granule is partially crystalline exhibiting

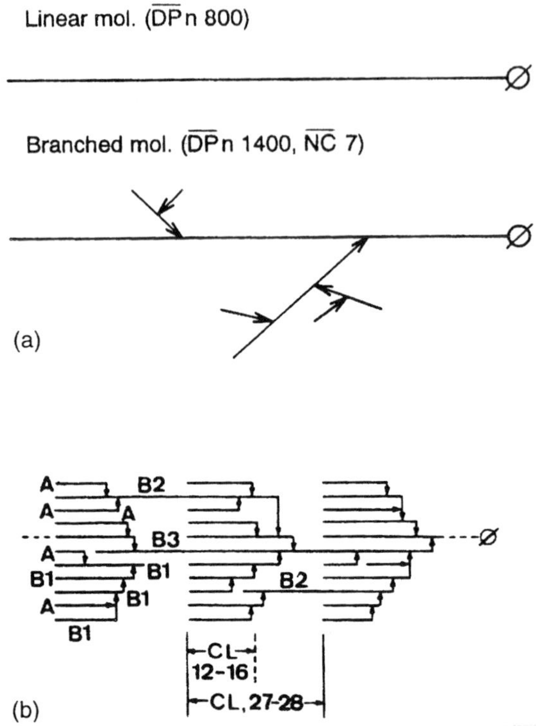

FIGURE 1 (a) Structural models for the molecules in rice amylose. (b) Structural model for three clusters in amylopectin. A, B1, B2, and B3 represent different chain lengths within the clusters: A and B1 chains make a single cluster; B2 and B3 chains extend into two and three clusters, respectively.

an x-ray diffraction pattern and birefringence. Most common cereal starches contain 20–30% amylose. Waxy starches (maize, rice, sorghum, barley) have no amylose and contain essentially 100% amylopectin. High-amylose starches (maize, barley) having 50–70% amylose are available. Waxy and high-amylose starches have properties different from normal starches that make them of use in certain food products.

Native starch, i.e. granules, are not water-soluble but easily hydrate in aqueous suspension, swelling about 10% in volume, but not losing their birefringence unless heated. When an aqueous suspension of granules is heated additional swelling occurs and a temperature is reached at which a transition from organization to disorganization occurs that is characterized by loss of birefringence and the x-ray diffraction pattern, and appearance of an endotherm in the differential scanning calorimetric thermogram. This is known as the gelatinization temperature and normally occurs over a range of about 10°C. Upon further heating (pasting or cooking), swelling continues and the amylose and portions of the amylopectin leach from the granule producing a viscous suspension. Cooling of this suspension leads to the formation of a gel. With further time, realignment of the linear chains of amylose and the short chains of amylopectin can occur in the process known as retrogradation. In food products based on starch gels, this can lead to liquid being expressed from the gel in the phenomenon known as syneresis—generally an undesirable occurrence. Retrogradation is most rapid with amylose and much slower and more incomplete with amylopectin due to the short chain length of its branches.

Starch granules are susceptible to the action of digestive enzymes (alpha-amylases) but the rate of enzymatic degradation is greatly increased when the starch is gelatinized. It is now recognized that a portion of the starch may not be digested and absorbed in the small intestine, but is passed into the lower intestine where it is fermented with production of short-chain fatty acids (SCFA). This fraction has become known as resistant starch.

CELLULOSE

Cellulose, the major cell wall structural component in plants, is an unbranched linear chain of several thousand glucose units with beta-D-(1 $\rightarrow$ 4)-glucosidic linkages. Hydrogen bonding occurs between hydroxyl groups on adjacent glucosyl units, causing the cellulose chain to exist in an extended, relatively inflexible conformation. In turn, this conformation favors the formation of hydrogen bonds between chains. These interchain hydrogen bonds are strong enough that formation of crystalline microfibrils up to 25 nm in diameter occurs. Cellulose's mechanical strength, resistance to biological degradation, low aqueous solubility, and resistance to acid hydrolysis occur because of the hydrogen bonding within the microfibrils (9). There is a portion, 10–15%, of the total cellulose, referred to as ''amorphous,'' that is more readily acid hydrolyzed. Controlled hydrolysis of cellulose, i.e. the amorphous fraction, yields microcrystalline cellulose. Cellulose has been used as a bulking agent in food due to its water-absorbing ability and low solubility. Some of the early ingredient sources of dietary fiber were based on cellulose powders or microcrystalline cellulose. Cellulose is not digested to any extent by the enzymes of the human gastrointestinal system.

HEMICELLULOSES

The cell wall polysaccharides of higher plants involve a number of non-starch polysaccharides that include cellulose, hemicelluloses and pectic substances. Historically, these have been defined by the extraction procedures used, i.e. hemicelluloses were those polysaccharides solubilized by aqueous alkali after water-soluble and pectic substances were removed (10). The situation is actually much more complex. Cell wall polysaccharides exist as heterogeneous mixtures of polysaccharides that are associated by hydrogen bonding and even covalently linked to varying extents. These include homopolysaccharides, those that contain only one type of carbohydrate monomer such as cellulose and mixed-linked beta-glucans, and heteropolysaccharides, those that contain more than one type of carbohydrate monomer such as arabinoxylans, galactomannans and xyloglucans.

Structural determination and characterization of these polysaccharides are made difficult by several factors. For each carbohydrate monomer involved, the following must be determined (11):

1. the identity of the monomer, i.e., D-glucose, D-xylose, L-arabinose;
2. the ring size (pyranose or furanose);
3. nature of the linkage (hydroxyl groups involved in linking monomer units), e.g., $1 \rightarrow 4$, $1 \rightarrow 3$, $1 \rightarrow 2$;
4. anomeric configuration, i.e., alpha or beta;
5. sequence of the different carbohydrate monomers in heteropolysaccharides; and
6. sequence of linkages in homopolysaccharides with multiple types of linkages.

Hemicelluloses may be present in soluble and insoluble forms and are comprised of a number of branched and linear pentose- and hexose-containing polysaccharides. In cereal grains, soluble hemicelluloses are termed ''pentosans.'' Hemicelluloses are of much lower molecular weight than cellulose. Component monosaccharide units may include xylose, arabinose, galactose, mannose, glucose, glucuronic acid and galacturonic acid.

Hemicelluloses are normally classified by the predominant carbohydrate monomer present. Illustrations are given in Table 1. The most abundant and widespread noncellulosic cell wall components are the xylans, polymers with a main chain of beta-D-($1 \rightarrow 4$)-linked D-xylose. The backbone structure may be substituted with single (4-O-methyl)-alpha-D-glucopyranosyluronic acid units, single alpha-L-arabinofuranose units or longer side chains in which the L-arabinofuranose residues have additional substituents. A general structure for xylans is shown below: some side chains (R) include D-galactose, L-galactose, and D-xylose units.

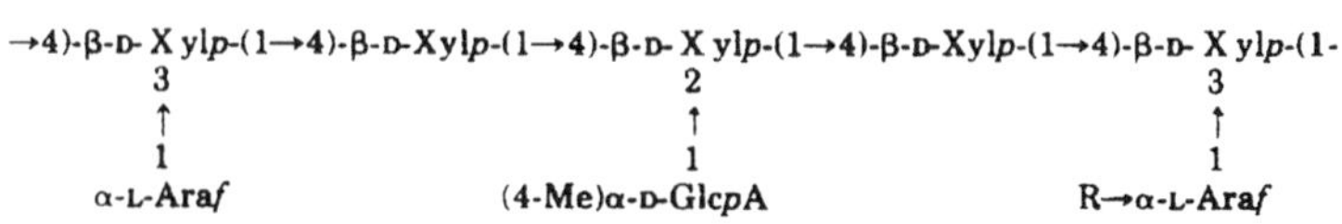

Xylans (5)

TABLE 1 Polysaccharides of Cell Walls in Higher Plants (11)

General category	Structural classification
Cellulose	β-D-Glucan (4-linked)
Pectic substances	Galacturonans and rhamnogalacturonans
	Arabinans
	Galactans and arabinogalactans I[1]
Hemicelluloses	Xylans [including arabinoxylans and (4-o-methyl)] glucuronoxylans
	β-D-Glucans (3- and 4-linked)
	Xyloglucans (4-linked-D-glucans with attached side chains)
Other polysaaccharides	Arabinogalactans II[1]
	Glucuronomannans

[1]Arabinogalactans of type I are essentially linear and contain 4-linked β-D-galactan chains, whereas those of type II contain branched 3- and 6-linked β-D-galactan chains. These polysaccharides may occur in part as proteoglycans or polysaccharide-protein conjugates.

While the arabinosyl residues play a major role in the solubility of the polymer and the shape of the molecule in arabinoxylans, there does not appear to be any consistent relationship between solubility and the amount of substitution with arabinose units. Water-soluble arabinoxylans (pentosans) are present in minor amounts in cereal grains, but they are of functional importance because of their water-binding capacity and ability to increase viscosity. In rye, the major portion of the arabinoxylans is water insoluble. The water-soluble arabinoxylans from rye exist as a range of polymer structures that differ in molecular weight, arabinose-to-xylose ratio, ferulic acid content, ratio of di- to monosubstituted xylose, and ratio of disubstituted xyloses that are isolated, paired, or present in longer sequences in the xylan chain (13).

The $(1 \rightarrow 3)(1 \rightarrow 4)$-beta-D-glucans, i.e. the mixed linkage beta-glucans, have generated considerable interest in recent years due to their physiological response as soluble dietary fiber. While these glucans are found in relatively small quantities in wheat, they are a major component of cell-wall material in barley and oats. These glucans form viscous aqueous solutions and have been shown to be effective in reducing serum cholesterol concentrations (13). Oat betaglucan is a linear polymer containing about 70% 4-O-linked beta-D-glucopyranosyl units and about 30% 3-O-linked beta-D-glucopyranosyl units. The $(1 \rightarrow 3)$ linkages appear to occur singly while the $(1 \rightarrow 4)$-linkages occur in groups of two or three. Thus the polysaccharide contains beta-$(1 \rightarrow 3)$-linked cellotriosyl and cellotetraosyl units. Oat bran, a rich source of the beta-D-glucan, has been incorporated into many food products, particularly cereals, as a source of the soluble fiber that has been touted for cholesterol reduction.

Both soluble and insoluble hemicelluloses play important roles in food products, the former functioning as soluble fiber. They are characterized by their ability to bind water and hence serve as bulking agents. The presence of acidic components in some hemicelluloses impart the capacity to bind cations. Hemicelluloses are digested/fermented to a greater extent than cellulose in the colon.

PECTIC SUBSTANCES

Pectic substances can be extracted with boiling water or with solutions of ammonium oxalate or ethylenedinitrilotetraacetic acid (EDTA) when they are present as salts in cell walls (11). They are normally considered as partially methyl esterified (pectins) or free (pectic acid) alpha-D-(1 $\rightarrow$ 4)-galacturonans. However, the situation is more complex since small amounts of rhamnose, galactose, arabinose and xylose are also present. At one time it was believed this indicated the presence of a mixture of galacturonans, galactans, and arabinans. This, too, appears to be an oversimplification. Rhamnose units are now known to be present in the main chain of alpha-D-(1 $\rightarrow$ 4)-galacturonic acid units to the extent of about 10% (11) while the neutral sugars are present in side chains. In some regions of the rhamnogalacturonan, rhamnose units may be adjacent or in alternate positions. Neutral polysaccharides such as beta-D-(1 $\rightarrow$ 4)-galactans, highly branched arabinans, and arabinogalactans containing 4-linked beta-D-galactan chains may be found in association with the rhamnogalacturonan. The nature of these associations is not clearly known.

The solubility of pectins increases with increasing extent of esterification. Pectins find widespread use in foods such as jams and jellies because of their ability to form stable gels. Completely esterified pectins do not require the addition of acid or electrolyte to form gels. The presence of calcium salts enhances the gelling capacity and decreases the dependence on pH and sugar concentration. Pectic substances are of importance as a component of dietary fiber because of their ion-exchange, due to the presence of the galacturonic acid units, and gelling (viscosity enhancing) properties.

HYDROCOLLOIDS (GUMS, MUCILAGES)

Hydrocolloids are used in food products for their thickening (viscosity increasing), gelling, stabilizing or emulsifying ability. They are derived from seaweed extracts, plant exudates, seeds and microbial sources.

Agar, carrageenan, furcellaran and alginates are obtained from seaweed extracts. The first three are galactose polymers that exhibit thermoreversible gelation and form gels having helix cross-linkages in their gel frameworks (14, 15).

The structures of furcellaran and alginates also contain sulfate esters. Three carrageenan fractions exist: one (kappa) does not gel, one (lambda) forms brittle gels in the presence of potassium ions, and one (iota) yields a more elastic gel in the presence of calcium ions. Alginates are linear copolymers of D-mannuronic acid (M-blocks) and L-guluronic acid (G-blocks) with regions (blocks) containing only one of the acids. Solubility properties are controlled by the ratio of mannuronic acid blocks to guluronic acid blocks. Alginate gels can be formed in the cold in the presence of calcium which induces intermolecular associations in the G-block regions and have sufficient stability to withstand heat processing.

Gums arabic, karaya and tragacanth are complex heteropolysaccharides derived from plant exudates. Guar and locust bean (carob) gums, obtained from seeds, are galactomannans where the mannan is made soluble by single galactose unit side chains. Guar gum (mannose to galactose ratio of 2:1) is more substituted than locust bean gum (4:1 ratio), and is cold water soluble. Locust bean gum requires hot water. An example of a mucilage not commercially available but used to thicken foods during cooking, particularly in the southeastern part of the United States, is that from okra. This is a rhamnogalacturonan in which L-rhamnose is linked to D-galacturonic acid units in the interior chain of the polymer.

Xanthan gum, produced by microbial fermentation, has a cellulose main chain that is made soluble by the presence of short side chains on every second glucose unit. These side chains contain glucose, mannose, and glucuronic acid units in a 3:3:2 ratio. Xanthan has a molecular weight in the millions and forms a synergistic gel with locust bean gum but not with guar gum.

While these are used in small amounts in food products, their complex carbohydrate nature and structure cause them to function as a component of dietary fiber. They are not digestible by the enzymes of the human gastrointestinal system.

MODIFIED STARCHES

Many starches do not have the functional properties needed to impart or maintain desired qualities in food products. As a result, starches have been modified to obtain the functional properties required. The types of modified food starches, also known as "starch derivatives," are listed in Table 2 (16).

The starches most commonly modified for commercial use are those from normal maize, tapioca, potato, and waxy maize. The methods used to produce modified starches include dextrinization, acid-hydrolysis, oxidation, cross-linking, monosubstitution by esterification and etherification, and combinations of these processes. The manufacture of food starches (chemicals used, amount incorporated into the starch, amount of residues permitted) is regulated by the Food and Drug Administration (FDA) and listed in the Code of Federal Regulations (21CFR 172.892). Modified food starches must be approved by the FDA as food

TABLE 2 Types of Modified Starches (16)

Bleached	Oxidized
	Lighter in color, sterile
Converted	Hydrolyzed
	Reduces viscosity
(a) Thin boiling	Fluidity
(b) Dextrins	Dry roasted
(c) Oxidized	Creaminess, short body
Cross-linked	Strengthens granule
	Increases viscosity
	Tolerance to acidity
	Yields to shear resistance
	Heat penetration
Stabilized	Resist retrogradation
	Add specific functional properties
	Low temperature stability

additives before they can be used in food products. It has been many years since a new starch derivative has been developed and approved because of the time and cost involved in obtaining approval.

Food starches are modified to obtain one or more of the following improvements in functional properties (16):

1. Decrease viscosity
2. Increase dispersion stability
3. Increase gel formation and strength
4. Improve gelatinization properties (lower temperature, rapid cooking, less viscosity breakdown)
5. Affect cold-water dispersibility
6. Introduce functional group properties

Modified starches are used to improve viscosity, shelf stability, particulate integrity, processing parameters, textures, appearance and emulsification. While virtually all of the different types of modified starches find use in the food industry, substituted and cross-linked starches are particularly important. These two types of modified starches are produced by reactions in which a small number of hydroxyl groups on the glucose units of amylose and amylopectin, mostly in amorphous regions and on the surface of the granule, are modified without destroying the granular nature of the starch.

Substituted starches are produced by etherification or esterification. This reduces the tendency of chains to realign (retrograde) following gelatinization of starch during heat processing. Substitution lowers the gelatinization temperature, gives freeze-thaw stability, increases viscosity, increases clarity, inhibits gel formation, and reduces syneresis.

Cross-linked starches are produced by introducing a limited number of linkages between the chains of amylose and amylopectin using difunctional reagents. Cross-linking essentially reinforces the hydrogen bonding occurring within the granule. Cross-linking increases gelatinization temperature; yields acid stability, heat stability and shear stability; inhibits gel formation; and controls viscosity during processing.

RESISTANT STARCH

While starch was long thought to be completely digested, it is now recognized that there is a portion (resistant starch) which resists digestion, passes into the lower intestine, and is fermented there. Resistant starch has been defined as ''the sum of starch and products of starch degradation not absorbed in the small intestine of healthy individuals'' (17). Three types of resistant starch have been identified (17,18):

RS1—Physically Trapped Starch

These starch granules are physically trapped within a food matrix so that digestive enzymes are prevented or delayed from having access to them. This can occur in whole or partly ground grains, seeds, cereals, and legumes. The amount of type 1 resistant starch will be affected by food processing and can be decreased or eliminated by milling.

RS2—Resistant Starch Granules

Certain raw (native) starch granules, such as potato and green banana, are known to resist attack by alpha-amylase. This is probably related to the crystalline nature of the starch, i.e., crystalline regions of the starch granule are less susceptible to attack by acid and enzymes than the amorphous regions. The double helical nature of the chains in the cluster regions of amylopectin are known to confer added stability to attack by acid and enzymes. Native starches having a B-type x-ray diffraction pattern (tuber starches) appear to be more resistant to digestion than starches having an A-type pattern (cereal starches) or C-type (pea and bean starches)(19, cited in 17).

Gelatinization normally occurs during cooking and food processing, although the extent is dependent on the moisture content of the food product and may not be complete in water-limited systems, e.g. sugar cookies. Gelatinized starch is much more rapidly digested by enzymes than is raw starch. Gelatinized potato and green banana starch are digested by alpha-amylases.

High amylose maize starches have high gelatinization temperatures, requiring temperatures that are often not reached in conventional cooking practices, i.e., 154–171°C before the granules are completely disrupted. As a result, undigested starch granules were observed in the effluent from ileostomates fed a meal containing high amylose maize (17). Thus, these starches offer an important opportunity to manipulate the amount of resistant starch present in food products.

RS3—Retrograded Starch

The amylose and amylopectin components of starch undergo the process of retrogradation in a time dependent process after starch has been gelatinized/cooked. The rate at which amylose retrogrades is much higher than that for amylopectin which has much shorter chain lengths. Amylose can be retrograded to a form that resists dispersion in water and digestion with alpha-amylase (20–23, cited in 17). This form of resistant starch can be generated during food processing.

There is currently great interest in resistant starch because of its potential use as a food ingredient to increase the dietary fiber content of foods and also because it may be possible to manipulate the amount of resistant starch in food products through processing conditions.

Of special interest is the fermentation of resistant starch in the large intestine to short chain fatty acids. In both in vitro and in vivo studies, it has been shown that starch is a rich source of butyrate via fermentation (17). This has also been shown in humans. A recent human study indicated that diets containing resistant starch increased fecal bulk and concentrations of short chain fatty acids (acetate and butyrate, with butyrate increasing by the larger amount), and lowered fecal pH (24). Butyrate may play a role in reducing colon cancer.

RESISTANT OLIGOSACCHARIDES

The term ''resistant oligosaccharides'' has been proposed for those oligosaccharides that are resistant to hydrolysis by human alimentary enzymes. There is support for expanding the definition of dietary fiber to include this group of carbohydrates (6).

Commonly encountered examples of resistant oligosaccharides include the raffinose series of alpha-galactosides, i.e., the trisaccharide raffinose, the tetrasaccharide stachyose, and the pentasaccharide verbascose. These are commonly found in beans, lentils and peas, where they occur in amounts from 5–8% (dry matter basis), and are associated with the flatulence commonly encountered from the consumption of these foods.

Fructans, such as inulin, and fructooligosaccharides occur in a number of plants, such as Jerusalem artichokes, onions, asparagus, wheat, rye, and triticale. In Jerusalem artichokes and onions, they may represent up to 60–70% of the dry matter. Smaller amounts of fructooligosaccharides are present in cereal grains (25).

Fructooligosaccharides are industrially prepared enzymatically from inulin or sucrose. They have a taste profile similar to sucrose with about 30% of the sweetness. They do not undergo the Maillard browning reaction since they are non-reducing oligosaccharides (26).

Fructans and fructooligosaccharides are not digested by human alimentary enzymes, but they are fermented in the large intestine. Their lower molecular weight compared to many other components of dietary fiber do not make then any less a complex carbohydrate. They are of interest as potential ingredients in foods because of their effects on intestinal flora, their functionality and their reduced caloric value.

CONCLUSION

It is trite, but true, to note that the area of complex carbohydrates is truly complex. The components comprising this class of carbohydrates cannot clearly be defined on the basis of structure, physiological response, or analytical methodology used to measure them. They have traditionally been defined based on the extraction procedures used to isolate them. Whenever solubility is used as a major criterion for a definition, the result is a lack of clear separation and delineation. It is becoming clear that these carbohydrate components can be measured, although the difficulties are clearly those so frequently encountered and discussed for dietary fiber. Analytical chemists have established a good basis of agreement for these procedures, have conducted many collaborative studies and surveys, and are in the process of fine tuning the methods to be used. The definition still is elusive and of little value to the consumer. As long as the United States uses the term "complex carbohydrates" in dietary recommendations but not on food labeling, the consumer be confused.

REFERENCES

1. Dietary Goals for the United States, Second Edition, U.S. Senate Select Committee on Nutrition and Human Needs, U.S. Government Printing Office, Washington, D.C., 1977.
2. Healthy People, The Surgeon General's Report on Health Promotion and Disease Prevention, U.S. Department of Health, Education and Welfare, U.S. Government Printing Office, Washington, D.C., 1979.
3. S. C. Lee and L. Prosky, Dietary Fiber Analysis for Nutrition Labeling. Cereal Foods World 38:135 (1993).
4. Department of Health and Human Services, Food Labeling, Federal Register 55: 29476 (1990).

5. Food and Drug Administration, General provisions on food labeling, nutrition labeling, label format, nutrient content claims, ingredient labeling, state and local requirements and exemptions. Final rules. Federal Register 58:631, 2302 (1993).
6. S. C. Lee and L. Prosky, Perspectives on complex carbohydrate definition. Cereal Foods World 41:88 (1996).
7. J. C. Brand, Digestion and absorption of cereal products–fast or slow? In The Role of Cereals in the Human Diet, L. O'Brein and K. O'Dea (eds), p. 29, Cereal Chemistry Division, Royal Australian Chemical Institute, Parkville, Victoria, 1988.
8. S. Hizukuri, Polymodal distribution of the chain lengths of amylopectins and its significance. Carbohydrate Res. 147:342 (1986).
9. D. R. Lineback and V. F. Rasper, Wheat Carbohydrates. In Wheat: Chemistry and Technology, Y. Pomeranz (ed), Vol. 1, p. 277, American Association of Cereal Chemists, St. Paul, MN, 1988.
10. O. Theander and P. Aman, The chemistry, morphology and analysis of dietary fiber components. In Dietary Fibers: Chemistry and Nutrition, G. E. Inglett and S. I. Falkehag (eds), p. 215, Academic Press, New York, NY, 1979.
11. G. O. Aspinall, Analysis of polysaccharides. In Food Carbohydrates, D. R. Lineback and G. E. Inglett (eds), p. 356, AVI Publishing Co., Westport, CT, 1982.
12. C. J. A. Vinkx, H. R. Reynaert, P. J. Grobet, and J. A. Delcour, Physicochemical and functional properties of rye nonstarch polysaccharides. V. Variability in the structure of water-soluble arabinoxylans. Cereal Chem. 70:311 (1993).
13. J. W. Anderson and S. R. Bridges, Hypocholesterolemic effects of oat bran in humans. In Oat Bran, P. J. Wood (ed), p. 139, American Association of Cereal Chemists, St. Paul, MN, 1993.
14. Y. Pomeranz, Functional Properties of Food Components, p. 91, Academic Press, New York, NY, 1985.
15. P. Chinachoti, Carbohydrates: functionality in foods. Amer. J. Clin. Nutr. 61 (suppl): 922S (1995).
16. P. S. Smith, Starch derivatives and their use in foods. In Food Carbohydrates, D. R. Lineback and G. E. Inglett (eds), p. 237, AVI Publishing Co., Westport, CT, 1982.
17. J. G. Muir, G. P. Young, K. O'Dea, D. Cameron-Smith, I. L. Brown and G. R. Collier, Resistant starch—the neglected 'dietary fiber'? Implications for health. Dietary Fiber Bibliography and Reviews, 1:33 (1993).
18. H. N. Englyst, S. M. Kingman and J. H. Cummings, Resistant starch: Measurement in foods and physiological role in man. In Plant Polymeric Carbohydrates, F. Meuser, D. J. Manners, and W. Seibel (eds), p. 137, The Royal Society of Chemistry, Cambridge, U.K., 1993.
19. D. J. Gallant, B. Bouchet, A. Buleon, and S. Perez, Physical characteristics of starch granules and susceptibility to enzymatic degradation. European J. Clin. Nutr. 46 (suppl):S3 (1992).
20. M. J. Miles, V. J. Morris, and S. G. Ring, The roles of amylose and amylopectin in the gelation and retrogradation of starch. Carbohydrate Res. 135:257 (1985).
21. M. J. Miles, V. J. Morris, P. D. Orford, and S. G. Ring, The roles of amylose and amylopectin in the gelation and retrogradation of starch. Carbohydrate Res. 135:271 (1985).
22. S. G. Ring, P. Colonna, K. J. I'Anson, M. T. Kalichevsky, M. J. Miles, V. J. Morris,

and P. D. Orford, The gelation and crystallization of amylopectin. Carbohydrate Res. 152:277 (1987).
23. S. G. Ring, J. M. Gee, M. Whittam, P. Orford, and I. T. Johnson, Resistant starch: Its chemical form in foodstuffs and effect on digestibility in vitro. Food Chemistry 28:97 (1988).
24. J. Phillips, J. G. Muir, A. Birkett, Z. X. Lu, G. P. Jones, K. O'Dea, and G. P. Young, Effect of resistant starch on fecal bulk and fermentation-dependent events in humans. Amer. J. Clin. Nutr. 62:121 (1995).
25. N.-G. L. Asp, Classification and methodology of food carbohydrates as related to nutritional effects. Amer. J. Clin. Nutr. 61 (suppl):930S (1995).
26. R. J. Bornet, Undigestible sugars in food products. Amer. J. Clin. Nutr. 59 (suppl): 763S (1994).

11

Complex Carbohydrates: Definition and Analysis

Susan Sungsoo Cho
The Kellogg Company, Battle Creek, Michigan

Leon Prosky
Prosky Associates, Rockville, Maryland

DEFINITION

Introduction

Dietary recommendations in many Western societies promote the consumption of a diet rich in complex carbohydrates and fiber (1–5). Such dietary guidelines, issued by the U.S. Department of Agriculture (USDA), U.S. Department of Health and Human Services, and by a variety of public and private agencies, often serve as a basis of policy in public health nutrition, including nutrition labeling and allowable health claims. An increasing number of studies show high-fiber, low-fat diets to be protective against disease, including atherosclerosis, colon cancer, and gastrointestinal disease (6–8). Health claims for products high in fiber and complex carbohydrates need to be well supported by scientific evidence. Therefore, accuracy in the definition of complex carbohydrates and fiber for food labeling purposes is an issue of prime importance both to the food industry and the consumer (9).

There was little consensus on what complex carbohydrates are, how they should be defined, and what information about their content in foods is most appropriate for a nutrition label. It would be most helpful for regulatory agencies if researchers in nutrition and food science, industry representatives, and health professionals were all to agree on a common definition of complex carbohydrates with consumers being aware of their finding. The term complex carbohydrates acquired importance because of the 1977 dietary advice form the U.S. Senate Select Committee on Nutrition and Human Needs. However, there has been no general consensus whether the definition of complex carbohydrates should be limited to digestible polysaccharides, primarily starch, or should also include dietary fiber. Given a professional consensus on what complex carbohydrates are, standardized analytical methods could be developed to test this definition. The present survey aimed at establishing a professional consensus regarding the definition of complex carbohydrates for food labeling purposes.

In the United States, following the passage of the 1990 Nutrition Labeling and Education Act (NLEA), the U.S. Food and Drug Administration (FDA) issued in 1991 its proposed labeling regulations for the purpose of soliciting public comment. In response to this solicitation, AOAC International in 1992 assembled a Task Force on Nutrient Labeling Analysis to review the available methods for carbohydrate analysis. The Subcommittee on Carbohydrate Methodology, composed of representatives from the FDA, USDA, academia and the food industry, was specifically charged with recommending appropriate analytical methodology to be used in carbohydrate analysis of foods for labeling purposes. The Subcommittee was also charged with identifying both immediate and future needs in the area of carbohydrate analysis.

The Subcommittee's work revealed two basic questions. First, there was no clear definition of complex carbohydrates. Second, there was a lack of validated analytical methods for those definitions of complex carbohydrates that were put forth. The Subcommittee concluded that more work was needed to develop analytical methods for complex carbohydrates. The FDA also concluded that there was not sufficient professional consensus on the meaning of the term complex carbohydrate to justify developing a definition, and requiring mandatory nutrition labeling. The final food labeling regulations issued in January 1993 by the FDA and the USDA did not include the term complex carbohydrate (10,11). One question posed was whether complex carbohydrates could be well defined from the standpoint of structure, function, and contribution to health. The other concerned the methodology for the analysis of complex carbohydrates.

To further address these issues, AOAC International established a refereeship in the area of complex carbohydrates in 1993. The first step taken by the two referees, S. S. Cho (formerly S. C. Lee) and L. Prosky, was to initiate an international survey on complex carbohydrates, which was conducted under the auspices of AOAC International. The purpose of the survey was to determine if an international consensus could be reached on the definition of complex carbohydrates and the most appropriate methods for their analysis.

International Survey on Complex Carbohydrates Definition

Approximately 200 survey questionnaires were distributed to prominent professionals in carbohydrate science. The survey yielded 114 respondents, representing scientists from 29 different countries. Table 1 shows the geographic distribution of the survey participants. Fifty-one percent of respondents were from Europe; another 26% were from North America; 19% were from the Pacific Rim, including Australia, Japan and Korea; and the remaining 3% were from Latin America. The research interests of the respondents were reported as nutrition (43%), analytical chemistry (29%), medical research (13%), food technology (10%), and other (6%). The respondents affiliations were reported as university (30%), research institutes (30%), industry (16%), and government/state agencies (13%).

Respondents were first asked to select from a provided list of carbohydrate components those which, in their view, should be included in the definition of complex carbohydrates for food labeling purposes. The question was presented in a multiple choice format, with the possibility of writing in additional options. The various options are listed in Table 2. The 107 respondents were also asked to explain and justify their choices.

Most respondents felt that available starches (72%) should be included in the definition of complex carbohydrates. The majority of respondents also listed the terms non-starch polysaccharides (69%), total starches (58%), and unavailable or resistant starches (58%) to be included in the complex carbohydrate fraction. Approximately one-third of respondents included both available (33%) and un-

TABLE 1 Distribution of Survey Participants

Region and country	No. of persons	No. of countries
Europe	58	18
North America	31	2
Asia	21	5
Latin America	4	4

TABLE 2 Answers to Question 1: For nutrition labeling purposes, which should be included in the complex carbohydrate definition? Check all that apply.

Definition choices	No. N = 107	Percent
Available starches	77	72%
Non-starch polysaccharides (NSP)	74	69%
Total starches	62	58%
Unavailable starches (Resistant starches)	62	58%
Oligosaccharide, available	35	33%
Oligosaccharide, unavailable (Resistant oligosaccharides)	34	32%
Lignin	31	29%

available oligosaccharides (32%) and lignin (29%) in their definition of complex carbohydrates. Further data analyses showed that 62% of respondents indicated that both total starches and unavailable polysaccharides were complex carbohydrates.

The second survey question (Table 3) asked respondents to define complex carbohydrates using their own descriptions. This open-ended question was intended to elicit an unprompted definition of complex carbohydrates directly from the respondent. Of the 72 persons who replied, 63 provided a definition of complex carbohydrates, while 9 stated that they did not like the term and failed to provide a definition. Out of the 63 respondents, 52 (82%) included dietary fiber polysaccharides in addition to available starches in their own definition of complex carbohydrates. Table 3 shows the most common descriptions of complex carbohydrates as provided by the 52 respondents. While 19 (26%) respondents described complex carbohydrates simply as polysaccharides, 10 (14%) based their answers on the physiology of digestion, defining complex carbohydrates as glucose polymers that are slowly digested or not digested in the small intestine. Another 10 respondents (14%) included all carbohydrates except simple sugars in their definition, while 7 (9%) described complex carbohydrates as starch plus dietary fiber. Eight responses referred to complex carbohydrates as starches or available starches, and the remainder used such terms as unavailable starches or oligosaccharides, cell wall carbohydrates or lignin.

Results of the AOAC Survey indicate that a consensus exists among professionals that dietary fiber polysaccharides should be included in the definition of complex carbohydrate. However, the inclusion of unavailable carbohydrates and lignin in the definition of complex carbohydrates for labeling purposes does pose certain dilemmas.

TABLE 3 Answers to Question 2: Using your own description, please define complex carbohydrates.

Definition provided	No. of respondents providing the definition	Percent
Polysaccharides	19	26%
Glucose polymers which are slowly digested or not digested in the small intestine	10	14%
Carbohydrates minus simple sugars	10	13%
Don't like the term	9	9%
Starch and dietary fiber	7	5%
Available starches	4	5%
Starch + dietary fiber + oligosaccharides	4	5%
Glucans with a complex structure	2	3%
Dietary fiber + unavailable oligosaccharides	1	1%
NSP + lignin	1	1%
Starch and cell wall carbohydrates	1	1%
Unavailable carbohydrates	1	1%
Glucans not soluble in 80% ETOH	1	1%
Carbohydrates of plant origin (>DP4)	1	1%

International Survey Results on Dietary Fiber Definition

If the definition of complex carbohydrates is to include dietary fiber, results of two prior international surveys on fiber should be of major interest (11). One hundred forty-four experts participated in the first survey and 122 responded to the second, representing professionals from 30 countries. The results of the first survey were reported in Lee and Prosky (9, 12, 13). In these surveys (Table 4), respondents generally supported the definition of dietary fiber as those polysaccharides and lignin that are not hydrolyzed by the human alimentary enzymes. According to this definition, dietary fiber would include non-soluble polysaccharides, resistant saccharides and lignin. In general, fiber survey respondents also supported the idea that the definition of dietary fiber be expanded to include ROs, unavailable polysaccharides, resistant starch and lignin.

Resistant oligosaccharides were defined as oligosaccharides that are not hydrolyzed by the human alimentary enzymes or as oligosaccharides that escape digestion in the human upper GI tract, including the mouth, stomach and small intestine. In the second survey, some 66% of survey respondents supported the

TABLE 4 Answers to Question: How would you define dietary fiber? (Check only one.)[a]

No.	Percent	Option
34	22.2	a. Remnants of plant components resistant to human alimentary enzymes. These include undigestible polysaccharides, lignin, undigestible proteins and lipids, etc.
66	43.1	b. The sum of lignin and polysaccharides that are not hydrolyzed by human alimentary enzymes, i.e., the sum of non-starch polysaccharides, resistant starch, and lignin.
10	6.5	c. Polysaccharides that are not hydrolyzed by human alimentary enzymes, i.e., the sum of non-starch polysaccharides.
11	7.2	d. The sum of non-starch polysaccharides plus lignin.
5	3.3	e. Plant cell-wall components.
9	5.9	f. Non-starch polysaccharides only.
16	10.5	g. Other answers.
2	1.3	No answer.

[a]Up to 2 answers were accepted

inclusion of ROs in the definition of dietary fiber. Respondents cited the following reasons to include ROs in the definition: (1) ROs are difficult to distinguish from the non-hydrolyzable polysaccharides, whether they are part of the total dietary fiber or the soluble dietary fiber fraction, and (2) they have a physiological effect in the large intestine similar to those of other dietary fibers. Those respondents (34%) who felt that ROs should not be included in the dietary fiber gave the following reasons: (1) there are no validated methods for analyzing ROs (e.g., ROs precipitate incompletely in 80% ETOH), (2) ROs are not true polysaccharides, (3) ROs are not part of the plant cell-wall material, (4) there is a lack of knowledge about the physiological effects of high amounts of ROs, and (5) the inclusion of ROs would complicate the definition.

A large percentage of respondents (86%) indicated that lignin should also be included in the expanded definition of complex carbohydrates. Although lignin is a polyphenol, and not a carbohydrate, it is historically included for several reasons: lignin (1) is resistant to human digestion, (2) has a physiological effect similar to dietary fiber on intestinal transit and fermentation, (3) is closely related in function to dietary fiber, and (4) is of cell-wall origin. Those respondents (14%) who opposed including lignin in the definition of dietary fiber gave the following reasons: lignin (1) is not a carbohydrate, (2) does not ferment in the intestine, (3) has no proven health benefits, and (4) there is no suitable analytical methodology for the determination of lignin content.

The 1995 AOAC International Workshop Results

To conclude the results of the three international surveys, an AOAC International Workshop was also held in Nashville, Tennessee, on September 15–16, 1995, with 57 participants from the United States, Canada, and Europe. The foremost authorities in the world from industry, academia, and government participated. The Workshop is a follow-up to the international surveys as well as the activities of the Carbohydrates Subcommittee of the Nutrients Labeling Analysis Task Force of 1992–1993 and the International Life Science Institute (ILSI)-North American Workshop held in November 1994 in Washington, D.C. (14).

The workshop results indicated that there is a general agreement among industry that complex carbohydrates equal available starch and dietary fiber (15). There was a general agreement among the workshop participants that dietary fiber should be included in the definition of complex carbohydrates and that ROs are part of dietary fiber. Twenty-nine persons, representing 85% of the 34 people providing a definition for complex carbohydrates, agreed that the definition is the sum of dietary fiber and starch (technically speaking, available or enzyme available starch). For the nutrition label, complex carbohydrates could be derived as the sum of analytically measured starch and dietary fiber values or by the calculation as total carbohydrates—(sugar + available oligosaccharides). Among the 29 scientists supporting the definition of complex carbohydrates as the sum of starch and dietary fiber, 16 persons (corresponding to 55%) supported the labeling of analytically derived values (total dietary fiber and available starch) and 13 persons (45%) were of the opinion that the values calculated by the difference method would be acceptable. It was recommended that the associate referee continue study based on this definition of complex carbohydrates as the sum of available starch and dietary fiber. It is in agreement with the definition of complex carbohydrates used in recent U.S. Dietary Guidelines of 1995 (2). An interesting point to note is only two persons supported the FDA's 1991 definition of complex carbohydrates as total carbohydrates—dietary fiber—simple sugars. Other definitions considered were the sum of starch and non-starch saccharides (3 persons) and the sum of starch and non-starch polysaccharides (which correspond to polysaccharides; 0 person). Strong interest was shown in analytical methods for ROs. It was recommended to establish new associate refereeships in this area (15).

ANALYSIS

An analytical method was developed to measure complex carbohydrates (CC) in foods as the sum of available starch and total dietary fiber. Desugared food samples were subjected to sequential starch and protein digestion by using heat stable alpha-amylase, protease, and amyloglucosidase, and filtered. Filtrate containing enzymatic digestate of starch was analyzed for glucose and maltose by using a high pressure liquid chromatography (HPLC) technique. Residues were subjected to further analysis of dietary fiber by using a gravimetric method. The available starch values obtained by the HPLC method were precise and in agreement with those derived by the calculation method (%Available Starch = %Total Carbohydrate − %Total Dietary Fiber − %Sugars − %H_2O − %Protein − %Fat − %Ash). The complex carbohydrates values generated as the sum of analytically measured available starch and total dietary fiber were precise and agreed with those calculated by the difference method (%CC = %Total Carbohydrates − %Sugars − %H_2O − %Protein − %Fat − %Ash).

Sample

Samples included the following products: (1) corn cereal; (2) rice cereal; (3) wheat cereal; (4) wheat bran cereal; (5) fat-free cracker; (6) high-fiber cereal; (7) green bean; and (8) wheat bran. The samples were purchased at a local supermarket, with the exception of the green bean, which was freeze dried. The samples were ground in a Wiley mill with a 0.5 mm screen. If the fat content of any food exceeded 10%, the food was defatted with petroleum ether before milling.

To test the sugar extraction efficiency, the following known standards were included: (1) standard mix, consisting of 40% sucrose, 30% corn starch, and 30% cellulose; (2) wheat starch standard; and (3) cellulose standard.

Method

Complex carbohydrates are determined as the sum of available starch and dietary fiber. Duplicate samples of dried foods, fat-extracted if containing >10% fat, undergo sequential enzymatic treatments by heat-stable α-amylase, protease, and amyloglucosidase to digest starch and protein. Enzymatic digestion steps have been adopted from AOAC official final action methods 991.43 (17, 18) and 985.29 (18, 19). For available starch, the enzyme digestate, containing mostly monosaccharides and some disaccharides, is analyzed by HPLC. Measured glucose and maltose are converted into a starch unit and reported as available starch. HPLC conditions have been adopted from AOAC official final action method 982.14 (18) for sugar determination. For total dietary fiber (TDF), the enzyme digestate is treated with alcohol to precipitate soluble dietary fiber before filtering, and TDF residue is washed with alcohol and acetone, dried, and weighed. TDF residue values are corrected for protein, ash, and blank. TDF determination is the same for method 991.43.

Analytical Column:	Zorbax NH_2, 4.6 mm I.D. x 25 cm
Guard Column:	Supelco, 10 cm, aminopropylsilyl
Mobile Phase:	70% acetonitrile, 30% water (v/v)

Flow Rate:	1.0 mL/min.
Injection Temperature:	room temp.
Elution Mode:	Isocratic
Detector:	Refractive index
Detector Sensitivity:	0.020 x 10^{-3}
Response Time:	2.0 min.
Run Time:	25 min.
Injection Volume:	15 µL

Note: Parameters may vary in order to optimize the chromatography.

Sugar extraction efficiency was calculated by comparing the sugar content of ethanolic extract prepared by the method described in this paper and the sugar content of the original sample analyzed by AOAC sugar method 982.14.

$$\% \text{ Sugar extraction efficiency} = \frac{\text{sugar extracted, } \%}{\text{sugars in samples, } \%} \times 100$$

Analytical Results

The HPLC method described in this paper is a quantitative method for available starch in foods. A variety of samples, such as grains, ready-to-eat breakfast cereals, breads, crackers, fruits, vegetables, and mixed diets can be analyzed by using this method. Complex carbohydrates are determined as the sum of available starch and dietary fiber; available starch by high performance liquid chromatography determination of glucose and maltose present in the enzymatic hydrolysates of desugared sample; and dietary fiber by enzymatic gravimetric method, official final action method 991.43.

It is important to remove simple sugars prior to enzymatic hydrolysis of starches, so that simple sugars do not carry over in the sugar analysis for available starch determination. For the efficient desugaring, we used 49% ethanol in water initially for easier dissolution of sugars. Additional 95% ethanol was added to make the final concentration of 78% ethanol to precipitate dietary fiber extraction. This procedure would ensure that simple sugars are efficiently removed without eliminating water soluble dietary fiber components. Table 5 indicates that the extraction efficiency is generally excellent, ranging from 90% to 99%. One cereal sample which showed 90% desugaring efficiency had a low sugar content (6.2%) in the original sample to begin with. Ethanolic extract of that sample contained 5.6% sugars. We consider both 6.2% and 5.6% to be in the normal analytical variability range for sugar determinations. Thus, overall efficiency of the desugaring step is considered excellent.

The elution orders of standard sugars in this HPLC method, using an amino-bonded silica column packing and acetonitrile-water mobile phase, follow the expected saccharide polarity: fructose, glucose, sucrose, and maltose. The enzy-

TABLE 5 Sugar Extraction Efficiency

Source	Sugar extracted, %	Sugars in sample, %	% Extraction efficiency
Standard Mix	39.8	40.0	99.0
Green Bean	15.6	16.2	96.3
Wheat Bran Cereal	15.9	17.0	92.9
Prune	53.5	56.2	95.2
Bread	5.6	6.2	90.3
Cellulose	0	0	0
Wheat Starch	0	0	0
Cracker	<1.0	<1.0	0

matic digestate of the desugared sample showed mostly glucose peaks and negligible peaks from maltose and sucrose. The sample chromatograms demonstrated that the starch digestion steps using three enzymes, heat stable alpha-amylase, protease, and amyloglucosidase, were near completion, producing mostly glucose. The glucose values in the enzyme hydrolysate were multiplied by the factor 0.9 to convert into starch values.

The Final Food Labeling Regulations in the United States (6) have recognized that HPLC methods are the most appropriate for nutrition labeling purposes among all the sugar determination techniques. The HPLC approach offers the most accurate and specific determinations of mono- and di-saccharides. Thus, the HPLC technique can give the most accurate figures for available starch, which is derived from glucose and maltose values of the starch hydrolysates. However, the method requires a high capital investment and trained personnel for troubleshooting. The presence of salt, especially in the hydrolysate of processed foods, interferes with the analysis because chloride ions elute quickly after glucose. It is important to wash the column for 2 hours at 1.5 mL/min with a solution of 0.1% tetraethylenepentamine (TEPA) (pH approximately 7 with acetic acid) in 78% acetonitrile in water and finally with normal mobile phase (20).

Table 6 shows the percent recovery of several standards. Percent recoveries of available starch and DF for these known standards are excellent. The starch digestion in our method was done by heat stable alpha-amylase and amyloglucosidase, which are more specific to glucose-glucose bonds. Thus, most of the sucrose in the sample (99%) was recovered as sucrose in the enzyme hydrolysate.

In Table 7 are the reported available starch data generated by HPLC and

Table 6 Percent Recovery of Standards

Source	TDF	Available starch
Cellulose	105.8	0.5
Wheat Starch	0.4	99.0
Corn Starch	0.5	100.8
Standard Mix	108.9	99.9

the difference methods. The samples tested were corn cereal, rice cereal, wheat and wheat bran cereals, crackers and bread, wheat bran and green beans.

Complex carbohydrate values derived analytically as the sum of DF and available starch were precise (Table 7). The current TDF methods do not fully recover RO. For the samples containing added RO sources such as inulin and polydextrose, the supplemental method should be used (21, 22). On the other hand, the difference method cannot be used for the samples containing significant amounts of available oligosaccharides, such as malto-triose and malto-tetrose, present in candies. The difference method would significantly overestimate complex carbohydrate content in these types of products.

Based on the results, we suggest that this HPLC method for analysis of available starches be collaboratively validated by different laboratories.

Table 7 Determination of Available Starch in Foods (by HPLC) and Complex Carbohydrates*1*2

Sample	% Available starch	% Complex CHO
Corn Cereal	76.2 ± 2.59	78.8 ± 2.59
Rice Cereal	72.5 ± 0.27	73.5 ± 0.27
Wheat Cereal	22.6 ± 0.86	53.5 ± 0.86
Wheat Bran Cereal	49.3 ± 0.50	67.0 ± 1.10
Cracker	71.4 ± 0.59	74.6 ± 0.37
Bread	57.7 ± 1.01	64.9 ± 0.89
Green Bean	16.6 ± 0.30	46.7 ± 0.30
Wheat Bran	19.6 ± 1.03	62.8 ± 0.14

*1 N = 4

*2 Available starch (calculation) = 100 − %H_2O − %protein − %ash − %fat − %sugar − %TDF.

Relative values comparing analytical and calculated values = (analytical values/calculated values) × 100.

REFERENCES

1. USDA's Food Guide Pyramid. Human Nutrition Information Service (1992) Home and Garden Bulletin No 249, USDA and USDHHS, Washington, D.C.
2. Nutrition and Your Health: Dietary Guidelines For Americans (1995) Home and Garden Bulletin No 232, 3rd Ed., USDA and USDHHS, Washington, D.C.
3. National Research Council (1989) Diet and Health: Implications for Reducing Chronic Disease Risk. Report of the Committee on Diet and Health, Food and Nutrition Board, National Academy Press, Washington, D.C.
4. U.S. Dept of Health and Human Services (1991) Healthy People 2000. National Health Promotion and Disease Prevention Objectives, PHS Publ 91-50212, Washington, D.C.
5. U.S. Department of Health and Human Services (1988) Surgeon General's Report on Nutrition and Health. USDHHS Publ. No. 88-50210, Washington, D.C.
6. Anderson, J. W., et al. (1984) Hypocholesterolemic Effects of Oat-bran or Bean Intake for Hypercholesterolemic Men. American Journal of Clinical Nutrition 40: 1146–1155
7. Klurfeld, D. M. (1987) The role of dietary fiber in gastrointestinal disease. Journal of the American Dietetic Association. 87:1172–1177
8. Greenwald, P., Lanza, E., and Eddy, G. A. (1987) Dietary Fiber in the Reduction of Colon Cancer Risk. Journal of the American Dietetic Association. 87:1178–1188
9. Lee, S. and Prosky, L. (1995) International Survey on Dietary Fiber: Definition, Analysis, and Reference Materials. Journal of AOAC International 78:22–36
10. Food and Drug Administration (1993) Food Labeling, General Provisions: Nutrition Labeling: Label Format: Nutrient Content Claims: Ingredient Labeling: State and Local requirements; and Exemptions: Final Rules. Fed. Register 58:2302–2941, 1993
11. Department of Agriculture (1993) Food Labeling; General Provisions: Nutrition Labeling: Label Format: Nutrient Content Claims: Ingredient Labeling: State and Local requirements; and Exemptions: Final Rules. Fed. Register 58:631–691.
12. Lee, S. C., and Prosky, L. Summary of AOAC International Survey on Complex Carbohydrates. International Life Sciences Institute. North American Workshop on Complex Carbohydrates, Washington, D.C. November 2, 1994
13. Lee, S. C. and Prosky, L. (1994) Perspectives on New Dietary Fiber Definition. Cereal Foods World. 39:767–768
14. Anonymous. (1995) Special Report: Complex Carbohydrates: The Science and the Label. Nutr. Rev. 53:186
15. Anonymous. (1995) International Workshop on Complex Carbohydrates Definition. The Referee 19(10), 15
16. Lee, S. C., Vincent, R., Prosky, L., Sullivan, D. M. (1996) Evaluating an analytical method for complex carbohydrate determinations. Cereal Foods World. 41:64–70.
17. Lee, S. C., Prosky, L., DeVries, J. W. (1992) Determination of Total, Soluble, and Insoluble Dietary Fiber in Foods-Enzymatic- Gravimetric Method, MES-TRIS Buffer: Collaborative Study. J. AOAC Int. 75:395–416
18. Association of Official Analytical Chemists International, Official Methods of Analysis, 16th Ed. The Association, Arlington, VA, 1995.

19. Prosky, L., Asp, N.-G., Schweizer, T. F., DeVries, J. W., Furda, I. (1988) Determination of Insoluble, Soluble and Total Dietary Fiber in Foods and Food Products: Interlaboratory Study. J. Assoc. Off. Anal. Chem. 71:1017–1023.
20. DeVries, J. W., Chang, H. L., Heroff, J. C., and Johnson, K. D. (1983) High Pressure Liquid Chromatography Determination of Carbohydrates in Food Products: Evaluation of Methods. J. Assoc. Off. Anal. Chem. 66:197–198.
21. Craig, S. A. S., Holden, J. F., Troup, J. P., Auerbach, M. H., and Frier, H. (1995) Polydextrose as Soluble Fiber and Complex Carbohydrates. AOAC International Workshop on Definition and Analysis of Complex Carbohydrates, Dietry Fiber, Nashville, TN, September 15–16, 1995.
22. Quemener, B., Thibault, J. F., and Coussement, P. (1994) Determination of Inulin and Oligofructose in Food Products, and Integration in the AOAC Method for Measurements of Total Dietary Fiber. Lebensm. Wiss. U. Technol. 27:125–132.

12

Determination of Complex Carbohydrate Fractions in Foods

Betty W. Li
Beltsville Human Nutrition Research Center, Agricultural Research Service, U.S. Department of Agriculture, Beltsville, Maryland

INTRODUCTION

A general scheme has been developed to determine sugars, starches, total dietary fiber, and dietary fiber polysaccharides in a half-gram freeze-dried food sample. Triplicate samples are weighed into teflon tubes; free sugars (mono- and disaccharides) are extracted into 80% methanol and analyzed on a gas-liquid chromatograph (GLC). The residues after 80% methanol extraction are incubated with amyloglucosidase and hydrolysates are removed for glucose determination by GLC. Starch content is calculated as glucose (g/100 g) $\times$ 0.9. The remaining hydrolysates are diluted with 95% ethanol, filtered through glass crucibles matted with Celite filter aid. The residues are dried and weighed. One of the triplicate residues is analyzed for crude protein, and the second one for ash. The third residue is hydrolyzed in H_2SO_4; analyzed for neutral sugars on GLC and uronic acids spectrophotometrically. Total dietary fiber content is calculated as the residue weight corrected for residual protein and ash, and dietary fiber polysaccharides are the sum of neutral sugars and uronic acids. According to this scheme, complex carbohydrates are found in the fractions represented by starch, total dietary fiber, and dietary fiber polysaccharides. Data will be presented on the contents of these complex carbohydrate fractions of some frequently consumed foods.

In the National Research Council's ''Recommended Dietary Allowances'' (1), dietary carbohydrates are defined as sugars and complex carbohydrates. Sugars include monosaccharides, such as glucose and fructose, and disaccharides, such as sucrose, maltose, and lactose. Complex carbohydrates (polysaccharides) comprise starches and dietary fibers. While starches are polymers of glucose that are known to be digestible by human gastrointestinal enzymes, dietary fibers are mainly indigestible complex carbohydrates in plant cell walls and a variety of gums, mucilages, and algal polysaccharides. Adopting the above definitions, we have developed and tested a method for determining sugars, starches, total dietary fiber, and dietary fiber polysaccharides in half-gram replicates of freeze-dried food samples.

METHOD

Triplicate samples (0.5 g) of freeze-dried foods are weighed into teflon tubes and extracted with 15 mL of n-hexane if the samples contain >5% fat; residues are ex-tracted with 10–15 mL of 80% methanol (Figure 1). The alcohol extract is used for the separation and quantitation of individual sugars using GLC (Figure 2). Residues after the alcohol extraction are suspended in 25 mL deionized water and autoclaved at 121°C for 1 h, cooled and mixed with a solution of amyloglucosidase (No. 208-469, Boehringer-Mannheim Corp.) in acetate buffer; the mixture is incubated at 55°C for 2 h. Aliquots (0.1 mL) of the hydrolysate are removed, dried, and derivatized for GLC analysis for glucose. Starch content is calculated as glucose × 0.9 (Figure 3). To the remaining hydrolysate and suspensions is added 4 × volume of 95% ethanol. After 1 h, the mixtures are filtered through glass crucibles matted with Celite (CAFA); residues are dried at 105°C and weighed. One of the triplicate residues is analyzed for crude protein as nitrogen × 6.25, the second is heated in a muffle furnace at 525°C for 5 h for ash determination (Figure 4). The third is hydrolyzed in H_2SO_4; aliquot of the acid hydrolysate is derivatized to alditol acetates and analyzed for neutral sugars by GLC, and for uronic acid colorimetrically (Figure 5) (2). Total dietary fiber (TDF) is the weight of residue after enzyme hydrolysis corrected for the weights of crude protein and ash. Dietary fiber polysaccharides (DFP) is the sum of neutral sugars and uronic acid in the residue.

RESULTS AND DISCUSSION

According to the method described above, complex carbohydrate fractions (starches and dietary fiber) are determined after the removal of alcohol soluble

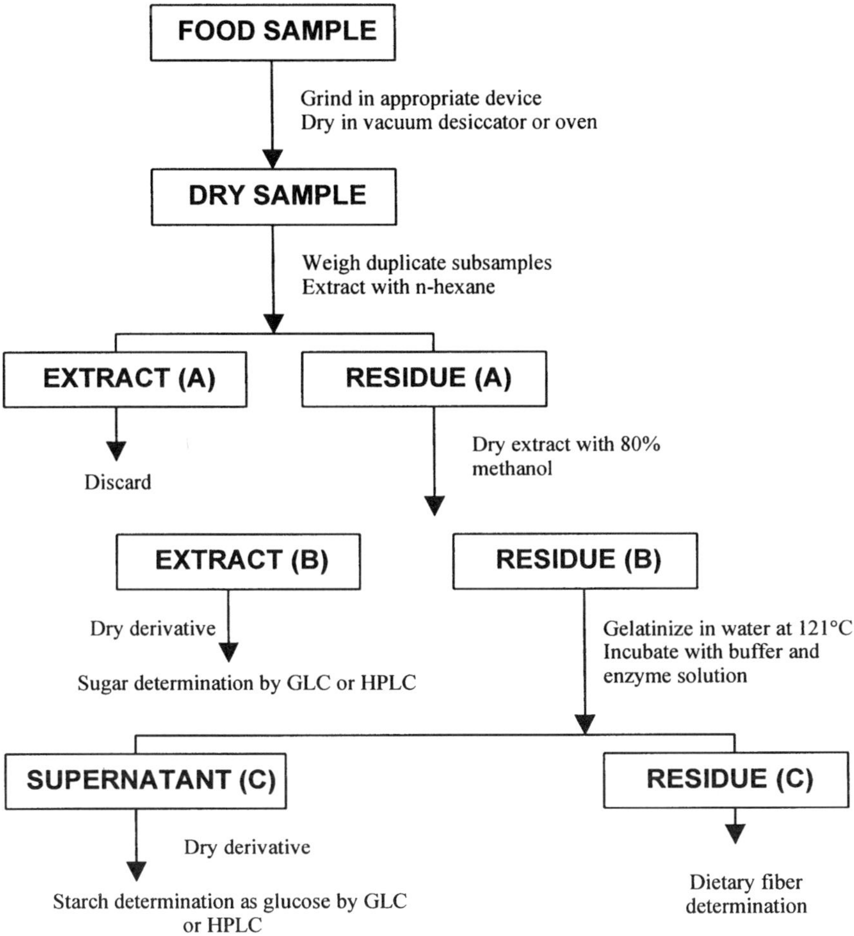

FIGURE 1 Sample Preparation and Extraction for Sugars, Starches, and Dietary Fiber Determination

sugars (mainly mono- and disaccharides). The procedures for the enzymatic hydrolysis of starches are essentially those we have reported earlier as a single enzyme method for total dietary fiber (3). It differs from AOAC method 985.29 and method 991.43 as follows: a) an autoclave is used to gelatinize starches in the sample, b) only one enzyme—amyloglucosidase—is used, and c) the protease treatment of samples has been eliminated. Since the amount of protein remaining in the gravimetrically isolated residue is usually much higher than that in a similar

80% METHANOL EXTRACT
(Containing Sugars)
↓
Take 0.5 or 1 mL to complete dryness
Add 0.5 mL of pyridine reagent containing internal standard and hydroxylamine HCl
↓
Keep at 75°C for 30 minutes
↓
Cool to room temperature
Add 0.5 mL hexamethyldisilazane and 4 drops of triflouroacetic acid
↓
Centrifuge
↓
TMS OXIMERS
and
TMS ETHERS

FIGURE 2 Sugar Derivation Procedure for GLC

RESIDUE FROM 80% METHANOL EXTRACTION
↓
25 mL deionized H_2O
Autoclave at 121°C for 1 hour
Cool to 60°C
↓
3 mg amyloglucosidase, 1 mL H_2O, 1mL acetate buffer (pH 4.8)
↓
Incubate at 55°C for 2 hours
Centrifuge
↓

HYDROSYLATE (supernatant + residue)	SUPERNATANT (0.1 mL)
↓	↓
4 Volumes of 95% ethanol	Dry derivative
↓	↓
TDF OR DFP DETERMINATION	**GLUCOSE TMS-OXIME (starch = glucose × 0.9)**

FIGURE 3 Determination of Starches

HYDROLYSATE
IN DILUTE ALCOHOL
↓
Leave at room temperature for 1 hour
↓
Filter through crucible
Rinse with ethanol and acetone
↓
Dry in oven at 105°C overnight
Weigh crucible + content
↓
DIETARY FIBER RESIDUE
(containing protein and ash)
↓

↓	↓
PROTEIN DETERMINATION (nitrogen × 6.25)	**ASH DETERMINATION** (525°C for 5 hours)

FIGURE 4 Determination of Total Dietary Fiber

residue obtained using either one of the AOAC methods, the determination of nitrogen for crude protein correction is especially critical with this method. However, the method is less labor intensive and more cost effective. The quantitation of glucose in starch hydrolysate can be done using GLC, HPLC, or other enzymatic methods. The above method was used to analyze a number of frequently consumed foods that had been stored at −20°C after they had been analyzed for sugars by HPLC, soluble and insoluble dietary fiber by AOAC method 991.43. The earlier analyses were done in a commercial laboratory (4) with a contract from the Nutrient Data Laboratory, ARS, USDA (formerly the Human Nutrition Information Service, USDA). Detailed procedures of our method and comparisons between the two laboratories of the data on sugars and dietary fiber contents of the same 34 foods are given elsewhere (3). Sample data from our laboratory on total sugar, starches, and total dietary fiber are presented here for 4 groups of foods. Table 1 gives the values for baked products; Table 2 for cereal grains and pasta; Table 3 for legumes, and Table 4 for vegetables. Table 5 gives the values for individual sugars, neutral sugars [(arabinose + fucose + galactose + glucose + mannose + rhamnose + xylose) × 0.89], uronic acid, dietary fiber polysaccharides (neutral sugars + uronic acid) and total dietary fiber of 12 selected foods.

Based on the dry weight of selected foods, baked products contain between 50 and 70 g/100 g of starch, 6 and 18 g/100 g of TDF; cereal grains and pastas contain between 55 and 90 g/100 g of starch, 2 and 10 g/100 g of TDF; canned legumes contain between 20 and 40 g/100 g of starch, 20 and 30 g/100 g of

DIETARY FIBER RESIDUE

↓

add 5 mL H_2SO_4, 12 M

↓

35°C for 1 hour

↓

add 25 mL H_2O

↓

100°C for 1 hour

↓

HYDROLYSATE

Left branch:

add to 3 mL; 1 mL internal standard
1 mL NH_4OH, 12.5 M, 5µL octan-2-ol,
0.2 mL NaBH4 solution

↓

40°C for 30 min

↓

add 0.4 mL acetic acid

↓

Take 0.5 mL
Add 0.5 mL of N-methylimidazole and
0.5 mL acetic anhydride

↓

20°C for 10 minutes

↓

Add 0.6 mL of ethanol and 5 mL of H_2O
2 × 5 mL of 7.5 M KOH

↓

ALDITOL ACETATES OF NEUTRAL SUGARS

Right branch:

Add to 0.3 mL; 0.3 mL $NaCl/H_3BO_4$
5 mL H_2SO_4

↓

70°C for 40 min

↓

add 0.2 dimethylphenol

↓

URONIC ACIDS

FIGURE 5 Englyst Procedure for Neutral Sugars and Uronic Acid Determination

TABLE 1 Total Sugar, Starches, and Total Dietary Fiber Content of Baked Products

Foods	Total sugar	Starch	Total dietary fiber
Bread, white, soft	3.03 ± 0.09	70.78 ± 0.77	5.82 ± 0.07
Bread, white, red. cal. soft	2.63 ± 0.18	48.87 ± 0.90	18.13 ± 0.34
Bread, rye, w/seed	3.41 ± 0.33	57.96 ± 4.92	7.05 ± 0.05
Bread, wheat, soft	5.02 ± 0.04	56.55 ± 2.40	11.43 ± 0.97
Tortilla, corn, RTE	0.12 ± 0.01	72.42 ± 1.96	8.75 ± 0.10

TABLE 2 Total Sugar, Starches, and Total Dietary Fiber Content of Cereal Grains and Pasta

Foods	Total sugar	Starch	Total dietary fiber
Rice, white, long grain		89.33 ± 0.51	1.79 ± 0.06
Rice, brown, long grain	0.55 ± 0.03	74.90 ± 7.90	5.08 ± 0.03
Spaghetti, regular	1.14 ± 0.05	67.20 ± 2.12	4.86 ± 0.05
Oats, quick	0.54 ± 0.03	72.55 ± 1.34	8.36 ± 0.01
Oatmeal, regular	0.82 ± 0.01	55.50 ± 1.55	10.73 ± 0.12

TABLE 3 Total Sugar, Starches, and Total Dietary; Fiber Content of Legumes

Foods	Sugar	Total starch	Total dietary fiber
Pork+beans w/tomato sauce	14.18 ± 0.12	18.58 ± 1.32	22.77 ± 0.63
Red kidney beans	6.27 ± 0.15	42.00 ± 0.17	23.15 ± 0.75
Chickpeas (garbanzo beans)	1.59 ± 0.02	27.81 ± 1.07	24.06 ± 0.33
Pinto beans	1.70 ± 0.05	33.11 ± 1.09	20.79 ± 0.71
Split peas	1.66 ± 0.09	34.18 ± 2.45	28.19 ± 0.62

TABLE 4 Total Sugar, Starches, and Total Dietary Fiber Content of Vegetables

Foods	Sugar	Total starch	Total dietary fiber
Beans, green, fresh steamed	28.48 ± 0.24	4.74 ± 0.12	28.48 ± 0.24
Potato, white, boiled, peeled	1.20 ± 0.12	77.12 ± 0.63	6.82 ± 0.14
Corn, yellow, from cob; store	21.89 ± 0.23	23.32 ± 0.47	25.19 ± 0.44
Corn, yellow or white, from cob; farmers' market	18.62 ± 0.38	46.90 ± 1.35	11.18 ± 0.67
Peas, green frozen, microwaved	25.34 ± 0.33	15.02 ± 0.04	18.01 ± 0.74

TDF; cooked vegetables contain between 5 and 80 g/100 g of starch, 7 and 30 g/100 g of TDF. When the sum of these two fractions is expressed as complex carbohydrates (CC), the range for all the foods shown in Tables 1 through 4 is between 33 and 90 g/100 g, with green beans having the lowest CC but the highest TDF, and rice having the highest CC but the lowest TDF. For other foods, a value for complex carbohydrates does not provide any information as to the ratio of starch to total dietary fiber. The acid hydrolysates of the dietary fiber

TABLE 5 Neutral Sugar and Uronic Acid Contents of Selected Foods

Foods	Rha	Fuc	Ara	Xyl	Man	Gal	Glu	Neutral sugar	Uronic acid	DFP	TDF	DFP as % TDF
Bread, reduced calorie	ND	ND	1.22	3.01	0.70	1.14	9.85	14.15	0.70	14.85	18.13	81.92
Bread, wheat	ND	ND	1.10	1.61	0.37	0.27	5.23	7.59	0.64	8.23	11.43	71.99
Tortilla, corn	ND	ND	1.17	1.60	0.18	0.29	3.00	0.58	0.21	5.79	8.75	66.14
Spaghetti, cooked	ND	ND	0.88	1.11	0.21	0.21	2.59	4.45	0.16	4.61	4.86	94.86
Grits, quick	ND	ND	0.59	0.69	0.15	0.13	5.77	6.62	0.17	6.79	8.36	81.27
Oatmeal, cooked	ND	ND	1.00	1.23	0.22	0.23	6.59	8.26	0.33	8.58	10.73	80.00
Kidney beans, canned	ND	0.22	3.19	1.93	0.76	0.97	13.00	17.94	0.46	18.40	23.15	79.50
Chick peas, canned	0.11	ND	2.72	0.49	0.27	0.54	17.29	19.00	1.38	2.00	24.06	85.11
Pinto beans, canned	0.12	0.12	1.88	0.96	0.49	0.47	1.00	12.77	0.61	13.38	20.79	64.36
Beans, green, steamed	0.42	0.14	1.35	1.57	1.51	2.80	11.18	16.89	5.52	22.41	28.48	78.68
White potato, boiled	0.09	ND	0.24	0.10	0.17	1.48	3.38	4.87	0.55	5.42	6.82	79.45
Peas, green, microwaved	0.29	ND	2.62	0.74	0.25	0.52	13.30	15.77	2.10	17.87	18.11	99.22

residues of 6 baked products, cereal grains and pasta contain arabinose, galactose, glucose, mannose, and xylose, but no detectable amount of rhamnose or fucose, the amount of dietary fiber polysaccharides (DFP) corresponds to the percentage of total dietary fiber range from 65 to 99%. Legumes and cooked vegetables shown here contain varying amounts of rhamnose and fucose along with the other sugars usually found in polysaccharide hydrolysates. All 12 foods, except chickpeas, contain uronic acids. Analytically, we can define complex carbohydrates as the sum of enzymatically hydrolyzable starch and enzymatic-gravimetrically obtained total dietary fiber as shown above. However, nutritionally, it may be important to know the actual amount of each of the fractions and the composition of neutral sugars and uronic acid in the dietary fiber fraction.

REFERENCES

1. National Research Council (1989) Recommended Dietary Allowances, 10th Ed., National Academy Press, Washington, D.C., p. 39.
2. Englyst, H. N. & Cummings, J. H. (1988) J. Assoc. Off. Anal. Chem. 71, 808–814.
3. Li, B. W. (1996) J. AOAC International, 79, 718–723.
4. Southern Testing and Research Laboratories, Inc. (1994) Final Report USDA/HNIS Requisition No. H393004600, pp. 1a–11b.

III

RESISTANT STARCH—ANALYSIS

13

In Vivo Techniques to Quantify Resistant Starch

M. Champ, L. Martin, L. Noah, and M. Gratas
I.N.R.A., Laboratoire de Technologie Appliqué la Nutrition, Nantes, France

INTRODUCTION

The physiological definition of resistant starch, which is largely adopted, implies the analytical methods of resistant starch in foods to be validated with in vivo data obtained from healthy individuals. The intubation technique is the only one to be applicable to healthy volunteers. The main drawback of the method is the presence of the tube along the small intestine (direct collection of ileal content) and its possible influence on the transit. Several other methods are available to assess physiologically resistant starch in vivo. Resistant starch can be quantified directly, by collecting ileal samples in human ileostomates or animals, or indirectly by estimating the amount of starch fermented in the colon. The ileostomy model allows direct and quantitative determination of small bowel excretion, provided the bacterial degradation of the effluent can be minimized. Hydrogen breath test is also used to quantify malabsorption of starch. It is rapid and simple but indirect and consequently semi-quantitative. Rats (antibiotic treated, germ-free or colectomized) and pigs (ileum cannulated or with ileorectal anastomosis) are considered as useful models for estimating starch digestion in humans. However

TABLE 1 Main In Vivo Techniques to Quantify RS

Animal models	Humans
Pigs	Indirect
Ileum cannulated	H_2 Breath test
Anastomosis	Direct
Rats	Ileostomy model
Antibiotic treated	Intubation of healthy subjects
Germ-free	Caecectomized
Colectomized	
H_2 excretion	

it cannot be expected from these animal models to predict accurate values of ileal digestibility.

Resistant starch (RS) is present in a number of foods and constitutes up to 15% of the dry matter of the product. Recent studies indicate that its presence in foods might be beneficial for health. RS is by definition not absorbed in the small intestine, thus it does not contribute to postprandial hyperglycemia (1,2). Its effect on lipid metabolism has recently been investigated. RS, added to the meals, might be beneficial for patients with subnormal or abnormal level of lipemia (3). Moreover, some animal studies indicate a serum cholesterol lowering effect but no evidence of similar effect on humans has been demonstrated. RS is largely fermented, producing short-chain fatty acids and bacterial cells. It may be important in determining colonic epithelial cell health through effects on bile acids, butyrate production and moderation of nitrogen metabolism (4). A number of studies of the effect of RS on bowel habit have been reported but findings are somewhat inconsistent (4).

The interest in RS has led to the need for a valid analytical method to quantify it in foods. The definition of RS being physiological, any analytical method should be validated on the basis of in vivo data obtained preferably on healthy subjects. Until now, all the methods available to quantify RS in healthy humans being criticizable, several methods applicable to animal models or humans have been proposed (Table 1).

STARCH DIGESTION IN HUMANS

Starch is mainly digested in the upper part of the digestive tract and absorbed as glucose in the duodenum and jejunum. Starchy foods are first chewed in the mouth and prehydrolyzed by salivary amylase. The salivary amylolysis is efficient in the stomach until it is inhibited by acidification due to hydrochloric acid secretion. The mechanical action of the stomach can disrupt the structure of most food. It thus increases the accessibility of the starch to α-amylase when it is entrapped in a protein network or in cell walls in unrefined seeds and grains. Pancreatic secretions at the duodenal level are very efficient and hydrolyze most of the starch. Glucoamylase, maltase and isomaltase of the brush border disrupt the small oligosaccharides into glucose which is absorbed in the portal blood to be delivered to the liver. A small fraction of the glucose is first metabolized by the intestinal cells. Most of it is metabolized by the liver and the peripheral cells.

A small part of the starch might be hydrolyzed later in the ileum and also be absorbed as glucose. Finally, another fraction can escape this endogenous hydrolysis and become a substrate for the bacterial flora. At this level, the final products of this fermentation are mainly short chain fatty acids (acetic, propionic and butyric acids) and gases (CO_2, H_2, and in some cases CH_4).

QUANTIFICATION OF RS IN ANIMAL MODELS

Pigs and rats are traditional models of humans in nutritional studies. Both species are omnivorous. Rats are useful animal models because of their size and small intake. Digestive physiology of pigs is closer to that of humans, however the digestive capacity of pigs is much higher than that of humans. Indeed, a piglet of 25 kg has been shown to have the digestive capacity of a man of 65 kg.

The Pig Model

It is possible to determine directly ileal digestibility in the pig. Two categories of techniques are available: ileum cannulations and ileo-rectal anastomosis. The main advantages and shortcomings of these methods are summarized in Table 2.

TABLE 2 Advantages and Shortcomings of the Pig as an Animal Model

Advantages	Shortcomings
❒ Digestive physiology close to that of humans ❒ Digestibility can be measured in the small and large intestine of the same animal (cannulations)	❒ Requires surgery ❒ Stomach and small intestine more heavily colonized by microflora than in humans ❒ Requires a marker technique to measure ileal digestibility (when the collection is not complete) ❒ Relatively expensive to use

Ileum cannulated pigs: simple T-cannulations, postvalvular T-caecum cannulation, ileoileal and ileo-caecal re-entrant cannulation, ileo-colic post-valvular cannulation
Anastomosis: ileo-rectal anastomosis
Adapted from (5)

TABLE 3 Digestibility of Plant Polysaccharides from Barley in the Small Intestine of Pigs (ileum cannulated pigs)

		Digestibility		
Diet	Intake (g/d)	Starch	NSP	Ref.
Basal diet	380	95.5	35	(6)
+β-Glucanase	380	96.7	41	(6)
Barley, raw	190	83.7	28	(7)
Barley, extruded	208	96.9	25	(7)
Barley, hull-less, raw		94.8	50	(8)
Barley, hull-less, baked		98.6	62	(8)

An example of such a study is presented in Table 3. It confirms that the hydrolysis of the viscous β-glucans by β-glucanase slightly increases the starch digestibility. However, hydrothermic treatments significantly improve starch digestion.

The Rat Model

Several methods utilizing the rat as a model are potentially available. Their main advantages and shortcomings are presented in Table 4.

The Nebacitin (antibiotic) treated rats have extensively been used by Asp and collaborators. They have been used in the validation of an in vitro method developed by this group (9,10) (Table 5).

Digestibility of starchy foods has also been determined in surgically modified rats. The aim of these surgeries is to remove most or all the large intestine. None of these methods eliminate enough bacteria to quantify properly the digestiblity of starch in the small intestine of the rat. Indeed, a large fraction of the most fermentable fiber disappears in the gastrointestinal tract of such animals confirming the lack of interest of the caecectomized rat to estimate RS (Table 6). The colectomized rat is potentially a more appropriate animal model to estimate RS in humans than is the caecectomized rat.

QUANTIFICATION OF RS IN HUMANS

One indirect and two direct methods have been used to estimate RS in humans. They are presented in Table 7.

H_2 Breath Test

Hydrogen is one of the end-products of carbohydrates fermentation. It is exclusively formed in the colon by the bacterial fermentation, partly absorbed and

TABLE 4 Advantages and Shortcomings of the Rat as an Animal Model

Advantages	Shortcomings
Antibiotic treated rats	
Treatment: 0.7% Nebacitin (2/3 Bacitracin, 1/3 Neomycin) → microbial density & activity: −80–90%; Starch digestibility performed on faecal sample	
Advantages	**Shortcomings**
Low cost	Efficiency of Nebacitin ±
Easy to use and standardize	Endogenous α-amylase in the large intestine
Germ-free rats kept in sterile isolators	
Advantages	**Shortcomings**
No microflora	Requires specific equipments
Non-invasive	High cost
	Correlation with data/humans?
H_2 excretion in rats	
Measurement of total H_2 excretion (breath and flatus) in a respiration chamber	
Advantages	**Shortcomings**
Non-invasive	Requires specific equipments
	Not suited as a quantitative model
Surgically modified rats	
Caecectomized (Cc): resection of the colon; Colectomized (Cl): ileorectal anastomosis	
Advantages	**Shortcomings**
Eliminate 70–80% (Cc) and 90% (Cl) of the microflora without the use of drugs	Requires skilled persons to perform surgery
	Microflora not completely eliminated (Cc)
	Digestibility of starch overestimated (Cc)

cleared in a single passage of the lungs, then excreted in the expired lungs. The results of gas perfusion techniques have suggested that a rather constant fraction of the total H_2 production is excreted by the lungs, and that rates of breath H_2 and H_2 production correlate well (15). Using a non-absorbable but quickly fermented oligosaccharide (the lactulose) to ''calibrate'' the subject, it can be expected to quantify a malabsorbed carbohydrate. Whereas this procedure remains quantitative for oligosaccharides it is only qualitative for insoluble or slowly fermented substrates. Table 8 illustrates the finding that in many cases, the method is inappropriate to quantify RS. The comparison of the RS values obtained by the H_2 breath test and by intubation of healthy subjects (direct measurement) when the

TABLE 5 In Vivo Recovery of RS in Nebacitin Treated Rats Compared to In Vitro Values

Source of starch	In vivo	In vitro (ASP method)	Ref.
Peas purée, autoclaved	29.2	23.4–29.0	(10)
Potato purée, autoclaved	7.5	7.0–9.2	(10)
Infant purée, canned	18.1	13.9–17.5	(10)
Dent corn arepas	4.1	4.2	(11)
High amylose arepas	32.5	32.2	(11)
Red bean, precooked flour	10	8.7	(12)
Red bean, coarse precooked flour	8	11.9	(12)
Lentil, precooked flour	11	8.3	(12)

volunteers were fed the same starch (high amylose corn starch retrograded and complexed) is characteristic of the discrepancy between the two methods.

Sample Test

An example of a protocol described in the literature (31) is the following:

Twelve young healthy volunteers first submitted to a lactulose test then took part in three experimental tests. Each H_2 breath test was at least one week apart.

The lactulose test, consisting of 10 g lactulose syrup in 100 ml water, was

TABLE 6 Digestibility of Plant Polysaccharides in Surgically Modified Rats

Diet	Intact rats	Modified rats	Ref.
Caecectomized rats*			
Digestibility (%) (barley diet)			
Starch	100	99.4	(13)
β-Glucans	100	79–88	(13)
Arabinoxylans	32–59	7–27	(13)
Cellulose	18–31	5–11	(13)
Colectomized rats**			
Digestibility of starch (%)			
Rice		99.8	(14)
Peas		84.8	(14)

*Resection of the caecum; **ileorectal anastomosis

TABLE 7 Advantages and Shortcomings of the Studies Performed with Humans

H_2 breath test

Determination of the increase in hydrogen in the breath after the consumption of malabsorbed carbohydrates

Advantages	Shortcomings
Simple and non-invasive	
Healthy subjects	Semi-quantitative
	Strict standardization necessary
	Large intra- and inter-individual variation in H_2 excretion

Ileostomy model

Patients who had had a colectomy for ulcerative colitis and Crohn's disease

Advantages	Shortcomings
Direct collection of the ileal effluent → quantitative	Cannot be considered as healthy
Easy to perform	Physiological adaptation
	water & electrolytes absorption
	bacterial overgrowth
	Transit time (not normal)

Intubation of healthy subjects

Collection of the ileal content in healthy subjects after intubation using a constant perfusion technique of solution containing an unabsorbable marker

Advantages	Shortcomings
Healthy subjects	Disturbance of the normal physiology by the long triple lumen tube
Direct collection of the ileal effluent	Quantification of the flow rate using a liquid phase marker
	Risk of selectivity of the tube in case of heterogeneous food
	Expensive and long

Adapted from (5)

done at 0900 h after suitable oral hygiene. Breath samples were collected at 15-min intervals from 30 min before lactulose ingestion until 6 h afterwards.

The meals were eaten at 0900h within 6 min after an overnight fast and immediately followed by meticulous oral hygiene. Each evening meal preceding the morning test was standardized to contain a low level of indigestible material.

TABLE 8 Malabsorption of Starch Estimated by Different Techniques

Source of starch	Starch ingested (g)	Malabsorption %	Ref.
H_2 breath test			
HACS, raw	30	9.2	(16)
HACS, complexed	30	9.5	(16)
HACS, retrograded	30	5.5	(16)
Cooked potatoes	60	6.7	(17)
Cooked & cooled potatoes	60	22.8	(17)
Cooked, cooled, and warmed-up potatoes	60	5.0	(17)
White bread	120	10.7	(18)
Whole meal bread	120	8.3	(18)
Wheat flour	50	2.8	(19)
Whole meal	50	13.6	(19)
Oat flakes (raw)	35	7.8	(20)
Oat flakes (cooked)	35	5.8	(20)
Lentils	120	17.6	(18)
Beans	100	38.0	(19)
Green banana	100	38.6	(21)
Banana + rice	n.m.	0.0	(22)
Ileostomy model			
Rice + bread	98–127	0.5	(23)
Bread	107	0.8	(24)
White bread	100	13	(18)
White bread	61.9	2.5	(25)
Whole meal bread	100	11	(18)
Oat flakes	57.8	2.2	(25)
Corn flakes	74.2	5.0	(25)
Cooked potatoes	45.4	3.3	(25)
Cooked & cooled potatoes	47.2	12.9	(25)
Cooked, cooled, and warmed-up potatoes	47.2	7.6	(25)
Banana (ripe)	2.1	66.7	(26)
Banana (unripe)	20.1	95.0	(26)
Lentils	100	21	(18)
Intubation of healthy subjects			
HACS, complexed	32.5	21.1	(27)
HACS, retrograded	32.5	50.9	(27)
Banana (unripe)	23.1	83.7	(28)
Banana + rice	20	10.5	(22)
Banana + rice + potatoes	61	8.0	(22)
Bread + pasta + potatoes	100	5.2	(29)
Bread + pasta + potatoes	200	4.1	(29)
Beans	68.5	16.5	(30)

Breath samples were collected at 15-min intervals from 30 min before to 9 h after ingestion of the test meal.

Alveolar air samples were obtained by having the subjects exhale through a mouthpiece into two bags connected by a three-way valve. When the first 500 ml of expiratory air filled one plastic bag, the end alveolar air was then collected in a second bag (1-L rubber anesthesia bag adapted with a one-way valve). The end alveolar air was then immediately transferred into 50 ml plastic syringes fitted with three-way stopcocks, and was usually analyzed within 2 h of collection. The hydrogen concentrations in breath samples were determined with a Microlyze DP gas chromatograph (Quintron Instrument Company, Milwaukee, WI).

A sample of gas was then injected in the GC and the quantitative data were available very quickly.

During the 9-h period after the test meal, an increase in hydrogen concentration of >10 ppp over baseline, measured upon two consecutive 15-min interval breath samplings, was considered to represent significant starch malabsorption.

Other procedures to collect and store the H_2 samples are described in the literature and are summarized by Rumessen (32). The calculations are performed usually by determining a ratio between the areas under the curves after the test meal and the lactulose. Knowing the amount of lactulose fermented, the amount of carbohydrate from the experimental meal which has been theoretically fermented can be calculated. Even if the principle appears as quite simple, there are several theories on the best way to do this quantification (32).

Ileostomy Model

The ileostomy model offers a method for direct and quantitative determination of small bowel excretion provided the bacteriological degradation of the effluent can be minimized. The subjects who take part in these studies had a conventional ileostomy after proctocolectomy for ulcerative colitis. This surgery is performed by eversion of the distal 5–10 cm of the small bowel pulled onto the abdominal wall as a fistula (33). These people can easily collect their effluent in a bag which is usually changed every second hour during daytime. The ileostomy bags are immediately deep frozen on carbon dioxide ice when possible. After the experimental meal, the subjects fast for 4 h, then they are given several snacks (plant polysaccharide-free) (34).

Intubation Technique (28)

Healthy volunteers are intubated with a triple-lumen polyvinyl tube whose transit down the gut is aided by a terminal inflatable bag containing mercury. When the bag reaches the cecum, as confirmed fluoroscopically, it is deflated and the subjects must remain in a semirecumbent position. One lumen is used to sample ileal content 5 cm above the ileocecal junction, and the other lumen, 25 cm proximal to the aspiration port, is used for perfusion. The perfusate contained NaCl and polyethylene glycol 4000 as a recovery marker to estimate water flow through the distal ileum. The solution is maintained at 37°C and stirred until the end of perfusion. The day after the intubation, the subjects are given the experimental meal as a breakfast. A second marker (previously (^{14}C)PEG, now indium) is added to the meal, and the intestinal contents are aspirated for 14 h, while subjects do not eat or drink. Intestinal contents are continuously collected on ice by manual aspiration to aspirate as much fluid as possible. Samples are divided into 30-min aliquots which are frozen in liquid nitrogen and then freeze-dried. Maintenance of tube position is confirmed fluoroscopically at the end of all experiments.

COMPARISON OF THE IN VIVO MODELS

Pigs/Humans

Two recent studies performed with the same meal based on beans on pigs (T-cannulation) and healthy humans (intubation) confirmed the greater digestive capacity of the pig compared to human subjects. Indeed with the same starch intake, malabsorption of starch was lower (11.2 ± 3.6%) for pigs (Gratas, personal communication) than for humans (16.5 ± 1.3%) (21). Mougham et al. (35) recently estimated that the digestive capacity of a man of 65 kg was equivalent to the one of a piglet of 25 kg.

H_2 Breath Test/Ileostomy Model/Intubation

It is difficult to compare the data obtained within different studies with different types of meal and different starch intakes. However one comparison can be made between two studies performed with the ileostomy model (34) and the ileal intubation in healthy subjects (20) with the same meal containing 30 g of starch from green banana. The ileal excretions of starch (=RS) were respectively 15.8 ± 0.7 and 19.3 ± 0.7 g/day for the ileostomates and the healthy subjects.

Such a difference can be explained by an underestimation of RS in ileostomates and/or by an overestimation of RS when intubation techniques is used. Indeed, on one hand, there is evidence of a bacterial overgrowth in the distal ileum of the ileostomates as well as in the collection bags. On the other hand, the intubation is thought to be the cause of a decrease of the oroileal transit time due to the tube which could decrease the efficiency of the intestinal digestion.

CONCLUSIONS

Several methods are available to evaluate RS in vivo in humans and animal models. It cannot be expected from any of the animal models to predict accurate values of human ileal digestibility, however they can be used for screening or for a qualitative evaluation.

The only direct technique to be appliquable to healthy volunteers is the intubation technique. The main drawback of the method is the presence of the tube along the small intestine and its possible influence on the transit. It might thus slightly overestimate the RS content of the foods. Resistant starch can also be quantified directly, by collecting ileal samples in human ileostomates. The determination of small bowel excretion is quantitative, provided the bacterial degradation of the effluent can be minimized. This technique probably slightly underestimates RS content of the foods. Hydrogen breath test is also used to quantify malabsorption of starch. It is rapid and simple but indirect and consequently semi-quantitative. However the use of an appropriate standard for the "calibration" of the subject could improve the quality of the method.

In conclusion, the two direct methods performed on humans undoubtedly are the best techniques to quantify RS as it has been defined in 1992 as ". . . the sum of starch and products of starch degradation not absorbed in the small intestine of healthy individuals." (1)

REFERENCES

1. Asp, N. G. (1992) Eur. J. Clin. Nutr. 46(S2), S1.
2. Ranganathan, S., Champ, M., Pechard C., Blanchard P., N'Guyen, M., Colonna P., Krempf, M. (1994) Am. J. Clin. Nutr. 59, 879–883.
3. Faisant, N., Champ, M., Ranganathan, S. S., Azoulay, C., Kergueris, M. F., Krempf, M. (1995) in Proceedings of the concluding plenary meeting of EURESTA, N. G. Asp, J. M. M. van Amelsvoort & J.G.A.J. Hautvast (Eds), European Flair-Concerted Action on Resistant Starch—No. 11 (COST 911), pp. 113–114.
4. Cummings, J. H., Edwards, C., Gee, J., Nagengast, F., Mathers, J. (1995) in Proceedings of the concluding plenary meeting of EURESTA, N.G. Asp, J.M.M. van Amelsvoort & J. G. A. J. Hautvast (Eds), European Flair-Concerted Action on Resistant Starch–No. 11 (COST 911), pp. 38–55.
5. Bach Knudsen, K. E. (1991) in Methodological aspects of in vivo methods for measurement of starch digestibility, Gudmand-Hoyer, E. (Ed), Report of the European Flair Concerted Action Workshop (EURESTA, Contract no. AGRF/0027), Velbaek, Copenhagen, 10–12 November 1991, 40–54.
6. Graham, H., Hesselman, K., Jonsson, E., Aman, P. (1986) Nutr. Rep. Int. 34, 1089–1096.
7. Fadel, J. G., Newman, C. W., Newman, R. K., Graham, H. (1988) Can. J. Anim. Sci. 68, 891–897.
8. Fadel, J. G., Newman, R. K., Newman, C. W., Graham, H. (1989) J. Nutr. 119, 722–726.
9. Bjôrck, I., Nyman, M., Pedersen, B., Siljestršm, M., Asp, N. G., Eggum, B.O.(1986) J. Cereal Sci. 4, 1–11.
10. Bjôrck, I., Siljestršm, M. (1992) J. Sci. Food Agric. 58, 541–553.
11. Granfeldt, Y., Drews, A., Bjôrck, I. (1993) J. Nutr. 123, 1676–1684.
12. Tovar, J., Bjôrck, I. M., Asp, N. G. (1992) J. Nutr. 122, 1500–1507.

13. Bach Knudsen, K. E., Agergaard, N., Olesen, H. P. (1991) J. Anim. Physiol. Anim. Nutr. 66, 190–203.
14. Hildenbrandt, L. A., Marlett J. A. (1991) J. Nutr. 121, 679–686.
15. Levitt, M. D. (1969) N. Engl. J. Med. 284, 1394–1398.
16. Bornet, F., Cloarec, D., Gouilloud, S., Champ, M., Colonna, P., Barry, J. L., Galmiche, J. P. (1990) Gastroenterol. Clin. Biol. 14, A90.
17. Scheppach, W, Bach, M., Bartram, P., Christl, S., Bergthaller, W., Kasper, H. (1991) Dig. Dis. Sci. 36, 1601–1605.
18. Wolever, T. M. S., Cohen, Z., Thompson, L. U., Thorne, M. J., Jenkins M. J. A., Prokipchuk, E. J., Jenkins, D. J. A. (1986) Am. J. Gastroenterol. 81, 115–122.
19. Levitt, M. D., Hirsch, P., Fetzer, C. A., Sheahan, M., Levine, A. S. (1987) Gastroenterol. 92, 383–389.
20. Lund, E. K., Johnson, I. T. (1991) J. Nutr. 121, 311–317.
21. Christl, S. U., Murgatroyd, P. R., Gibson, G. R., Cummings, J. H. (1992) Gastroenterol. 102, 1269–1277.
22. Stephen, A. M., Haddad, A. C., Phillips, S. F. (1983) Gastroenterol. 85, 589–595.
23. Sandberg, A. S., Andersson, H., Hallgren, B., Hasselblad, K., Isaksson, I. (1981) J. Nutr. 45, 283–294.
24. Sandberg, A. S., Andersson, H., Kivistš, B., Sandstrŝm, B. (1986) Br. J. Nutr. 55, 245–254.
25. Englyst, H. N., Cummings, J. H. (1985) Am. J. Clin. Nutr. 42, 778–787.
26. Englyst, H. N., Cummings, J. H. (1986) Am. J. Clin. Nutr. 44, 42–50.
27. Molis, C., Champ, M., Flouri, B., Pellier, P., Bornet, F., Colonna, P., Kozlowski, F., Rambaud, J. C., Galmiche, J. P. (1992) Eur. J. Clin. Nutr. 46, S131–S132.
28. Faisant, N., Bulon, A., Colonna, P., Molis, C., Lartigue, S., Galmiche, J. P., Champ, M. (1995) Br. J. Nutr. 73, 111–123.
29. Flouri, B., Leblond, A., Florent, F., Rautureau, M., Bissalli, A., Rambaud, J. C. (1988) Gastroenterol. 95, 356–363.
30. Noah, L., Guillon, F., Bouchet, B., Bulon, A., Gallant, D. J., Colonna, P., Molis, C., Faisant, N., Galmiche, J. P., Champ, M. (1995) in Proc. Eur. Assoc. for Grain Legume Research Conf. July 9–13, pp. 276–277.
31. Bornet, F. R. J., Cloarec, D., Barry, J. L., Colonna, P., Gouilloud, S., Delort-Laval, J., Galmiche, J. P. (1990) Am. J. Clin. Nutr. 51, 421–427.
32. Rumessen, J. J. (1992) Eur. J. Clin. Nutr., 46(S2), S77–S90.
33. Andersson, H. (1992) Eur. J. Clin. Nutr., 46(S2), S69–S76.
34. Langkilde, A. M., Andersson, H., Faisant, N., Champ, M. (1995) in Proceedings of the concluding plenary meeting of EURESTA, N. G. Asp, J. M. M. van Amelsvoort & J. G. A. J. Hautvast (Eds), European Flair-Concerted Action on Resistant Starch—No. 11 (COST 911), pp. 28–30.
35. Mougham, P. J., Cranwell, Darragh, A. J., Rowan, A. M. (1994) in Proc. VIth International Symposium on Digestive Physiology in Pigs. Souffrant W.-B. & Hagemeister H. (Eds), Bad Doberan, D, 4–6 October 1994. pp. 389–396.

14

Analytical Methods for Resistant Starch

M. Champ, L. Martin, L. Noah, and M. Gratas
I.N.R.A., Laboratoire de Technologie Appliqué la Nutrition, Nantes, France

INTRODUCTION

Resistant starch has recently been defined as ". . . the sum of starch and products of starch degradation not absorbed in the small intestine of healthy individuals" (1). An analytical method for RS should then take into account all the starch and α-dextrins covering this physiological definition. Furthermore, it should be validated using in vivo data from human healthy subjects. The general principle of the method is the following: 1) the samples are digested by a pancreatic α-amylase then 2) resistant starch content is determined by direct analysis of the residual starch after hydrolysis or by substracting to the total starch of the sample, the amount of starch which has been digested. None of the "European methods" (Englyst et al., 1992, Bjôrck et al., 1986, Champ, 1992, Faisant et al., 1995) are exempt of criticism. Moreover, none of them are able to analyze resistant starch as defined because they do not consider potentially digestible starch arriving at the end of the ileum. The last two methods appeared to be more quickly and easily reproduced than Englyst's method. However Englyst's method is the only one which has been validated in vivo on humans. Besides these European methods, Muir and O'Dea (1992, 1993) developed another procedure, validated in vivo, that is supposed to mimic physiological conditions for starch digestion.

Resistant starch should then be analyzed using a method which mimics the digestion of starchy food in the upper part of the digestive tract. Several methods have been published during the past 15 years, some of them being validated on the basis of in vivo measurements.

CLASSIFICATION OF RS

The increasing knowledge of starch digestion in humans has allowed a new classification of RS which is commonly approved (2). Three classes of RS are identified:

RS1

Physically inaccessible starch (RS1) is found in partly milled grains and seeds. Legumes such as beans or lentils are known to be one of the main sources of RS. The preparation and cooking process is of great importance in the RS content of the food.

RS2

B-type starch when uncooked is known to be very resistant to enzymatic hydrolysis. B-type refers to the X-ray diffraction pattern of the starch. Raw starches are classified in 3 main types: A (ex: most cereal starches, cassava starch), B (ex: potato and banana starches) and C (most legume starches). Banana is the main source of RS2 in the human diet. During ripening of the fruit, starch is being converted into simple sugars and sucrose and in ripe bananas still have a significant amount of starch. Most of the cooking procedures are able to gelatinize raw starches allowing the disappearance of RS2 in the food.

RS3

Retrograded starch is present in most starchy foods which have been cooked then cooled and stored from several hours to several months. The retrogradation is a recrystallization of starch granules which occurs after the gelatinization and which implies mostly the linear fraction of the starch: the amylose. However, amylopectin can also retrograded on a much longer term than for amylose. Potatoes cooked then cooled have been shown to contain RS (3). Reheating of starch

TABLE 1 RS (g/100 g total starch) from Different Sources of RS Determined In Vitro

Source of starch	TS % DM	RS % TS
Beans, canned	43.6	17.1
Lentils, canned	50.7	12.1
Chickpeas, canned	46.3	11.0
Lasagne	69.9	3.6
Spaghetti	70.6	3.0

reduces RS content of the potato showing that the retrogradation is partly reversible. Several cycles of heating then cooling allow an increase of RS.

RS1, RS2 and RS3 can coexist in the same food. Indeed a meal of beans contains both RS1 and RS3 (4) whereas RS1 and RS2 are both present in bananas (5).

ANALYSIS OF TOTAL STARCH

RS is often expressed as percentage of total starch or in in vivo studies as a percentage of malabsorbed starch. Therefore an analysis of total starch prior to RS analysis is usually needed. Moreover, some of the methods need a preliminary total starch analysis to allow the suited weight of sample to respect the right enzyme/starch ratio in the determination of RS.

Starch has long been analyzed using polarimetric methods. This method is still used in feed industry because it allows a quick analysis of the starchy material then of the feed at the different steps of the process. However these methods were mostly abandoned for precise analysis of starch in food and feed because of numerous artifacts (amino acids, oligosaccharides, simple sugars etc.).

Any analysis of starch implies 4 major steps:

Preparation of the Samples: To allow a proper analysis of starch, it has to be fully accessible to amylolytic enzymes. Therefore grinding should be efficient enough to disrupt the cell walls and/or protein network surrounding the starch granules.

Dispersion of the Starch: In order to be completely hydrolyzed by the amyloglucosidase, the starch must be decrystallized and amylose and amylopectin must be accessible to the enzyme. This step was performed using boiling water and autoclaving. Then the use of dimethylsulfoxide (DMSO) was proposed but now most methods suggest the use of alkali such as sodium and potassium hydroxide (2M as a final concentration in the dispersion medium).

Hydrolysis of Starch: Starch is hydrolyzed by an amyloglucosidase into glucose. The enzyme is an endoenzyme able to hydrolyze both $\alpha 1-4$ and $\alpha 1-6$ linkages.

Quantification of Glucose: If properly ground, dispersed then hydrolyzed, starch should be totally analyzed as glucose. The choice of the analytical method for glucose should be guided by the expected concentration of glucose as well as by the possible presence of pigment(s) in the sample. Indeed, the complex hexokinase/glucose-6-P-deshydrogenase is very sensitive and does not have any contraindication whereas the use of the glucose-oxidase/peroxidase complex should be prohibited in the presence of pigments such as biliary pigments (digestive contents, for example).

GOD-POD or GOD-PAP: glucose-oxidase/peroxidase

$$\text{D-glucose} + H_2O + O_2 \xrightarrow{\text{GOD}} H_2O_2 + \text{gluconic acid}$$

$$H_2O_2 + DH_2 \xrightarrow{\text{POD}} 2H_2O + D$$

DH_2: 4-aminoantipyrine + 4-hydroxybenzoic acid
(Merckotest, ref. 14365,Darmstadt, Germany)
D: N-(4-antipyryl)-p-benzoquinone imine

HK-G6PDH: hexokinase/glucose-6-phosphate-deshydrogenase

$$\text{D-glucose} + \text{ATP} \xrightarrow{\text{HK}} \text{glucose-6-phosphate}$$

$$\text{G6PDH glucose-6-P} + \text{NADP}^+ \longrightarrow \text{gluconate-6-P} + \text{NADPH} + \text{H}^+$$

NADPH absorbance is determined at 340 nm. It is proportional to the amount of glucose present in the sample after the complete hydrolysis of starch.

ANALYTICAL METHODS FOR RS

During recent years, a lot of effort has been put into the evaluation, then into the improvement of the existing methods of RS. Roughly, two analytical methods are now proposed in the literature: one was described by Englyst et al. (1992)(2), the other was obtained during the European Research Program EURESTA (6). They provide very similar data for most starch samples however they both probably underestimate RS as defined above. Indeed, RS collected in vivo in humans (ileostomates or healthy subjects using the intubation technique) is composed of oligosaccharides (including glucose), α-glucans of high molecular weight (mainly starch granules) and a crystalline fraction whose size depends on the origin and the treatment of the starch. None of the analytical methods of RS takes into account the potentially digestible starch (oligosaccharides and part of the high molecular weight fraction) (7,8).

General Principle

In order to quantify RS, the first step is to remove the digestible starch from the sample. This is performed using a pancreatic (α-amylase. In some of the methods, an amyloglucosidase is added in order to avoid a possible inhibition of the α-amylase by the products of the digestion (mainly maltose, maltotriose). The amylolysis is also sometimes preceded by a proteolysis which is supposed to reflect the action of the pepsin inside the stomach and of the trypsin which is secreted in the pancreatic juice together with the α-amylase.

After the hydrolysis of the digestible starch, RS is quantified directly in the residue (isolated most of the time by 80% ethanolic precipitation) (6,9) or by difference between total starch and digestible starch which are quantified separately (2).

Main Analytical Methods

The main methods proposed in the literature will be briefly described and criticized.

The Method of Bjôrck et al., 1986 (10)

Principle

It quantifies the starch residue present in the dietary fiber residue obtained by the methods of Asp et al. (1983) (11) or Prosky et al. (1988) (12).

Procedure (Figure 1)

Main Characteristics

- Some of the samples such as bread can be analyzed as eaten without further drying. All the samples have to be milled (<0.5 mm).
- The samples are then submitted to a triple hydrolysis by Termamyl (100°C, 15 min), pepsin and pancreatin. The main consequence of this procedure is the gelatinization of all raw starch present in the sample which cannot be quantified as resistant starch.

Advantages and Drawbacks

- Can be performed with total dietary fiber analysis
- Analyze mostly retrograded starch
- Validated with a rat model (antibiotic treated rat). Figure 2 shows the

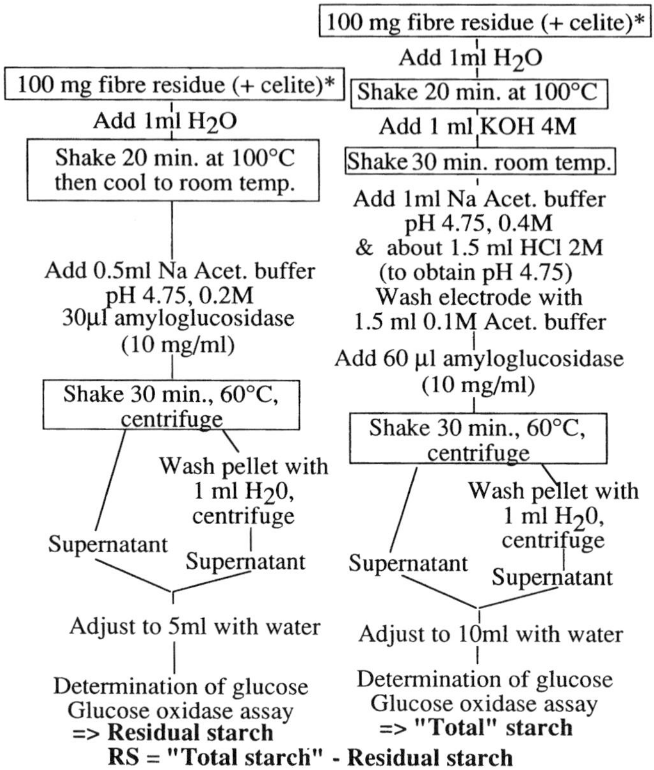

FIGURE 1 Determination of resistant starch according to Bjôrck et al., 1986 (10) (From Ref. 6).

good correlation between this in vitro method and the determination of the digestibility in antibiotic (Nebacitin) treated rats (13).

The Method of Englyst et al., 1992 (2)

Principle

The various types of starch are determined by controlled enzymic hydrolysis and measurement of the released glucose using glucose oxidase. Resistant starch is defined as the starch not hydrolyzed after 120 min incubation with pancreatic amylase and amyloglucosidase at 37°C. It is calculated by deducting from total starch content, the slowly digestible starch and the rapidly digestible starch contents of the sample hydrolyzed respectively after 120 and 20 min incubation.

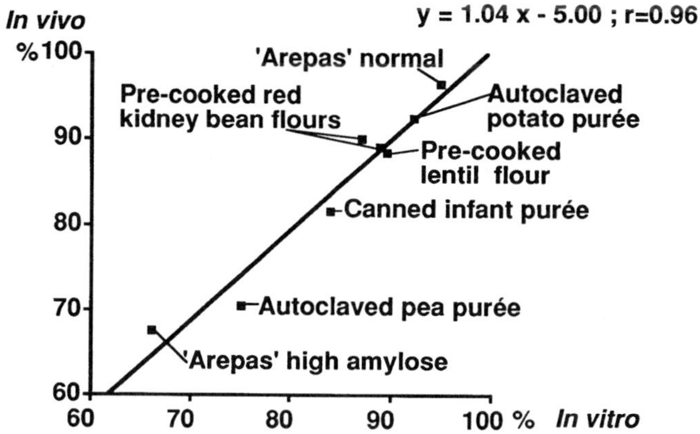

FIGURE 2 Correlation between in vitro method (10) and the determination of the digestibility in antibiotic (Nebacitin) treated rats (From Ref. 13).

Procedure (Figure 3)

Main Characteristics

- Fresh foods can be analyzed as eaten. They are passed through a mincer. The hydrolysis is performed in presence of glass ball and guar gum (to prevent mechanical alteration of very sensitive starch such as raw potato starch).
- The samples are hydrolyzed with pancreatin, amyloglucosidase and invertase. The pancreatin contains several enzymic activities including α-amylase and proteolytic enzymes which allows the digestion of the digestible material (starch and proteins). In contrast, the lipolytic activity of the pancreatin might be ineffective due to the absence of bile in the medium, into glucose and fructose. The invertase is added in order to hydrolyze all the sucrose present in the sample. The sucrose must then be quantified separately. This step has been introduced in the method because of the presence of an invertase contaminating activity in the amyloglucosidase. This activity could lead to an overestimation of the starch content of the sample.
- The digestible starches (starches hydrolyzed after 20 and 120 min hydrolysis) are quantified on an ethanolic extract (64.4% ethanol). The extract is hydrolyzed into glucose by amyloglucosidase. Then the glucose is quantified using GOD-PAP kit.
- RS content is determined by difference between total starch and digestible starch contents.

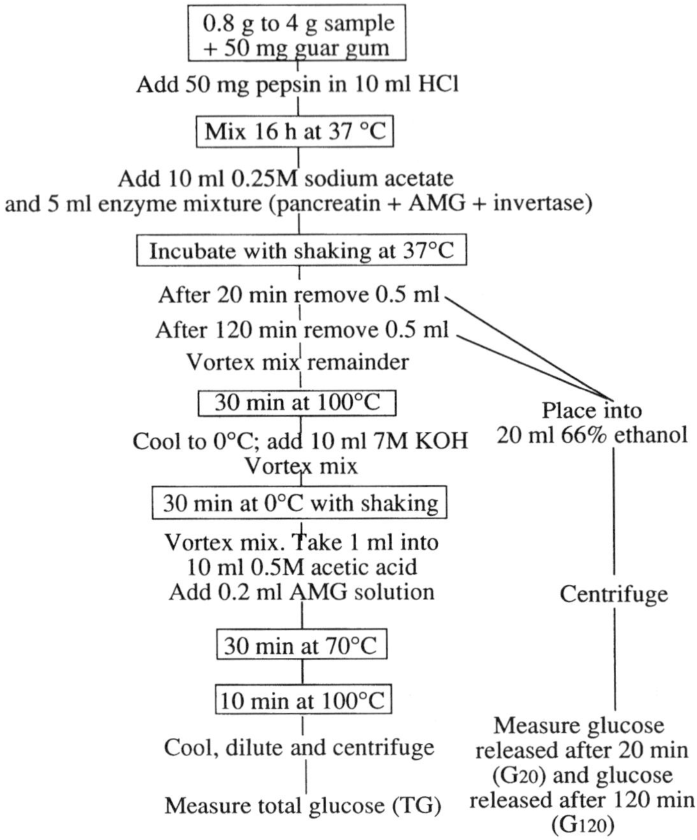

=> Resistant starch = (TG - G_{120}) x 0.9

Figure 3 Determination of resistant starch according to Englyst et al., 1992 (2).

Advantages and Drawbacks

- Optimization of the conditions of hydrolysis
- Adapted to a large variety of substrates
- Long and poor reproducibility without long training
- Need for very specific equipment (mincer, shaking water-baths)
- Enzymes not all commercially available

The Method of Muir & O'Dea, 1992 & 1993 (14, 15)

Principle

The chewed food sample is incubated with pepsin, then hydrolyzed by α-amylase and amyloglucosidase. The insoluble residue represents RS.

Procedure (Figure 4)

Main Characteristics

- The food is first chewed by a volunteer in standardized conditions. The sample weighed for the analysis contains about 100 mg carbohydrate.
- Pepsin, α-amylase and amyloglucosidase are used for the hydrolysis of the digestible fraction of the sample.
- RS is recovered by centrifugation followed by aqueous washing of the pellet.
- Starch in the residue is hydrolyzed into glucose by Termamyl then pancreatin and amyloglucosidase. Dimethylsulfoxide is used prior to the second hydrolysis step to allow a complete dispersion of the RS. Glucose is then quantified using a GOD-PAP kit.

Advantages and Drawbacks

This method has been validated with in vivo studies on ileostomates (15,16). From the 7 comparisons available, it seems satisfactory. No comparison with other in vitro have been published. Being used, until now, only by the authors, difficulties and reproducibility cannot be evaluated.

The Method of Champ et al., 1992 (6)

Principle

In vitro RS was defined as the starch not hydrolyzed by incubation with α-amylase. Hydrolysis products are extracted in 80% ethanol and discarded. RS is then solubilized with 2N KOH and hydrolyzed with amyloglucosidase. In the new procedure, amyloglucosidase is added to the pancreatic α-amylase to avoid inhibition of the amylase by the products of the digestion.

Procedure (Figure 5)

Main Characteristics

- In the first two methods, the sample has to be dried (freeze-dried when possible) and ground into fine particles. In the new procedure, fresh

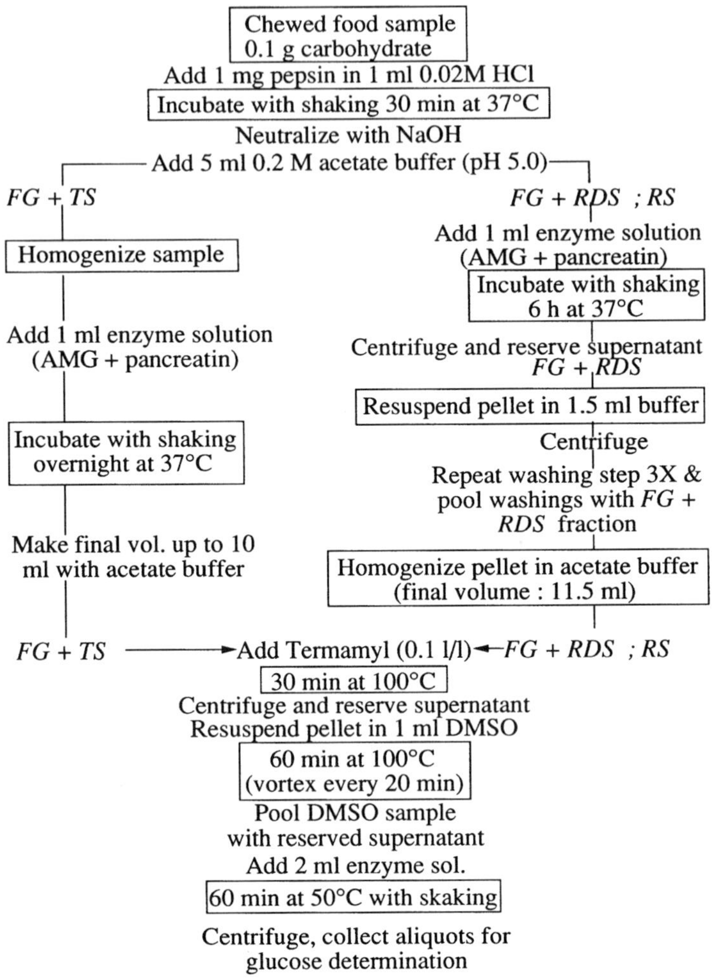

Figure 4 Determination of resistant starch according to Muir & O'Dea (14, 15).

samples can be analyzed after a grinding in a mincer which is supposed to simulate chewing of the food.

- 100 mg of test material are weighed for the analysis, in Faisant et al. (1995)(9). In the new procedure, the sample must be weighed to contain about 50 mg starch.

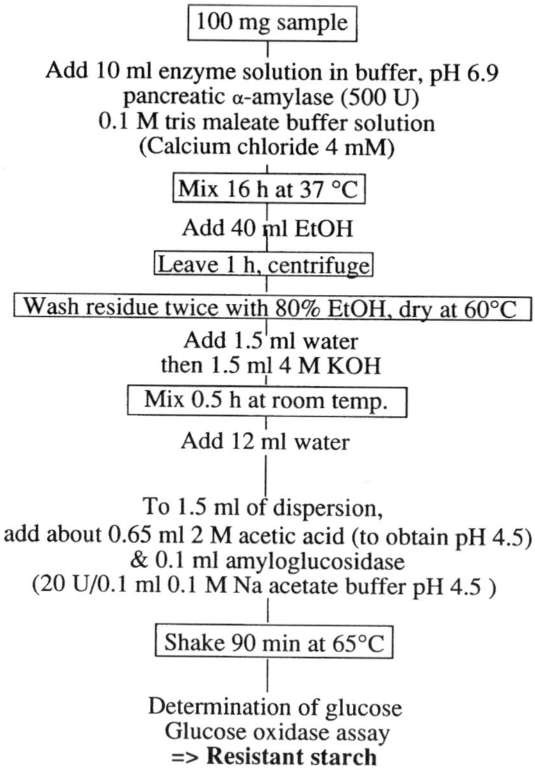

FIGURE 5 Determination of resistant starch according to Champ (1992) (Method A) (From Ref. 6).

- Only pancreatic α-amylase is used for the hydrolysis of the digestible starch in the first two methods whereas amyloglucosidase is introduced in the new method. Sodium azide is used in the last two methods to prevent bacterial proliferation (and degradation) during the overnight hydrolysis.
- RS is recovered by ethanolic precipitation. In Champ method (1992)(6) the precipitate was washed then dried with acetone. The drying has been suppressed in the last two methods.
- RS is then dispersed using potassium hydroxide before the amyloglucosidase hydrolysis into glucose. A first step of gelatinization has been added in the last two methods to facilitate starch dispersion. Glucose is analyzed with GOD-PAP kit.

Advantages and Drawbacks

- Simple and relatively rapid
- Ten samples can easily be analyzed (in duplicates) in a normal day of work

No particular training is needed. The first methods were optimized using values provided by Englyst et al. (2). The new procedure has recently been validated in collaboration with Dr. Langkilde and Prof. H. Andersson using in vivo values obtained from ileostomates. More comparisons will be performed between in vitro and in vivo values.

COMPARISON OF THE MAIN METHODS

Few comparisons have been performed using exactly the same samples. However, one has been published by Champ (6) and Englyst et al. (2) within EURESTA program (Table 2).

As expected, the method of Bjôrck et al. (10) provides the lowest values however the significant underestimation is observed only for native and treated pure starches. Englyst et al. (2) and Champ (6) methods give very similar values. The method modified by Faisant et al. (9) provides a significantly higher value of RS for the raw potato starch. This value is closer to the in vivo value obtained with ileostomates. This was later confirmed by the data published by Langkilde and Andersson (19). The comparison of the new Champ method (Appendix) with Englyst's method has been performed on a sample of fresh and mashed beans. Both methods provided exactly the same result: 7.3 g RS/100 g dry matter.

TABLE 2 Analysis of RS (g/100 g dry matter) in Different Sources of Starch with Different in Vitro Methods

Source of starch	Bjorck et al., 1986	Englyst et al., 1992	Champ, 1992 (method A)	Faisant et al., 1995
Reference	(10)	(2)	(6)	(9)
Potato starch, raw	0.2	64.9	6602	85.3
HACS,[1] raw		68.8		67.3
HACS, retrograde		30.0		35.3
HACS, pregelatinized	9.6	16.3	15.7	
Bean flakes	4.3	5.0	5.0	4.5
Corn flakes	2.3	2.4	2.8	2.8

[1]HACS: High amylose corn starch

TABLE 3 In Vivo Recovery of RS in Nebacitin Treated Rats Compared to In Vitro Values

Source of starch	In vivo	In vitro (10)–(20 meth. C)	Ref.
Peas purée, autoclaved	29.2	23.4–29.0	(20)
Potato purée, autoclaved	4.5	7.0–9.2	(20)
Infant purée, canned	18.1	13.9–17.5	(20)
Dent corn arepas	4.1	4.2	(21)
High amylose arepas	32.5	32.2	(22)
Red bean, precooked flour	10	8.7	(22)
Red bean, coarse precooked flour	8	11.9	(22)
Lentil, precooked flour	11	8.3	(22)

Comparison Between In Vitro and In Vivo Measurements

Some of the in vitro methods have been validated using in vivo data which are in most cases obtained with ileostomates (Tables 2–4). However, Bjôrck and collaborators compared their in vitro values to data obtained in rats (Nebacitin treated rats).

This comparison appears relatively satisfactory. However RS in potato biscuit is probably, as expected, underestimated. It is unexpected not to have the same discrepancy with banana biscuit if it is made from green banana as the main ingredient.

The predicting power of the in vitro method is satisfactory. However a slight discrepancy appears with some of the samples: baked beans, low and high RS meals.

TABLE 4 In Vivo Recovery of RS (g/100 g dry matter) from Different Sources of RS in Ileostomates (from (2))

	Resistant starch		
Source of starch	Fed (g)	Recovered (g)	Mean recovery (%)
Wheat Biscuit	0	0.3	—
Wheat RS Biscuit	8.5	9.0	106
Maize RS Biscuit	8.5	8.6	101
Potato Biscuit	11.7	13.7	117
Banana Biscuit	15	13.7	91

TABLE 5 In Vivo Recovery of RS (g/100 g dry matter) from Different Sources of RS in Ileostomates (from (15) and (16))

	G starch		% RS		
Source of starch	Ingested	Recovered	In vivo	In vitro	Ref.
High RS meal	52.7	19.9	37.8	35.1	(16)
Baked beans	22.7	1.3	5.7	6.9	(15)
Pearl barley	41.0	2.3	5.5	5.5	(15)
Low RS meal	51.8	2.4	4.6	3.1	(16)
Corn flakes	44.1	1.4	3.1	2.9	(15)
Whole rice	48.9	1.5	3.1	2.7	(15)
Ground rice	46.1	0.3	0.7	0.8	(15)

In Vitro Data from Champ and Collaborators and In Vivo Data from Langkilde and Andersson

The new method described in Annex 1 appears to be satisfactory when compared to in vivo data obtained on ileostomates with the same starchy foods (Table 6). However it underestimates the RS values, when compared to data obtained in healthy subjects by the intubation technique, except in the case of canned beans. Indeed, intubation technique always provides higher RS values than the ileostomy model; the exception of canned beans is probably due to a partial collection of the bean residues due to the presence of large particle in the ileum.

TABLE 6 Comparison of Resistant Starch (RS % total starch) Data Determined In Vivo and In Vitro

	In vitro RS			In vivo RS	
Source of starch	Englyst et al., 1992 (2)	Faisant et al., 1995 (9)	Champ et al.	RS	Ref.
Potato starch, raw	66.5	83.0	77.7	78.8	*
HACS,[1] raw	71.4	72.2	52.8	50.3	*
HACS, retrograded	30.5	36.4	29.6	30.1	*
Bean flakes	10.6	12.4	11.2	9–10.9	23
Corn flakes	3.9	4.9	4.3	3.1–5.0	14,2
Beans, raw	17.1		17.1	16.5	4

[1]HACS: High amylose corn starch
*Langkilde et al., personal communication

TABLE 7 RS Content of Some Samples Fed to Antibiotic Treated Rats and Compared with Two In Vitro Methods (g/100 g dry matter) from Different Sources of RS in Ileostomates (from (24))

	Resistant starch (%, dry matter basis)		
		In vitro	
Source of starch	In vivo	Englyst et al., 1992 (2)	Champ, 1992 (6) (method A)
Raw potato starch	45	65	68
Pregelatinized potato starch	1	Nd	Nd
Bean flakes	4	5	5
Raw green banana	4	54	47
Cooked green banana	3	4	5
Raw HACS[1]	37	69	Nd
Extruded retrograded HACS	22	30	29

[1]HACS: High amylose corn starch

The in vitro methods described by Englyst et al. (2) and Champ (6) provide much higher values of RS than the antibiotic treated rat (Table 7).

CONCLUSIONS

Resistant starch, as defined in the physiological definition, is composed of strictly resistant starch but also of potentially digestible fractions. None of the methods presently available have been shown to analyze all RS as defined. However several methods are proposed in the literature, some of them being validated on a quantitative basis with in vivo data obtained from healthy subjects, ileostomates or antibiotic treated rats. Main methods which are validated with digestibility values obtained from human volunteers provided acceptable values but are never exempt of criticism.

The method proposed by Englyst and collaborators has been optimized to be appliable to any food, however it is long and offers a bad reproductibility when technicians don't undergo a specific training.

Muir & O'Dea provided a new method derived from Englyst's method. Unfortunately, until now no comparison with other methods is available and it has not apparently been used outside Australia. The number of comparisons with in vivo data is still too limited to conclude as to its validity.

We suggest the use of our own method (Annex 1) which provides similar values to those obtained with Englyst's method but is much simpler and easy to use. Some comparisons have been performed with in vivo values obtained in ileostomates and in healthy subjects but more comparisons are necessary.

APPENDIX

Analysis of Resistant Starch in Dry and Fresh Samples (Champ et al., New Procedure)

Principle

Resistant starch is the starch not hydrolyzed by pancreatic α-amylase. Hydrolysis products, solubilized in 80% ethanol, are discarded. Resistant starch, present in the pellet, is solubilized in 2N KOH then hydrolyzed into glucose with an amyloglucosidase. Glucose is then quantified with a glucose oxidase/peroxidase analysis kit.

Reagents

- Tris maleate buffer 0.1M pH 5.25 containing $CaCl_2$ 4 mM and sodium azide (0.02%).
- A: 0.2M tris maleic acid (24.2 g of tris hydroxymethylaminomethane and 23.2 g of maleic acid in 1 L)
- B: 0.2M NaOH
- (250 ml of A + 48.5 mL of B) then 588 mg $CaCl_2$, $2H_2O$ and 200 mg NaN_3 diluted with water to 1000 mL final volume
- Pancreatic α-amylase Sigma ref A-3176 (500U)
- 10 mg/mL of tris maleate buffer
- Acetic acid 0.5M, $CaCl_2$, $2H_2O$ 4 mM
- 28.6 mL pure acetic acid and 4 ml $CaCl_2$, $2H_2O$ 1M (1.47 g in 10 mL H_2O) diluted with water to 1000 mL final volume
- Solution of saturated benzoic acid
- 4 g/L filtered at 25°C
- Glucose standard 2.5 mg/mL (2.5 g of anhydrous glucose dehydrated under vacuum) in 1L with 50% saturated benzoic acid solution
- Potassium hydroxide 4M (224.4 g/L)
- Amyloglucosidase Novo Nordisk Bioindustries AMG 400L, 400 AGU/mL
- Sol. 1: 6 AGU/mL. Dilute the enzyme solution: 0.15 mL + 9.85 mL H_2O
- Sol. 2: 14 AGU/mL. Dilute the enzyme solution: 0.14 mL + 3.86 mL H_2O
- GOD-PAP kit Merckotest ref Merck 14365

Method

Determine total starch content of the sample

- Weigh the amount of sample containing 50 mg of starch in centrifugation tubes of 100 mL.
- Add 5.8 mL of tris maleate buffer and 4 mL of enzymatic solution (10 mg of pancreatic α-amylase/mL of buffer) and 0.2 mL amyloglucosidase 6AGU/mL (Sol. 1)
- Mix and incubate in a shaking bath at 37°C during 16 h.
- Add 40 mL absolute ethanol, mix and leave 1 h at ambiant temperature.
- Centrifuge 10 min at 3000 g.
- Discard the supernatant and rinse the pellet with 10 mL 80% ethanol, centrifuge and discard the supernatant (twice).
- Collect the pellet with 10 mL H_2O.
- Leave in a shaking bath during 30 min.
- Cool in ice.
- Add 10 mL KOH 4M and shake under magnetic shaking at 0°C during 30 min.
- Transfer 1 mL in 10 mL acetic acid solution 0.5M containing $CaCl_2$ and add 0.2 mL amyloglucosidase 14 AGU/mL (Sol. 2).
- Incubate 30 min in a bath at 70°C then 10 min at 100°C.
- Cool
- Neutralize with 0.6 mL KOH 4M.
- Centrifuge 10 min at 4000*g*
- Collect 0.1 mL of supernatant in 2 mL of GOD-PAP reactant.
- Shake, leave 20 min at 37°C and read the absorbance at 510 nm.
- In parallel, prepare 2 glucose standards and 2 enzyme blanks in the same conditions: 0.5 mL of glucose standard or 0.5 mL H_2O diluted in a same volume of 4M KOH are transferred to tubes containing 10 mM acetic acid solution, incubate 30 min at 70°C then 10 min at 100°C, cool, neutralize, centrifuge and then analyze the glucose as previously described.
- The samples are analyzed in duplicates.

Calculation

Resistant starch % of the dry matter = Ae*Vt*C*D*0.9/(Ast*We)
Ae = Absorbance of the sample corrected from the absorbance of the enzyme blank
Vt = Volume of the test (10)
D = Dilution factor
C = Concentration in mg/mL of glucose standard (2.5)

Ast = Absorbance of the standard corrected from the absorbance of the enzyme blank and diluted like the sample
We = Weight of dry sample in mg
0.9 is the correction factor glucose → starch

Remark

Fresh samples like canned lentils or beans or cooked pasta have to be passed through a mincer (Plate of 9 mm diam. holes) before weighing (equivalent of 50 mg starch).

REFERENCES

1. Asp, N. G. (1992) Eur. J. Clin. Nutr. 46(S2), S1.
2. Englyst, H. N., Kingman, S. M., Cummings, J. H. (1992) Eur. J. Clin. Nutr. 46(S2), S33–S50.
3. Englyst, H. N., Cummings, J. H. (1987) Am. J. Clin. Nutr. 45, 423–431.
4. Noah, L., Guillon, F., Bouchet, B., Bulon, A., Gallant, D. J., Colonna, P., Molis, C., Faisant, N., Galmiche, J. P., Champ, M. (1995) in Proc. Eur. Assoc. for Grain Legume Research Conf. July 9–13, pp. 276–277.
5. Faisant, N., Bulon, A., Colonna, P., Molis, C., Lartigue, S., Galmiche, J. P., Champ, M. (1995) Br. J. Nutr. 73, 111–123.
6. Champ, M. (1992) Eur. J. Clin. Nutr. 46(S2), S51–62.
7. Faisant, N., Champ, M., Colonna, P., Bulon, A. (1993) Carboh. Polym. 21, 205–209.
8. Faisant, N., Champ, M., Colonna, P., Bulon, A., Molis, C., Langkilde, A. M., Schweizer, T., Flouri, B., Galmiche, J. P. (1993) Eur. J. Clin. Nutr. 47, 285–296.
9. Faisant, N., Planchot V., Kozlowski F., Pacouret, M. P., Colonna, P., Champ, M. (1995) Sci. Alim. 15, 83–89.
10. Bjôrck, I., Nyman, M., Pedersen, B., Siljestrsvm, M., Asp, N. G., Eggum, B. O. (1986) J. Cereal Sci. 4, 1–11.
11. Asp, N. G., Johansson C. G., Hallmer, H., Siljestrsvm, M. (1983) J. Agric. Fd Chem. 31, 476–482.
12. Prosky, L., Asp, N. G., Schweizer T. F., De Vries, J. W., & Furda, I. (1988) J. Ass. Off. Analyt. Chem. 71, 1017–1023.
13. Bjôrck, I., Asp, N. G. (1991) in Methodological aspects of in vivo methods for measurement of starch digestibility, E. Gudmand-Hoyer (Ed), European Flair-Concerted Action on Resistant Starch–Contract No. AGRF/OO27, pp. 35–39.
14. Muir, J. G., O'Dea K. (1992) Am. J. Clin. Nutr. 56, 123–127.
15. Muir, J. G., O'Dea K. (1993) Am. J. Clin. Nutr. 57, 540–546.
16. Muir, J. G., Birkett A., Brown, I., Jones, G., O'Dea, K. (1995) Am. J. Clin. Nutr. 61, 82–89.
17. Englyst, H. N., Wiggins, H. S., Cummings, J. H. (1982) Analyst 107, 307–318.
18. Berry, C. S. (1986) J. Cereal Sci. 4, 301–314.
19. Langkilde, A. M., Andersson, H. (1995) in Proceedings of the concluding plenary

meeting of EURESTA, N.G. Asp, J. M. M. van Amelsvoort & J. G. A. J. Hautvast (Eds), European Flair-Concerted Action on Resistant Starch–No. 11 (COST 911), pp. 31–32.
20. Bjôrck, I., Siljestrôm, M. (1992) J. Sci. Food Agric. 58, 541–553.
21. Granfeldt, Y., Drews, A., Bjôrck, I. (1993) J. Nutr. 123, 1676–1684.
22. Tovar, J., Bjôrck, I.M., Asp, N.G. (1992) J. Nutr. 122, 1500–1507.
23. Schweizer, T. F., Andersson, H., Langkilde A. M., Reimann, S., Torsdottir, I. (1990) Eur. J. Clin. Nutr. 44, 567–575.
24. Ekwall, H., Bjôrck, I., Asp, N. G. (1995) in Proceedings of the concluding plenary meeting of EURESTA, N. G. Asp, J. M. M. van Amelsvoort & J. G. A. J. Hautvast (Eds), European Flair-Concerted Action on Resistant Starch–No. 11 (COST 911), pp. 105–107.

IV

RESISTANT OLIGOSACCHARIDES—ANALYTICAL METHODOLOGY

15

A Sensitive and Reproducible Analytical Method to Measure Fructooligosaccharides in Food Products

F. Ouarne and A. Guibert
Béghin-Say, INSA, Toulouse, France

D. Brown
Golden Technologies Co., Johnstown, Colorado

F. Bornet
Eridania Béghin-Say, Vilvoorde Research and Development Centre, Vilvoorde, Belgium

INTRODUCTION

Short-chain fructooligosaccharides (DP5) (Actilight®, Nutraflora®) are undigestible oligosaccharides industrially produced from sucrose. A recent survey (1) was conducted to get the views of professionals in the field concerning the definition of dietary fibers (DF). The majority felt that the definition of DF should be revised to include oligosaccharides which are resistant to hydrolysis by the alimentary tract. The AOAC DF analytical method does not measure short-chain fructooligosaccharides (FOS) because of their ethanol/water mixture solubility.

In order to overcome this problem, we developed an analytical method to measure short-chain FOS in food products (small cakes, dairy products). This method is based on an extraction step, followed by anion exchange liquid chromatography (Dionex) associated with an hydrolysis step using invertase. This method has been applied to two types of small cake and three dairy products. In all cases 100% of added FOS has been recovered and measured. The results demonstrated the validity and reliability of the method for determining FOS in food products.

Fructooligosaccharides are naturally occurring molecules present in numerous edible plants. For example, they have been found in asparagus (2), banana (3) and onion (4). With a polymerization degree lower than 5, FOS are composed of one sucrose molecule to which is bound one to three fructose molecules. The resulting compounds are 1-kestose or GF2, nystose or GF3, and fructosylnystose or GF4. The production of these FOS from sucrose is protected by patents owned by the Japanese company Meiji Seika Kaisha. In Europe, these patents are exploited through a Béghin-Say-Meiji Seika Kaisha joint-venture: Béghin-Meiji-Industries.

The commercialization of such a new ingredient for human food involves the investigation of its nutritional properties. First of all, in vitro studies incubating FOS with human saliva, rat pancreas homogenates, rat and rabbit intestine mucosa (5), purified sucrase, α-amylase and isomaltase (3) have demonstrated that FOS are not hydrolyzed by digestive enzymes.

We did complementary in vitro and in vivo studies on humans (from stomach to stools). The first in vitro study showed the stability of FOS incubated with human gastric juice (personnal communication). The second in vitro study showed the stability of FOS incubated with small intestine mucosa (6). The third study, in vivo, concerning the adsorption of FOS along the small intestine, showed the non-adsorption in this part of the intestine and allowed us to determine the energy value of FOS: 2 Kcal/g.

In another we have demonstrated that FOS were fermented preferentially by bifidobacterium microflora and thus increased this population as well as the fructooligohydrolase activity of stools.

Therefore FOS, like dietary fibers, enter the large intestine without any change in their structure. At this stage, they are totally fermented by the resident microflora and not directly used as an energy source.

As a conclusion of all these studies, in 1994, the French "Conseil Supérieur d'Hygiène Publique" (Council for Public Health) admitted for the first time a functional claim for a food ingredient. Industrial users can now claim the stimulating effect of FOS on the growth of bifidobacteria microflora in the human colon. It must be noted that the use of this claim is limited to G(F)n type molecules for which n is lower than 4.

Furthermore, a recent survey by Lee and Prosky (1) in 1995 conducted to obtain the view of professionnals concerning the definition of dietary fibers supports that dietary fibers should be re-defined to include short chain FOS resistant to hydrolysis by the alimentary tract.

The AOAC procedure for the determination of total dietary fiber involves three enzymatic digestion steps with (α-amylase, protease and amyloglucosidase.

These enzymatic treatments do not modify the FOS structure. The obtained solution then undergoes an ethanol precipitation. Only the resulting precipitate is used for the determination of total dietary fibers with the AOAC method. FOS are soluble in an ethanol/water mixture, and because of this, the AOAC dietary fiber analytical method does not measure short chain FOS.

This is why we needed to develop an analytical method to measure short chain FOS in food products. Our aim was to determine the validity and the repeatability of a method to quantify FOS in dairy products and cakes.

MATERIALS AND METHODS

Products

The concentrations of FOS which were determined in food products came from the Actilight* P powder which had a mass composition of quantifiable sugars as follows: glucose (G) 1.0%, fructose (F) 0.8%, sucrose (GF) 3.3%, GF2 38.8%, GF3 46.6% and GF4 9.5%.

Food Products

A Danone plain yogurt
Composition: milk of 13 g fat per liter, powder skimmed milk, yogurt starters. Mean nutritional value per 100 g: proteins 4.4 g, lipids 1.2 g, glucides 6.4 g, calcium 164 mg, sodium 57 mg, potassium 210 mg, phosphorus 114 mg.

A Danone Bio yogurt
''Plain fermented milk with active bifidus''. Composition: milk of 3.5% fat per liter, powder skimmed milk, Bifidobacterium (ACTIVE BIFIDUS). Mean nutritional value per 100 g: proteins 4.5 g, lipids 4.4 g, glucides 6.5 g, calcium 166 mg.

A Lactel fruit yogurt (strawberry)
Composition: full fat milk, sugar (11.5%), strawberry (8%), powder skimmed

milk, selected yogurt starters. Mean nutritional value per 100 g: proteins 3.4 g, lipids 2.6 g, glucides 15.4 g, calcium 129 mg.

A LU ''Petit Brun Extra'' biscuit
Composition: wheat flour, sugar, vegetable fat, invert sugar, powder skimmed milk, baking powder, salt, artificial aroma, antioxidant.

A J. PASQUIER Pâtissier ''Madeleine Superstar'' small cake
Composition: wheat flour, egg, sugar, butter, stabilizing agent E420, glucose, powder skimmed milk, baking powder, salt, artificial aroma.

Sample Preparation

The product was diluted 5 times (Md: final mass of dilute yogurt) with a solution of Actilight P (final concentration of approximately 1.5 g FOS per 100 g yogurt and 20 g FOS per 100 g bakery product). The suspension thus obtained was homogenized 5 min at 4°C with a high speed mixer (Ultraturax: Labortechnik, Saufer, Germany). Aliquots were taken (10 aliquots of a known mass Mk of approximately 10 g) and centrifuged 20 min, 2500 *g* at 4°C. A known volume, Vs, was filtered on a 0.45 μm porous filter, ultrafiltered by centrifuging 25 min at 2500 *g* on a 30 kD porous membrane (Microsep, Filtron, Northborough, MA), diluted, and then analyzed by anion exchange chromatography (Dionex). The pellet was weighed and dried in order to determine the volume (Vp) of liquid it contained.

Determination of Recovery of FOS Contained in Yogurt

The quantity of FOS determined is calculated as follows:

$$\text{FOS quantity in g} = C(Vs + Vp)(Md/Mk)$$

where

- C = FOS concentration in sample (g/L), determined by anion exchange chromatography
- Vs = volume of supernatant (L)
- Vp = volume of liquid in pellet (L)
- Md = mass of dilute yogurt (g)
- Mk = sample known mass (g)

The recovery corresponds to 100 times the ratio of the amount of FOS determined to the amount of FOS added to the yogurt.

Validity of the Analysis

To establish the sugar composition of products without FOS addition, they were diluted 5 times with ultra pure water. The suspension thus obtained was treated and analyzed as previously described.

To determine the nature of the oligosaccharides present in FOS containing samples, the supernatants obtained during sugar extraction were incubated 6 hours at 40°C in the presence of invertase (Max Invert, Gist Brocade, Delft, Netherlands, final activity: 1326 U/L reaction medium). One U of invertase activity was defined as the amount of enzyme which produced one mole of fructose per min at 60°C in a 0.5 mol/L sucrose solution in 0.1 mol/L acetate buffer at pH 4.5.

Invertase is an enzyme hydrolyzing the $\beta 1 \rightarrow 2$ linkage between glucose and fructose in sucrose, as well as the $\beta 1 \rightarrow 2$ linkages between fructoses in FOS. This step allows us to confirm the results of the direct analysis, by comparing them to the amount of glucose and fructose produced during hydrolysis. The solutions obtained before and after treatment by invertase were injected directly on the Dionex Ion Chromatograph.

Analysis of the Products by Dionex Ion Chromatograph

Principle of the Determination of Sugars by Dionex Ion Chromatograph

The determination of sugars was carried out on a Dionex (Sunnyvale, Ca, USA) chromatograph equipped with a gradient pump, a degas module and a pulsed amperometric detector (p.a.d.). The column used was a Dionex, Carbopac TM PA1 (4 × 250 mm) with a precolumn Carbopac PA (3 × 25 mm). The p.a.d. sensitivity was set at 3K. Results were recorded on a Hewlett-Packard H.P. 3365 integrator, series II. The volume of the injection loop was 25 μL. Detection was performed by a gold electrode under three alternating potentials. The values and duration of these potentials are: $E1 = 0.05$ V, $t1 = 480$ ms; $E2 = 0.65$ V, $t2 = 120$ ms; $E3 = -0.65$ V and $t3 = 60$ ms, respectively. The elution gradient was established by combining an eluent A (NaOH 150 mM) with an eluent B (NaOH 150 mM, NaOAc 600 mM). In the course of the analysis, sodium acetate concentration varied from 6 to 180 mM in 20 min with a constant flow rate of 1 mL/min. Eluents were prepared with ultra pure water which had been degassed by sparging with helium. Under these conditions, it was possible to separate all the products contained in Actilight*950P.

Calibration of the Pulsed Amperometric Response

FOS standard solutions were prepared from purified standards. Quantities of 300 μL were injected with a Spectra Physics SP8875 autosampler. A linear response was obtained on the integrator for concentration values ranging from 0.15 to 70 mg/L. The lower detection limit was based on a peak height at least three times that of the background noise.

RESULTS AND DISCUSSION

Validity of the Method and Determination of the Recovery

In order to establish the sugar composition of the control dairy products, a sample of each yogurt without FOS addition was treated and analyzed as previously described.

For all yogurts, the determination showed only a simple sugar, galactose, and a disaccharide, lactose. The retention times of these sugars differed from those of FOS and therefore should not interfere with the determination of FOS in yogurt.

Inversely, the determination of sugars in the control cake with no FOS addition showed two simple sugars, glucose and fructose, one disaccharide, sucrose, and two starch residues, Rs1 and Rs2, the retention times of which correspond respectively to those of GF2 and GF3 peaks (Figure 1).

As can be seen in Figure 2, the H.P.L.C. analysis of the supernatant of a

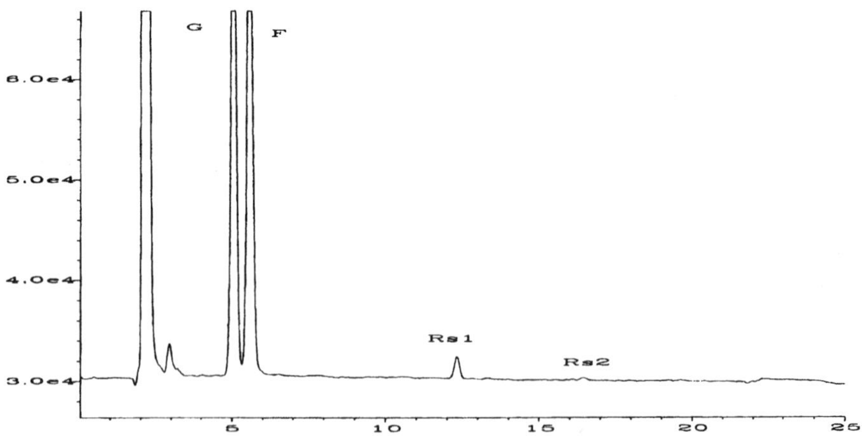

FIGURE 1 Determination of sugars in the control cake before FOS addition.

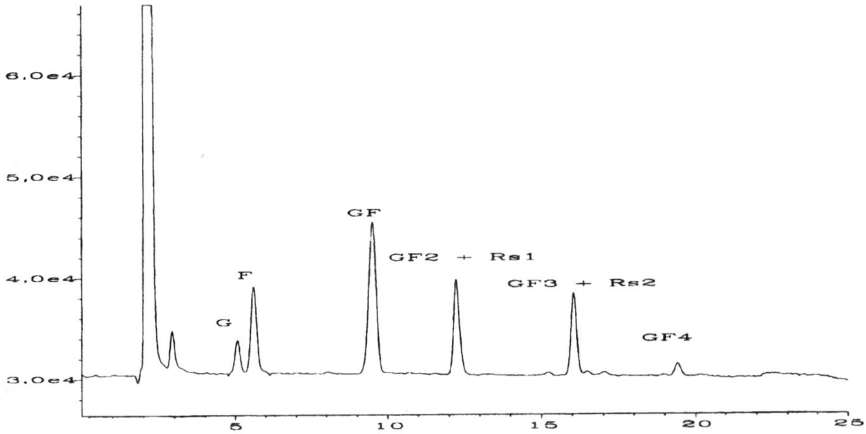

FIGURE 2 Determination of sugars in a small cake after FOS addition.

small cake (J. Pasquier pâtissier ''madeleine superstar'') after FOS addition showed glucose (G), fructose (F), sucrose (GF), GF2, GF3 and Rs1 and Rs2.

To investigate the nature of the oligosaccharides present in cakes containing FOS, the supernatants obtained during sugar extraction were incubated in the presence of invertase.

After the invertase action (Figure 3) the disappearance of oligosaccharides can be observed, correlated to an increase in glucose and fructose concentrations. On the other hand, Rs1 and Rs2 were not hydrolyzed, and appear on the chromatogram. If the specific areas of GF2 and GF3 were related to Rs1 and Rs2, respectively, the theoretical concentrations of these sugars in the supernatants analyzed could then be determined. The theoretical amounts (in g) of Rs1 and Rs2 in cakes can be calculated from the chromatogram corresponding to Figure 3. The recovery is then calculated as follows:

$$\frac{[(GF2 + RS1) - RS1] + [(GF3 + RS2) - RS2] + GF4}{(GF2i + GF3i + GF4i)} \times 100$$

where:

- GF2i = quantity (in g) of GF2 introduced in cake
- GF3i = quantity (in g) of GF3 introduced in cake
- GF4i = quantity (in g) of GF4 introduced in cake
- GF2 + RS1 = quantity (in g) of GF2 + RS1 determined in cake containing FOS

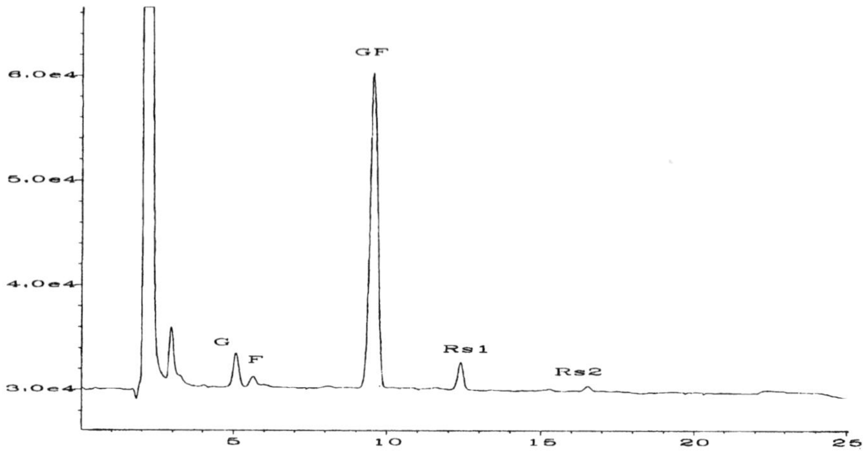

FIGURE 3 Determination of sugars in a supernatant of a small cake after invertase addition.

- GF3 + RS2 = quantity (in g) of GF3 + RS2 determined in cake containing FOS
- RS1 = quantity (in g) of RS1 determined in control cake without FOS
- RS2 = quantity (in g) of RS2 determined in control cake without FOS

With the invertase treatment, sucrose and FOS could be specifically hydrolyzed and the recovery of fructooligosaccharides calculated. The results obtained during direct analysis could also be verified by measurement of the glucose and fructose produced during hydrolysis (Table 1). Indeed, a quantitative study

TABLE 1 Sugar Concentrations in a Small Cake After FOS Addition

Calculated sugar concentration before inverse hydrolysis:								
Sugars	G	F	GF	GF2 + RS1	GF3 + RS2	GF4	Total glucose	Total fructose
g/L	2.3	7.6	38	11	12.1	3.2		
mM	13.3	42.2	111	21.8	18.2	3.9	168.2	267.3

Concentration of glucose and fructose produced during the hydrolysis step:		
Sugars	G	F
g/L	30.4	47.221
mM	168.7	261.9

demonstrated a direct correlation between the concentrations of FOS analyzed, and the quantities of glucose and fructose produced (Table 1).

The results demonstrated with certainty the validity of the method for determining FOS levels in cakes.

Recovery of FOS in Food Products

The final FOS concentration studied was 1.5 g fructooligosaccharide per 100 g of yogurt. The extraction rates of FOS are listed in the table. As can be seen, for each sample, the study of the repeatability of the extraction method was done by treating each sample ten times. For plain yogurt, the mean recovery is equal to 99.7% of initial FOS, with a standard deviation of 1.9%. The recovery of FOS from Bio yogurt is equal to 99.2% of initial FOS with a standard deviation of 2.4%. For fruit yogurt, the mean extraction rate is equal to 99.2% of initial FOS with a standard deviation of 1.3%. The results obtained for cakes can be observed in Table 3. Here, the final fructooligosaccharide concentration studied was 20 g FOS per 100 g of cake.

We studied the repeatability of the extraction method in the same way as for dairy products. For cookies ''Petit Brun'' LU, the mean recovery was 100.9% of the initial FOS with a standard deviation of 1.5%. For J. Pasquier pâtissier ''Madeleine Superstar'' cakes, the mean recovery was 99.7% of the initial fructooligosaccharide with a standard deviation of 1.1%.

The results obtained for yogurts can be observed in Table 2.

TABLE 2 Recovery of FOS Contained in Dairy Products

	Recovery of FOS in dairy products (%)		
Extraction	Plain yogurt	Bio yogurt	Fruit yogurt
1	97.4	100.4	101.1
2	99.1	102.6	99.9
3	97.6	97.8	100.4
4	98.0	97.5	99.7
5	100.3	102.1	100.0
6	103.9	98.1	97.7
7	100.9	99.8	99.0
8	99.8	94.4	100.0
9	98.9	98.4	98.3
10	101.2	101.4	96.4
Average	99.7	99.2	99.2
Standard deviation	1.9	2.4	1.3

TABLE 3 Recovery of FOS Contained in Bakery Products

	Recovery of FOS in cookies and small cakes (%)	
Extraction	Petit brun	Madeleine superstar
1	100.8	100.1
2	103.5	100.6
3	100.1	98.8
4	102.3	100.6
5	100.7	100.9
6	101.8	97.2
7	99.1	100.2
8	98.4	99.5
9	99.6	NA
10	102.5	NA
Average	100.9	99.7
SD	1.5	1.1

Sensitivity of the Method for Determining FOS in Cakes and Dairy Products

With the defined experimental protocol and with the sensitivity of the H.P.L.C. method used, the detection limit of quantifiable FOS is 0.04 g per 100 g of yogurt and 0.75 g per 100 g of cake. However, in these conditions, in cakes there is an excess of maltooligosaccharides in relation to FOS. In such a product, we introduced the extra step of hydrolysis of the maltooligosaccharides with α-glucosidase, followed by hydrolysis with invertase.

CONCLUSION

From the results of our work, we believe a valid, sensitive method, with good repeatability, has been established for the analysis of FOS in small cakes and dairy products. The methodology involves the analysis of the original product with the Dionex Ion Chromatograph, followed by analysis of the product after hydrolysis with invertase.

It should be a complementary method to the AOAC procedure for the determination of total dietary fibers, which does not take into account the water/ethanol soluble fibers such as short chain FOS.

REFERENCES

1. Lee S. S. & Prosky L. (1995) J. of AOAC, Vol. 78, 22–36.
2. Cairns A. J. (1992) New Phytol., 120, 463–473.
3. Fishbein L., Kaplan M. & Gough M. (1988) Vet. Mum Toxicol., 30(2), April, 105–107.
4. Shiomi N. (1978) Jour. Facul. Agri., Hokkaido Univ., Sapporo, 58, pt 4.
5. Oku T., Tokunaga T. & Hosoya N. (1984) J. Nut., 114, 1574–1581.

16

Inulin and Oligofructose as Dietary Fiber: Analytical, Nutritional and Legal Aspects

Paul Coussement
ORAFTI, Tienen, Belgium

INTRODUCTION

Inulin is a mixture of molecules with general structure GFn, in which G = glucose, F = fructose and n = number of fructosyl moieties linked by a β(2-1) bond. Oligofructose may contain both Fn-type and GFn-type molecules with a DP lower than 10. Both inulin and oligofructose are fructans.

Both inulin and oligofructose occur naturally in significant amounts in common vegetables and cereals. Inulin (Raftiline®) and oligofructose (Raftilose®) are used as food ingredients by the food industry for a variety of applications.

Both ingredients are metabolized in the same way as dietary fibers are and show significant 'dietary fiber' effects. Inulin and oligofructose have already been confirmed by the legal authorities in many countries as 'dietary fibers' for food labeling purposes.

The classical methods of analysis for dietary fibre cannot determine inulin or oligofructose accurately or reliably. Therefore, a modification of the AOAC method was elaborated. This was based on the use of a specific inulinase enzyme, resulting in the total elimination of all fructans from the AOAC TDF determination.

An overview of analytical methods that can be used for the determination of fructans is presented. The general method which can be used in all circumstances can be called the 'inulinase method for fructan determination'.

INULIN AND OLIGOFRUCTOSE

Inulin is a natural constituent of many common vegetables and cereals: for example onions, garlic, artichokes, leek, asparagus and wheat all contain significant amounts of inulin (Table 1). As a consequence, the daily consumption of inulin has been estimated to be a few grams per day (1).

Chemically speaking, inulin is a mixture of poly- and oligosaccharides which almost all have the chemical structure GFn (G = glucose, F = fructose and n = number of fructose units linked to one another). The links between the molecules are of a very special type: the β(2-1) form (2), which makes these molecules indigestible for all higher animals.

The degree of polymerization (DP) of inulin is variable: it is a function of many factors such as the source from which it was extracted, the climate and growing conditions, the harvesting time and storage conditions (1). Table 2 gives an overview of a number of inulin compositions. This makes clear that the DP range and distribution of inulin can be variable, which makes its analytical determination more complicated.

The commercial inulin is obtained by hot water extraction from chicory

TABLE 1 Natural Occurrence of Inulin and Oligofructose

Source	Inulin (%)	Oligofructose (%)
Wheat	1–6	1–4
Onion	2–10	2–6
Leek	3–16	2–5
Garlic	9–11	3–6
Salsify	4–10	2–5
Artichoke	2–9	<1
Asparagus shoot	1–4	2–3
Banana	0.3–0.7	0.3–0.7
Jerusalem artichoke	16–20	16–20
Murnong	8–13	
Yacon	3–19	
Chicory	15–20	5–10

TABLE 2 Overview of a Number of Inulin Compositions

Substance	Basic structure	DP range	DP	DP < 10 (%)	DP < 20 (%)	F/G ratio
Oligofructose	GFn	3–10	~4	100	100	3–40
	Fn	2–10		100	100	
Inulin						
Chicory	GFn	3–60	~10	~30	55	~9
Topinambour		3–50	~6*	50	75	~5*
Onion		3–12	~4*	100	100*	~3*
Artichoke		3–200	~40*	0*	0*	~40*
As in Raftiline®ST		3–60	~10	30	55	~9
As in Raftiline®HP		6–60	~25	~10	~45	~25

*Estimations

roots. It exists in five different forms. Each of these forms was specifically developed to suit a particular end use.

Oligofructose is the common (labeling) name for fructooligosaccharides. Their chemical composition is noted as Fn, indicating n fructose units linked by β(2-1) linkages. Molecules with the structure GFn are also commonly considered as fructooligosaccharides or oligofructose. Depending on the definition of 'oligosaccharides' that one accepts, their DP can go up to 10 or 20.

Oligofructose obtained commercially by enzymatic hydrolysis from inulin (Raftilose®) has a DP range as indicated in Table 2. It is a mixture of GFn and Fn molecules where the F/G ratio may vary between 3 and 40. Oligofructose obtained by enzymatic synthesis from sucrose contains mainly GFn molecules within the same DP range and with low F/G ratios. Both inulin and oligofructose are 'fructans', which are defined as β(2-1) linked fructose polymers and oligomers (1).

Raftiline® and Raftilose® are recognized, confirmed and used as 'food ingredients' (not as food additives) in most industrialized countries in a variety of food products, with the dairy sector as their most successful field of application.

INULIN AND OLIGOFRUCTOSE: DIETARY FIBERS

In this chapter, I would summarize that both inulin and oligofructose are indigestible, have significant 'dietary fiber effects' often comparable to pectins, are carbohydrates of plant origin, naturally occurring in significant amounts and show beneficial effects on the gut flora. For these properties, no significant differences have been found between inulin and oligofructose.

Consequently it cannot be considered 'misleading' to the consumer to present inulin and oligofructose as dietary fiber for labeling purposes from a nutritional viewpoint. This classification has been proposed by many authors (3–9).

Often it is questioned whether indigestible oligosaccharides should not be excluded from the dietary fiber group. The 'cutting point' could lie at DP = 10. However such a distinction would be very artificial. There are no nutritional grounds which would allow one to state that oligosaccharides with a DP of 9 would not be fibers, while those with the same structure but a DP of 11 would. Dietary fiber effects are not limited by the DP of the molecules.

It is hard to sustain that oligosaccharides should be excluded for historical reasons. Nutritional knowledge and progress should never be fixed by historical findings. Also, the first scientists who identified a food fraction which they called 'dietary fiber' characterized it as 'polysaccharides' indeed. This characterization was probably meant to describe the fraction, and not to exclude the oligosaccharide fraction which they most probably were not aware of. Moreover, even Trowell and Burkitt included oligosaccharides in the DF definition (10).

Some people believe oligosaccharides should be excluded from the dietary fiber fraction because of an assumed laxative effect. It is obvious that the borderline DP of 10 is not determining a laxative potential. Normal doses of non-digestible oligosaccharides cause no laxative effects, as is witnessed by already more than 150 commercial products containing inulin and oligofructose on the market. And after all, is the laxative effect not an inherent property of dietary fiber?

LEGAL STATUS

Inulin (Raftiline®) and oligofructose (Raftilose®) are confirmed as food ingredients, not food additives, in most industrialized countries. In the U.S.A., they were determined generally recognized as safe (GRAS) by a panel of experts. In Europe, the nutrition labeling system is not clear at all for dietary fibre. The absence of a definition for dietary fibre has created a legal grey zone.

By the end of 1994, the Scientific Committee for Foods of the European Commission rejected a report that proposed dietary fibre to be defined as 'Non-Starch Polysaccharides of the Cell Wall', and admitted it could not come to a consensus on the matter. As a consequence, the Standing Committee for Foodstuffs decided that AOAC methods 985.29 (Prosky) and 991.43 (Lee) and Englyst methods could be used for food labeling purposes, at there may be also other substances that can be considered as dietary fiber which have to be measured by other methods (11). This position is not final and not even very useful directly, but it allows the European member states to create their own guidelines for the food industry.

Some EU member states (Belgium, Germany, Italy) have legal definitions which include inulin and oligofructose. In the United Kingdom, inulin was al-

TABLE 3 Recovery by Dietary Fiber (DF) Methods

Sample	AOAC 991.43 Range (%)	AOAC 991.43 Average (%)	Englyst Range (%)	Englyst Average (%)
Oligofructose, all concntrt.	0	0	0	0
Raftilin®ST, pure	7–17	14	1.6–1.8	1.7
Raftilin®HP, pure	48–74	54	22.8–23.2	24
Raftilin®ST, 10% in foods	2–15	10	NA	NA
Raftilin®HP, 10% in foods	10–45	30	NA	NA

ready classified as a non-starch polysaccharide, thus accepting it as dietary fiber (3). Other countries are preparing new definitions which will include these fructans (the Netherlands). Denmark has confirmed that inulin and oligofructose are DF after evaluation. In France, the Superior Health Counsel has done the same. Similar evaluation processes are now going on in Spain, Ireland, the United States, Canada, Australia and other countries. We believe we are slowly growing towards a large legal acceptance of inulin and oligofructose as dietary fibers for labeling purposes.

FRUCTANS: RECOVERY BY DF METHODS

Using the classical AOAC or Englyst methods for analysis of dietary fiber (DF), it is impossible to detect oligofructose (12) (Table 3). For inulin, the results can vary considerably in function of the food sample composition and the lab. Figure 1 illustrates the range of results obtained for the same sample by a small number

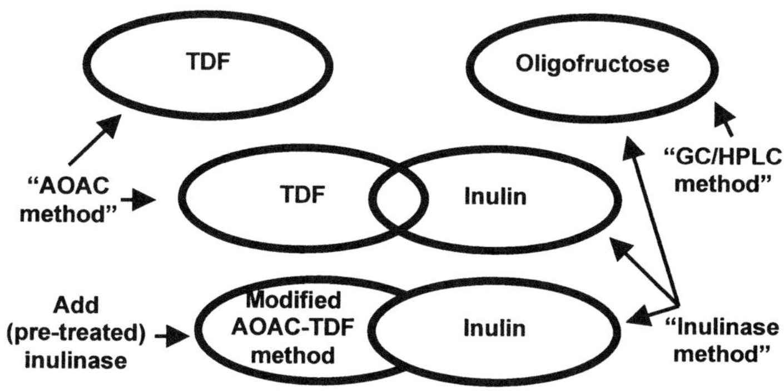

FIGURE 1 Recovery by dietary fiber (DF) methods

of labs in a short test (unpublished results). It is clear from these results that, for the pure standard inulin, both methods do detect some inulin. However these results are very unreliable and the fraction recovered is too low.

For pure inulin, in which part of the smaller molecules are removed, the recovery can be significantly higher but is never complete. These results are even worse when concentrations of 10% or lower in real foodstuffs are measured.

Consequently, it is clear that the existing methods for DF analysis do not determine inulin or oligofructose. Also, it can be concluded that these methods will give unreliable results for the total DF fraction when used for foodstuffs which contain significant amounts of inulin (1).

MODIFIED AOAC METHOD

We have tested several modifications to the existing AOAC methods for DF in order to increase the recovery of inulin and oligofructose. Although it is possible to increase the inulin recovery by small modifications, it was not possible to us to improve the oligofructose recovery. Moreover, we assumed that any modification of the AOAC method would have negative influences on the accuracy of the method as a whole.

Therefore, another approach was necessary. We found that it was possible to modify the AOAC method 991.43 (Lee et al., Ref. 12) in such a way that no more inulin or oligofructose was recovered, without affecting the recovery of the 'other fibers'. The remaining problem is then only, to have an accurate method for the fructans (Figure 2).

The modification consists of the addition of an inulinase enzyme to the amyloglucosidase treatment (13). This inulinase removes the fructans from the sample right from the start. A slight pectinase side-activity of the inulinase can

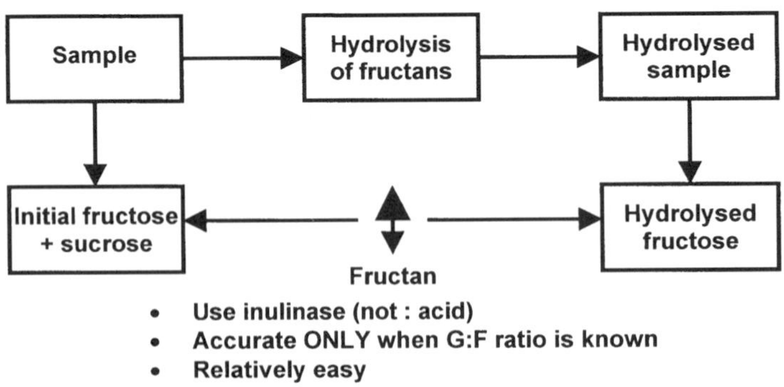

FIGURE 2 Fructose determination method

be depressed by a temperature treatment of the inulinase enzyme (INRA Nantes, unpublished results).

Different methods can be used to measure fructans, as will be summarized in the next chapter. The final method was optimized both by INRA Nantes (F) and Institut Meurice (B) and is presented by Dr. Dysseler.

ANALYTICAL METHODS: AN OVERVIEW

In this chapter, we will shortly list available methods with their advantages and disadvantages.

Direct HPLC

Direct HPLC (2) can be used reliably for quantitative determination of oligofructose, but not for inulin except for pure samples. The procedures are relatively simple and straightforward. The DP information is not very reliable: peaks do not represent one single DP fraction (example: the F4 fraction mixes with the GF2 fraction) and from DP 4 the accuracy and separation are low. There can be significant interferences with other oligosaccharides (maltodextrins, galactooligosaccharides, others) and other organic components.

Direct GC

Although these methods are more complicated, they provide the most accurate information on the oligosaccharide fraction (2). They cannot be used for inulin. These methods provide well separated chromatographic peaks for the GFn and Fn fractions, thus allowing their accurate measurement up to about DP 10. There are almost no interferences with other oligosaccharides, allowing the differentiation of different types of oligosaccharides in the same mixture. The sample preparation can be standardized to such an extent that very accurate and reliable measurement is possible.

HPAEC/PAD Methods

These methods, although providing interesting qualitative results, are difficult to use for quantitative determinations. However, also here significant progress has been achieved recently (non-published results).

Fructose Determination Method

This method (Fig. 2) is based on the hydrolysis of fructans. Since this gives mainly fructose, the measurement of fructose before and after hydrolysis allows the calculation of the fructan content. However, accuracy can only be achieved when the hydrolysis is complete and the average DP and F/G ratio of the fructan are known, which is not often the case in foodstuffs. Therefore, these methods are mainly used for production control reasons.

Inulinase Method

This method (Fig. 3) allows the accurate determination of the total fructan content of any nature in foodstuffs (12). The principle of the method is the specific hydrolysis of fructans using an inulinase enzyme. The calculation is done based on a comparison of the glucose, fructose and sucrose determinations before and after hydrolysis. The analysis of these mono- and disaccharides can be done by any reliable method (not with enzymatic methods). To avoid interference with, e.g., lactoses, maltitol and isomalt a GC method is preferred.

The method has been used in many laboratories for quite some time, and has been perfected. In our experience, it has proven to be reliable and accurate in practice. A more thorough inter-laboratory comparison is being prepared now.

The inulinase method does not allow one to distinguish between inulin and oligofructose, and does not give information on DP fractions. The method is accurate in all food samples and requires no significant sample pretreatment. There are almost no interferences with other substances.

The method can be combined with the modified AOAC method as described in Chapter 5 (Figures 4 and 5). It can also be combined with any of the other methods described above to allow the differentiation between inulin and oligofructose.

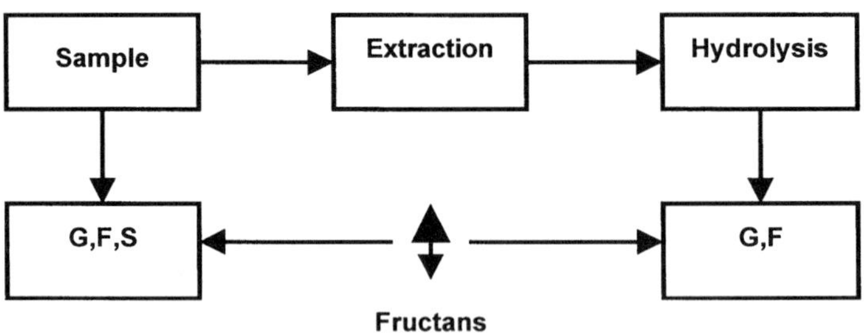

- **Accurate total inulin + oligofructose content**
- **Works in all food samples**
- **Very little interference**
- **No DP information**

Figure 3 Inulinase method (fructan method)

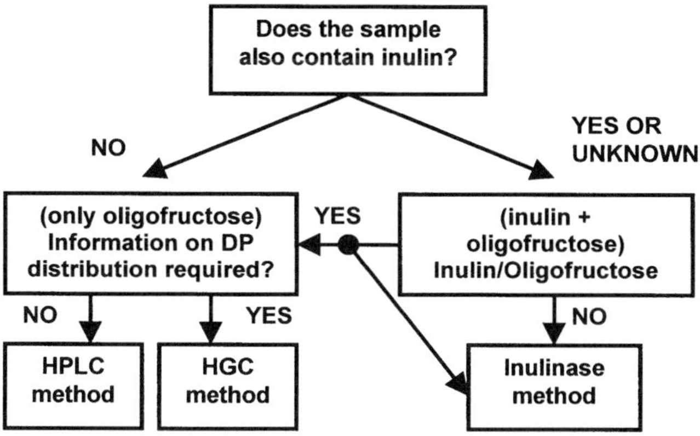

FIGURE 4 Inulin method combined with the modified AOAC method

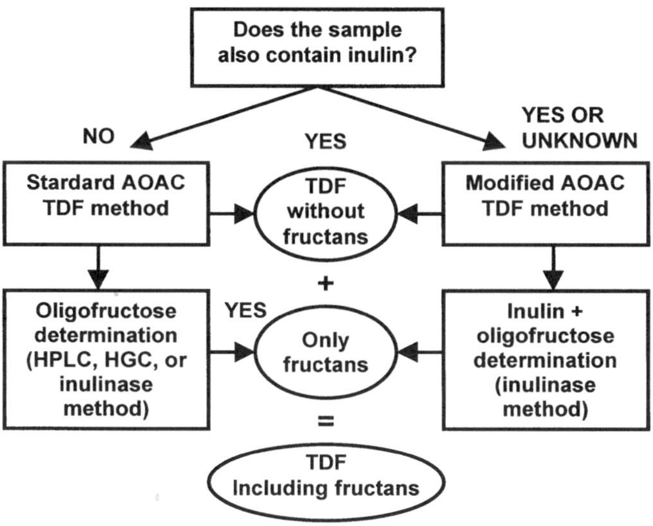

FIGURE 5 Combination with AOAC method for total dietary fiber

SUMMARY AND CONCLUSION

There are no nutritional grounds to exclude inulin and oligofructose from the dietary fraction for nutrition labeling. Both substances cannot be measured using the existing methods for dietary fiber determination, but accurate methods do exist which allow their analytical determination in foodstuffs. Many legal authorities have already confirmed that inulin and oligofructose can be labeled as dietary fiber. In some countries, this will require modifications of the food labeling laws. Both inulin and oligofructose are gaining wide acceptance as dietary fibers for use in industrial food preparation.

ACKNOWLEDGMENT

Special thanks to L. De Leenheer and H. Hoebregs for their assistance in writing this manuscript.

REFERENCES

1. Van Loo J., Coussement P., De Leenheer L., Hoebregs H., Smits G. (1995) Critical Reviews for Food Science and Nutrition 35, 525–552.
2. De Leenheer L. and Hoebregs H. (1994) StŠrke, May 1994.
3. COMA Report of the Panel on Dietary Reference Values of the Committee on Medical Aspects of Food Policy, nr. 41, Chapter 4, 1991.
4. COST 92 Group, 1994, Letter to the EC Commission.
5. Delzenne N. and Roberfroid M. (1994) Lebensm.-Wiss. u. Technol. Vol. 27, 1–6.
6. Nilsson and Bjšrck (1988) J. Nutr. 118, pp. 1482–1486.
7. Remesy C., Demigne C., Levrat M. A. (1994) Md. et Nut.–T. 30(4), 189–198.
8. Roberfroid M. (1993) Critical Reviews in Food Science and Nutrition 32(2), 103–148.
9. Lee, Sungsoo C. and Prosky, Leon (1994) Cereal Foods World, Vol. 39, No. 10, pp. 767–768.
10. Trowell H. and Burkitt D. (1986) Bol. Asoc. Med. P. Rico, pp 541–544.
11. EU Standing Committee for Foodstuffs, Report of the Meeting on 19–20/12/94.
12. Lee, S. C., Prosky, L, DeVries, J. W. (1992) JAOAC Int. 75, 396–416.
13. Quemener B., Thibault J. F. and Coussement P. (1994) Lebensm.-Wiss. u.-Technol., 27, 125–132.

17

Determination of Inulin and Oligofructose in Food Products (Modified AOAC Dietary Fiber Method)

P. Dysseler and D. Hoffem
Institut Meurice, Brussels, Belgium

J. Fockedey
Sucrerie de Warcoing, Pecq-Warcoing, Belgium

B. Quemener and J.-F. Thibault
INRA, Nantes, France

Paul Coussement
ORAFTI, Tienen, Belgium

INTRODUCTION

Inulin is a polymer of fructans with a degree of polymerization of 2 to 60. It consists principally of linear chains of fructosyl units linked by β(2-1) bonds ended by a glucosyl unit. Due to this structure, both inulin and oligofructose resist hydrolysis by human digestive enzymes but are fermented by the caecocolonic microflora. Thus, they have quite the same physiological action as dietary fiber. Finally, as the term dietary fiber doesn't cover a single entity, in the point of view of food analysis, it is more practical to analyze inulin or oligofructose with a specific method which involves enzymic hydrolysis followed by high performance liquid chromatography (HPLC) (done by CERIA, Belgium) or by high performance anion exchange chromatography (HPAEC) (done by INRA, France). In conclusion, a modification of the AOAC method is proposed to include these fructans in the determination of the soluble dietary fiber fraction.

The concept of dietary fiber, first described in the context of the hypothesis developed by Burkitt and Trowell in 1975, covers actually a series of complex compounds which are, according to the current most widely accepted physiological definition, "The sum of polysaccharides and lignins that are not hydrolyzed by the endogenous secretion of the human digestive tract" (1).

Within the last 5 years attention is increasingly drawn towards fiber isolates to be used as dietary fiber-enriched ingredients, and more specifically towards the group of indigestible poly- or oligosaccharides. This group of products, which cannot be assessed as dietary fiber by means of any currently available method, includes mainly polydextrose and inulin. These products are not absorbed by the small intestine of the human digestive tract and therefore show such physiological properties as are generally attributed to dietary fiber (2).

Chemically speaking, the inulin molecule is represented by the simple formula G-F-(F)n (where G-F denotes a sucrosyl group and n the number of fructose units present in the molecule) is a linear β(2-1) linked fructose polymer terminated by a sucrose unit residue; n varies from 2 to 60 or more. The hydrolysis of inulin by endoglycosidase produces linear oligomers. They are called GFn, in which n represents the number of fructosyl moieties.

This hydrolysis of inulin produces linear oligomers both of GFn and Fm types. This last type is composed of homopolymers of fructose bound by a β(2-1) linkage. m represents the number of fructosyl moieties in the homopolymers. These products of the hydrolysis of inulin are a mixture of oligomers in which n or m varies from 2 to 9.

Because of their relatively smaller molecular weight, as compared to the compounds conventionally accepted as dietary fiber, they are not completely precipitated by 95% ethanol. This is the reason why they cannot be assessed by the A.O.A.C. method used for dietary fiber analysis. We have therefore developed a reliable method to be used in routine analysis of inulin and oligofructose (3, 4).

QUANTITATIVE ANALYSIS OF INULIN AND OLIGOFRUCTOSE

Though the general properties of inulin are in line with those of the traditional dietary fiber, it cannot be assessed by the standard AOAC dietary fiber method

(5) wherein the soluble fibers precipitate at 60°C in ethanol. Because inulin has a relatively low average molecular weight (MW 6,000) as compared to the traditional soluble fiber (MW 10,000 to 50,000) it does not precipitate completely under these conditions.

HPLC Method for Inulin (CERIA-BELGIUM)

To supply the manufacturers with an appropriate means for production, food labeling, and quality control of inulin and inulin-containing products, the merits of an enzymatic digestion method followed by HPLC have been tested for the quantitative assessment of inulin. Moreover, if total soluble dietary fiber is wanted, the standard AOAC method has to be modified by including an enzymatic treatment with inulinase in addition to the amyloglucosidase incubation step in order to remove the residual β-fructans from the soluble fiber fraction (Figures 1 and 2). In these conditions these β-fructans directly determined have to be added to the ''soluble fiber fraction'' obtained with the AOAC modified method.

Enzymatic Digestion

Inulin can be hydrolyzed chemically or enzymatically to yield fructose and glucose (7). In the enzymatic digestion step, Novozym SP 230® Novo Nordisk enzyme hydrolyzes inulin totally. As shown in Figure 1, the enzymatic digestion yields the total amount of fructose, which is then quantified by HPLC (R1).

A blank test is run to account for any free fructose (R2) and the result is substracted from the value of the assay. To compute the inulin equivalent, (R1-R2) is multiplied by the correction factor 1.1 (assuming that the ratio of fructose/glucose is 85/15 in inulin). Since inulin is a natural product, this ratio fluctuates somewhat in practice according to the origin of the raw product from which inulin is obtained.

For samples containing sugar (sucrose), a correction has to be made since the Novozym SP 230® enzyme also totally splits sucrose, producing 50% glucose and 50% fructose. This problem can be alleviated by analyzing a duplicate sample of identical weight and followed likewise by HPLC analysis, the fructose originating from sucrose (R3) can thus be assessed and substracted also from the amount of fructose (R1) obtained by the Novozym SP 230® digestion. This method gives the β-fructan dietary fiber (see Equations (1) and (2)).

Removal of β-Fructans

This is usually achieved with Novozym SP 230® inulinase after the treatment with amyloglucosidase. This procedure yields the total dietary fiber content except for β-fructan dietary fiber.

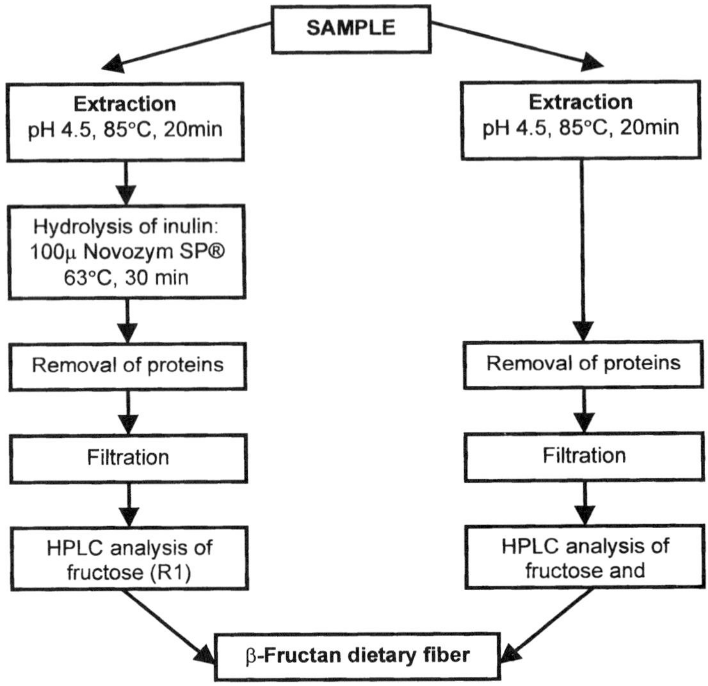

FIGURE 1 β-Fructan determination

Materials and Methods: β-Fructan Dietary Fiber Method

Apparatus

HPLC

High pressure pump, Millipore Waters (type 510)
Automatic sample injection device, Waters (type 712)
Oven with temperature control, Millipore Waters TCM
Refractometer detector, Millipore WATERS (type R401) with thermostatic water bath (30°C) for the refractometer cell
Integrator, Millipore WATERS (type 740)
HPLC column Hypersil APS NH2 (Chrompack), 20 cm

HPLC working parameters

Mobile phase: Water-acetonitrile: 15%–85% (V/V)

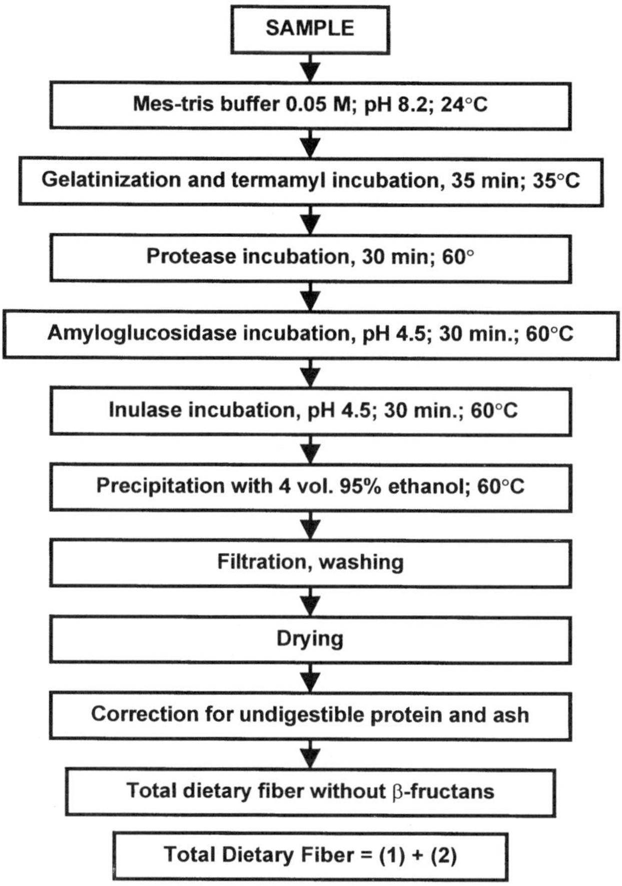

FIGURE 2 Flow diagram of the AOAC dietary fiber method (991.43: Lee et al., Ref. 5) modified for total dietary fiber to assure total removal of β-fructans

Flow rate: 0.4 ml/min.
Column temperature: 30°C

Test Samples

1. Standards: fructose, glucose, saccharose and sorbitol MERCK GLC grade (calibration samples)
2. Inulin
3. Inulin (for biochemical use, Merck n°4733)
4. Fibrulin (Cosucra company) batch 1

5. Fibrulin (Cosucra company) batch 2
6. Raftiline® (Raffinerie Tirlemontoise)
7. Raftilose® (Raffinerie Tirlemontoise)
8. Yogurt
9. Commercial samples, dosed with known amounts of inulin
10. Plain yogurt from skimmed milk and yogurt from skimmed milk with fruit ingredients

Method

Duplicate samples are required for this analysis:

1. Sample to be digested by Novozym SP 230®
2. Blank sample

Hydrolysis of fructans by Novozym SP 230® enzyme

1. Weigh accurately a sample of ca 10 g containing ca 1 g ''Fructan'' into 400 ml beaker
2. Add 150 ml acetate buffer solution 0.1 M, pH = 4.5
3. After homogenizing, cover beaker with aluminium foil. Place the beaker in the shaking water bath at 85°C for 20 minutes, to dissolve the sample
4. Remove the beakers from the bath and cool down to 60°C
5. Add 100 μl Novozym SP 230® enzyme and incubate in shaking water bath at 60°C for 30 minutes for total digestion of the inulin
6. Cool to room temperature and transfer quantitatively to 200 ml volumetric flask
7. Add 3 ml of lead hydroxy acetate to precipitate the protein and make up to
8. 200 ml with water
9. After homogenizing, filter through filter paper
10. Transfer a small amount of the solution into a capped vial
11. Carry out the HPLC assay with this solution.
12. The quantity of fructose obtained by HPLC (R1) represents the total amount of fructose in the sample.
13. Weigh accurately (within 20 mg) a duplicate sample of ca 10 g of the sample used for enzyme digestion; proceed exactly in the same manner as for the test sample, but without addition of Novozym SP 230®.

The quantity of fructose obtained by HPLC (R2) represents the amount of free fructose in the sample. (R3) represents the amount of fructose obtained in the sample by HPLC.

Calculation and Expression of Results

The amount of "fructan dietary fiber" (FDF) is given by:

$$\% \ \beta\text{-FDF} = \frac{1.1\ (R1 - R2)\ 100}{P}$$ (1) for samples containing no sucrose, and

$$\% \ \beta\text{-FDF} = \frac{1.1\ [R1 - (R2 + R3)]\ 100}{P}$$ (2) for samples containing sucrose,

where:

R1 = concentration of the total fructose (g/l)
R2 = concentration of the free fructose (g/l)
R3 = concentration of the fructose (g/l) from sucrose
P = mean mass (g/l) of the duplicate test samples,where P = 5 times the mean dry mass of the test sample taken

Empirical conversion factor for fructose to fructan, assuming a ratio of 80 to 85% fructose and 15% glucose in the fructan polymer.

Modified A.O.A.C. Dietary Fiber Method 991.43 Without β-Fructan Dietary Fiber

As shown in Figure 2, we apply A.O.A.C. TDF method 991.43 (Lee et al., Ref. 5), but with some modification. This minor modification includes only a stage of inulinase digestion performed, after the amyloglucosidase digestion. It aims to eliminate the fructans, under the following conditions:

inulinase: Novozym SP 230® 1800 inu/g, 100 ml
temperature: 60°C; pH: 4.5

The pH adjustment step for the inulinase is the same as for amyloglucosidase.

Results

Inulin Assay—Samples Without Sugar

Inulin samples were digested with Novozym SP 230® to check the performance of the hydrolysis according to the HPLC procedure for samples without sugar. As shown in Table 1, the enzymatic digestion recovery is higher than 95%.

The moisture contents of all the samples, as determined separately, were ca 5%. The correction factor applied to compute the amount of inulin in the sample varies between 1.0 and 1.2 for the different fructans. However, in practice, a correction factor 1.1 for routine analyses should procure fairly accurate results.

TABLE 1 Analysis of Inulin and Oligofructose Samples With and Without Added Sugar

Sample	P (g/l)	R1 (g/l)	R2 (g/l)	R3 (g/l)	Concentration fructans (g/l)	% recovery
Samples without sugar						
Inulin (Merck)	4.82	4.72	0.00		5.19 (0.29)	107.7
Fibrulin–1*	4.84	4.43	0.04		4.83 (0.35)	99.7
Fibrulin–2*	4.82	4.45	0.07		4.82 (0.38)	99.9
Raftiline®*	4.83	4.57	0.04		4.98 (0.31)	103.2
Raftilose®*	4.85	4.29	0.01		4.71 (0.28)	97.1
Sugar-dosed samples						
Fibrulin–1 + sugar	3.24	4.08	0.05	0.98	3.35 (0.14)	103.5

*Indicates industrial product
The analytical data are mean values of four series of analyses each, the confidence limits are computed for a probability 0.05.

Inulin Samples Containing Sugar

The influence of the presence of sugar has been checked on one of the industrial inulin samples. To this effect, 60% Fibrulin-1 was dosed with 40% sucrose, weighed accurately.

The digestion procedure was carried out with Novozym SP 230® according to the given procedure. The recovery is close to 100% (as in Table 1). Thus, the interference of sugar can be considered as negligible for practical purposes.

Inulin Assay with Yogurt

After having ascertained the suitability of the Novozym SP 230® for the assessment of fructans, inulin was assessed on commercial yogurt samples dosed with known amounts of inulin.

Two commercial yogurt samples, (ca 150 g) plain yogurt and yogurt, which contains sugar sweetened fruit, were each blended homogeneously with 6.6% of accurately measured inulin (ca 10 g). This represents ca 40% inulin on dry matter basis. The yogurt with fruit contains ca 4% sugar. The data shown in Table 2

TABLE 2 Analysis of Inulin in Yogurt

Sample	P (g/l)	R1 (g/l)	R2 (g/l)	R3 (g/l)	Concentration fructans (g/l)	% recovery
Plain yogurt	3.00	2.80	0.03	0.01	3.03 (0.09)	101.2
Fruit yogurt	3.00	5.81	0.35	2.84	2.88 (0.12)	96.1

are mean values of 4 analyses. The results show that for plain yogurt (which contains only very small amounts of sucrose) the recovery is 101%, a very good result for practical purposes. For fruit yogurt (where the sucrose content is significantly higher) the 96% recovery value is also quite acceptable.

HPAEC-PAD Analysis (INRA-Nantes) for Inulin and Oligofructose

High performance anion exchange chromatography was performed on a Dionex (Sunnyvale, CA, USA) 4500i LC gradient pump equiped with a pulsed electrochemical detector working in pulsed amperometric detection mode (PAD). The column was thermostated to 20°C excepted for the analysis of chocolate bar (15°C). The eluent was NaOH, 0.16 mol/l, at a flow rate of 1 ml/min. Detection was by triplepulsed amperometry with a goldworking electrode. The working pulse potentials and duration were as followed: E1 = 0.40 V (t1 = 500 ms), E2 = 0.90 V (t2 = 90 ms), E3 = −0.3 V (t3 = 50 ms).The sensitivity range used was 0.3 mC or 1 mC. The output was recorded by a CR4AX chromatopac (Shimadzu, Kyoto, Japan) with attenuation 10 (1024 mV/full scale).

Materials and Methods

Reference sugars (glucose, fructose, lactose, sucrose and rhamnose) were from Fluka AG (Buchs, Switzerland). Raffinose (5H2O) was from Merck (West Germany) and stachyose (4H2O) from Koch-Light Laboratories Ltd (England). Commercial inulin (Raftiline® ST) and oligofructose (Raftilose®) from chicory root were products of Raffinerie Tirlemontoise (Belgium). The tested food products were a Bifidus yogurt (oligofructose content of 1.5 g/100 g wet weight basis, dry matter 17.4 g/100 g), an orange-based jam filling for confectionery (oligofructose content 31.1 g/100 g wet weight basis); a ''cruesli bar'' (oligofructose content 11.9 g/100 g wet weight basis) and a chocolate bar (inulin content 16.8 g/100 g wet weight basis).

Pectibran® (Institut de Recherche Biologique Yves Ponroy, Bailly, France), All-Bran® (Kelloggs, Manchester, Great Britain), and Jacotte® (Pain Jacquet S.A., Bezons, France) were purchased from a local market.

Proposed Method for Determination of Inulin and Oligofructose

The samples (1 g) were extracted with 100 ml of hot water (85°C, 15 min). The chocolate sample (5 g) was preliminarily dispersed at about 40°C by hand using a glass rod and then extracted with 200 ml of water at 85°C. The extracts were cooled and made up to 100 ml. After homogenization and centrifugation (20,000 g, 10 min), an aliquot of 5 ml was incubated with about 100 μg of amyloglucosidase (100 U/mg of enzyme) for 30 min at 60°C. After dilution with an aqueous solution of rhamnose used as internal standard (final concentration of about 5-10 ppm), 25 ml were injected on the Carbopac PA1 column. This analysis gives the amount of the free sugars as fructose (Ff), sucrose (S) and glucose as the sum of free glucose (Gf) and glucose from maltodextrins (Gn). Another aliquot of 5 ml was treated with Novozym SP 230® (protein/substrate ratio of about 0,01) and amyloglucosidase (100 μg) at 60°C. This analysis leads to the amount of total glucose (Gt): $Gt = Gi + Gs + Gf + Gm$, with Gi = glucose from inulin or oligofructose and Gs = glucose released from sucrose (= S/1.9) and to the amount of total fructose (Ft): $Ft = Fi + Fs + Ff$ with Fi = fructose released from inulin or oligofructose and Fs = fructose from sucrose (S/1.9).

The inulin or oligofructose content (I) is obtained by: $I = k\ (Gi + Fi)$, with $k = [180 + 162\ (n\text{-}1)]/180\ n$, n being the sum of fructose and glucose residues per molecule of inulin or oligofructose. As the general formula of inulin is GFn and fructose and glucose have the same molecular weight, the number n may be calculated from the ratio of fructose/glucose amount measured after complete hydrolysis. The value for ''n'' of commercial inulin from chicory is around 10. For oligofructose, where the general formulae can be GFm and Fm, a value for ''n'' of about 4 can be safely used.

Results

Tentative determination of oligofructose and inulin in the soluble fiber fraction obtained by the AOAC method: Soluble and insoluble dietary fiber contents of two foods enriched in oligofructose (filling and yogurt) and of a food enriched in Raftiline® (chocolate bar) were measured by the AOAC method. Table 3 shows that very low values of fibers were obtained for filling and yogurt. The soluble dietary fiber amount of chocolate bar was higher (9.1 g/100 g wet matter). The respective amounts of oligofructose and inulin were measured in the soluble dietary fiber fraction. The recoveries of oligofructose in the case of filling and yogurt were extremely low. An average degree of polymerization n of 20 was calculated leading to a value of 0.905 for the factor k used for calculations of inulin content in the soluble dietary fiber fraction of the chocolate bar. The recovery of inulin, though more important, was less than 32 g/100 g demonstrating that the conditions used to eliminate starch and proteins and/or to extract the soluble fiber are too harsh for a quantitative recovery of inulin in the soluble fraction.

These results show that the AOAC method, in the case of inulin-rich products, seriously underestimates soluble dietary fiber amounts due to the loss of virtually all oligofructose and an important fraction of inulin.

TABLE 3 Determination of Dietary Fiber with AOAC Method and Recovery of Oligofructose and Inulin (% of theoretical amount) in the Soluble Dietary Fiber Fraction of Commercial Foods[a,b]

	Product		
Commercial foods	Filling	Yogurt	Chocolate bar
Insoluble dietary fiber (g/100 g DM)	0.1 (0.0)	0.7 (0.0)	0.4 (0.0)
Soluble dietary fiber (g/100 g DM)	2.0 (0.0)	4.4 (0.3)	9.1 (0.7)
Theoretical oligofructose amount (g/100 g DM)	44.5	8.6	
Oligofructose content (% soluble fraction)	0.5 (0.1)	0.2 (0.0)	
Oligofructose recovery (% theoretical)	0.0		
Theoretical inulin amount (%WM)	16.8		
Inulin content (% soluble fraction)	58.5 (1.3)		
Inulin recovery (% theoretical)	31.7		

[a]Values in parentheses are standard deviation (n = 5)
[b]Content expressed in g/100 g wet matter

DIRECT DETERMINATION OF OLIGOFRUCTOSE AND INULIN IN COMMERCIAL FOOD PRODUCTS

In Table 4 are shown the results of the determination of oligofructose in different commercial food products with Dionex system. The recovery values obtained are in most cases superior to 95%. Furthermore, the relative standard deviation values (4.4, 6.0, 4.1 and 2.4 for filling, yogurt, cruesli and chocolate bars respectively) give evidence of the acceptable accuracy of the proposed method using this HPLC system.

TABLE 4 Analysis of Oligofructose Content (g/100 g DM) in Industrial Food Products (HPAEC-PAD)[a,b]

	Product			
	Filling	Yogurt	Cruesli bar	Chocolate bar
Oligofructose	40.05 (1.8)	8.4 (0.5)	12.3 (0.5)	16.4 (0.4)
% Recovery	90.4	97.7	94.3	97.6

[a]Values in parenthesis are standard deviations (n =3)
[b]Content expressed in g/100 g wet matter

TABLE 5 Determination of Dietary Fiber (g/100 g DM) in Commercial Foods with the Modified and Non-modified AOAC Method[a]

Fiber		Product	
		All Bran®	Pectibran®
AOAC method	Insoluble dietary fiber	26.6 (2.5)	28.7 (0.5)
	Soluble dietary fiber	5.3 (0.8)	17.2 (0.3)
	Total dietary fiber	31.9 (3.1)	45.9 (0.8)
Modified AOAC method	Insoluble dietary fiber	30.3 (1.1)	28.9 (1.3)
	Soluble dietary fiber	8.5 (0.5)	14.2 (0.6)
	Total dietary fiber	38.8 (1.6)	43.1 (1.7)

[a]Values in parentheses are standard deviations

FIBER CONTAINING COMMERCIAL PRODUCTS

Additional assays were finally carried out on Pectibran® and All-Bran® by the modified AOAC method proposed in order to evaluate the potential losses (especially pectic substances) of the soluble dietary fiber fraction due to the combination of Novozym SP 230® with amyloglucosidase. The results obtained for these two commercial food products are compared to those obtained with the non-modified standard AOAC method 991.43 in Table 5. The losses of the soluble dietary fiber fraction were substantial in the case of Pectibran® (~50%) as a consequence of the contaminating pectolytic activities of Novozym SP 230®. There were no significative differences for All-Bran® which is devoid of pectic substances.

ELIMINATION OF THE PECTOLYTIC ACTIVITIES OF NOVOZYM SP 230® BY THERMIC TREATMENT

The commercial inulase used (Novozym SP 230®) contains some pectolytic activity (4). It is demonstrated that a thermic pretreatment of Novozym SP 230® at 60°C for 2 hours is sufficient to destroy this pectolytic activity (Table 6), while keeping sufficient inulinasic activity to hydrolyze residual inulin in the ''soluble fiber fraction'' (Table 7).

Preheated Novozym SP 230® (60°C, 2h) allows complete hydrolysis of pure Raftiline® with a 1.6% of enzyme/substrate ratio. This result was obtained by HPLC according to Quemener et al. (4). The amount quantified was equal to 101.8% (CV:0.5%) of that measured by active (non-treated) enzyme in the same conditions. In the same manner, the addition of preheated Novozym SP 230® in AOAC method for dietary fiber determination completely eliminates the residual

TABLE 6 Relative Activities* of Novozym SP 230® on Apple Pectin after Thermic Pretreatment

Inactivation time (min)	60°C	65°C	70°C	75°C
0	100	100	100	100
10	23	31	29	31
20	18	25	18	20
30	22	16	13	13
45	7	11	7	0
60	10	11	7	0
90	10	11	5	0
120	1	2	0	0

*Activities measured by the determination of reducing sugars according to the method of Nelson (9)

inulin amount of soluble fraction of a pudding containing 7% of Raftiline®. The Raftiline® content of this soluble fraction was 12.1% (of SDF) without addition of inulase as in standard AOAC method.

Determination of dietary fiber in Pectibran®, a product particularly rich in pectins, with non-modified and modified AOAC method using active Novozym SP 230® and partially inactivated Novozym SP 230® by preheating demonstrates that 1) with active Novozym SP 230®, losses in the soluble fraction are substantial as a consequence of the contaminating pectolytic activities and

TABLE 7 Relative Activities* of Novozym SP 230® on Raftiline® After Thermic Pretreatment

Inactivation time (min)	60°C	65°C	70°C	75°C
0	100	100	100	100
10	92.4	70.2	30.4	0.5
20	87.2	70.2	23.0	0
30	82.5	56.3	12.1	0.9
45	82.9	47.3	8.2	1
60	73.5	45.3	8.9	4
90	73.5	33.1	1.9	0
120	59.3	33.1	0	0

*Activities measured by the determination of reducing sugars according to the method of Nelson (9)

TABLE 8 Determination of Dietary Fiber (g/100 g DM) in Commercial Foods (Pectibran®) with the Modified and Non-modified AOAC Method[a]

Method		Pectibran®
AOAC	Insoluble dietary fiber	28.7 (0.5)
	Soluble dietary fiber	17.2 (0.3)
	Total dietary fiber	45.9 (0.8)
AOAC modified with active Novozym SP 230®	Insoluble dietary fiber	28.9 (1.3)
	Soluble dietary fiber	14.2 (0.6)
	Total dietary fiber	43.1 (1.7)
AOAC modified with preheated Novozym SP 230®	Insoluble dietary fiber	28.7 (0.2)
	Soluble dietary fiber	18.2 (0.6)
	Total dietary fiber	46.9 (0.4)

[a]Numbers in parentheses are standard deviation (n = 3)

2) there is no significative decrease in this soluble fraction with preheated Novozym SP 230® (Table 8).

CONCLUSION

Because of the diversity of dietary fiber like products, it would be difficult to elaborate a single analytical method capable of quantifying each type of dietary fiber, and more especially in case of mixed fiber components. It must be pointed out that inulin or oligofructose cannot be quantitatively measured in the soluble fiber fraction of food as obtained by the standard AOAC Dietary Fiber Method. This indicates that inulin and oligofructose (fructans) have to be directly determined on the food products. This method gives good accuracy and repeatability of the results and is easily applicable for routine analysis. The analysis takes three hours, but it can be serialized and requires only minimum handling. The method has been tested on pure samples as well as on industrial food products, such as yogurt, chocolate bar, and Cruesli bar.

Furthermore, in case of inulin or oligofructose enriched fiber ingredients the addition of an inulinase hydrolysis step to the standard AOAC method for the determination of total dietary fiber eliminates successfully the interference of the β-fructans, without unduly prolonging this analysis. For the experiments done by INRA-NANTES, the method developed for the determination of inulin or oligofructose in complex food products was efficient. Evidence is presented that the inulinase used (Novozym SP 230®) was strongly active on α-galactoside as raffinose and stachyose and slightly active on α-(1-4)-glucans as maltodextrins and on some polysaccharides such as pectins. The interference with glucose from starchy compounds can be eliminated by adding amyloglucosidase to the extracted sample.

Finally, a pretreatment of Novozym SP 230® by heating at 60°C for 2h is sufficient to eliminate the pectolytic activities of this enzyme and allows its utilisation in AOAC dietary fiber modified method for products rich in pectins.

REFERENCES

1. Asp, N. G., In: Dietary Fibre: Chemical and Biological Aspects. Ed. by Southgate D. A. T., Waldron K, Johnson L. T. and Fenwick G. R., Royal Soc. Chem. Special Publicat. 83, Cambridge, 1990, 327–336.
2. Roberfroid, M., Crit. Rev. Food Sci. Nutr., 1993, 33, 103.
3. Dyssler, P, Hoffem, D., In: Symposium COST 92: Topics in Dietary Fibre Research, Roma, May 1992.
4. Quemener, B., Thibault, J.-F. and Coussement, P., Lebensm.-Wiss. u. Technol., 1994, 27, 125–132.
5. Lee, S., Method 991-43, TDF, SDF and IDF method–Mes-Tris buffer. In: 3d supplement Official Methods of Analysis, 15th Edition, Arlington, Virginia.
6. Prosky, L., Asp, N.-G., Schweitzer, T. F., Devries, J. W., Furda, I. and Lee, S. C., J. AOAC Int., 1994, 77, 690–694.
7. Guiraud, J.-P. and GALZY, P., Ind. Alim. et Agric., 1981, 98, 45.
8. Asp, N.-G., In: Dietary Fibre. New developments in physiological effects and physicochemical properties, Furda, I. and Brine, C (Eds), New York, Plenum Publ. Corp., 1991, 227–236.
9. Nelson, N., Journal of Biological Chemistry, 1944, 153, 375–379.

18

Polydextrose as Soluble Fiber and Complex Carbohydrate

S.A.S. CRAIG, J.F. HOLDEN, J.P. TROUP, M.H. AUERBACH, AND H. FRIER
H.I. Cultor Food Science, Groton, Connecticut

INTRODUCTION

Foods containing resistant oligosaccharides (RO) are growing in popularity with health-conscious consumers. RO are resistant to hydrolysis by human alimentary enzymes and reach the lower intestine. Recent literature is focusing attention on the positive physiological effects of RO (1–6) as both fiber and complex carbohydrate.

Polydextrose is regarded as either a resistant polysaccharide (RP) or a RO, and is recognized in a number of countries as a soluble fiber. Physiological benefits of polydextrose as a soluble fiber and complex carbohydrate have been determined, including effects on lower gastrointestinal fermentation, production of short chain fatty acids (SCFA), fecal bulking, reduced transit time and glucose homeostasis (7). Additional studies are currently underway.

A recent international survey (8) on dietary fiber (DF) showed strong support for expansion of the definition of DF to include RO in all countries. The most appropriate basis for the definition of DF is from both the physiological and chemical perspectives (8,9). The Association of Official Analytical Chemists (AOAC) method of analysis for fiber (10,11) is the most widely accepted measurement of total dietary fiber (TDF). However, this procedure does not include RO (including polydextrose) as fiber. A number of HPLC-based analytical methods have been developed for quantifying polydextrose in foods (12–15). One method (12) has been applied to the determination of polydextrose as fiber, primarily in beverages. This chapter discusses issues surrounding these methods, including a study of the AOAC precipitation step on polydextrose.

POLYDEXTROSE STRUCTURE

Polydextrose is prepared by vacuum thermal polymerization of glucose, using sorbitol as plasticizer and citric acid as catalyst (89:10:1 ratio). This random polymerization and branching yields various types of glucosidic bonds in the structure (α-1,6 bonds predominate) (16,17). The R-groups may be hydrogen, glucose, sorbitol, citric acid or a continuation of the polydextrose polymer.

The representative structure is derived from characterizations that include methylation and periodate oxidation for degree of branching; Smith periodate degradation, methylation and acetolysis for linkage positions; Smith degradation and acetolysis for anomeric linkage configuration and 13C-NMR (17). Polydextrose is more highly branched than other carbohydrates, such as the amylopectin component of starch, which contains mainly α-1,4 linkages with about 4–5% of α-1,6 linkages as branch points. The structural compactness and complexity of

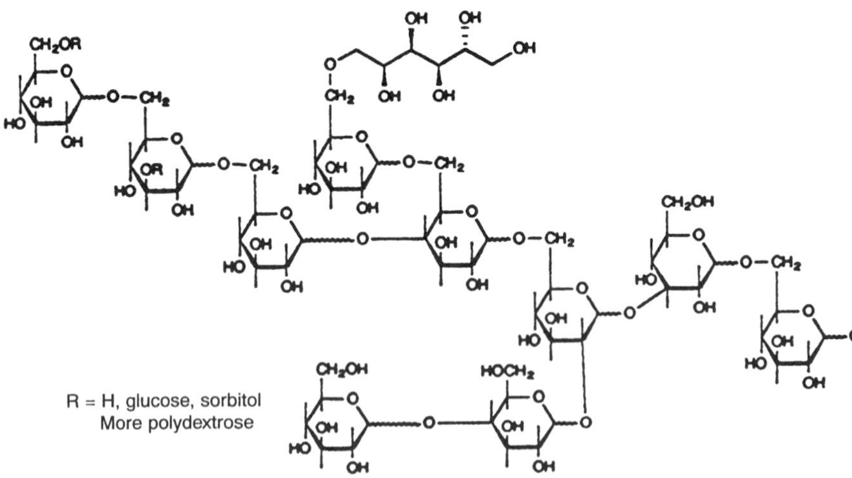

FIGURE 1 Representative structure for polydextrose.

polydextrose prevents mammalian digestive enzymes from readily hydrolyzing the molecule, imparting reduced caloric content. Thus, radiotracer studies in both rats and humans found that polydextrose was utilized at about one-fourth of that of sucrose (i.e., 1 kcal/g) (18,19). Recent studies have confirmed this value (20,21).

The average degree of polymerization (DP) of polydextrose is ~12 (weight average molecular weight of ~2000), although the range of molecular weight is 162 to about 20,000 (Figure 2). The calculation of an average DP of 12 is derived from three different techniques (Craig, S.A.S. and Auerbach, M.H., unpublished results). First, polydextrose was chromatographed by HPLC on a Synchropak GPC 100 column, calibrated with dextran standards. The average DP was 11.6 ± 0.5. Second, polydextrose was chromatographed by HPLC on 3 Shodex OHpak columns in series (802.5, 804, 806). The absolute average molecular weight by multiangle laser light scattering gave a DP of 12.3 ± 0.6 (data courtesy of Wyatt Technology Corp). Third, polydextrose was chromatographed by HPLC on a TSK PW 2000A column. The average DP by viscometry/light scattering detection was 14.2 (data courtesy of Viscotek Corp).

The DP range for RO is usually defined as 3-9, with polysaccharides >10

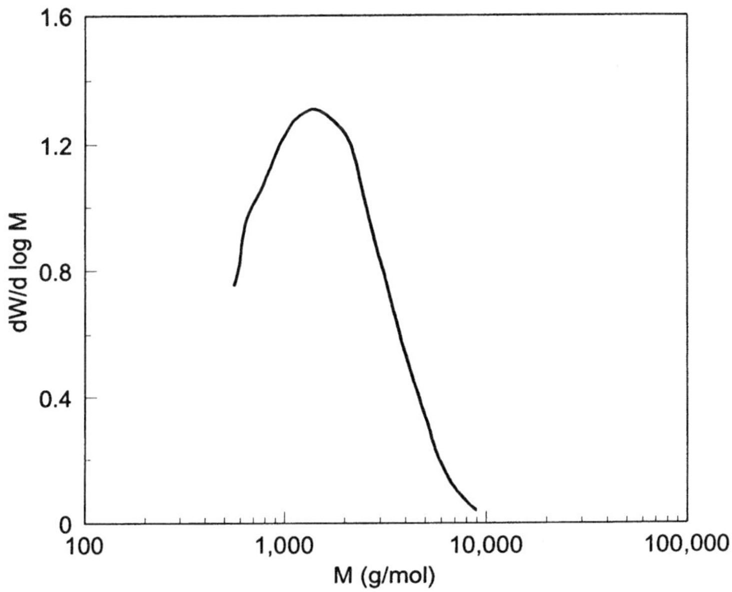

FIGURE 2 Differential molecular weight distribution of polydextrose. (Courtesy of Wyatt Technology.)

(5). Polydextrose is often regarded as an RO, although the majority of molecular species are of DP $>$ 10 and the average DP is 12. In Japan, RO are considered resistant to hydrolysis and mostly fermented in the large intestine (i.e. do not appear in feces). Resistant polysaccharides (RP) are also resistant to hydrolysis, but only partially fermented. In addition, RO tend to have lower laxation thresholds than RP. On this basis, polydextrose better fits the description, used in Japan, of RP (see later section on laxation thresholds and on fermentation). On the other hand, the RO classification fits the behavior of polydextrose in the current AOAC assay for TDF. Less than 10% of polydextrose is measured as TDF by this method (see analytical section for details). The highly branched structure of polydextrose prevents significant precipitation in the 80% ethanol step of the AOAC assay. Overall, polydextrose is more accurately classified as a RP.

REGULATORY STATUS AROUND THE WORLD

Polydextrose is an approved food additive in forty-six countries around the world, and is commercially accepted and sold in two others without requirement of formal approval. Both the Joint FAO/WHO Expert Committee on Food Additives (JECFA) and the European Commission Scientific Committee for Foods (EC/SCF) have reviewed the safety of polydextrose and given it an ADI "not specified," meaning they have no concerns about daily intake levels. The 1 kcal/g energy content of polydextrose is generally accepted for labeling purposes in all countries where it is approved.

In Japan, polydextrose is considered a food, not a food additive, and is widely used there in fiberfortified health beverages. It is also approved under the Japanese Foods for Specified Health Use (FSHU) law as an ingredient for which the label claim "provides improved intestinal function" may be made. Polydextrose can be labeled as fiber in seven countries (Japan, Korea, Taiwan, PR China, Argentina, Egypt and Poland). Because it is fermented in the colon like many other fiber sources, excessive consumption of polydextrose may cause symptoms of laxation in sensitive individuals. The mean laxation intake is 90 g/day, which is significantly greater than that of most other RO and sugar alcohols. Because of this effect, five countries require a laxation statement in the label of foods containing polydextrose when a single serving of the food contains more than 15 g of polydextrose (United States, Argentina, Brazil, PR China and Taiwan).

DIETARY FIBER DEFINITION

"Fiber" or "dietary fiber" (DF) is a variety of complex organic substances each having unique physical and chemical properties which in turn determine their physiological effect. Plant cell wall material containing cellulose, hemicellulose, pectin substances and lignin are major sources of DF. Additionally, mucilages, gums, algal and synthetic polysaccharides behave as DF. With the exception of lignin, dietary fibers are carbohydrates, and it has been suggested that the measurement of nonstarch polysaccharides is more accurate than determination of DF (22). On the other hand, it has been proposed that starch not digested in the small intestine and reaching the colon (i.e., resistant starch (RS)) is chemically and physically similar to other nondigestible polysaccharides and should therefore be included in the definition of DF (23). This definition describes polysaccharides and RS as a fiber by the AOAC assay (see later section).

There are a number of definitions for "fiber" or "DF" in countries around the world. In 1972 Trowell described DF as "the remnants of the plant cell walls that are not hydrolyzed by the alimentary enzymes of man" (24). In 1976 this definition was modified to include all ". . . plant polysaccharides and lignin which are resistant to hydrolysis by digestive enzymes of man"(25). These definitions were physiologically based, moving beyond the simple analytical definition of "crude fiber." In 1978 Trowell proposed that indigestible polysaccharides that had been added to foods should be excluded from "dietary fiber" (26). However, this proposal was not pursued because of the impossibility of differentiating, by analytical means, between "extrinsic" and "intrinsic" dietary fiber. In 1981 the term "non-starch polysaccharides" (NSP) was coined in a proposal to define DF as the sum of NSP and lignin (27). An expert panel of the Life Sciences Research Office (LSRO) for the Food and Drug Administration (FDA) used the following definition in 1987: "DF is the endogenous components of plant materials in the diet which are resistant to digestion by enzymes produced by man . . . predominantly NSP and lignin" (28). To include RS, which passes the small intestine undigested, the term "unavailable complex carbohydrate" (UCC) was developed. UCC comprises NSP and RS (29). A restriction to plant or plant cell wall origin was not made. This was to account for some compounds which behave as DF physiologically, but were not considered DF (e.g., polydextrose, inulin, chemically modified celluloses, isolated plant gums, etc.)

Debate regarding fiber definitions continues today. In Europe, the Scientific Committee for Food (SCF) could not agree on an EC definition of dietary fiber in 1994. Two views are held; one includes only cell-wall-NSP (i.e., not RS or RO). The other was proposed as: " 'Fibre' is the part of oligo and polysaccharides and their (hydrophilic) derivatives which by human digestive enzymes cannot be decomposed to absorbable components in the upper alimentary tract. It includes lignin" (30). Until agreement can be reached, EC member countries are pursuing individual definitions. Worldwide, definitions can be described as based either on analysis (e.g., AOAC, Englyst assays, etc.) or non-digestibility. This leads to inconsistencies regarding the inclusion of certain food fractions.

Recent papers (8,9) have discussed a change in the definition of DF. An international survey (8) found that the most accepted definition for DF is "polysaccharides and lignin that are not hydrolyzed by human alimentary enzymes" (i.e., DF is the sum of RS, nonstarch polysaccharides, and lignin, not requiring plant origin). Oligosaccharides that escape the human small intestine (RO) are considered DF by a majority of the survey participants. Therefore it was recommended to revise the definition of DF to ''. . . oligo- and polysaccharides and lignin that are resistant to hydrolysis by human alimentary enzymes.''

In conclusion, there is considerable interest and debate surrounding RS, RO and RP (including polydextrose as fiber/DF). Later sections will address physiological and analytical performance of polydextrose in this context.

COMPLEX CARBOHYDRATE DEFINITION

The term ''complex carbohydrates'' was proposed as a mandatory item on the U.S. food nutrition label in 1991. However, the final regulations in 1993 do not allow the use of the term on the nutrition label because of a lack of clear definition and methodology. At the end of 1994, ILSI North America's Technical Committee on Carbohydrates sponsored a workshop entitled ''Complex Carbohydrates: The Science and the Label.'' The following resulted:

1. Complex carbohydrates is a familiar term to consumers who are aware of the need to increase their consumption. However, consumers are unable to readily determine this information from the nutrition label.
2. Based on a recent AOAC International survey, complex carbohydrates definition includes both DF and digestible complex carbohydrates (e.g., starch). Since RO is generally considered part of DF, it is also a complex carbohydrate.
3. An AOAC assay for complex carbohydrates under development will measure both DF and digestible complex carbohydrates. However, an 80% ethanol precipitation step to remove sugars will discard RO. This is the same problem that occurs during the AOAC assay for DF (see later section).

Therefore an analytical method is required to measure polydextrose as complex carbohydrate.

DIETARY FIBER: PHYSIOLOGICAL EFFECTS

Disease Prevention/Intervention

In an attempt to clarify the concept of DF, individual fiber sources can be defined by their physical properties. A widely used classification is that of 1) water soluble or gelforming viscous fibers and 2) water insoluble fibers. This distinction is convenient since many of the physiological effects of fiber seem to be based on this property. Clearly, polydextrose would be referred to as a soluble fiber having similar physiological effects.

Soluble fibers are highly fermentable and are associated with carbohydrate and lipid metabolism, while insoluble fibers contribute to fecal bulk and reduced transit times (31). Particle size, water holding capacity, viscosity, cation exchange capability and binding potential are specific for every fiber source. These properties can change when a food undergoes cooking and digestion.

DF has been shown to play a role in the prevention and/or management of a wide variety of disease states and metabolic conditions (Table 1). Fiber has been implicated as important in various aspects of bowel function and can exert

TABLE 1 The Role of Dietary Fiber in the Prevention and Management of Disease States and Metabolic Conditions

Physicochemical property	Type of fiber	Physiological effect	Clinical significance
Viscosity	Gums, mucilages, pectins	↓ Gastric emptying ↓ Rate of small intestine absorption	Diabetes Hypercholesterol
Particle size and water-holding capacity	Wheat bran, pentosan content, polysaccharide-lignan mixtures	↑ Gastric emptying ↓ G.I. tract transit time ↓ Colonic intraluminal pressure ↑ Fecal bulk	Constipation Peptic ulcer Diverticular disease Dilute potential carcinogens
Adsorption and non-specific effects	Lignin, pectin-mixed fibers	↑ Fecal steroid output ↑ Fecal fat and nitrogen loss	Hypercholesterol
Cation exchange	Acidic polysaccharides (i.e., pectins)	↑ Small intestine losses of minerals, trace elements, heavy metals	Negative mineral balance Antitoxic effect
Antioxidant	Lignin (reducing phenolic groups)	↓ Free radicals in digestive tract	Anticarcinogenesis
Degradability (colonic bacteria)	Polysaccharides (free of lignan)	↑ Production of gas and volatile fatty acids ↓ Cecal pH	Flatus Energy production Serum cholesterol Carbohydrate/lipid metabolism

influence on several metabolic (e.g., diabetes) and inflammatory bowel diseases (e.g., diverticulitis). The control and/or prevention of a variety of carcinomas as well as certain diseases affecting the cardiovascular system have also been suggested to be influenced by DF intake.

Fermentation to Short Chain Fatty Acids (SCFA)

Studies in rats and man have shown that polydextrose is partially fermented in the large intestine (18–21, 32). Because not all fibers are degraded equally by bacteria, a range of 0 (nonfermentable, insoluble) to 4.0 (fermentable, soluble) kcal/g have been used for these fibers unless proven otherwise. As previously described, polydextrose has been determined to be 1 kcal/g. Many fibers can be fermented by bacteria in the large intestine to produce hydrogen, methane, carbon dioxide and SCFA (also referred to as volatile fatty acids, VFA). The SCFA are rapidly absorbed from the gastrointestinal tract through the hepatic portal vein and contribute to the energy balance of the body. These contributions include inhibition of hepatic cholesterol synthesis by propionate (33) and aptosis of cancer cells by butyrate (34,35). Qualitative measurement of SCFA was conducted in PDX studies (7) and revealed typical profiles of acetic, butyric and propionic acids. Of the total radioactivity recovered, 17% was from volatile fatty acids. A recent study (36) measured SCFA production from fermentation of 17 carbohydrates by slurries of mixed fecal bacteria. Polydextrose was found to have a molar ratio of acetate : propionate : butyrate of 61 : 25 : 14. Only 2 carbohydrates provided a higher proportion of propionate and only 3 provided a higher proportion of butyrate. Harada et al. (37) showed, in rats, that SCFA production from polydextrose increased epithelial cell turnover. This positive effect was more pronounced with polydextrose than with pectin.

Polydextrose causes a significant decrease in the pH of duodenal juices. Intestinal infusion of polydextrose (7) resulted in a drop of pH from 7.24 ± 0.45 to 6.44 ± 0.35 after 150 minutes ($p < .05$). Endo et al. (32) found a similar pH drop. This change can improve the composition of gut microflora by promoting growth of specific beneficial bacterial strains such as *Bacteroides* sp. (personal communication, Carmen, R.J., Techlabs, Virginia) or diminishing detrimental bacteria such as *Clostridium perfringens*. Polydextrose was found in one study to significantly increase *Bacteroides* sp. (36), and in another study to diminish *Clostridium perfringens* (32). The latter study also found that polydextrose reduced the levels of certain putrefactive/carcinogenic substances (indole and p-cresol) produced by bacterial fermentation.

These studies show that polydextrose is fermented in a similar way to other fibers, and even has advantages over some (e.g., butyrate/propionate production, beneficial bacteria).

Gastrointestinal Function

Changes in gastrointestinal function are most pronounced for insoluble fibers. However, Oku et al. (38) found that polydextrose fed to rats at a dose of 3% of the diet partially demonstrated the DF actions of increased fecal volume and weight, decreased transit time and increased moisture of fecal samples. Tomlin and Read (39) found that polydextrose increased fecal mass and softened stools. Nakagawa et al. (40) found that polydextrose ingestion led to softer stools. Also, Wang and Gibson (36) measured growth of colonic bacteria in batch fermenters with various carbohydrates added. Over 12 h, polydextrose caused an increase in total bacteria similar to the other carbohydrates (pectin, starch, inulin, oligofructose, fructose). This is important because bacteria form a significant portion of fecal bulk.

Glycemic Index

Although insoluble fiber has little to no effect on carbohydrate metabolism, water soluble fiber and foods rich in viscous fiber have been found to reduce and control postprandial glucose response and improve insulin profiles. The rate of glucose absorption and uptake in the body is dependent on the composition and structure of the food eaten. Jenkins et al. (41) proposed the concept of glycemic index which compares carbohydrate-containing foods on the basis of postprandial glucose profiles in relation to a standard glucose load or white bread. A combination of slowing of gastric emptying and reduced intestinal absorption appears to be responsible for the reductions in postprandial glucose concentrations. Although the specific design for measurement of glycemic index was not used, a measurement of the postprandial glucose response for polydextrose was determined in a diabetic patient group following a 50 gram intake level (7). The glucose response following polydextrose intake was modulated compared to the response of a standard glucose tolerance test, suggesting that the glycemic index would be lower for polydextrose.

Nutrient Interference

The small intestine is the site of the digestion and absorption of large quantities of food. DF has a significant influence on the rate and effectiveness of nutrient absorption. By binding and adsorbing water, enzymes, cations and inorganic micronutrients, fiber can make these dietary components unavailable for digestion and absorption. Binding of bile salts may interfere with intestinal lipid absorption. Nutritional interaction studies (7) show that intake of polydextrose does not interfere with nutrients (i.e., amino acids, potassium and calcium).

Overall, ingestion of polydextrose delivers a number of physiological effects consistent with other DFs. Additional studies are underway.

ANALYTICAL MEASUREMENT OF DF

AOAC Method

The AOAC assay for TDF is a widely accepted protocol in many countries (10,11). However, this enzyme-gravimetric procedure does not include RO (including polydextrose and inulin) as DF. A schematic of the critical steps in the AOAC assay is shown in Figure 3. Petroleum ether removes fat, enzymes remove starch, starch dextrins and protein. The ethanol step is designed to precipitate polysaccharides, leaving behind sugars and other small molecules. However, the ethanol precipitation step leaves most RO in the discarded supernatant, along with sugars. As RO is increasingly used in foods, this step becomes more problematical. In addition, studies (42–44) have indicated that a number of polysaccharides (pectin, arabinan and arabinogalactan) are not quantitatively precipitated by 80% ethanol.

Ethanol Precipitation Step of AOAC Method

An HPLC system was assembled to profile oligo- and polysaccharides. It consisted of an isocratic pump, injector, 2 columns (Biorad Aminex 42A and Supelco G2000 PW) and guards, detector (refractive index) and integrator.

An HPLC profile of Litesse® polydextrose is shown in Figure 4a. Four volumes of 95% ethanol were added to a polydextrose solution at 60°C, as described in the AOAC assay. Only 8% precipitated, and the HPLC profile of this material is shown in Figure 4b. The remaining polydextrose (92%) gave an HPLC profile shown in Figure 4b. As expected, only the high molecular weight component of polydextrose precipitated. Note the overlap of molecular profiles. This is typical of solvent precipitations.

Other solvents were evaluated in place of ethanol. Figure 5 shows a plot of dielectric constant vs. TDF (%) for 6 solvents. Isopropanol and acetone showed promise, by precipitating more polydextrose. HPLC profiles are shown in Figs. 6 (isopropanol) and 7 (acetone). Acetone was subsequently shown to precipitate sugars (10% of lactose and sucrose), so 80% acetone was tried. However, the precipitate from 80% acetone was extremely sticky, and proved impossible to transfer quantitatively. The precipitate from isopropanol was also somewhat sticky. Ultimately, solvents cannot be used to quantitatively precipitate polydextrose (90%+), without contamination from sugars.

For comparison, we evaluated the effect of the ethanol step on inulin (a RO or RP). Figure 8a shows a profile of Raftiline (sample courtesy of Orafti).

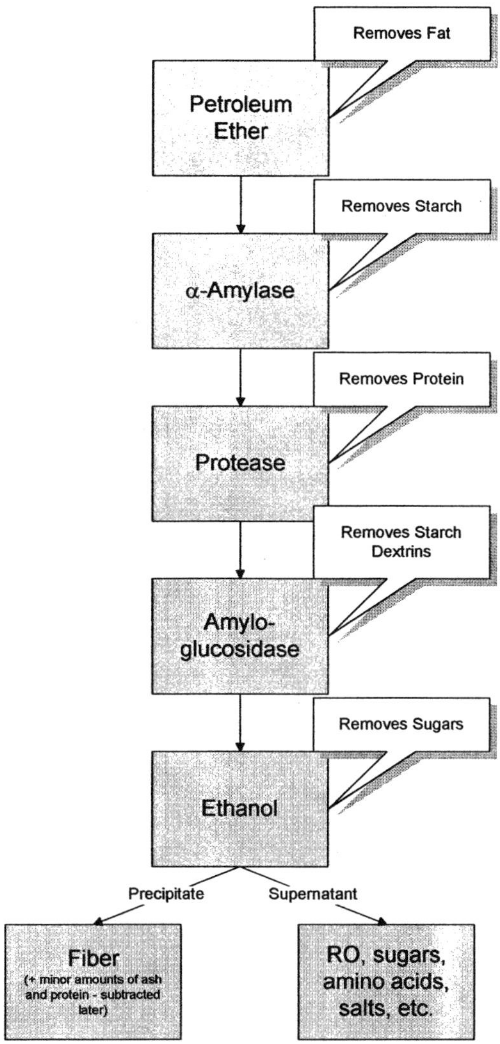

FIGURE 3 Schematic of some steps in the AOAC assay for TDF.

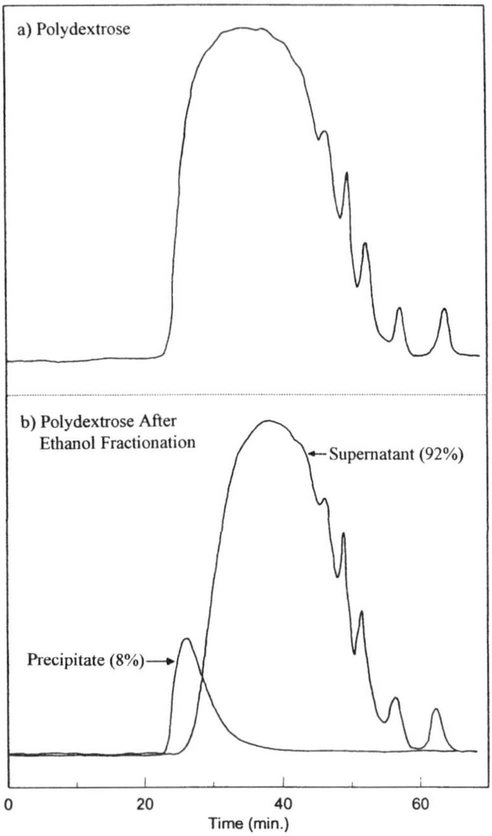

FIGURE 4 HPLC profile of litesse polydextrose (before and after ethanol fractionation).

About 35% precipitated (Fig 8b), leaving 65% in solution (Figure 8b). Fig. 9 compares Raftiline to inulin (from chicory root, Sigma) and to Raftilose (oligofructose). Orafti and INRA have published an HPLC method (45) to specifically measure β-fructans (inulin and oligofructose) in food. They propose that this value then be incorporated into the DF value.

HPLC Methods

An assay used currently in Japan to quantify polydextrose as fiber utilizes HPLC (12). Enzymes (α-amylase and amyloglucosidase) break down starch/maltodextrins in the sample, similar to the AOAC assay. The sample is then membrane

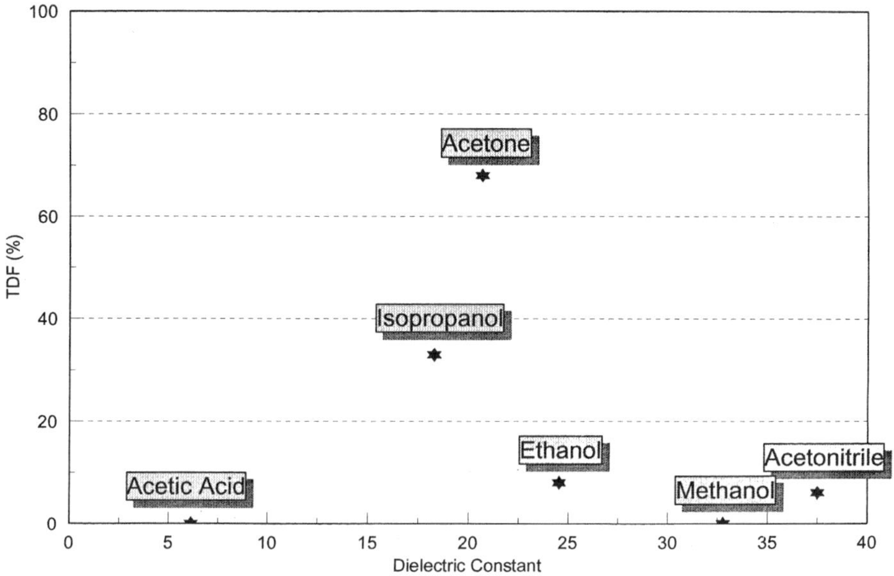

FIGURE 5 TDF of polydextrose using different precipitating solvents.

filtered, deionized and injected into the HPLC (Ultron PS-80 N column and refractive index (RI) detection). This assay works well in relatively simple food systems (e.g., clear beverages). However, contaminating substances (e.g., gums) might confound the chromatogram in other foods.

Other HPLC-based methods have been published that measure polydextrose in foods (13–15). Noffsinger et al. (14) used a polystyrene divinylbenzene (calcium form) column (Biorad Aminex HPX-87C) and RI. This method is useful for simple foods. Arrigoni and Amado (15) used a polystyrene divinylbenzene (lead form) column (Biorad Aminex HPX-87P) and RI. By using RI, both methods are relatively nonspecific for polydextrose. Stumm and Baltes (13) used an anion-exchange column (Dionex CarboPac PA1), mobile phase gradient and pulsed amperometric (PAD) detection. This provides greater selectivity, but is a more complex system. We have worked with the Stumm and Baltes method to improve the sample preparation step. Enzymes remove polysaccharides which might interfere with quantitation (e.g., α-amylase, amyloglucosidase, cellulase, mannanase, pectinase, etc.). Early results (Khaled, M., Craig, S.A.S., unpublished results) indicate good consistency of 1.6–2.7% RSD. Therefore, polydextrose can be accurately measured in foods and added to the TDF value. We are currently working towards an AOAC-approved procedure utilizing HPLC.

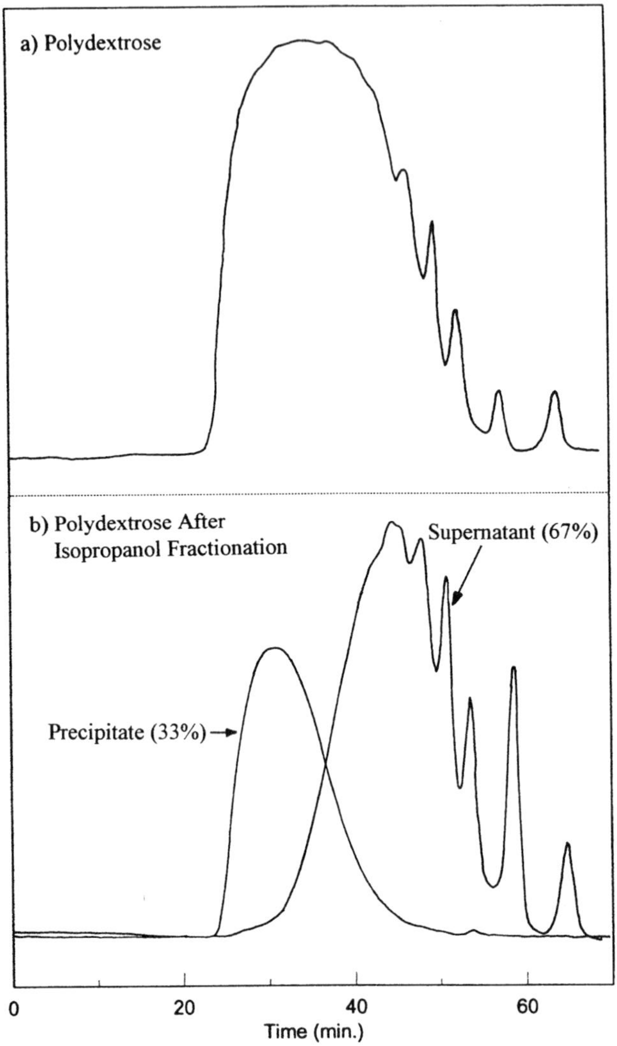

FIGURE 6 HPLC profile of litesse polydextrose (before and after isopropranolol fractionation).

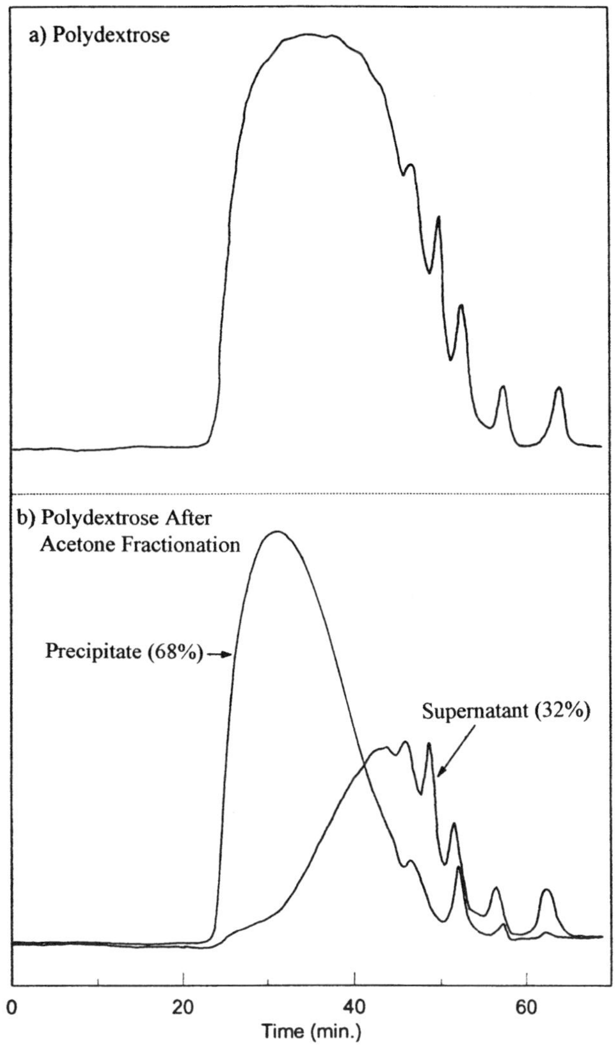

Figure 7 HPLC profile of litesse polydextrose (before and after acetone fractionation).

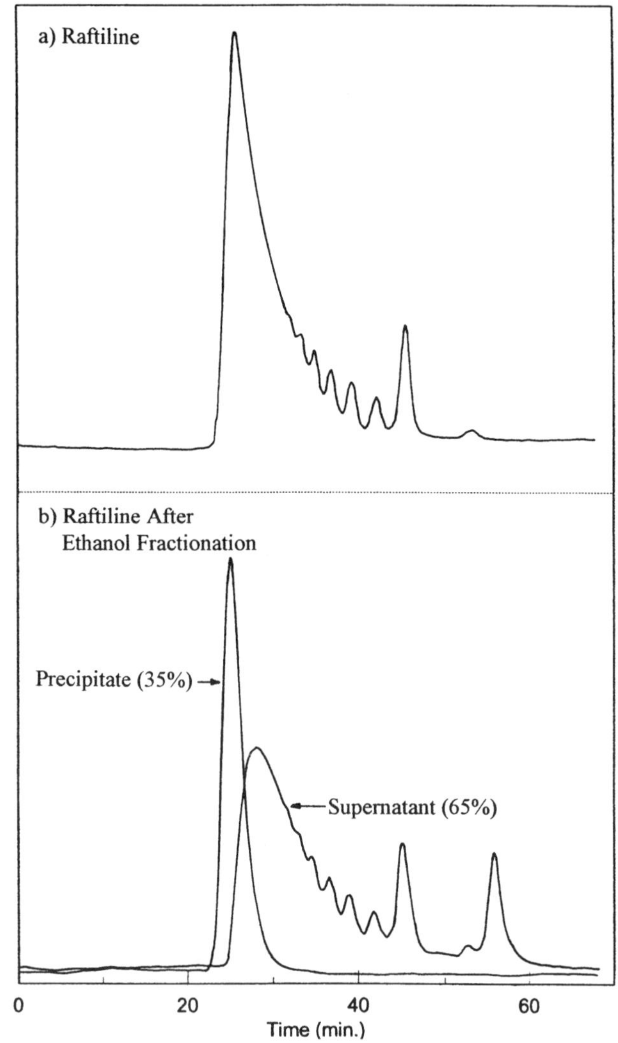

FIGURE 8 HPLC profile of raftiline inulin (before and after ethanol fractionation).

CONCLUSIONS

Polydextrose is an carbohydrate with a complex structure, resistant to mammalian digestive enzymes and partially fermented by intestinal microflora. It is widely used as a 1 kcal/g bulking agent in reduced-calorie and reduced-fat foods. In a

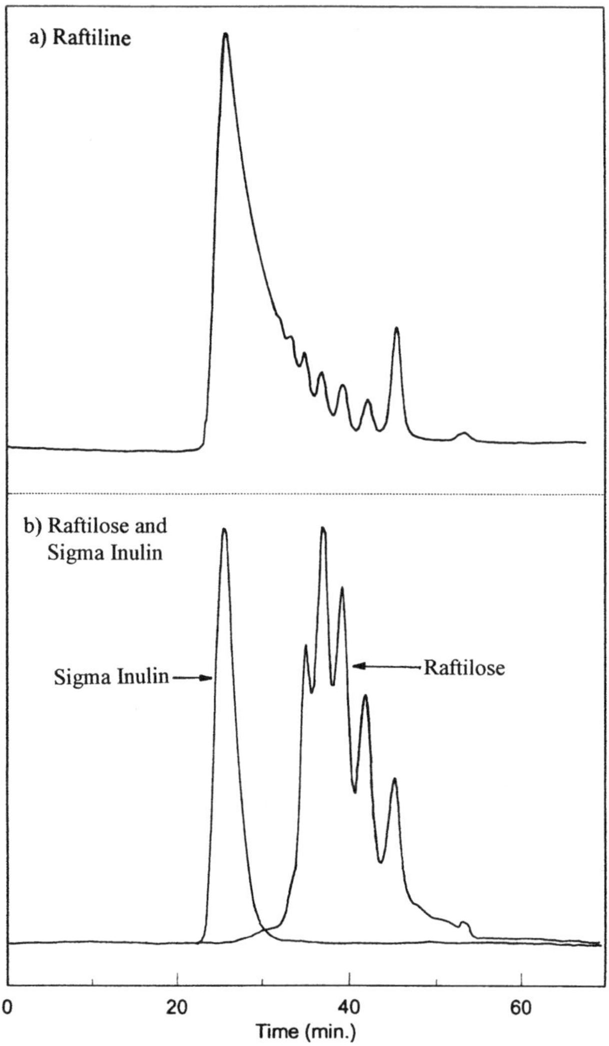

Figure 9 HPLC profile of β-fructans.

number of countries, polydextrose can be labeled as fiber. Studies demonstrate that some of the physiological effects of polydextrose are consistent with those expected of fiber. Recent surveys have shown that RO (including polydextrose and inulin) should be part of the definition of DF. However, the AOAC assay for DF does not account for RO due to the 80% ethanol step. Similarly, RO would be complex carbohydrate, but analytical methods might not account for it. Substituting other solvents for ethanol did not account for all of the polydextrose (without precipitating sugars). A number of HPLC methods are available to reliably quantify polydextrose in food. However, further work is required to develop an AOAC-approved method for addition of polydextrose and all RO to the TDF value. This method will probably utilize HPLC.

REFERENCES

1. Tomamatsu, H. (1995) Food Tech. Oct., 61–65.
2. Gibson, G. R. & Robefroid, M. R. (1995) J. Nutr. 125, 1401–1412.
3. Younes, H., Garleb, K., Behr, S., Remesy, C. & Demigne, C. (1995) J. Nutr. 125, 1010–1016.
4. Haastrecht, J. (1995) Int. Food Ingr. 1, 23–27.
5. Cummings, J. H. & Englyst, H. N. (1995) Am. J. Clin. Nutr. 61(suppl), 938S–945S.
6. Gibson, G. R. & Roberfroid, M. B. (1995) J. Nutr. 125, 1401–1412.
7. Polydextrose Food Additive Petition, Pfizer (1975).
8. Lee, S. C. & Prosky, L. (1995) J. AOAC Int. 78, 22–36.
9. Lee, S. C. & Prosky, L. (1994) Cereal Foods World 39, 767–768.
10. Prosky, L., Asp, N.-G., DeVries, J. W., Schweizer, T. F. & Harland, B. (1988) J. Assoc. Off. Anal. Chem. 71, 1017–1023.
11. Lee, S. C., Prosky, L. & DeVries, J. W. (1992) J. AOAC Int., 75, 395–416.
12. Kobayashi, T., Yoshino, H. & Mori, B. (1989) Nippon Nogeikagaku Kaishi 63, 1611–1613.
13. Stumm, I. & Baltes, W. (1992) Z. Lebensm. Unters Forsch 195, 246–249.
14. Noffsinger, J. B., Emery, M., Hoch. D. J. & Dokladalova, J. (1990) J. Assoc. Off. Anal. Chem. 73, 51–53.
15. Arrigoni, E. & Amado, R. (1990) Mitt. Gebiete Lebensm. Hyg. 81, 51–67.
16. Rennhard, H. H. (to Pfizer Inc.) (1973) US Patent 3 766 165.
17. Allingham, R. P. (1982) in Chemistry of Foods & Beverages: Recent Developments, Academic Press, New York, NY, pp. 293–303.
18. Figdor, S. K. & Rennhard, H. H. (1981) J. Agric. Food Chem. 29, 1181–1189.
19. Figdor, S. K. & Bianchine, J. R. (1983) J. Agric. Food Chem. 31, 389–393.
20. Juhr, N. & Franke, J. (1992) J. Nutrition. 122, 1425–1433.
21. Achour, L., Flourie, B., Briet, F., Pellier, P., Marteau, P. & Rambaud, J. (1994) Am. J. Clin. Nutr. 59, 1362–1368.
22. Englyst, H. N., Trowell, H. et al., (1987) Am. J. Clin. Nutr. 46, 873–874.
23. Asp, N. B. (1990) in New Developments in Dietary Fiber–Physiological, Physicochemical & Analytical Aspects, I. Furda & C. J. Brine (Eds), Plenum Press, New York, NY, pp. 227–236.
24. Trowell, H. (1972) Am. J. Clin. Nutr., 25, 926–932.
25. Trowell, H., Southgate, D. A. T., Wolover, T. M. S., Leeds, A. R., Gassull, M. A. & Jenkins, D. J. A. (1976) Lancet, 1, 967.
26. Trowell, H. (1978) Am. J. Clin. Nutr. 31(suppl 10), 3–11.

27. Cummings, J. H. (1981) Br. Med. Bull. 37, 65–70.
28. Life Sciences Research Office (1987) Physiological Effects and Health Consequences of Dietary Fiber, LSRO/FASEB, Bethesda, MD.
29. British Nutrition Foundation (1990) Complex Carbohydrates in Foods, Chapman and Hall, London, pp. 56–159.
30. Food Industry Ad-Hoc Working Group on Dietary Fiber (1994) Int. Food Ind. 1/2, 46–49.
31. Madar, Z., & Odes, H. S. (1990) in Dietary Fiber Research, R. Paoletti (Ed.), Kruger, Basel pp. 1–65.
32. Endo, K., Kumemura, M., Nakamura, K., Fujisawa, T., Suzuki, K., Benno, Y. & Mitsuoka, T. (1991) Bifidobacteria Microflora 10, 53–64.
33. Chen, W. L., Anderson, J. W., Plyley, M. A., Thomas, P. X. and Gibson, L. B. (1984) Proc. Soc. Exp. Biol. Med. 175, 215–218.
34. Cummings, J.H. (1991) Report of 10th Ross Conference on Medical Research, 11–17.
35. Scheppach, W. M. (1991) Report of 10th Ross Conference on Medical Research, 90–93.
36. Wang, X. & Gibson, G. R. (1993) J. Appl. Bacter. 75, 373–380.
37. Harada, E., Hashimoto, Y. & Syuto, B. (1995) Comp. Biochem. Physiol. 111A, 479–485.
38. Oku, T., Fujii, Y. & Okamatsu, H. (1991) J. Clin. Biochem. Nutr. 11, 31–40.
39. Tomlin, J. and Read, N. W. (1988) Aliment. Pharmacol. Therap. 2, 513–519.
40. Nakagawa, Y., Okamatsu, H. & Fujii, Y. (1990) J. Jpn. Soc. Nutr. Food Sci. 43, 95–101.
41. Jenkins, D. J., Wolever, T. M., Kalmusky, J., Guidici, S, Buckley, G. and Little, J. A. (1985) Am. J. Clin. Nutr. 42, 604–617.
42. Manas, E. & Saura-Calixto, F. (1993) Food Chemistry 47, 351–355.
43. Amado, R. & Neukom, H. (1985) in New Approaches to Research on Cereal Carbohydrates. R. D. Hill & L. Munck (Eds.), Elsevier, pp. 217–230.
44. Larm, O., Theander, O. & Aman, P. (1975) Acta Chem Scand. Ser. B. B29, 1011–1014.
45. Quemener, B., Thibault, J.-F. & Coussement, P. (1994) Lebensm.-Wiss. u. Technol. 27, 125–132.

V

DIETARY FIBER—ANALYTICAL METHODOLOGY

19

Progress in the Certification of Five New Food Reference Materials by AOAC, Englyst and Uppsala Methods of Dietary Fiber Analysis

ALAN W. PENDLINGTON
RHM Technology Ltd., High Wycombe, Bucks, England

The paper outlines progress on a project within the Third Framework Programme of the European Commission, Measurements and Testing (M&T) Programme (formerly Community Bureau of Reference–BCR). The aim of the work was to produce five new food reference materials from a range of food sources with different levels of dietary fiber and other components, and to certify them simultaneously by Englyst, Uppsala and AOAC methods of analysis. The use of several methods of analysis is desirable because no single method is universally used, and there is a lack of reference materials certified by methods other than AOAC. The new materials are dried haricot bean, dried carrot, dried apple, dried full fat soya flour and dried bran breakfast cereal. The paper includes a brief description of the preparation and packing of these materials and the steps taken to ensure their homogeneity and stability when tested by Englyst and AOAC methods. A preliminary intercomparison study was carried out among thirty-two European laboratories to ensure that the protocols for the methods gave accurate, repeatable and reproducible results that would be acceptable for certification. The materials used for intercomparison were four existing cereal based reference materials, and the methods which were examined were Prosky AOAC 985.29, Lee AOAC 991.43, the Englyst GC procedure, the Englyst Colorimetric procedure and the Uppsala procedure. As a result of this study, it was decided to attempt to certify the new materials using all five methods. The analysis for certification is complete but the results have not yet been evaluated in detail since the participants met to discuss them. The results in this paper are presented provisionally. The materials will not be certified and available until the certification report and the corresponding certificate have been accepted by the certification committee. An additional study was supported within this project to carry out further characterization analysis on the residues obtained from the AOAC and Englyst procedures. The main project is not intended to recommend which method should be used for dietary fiber analysis, nor to compare the merits of the methods. However, the work provides a unique opportunity to study the dietary fiber values of the five new reference materials and of four cereal based materials using five different methods of analysis.

INTRODUCTION

In the European Union it is difficult to compare the dietary fiber content of foodstuffs because of the use of different methods of analysis. The main problem is that the Directive on Nutrition Labelling of Foodstuffs (1) issued by the European Union requires quantitative information on the level of dietary fiber. The directive does not give a definition of dietary fiber and it does not specify a method of analysis so European laboratories use a range of methods, and this is worrying in the European Union where harmonization is an important aim. One consequence is a lack of certified reference materials for dietary fiber analysis The M&T Programme only has reference materials for dietary fiber certified by the Prosky (AOAC 985.29) method (2). These are available via the Institute for Reference Materials and Measurements, Geel, Belgium. Another general concern is that many laboratories do not use reference materials. A recent survey by Lee and Prosky (3) found that less than 30 out of 147 laboratories used them for dietary fiber analysis. This may be due to a lack of appropriate certified reference materials (CRMs).

The M&T Programme exists to enhance measurement and testing methods throughout the European Union, and provide CRMs for a wide range of purposes. The project described in this paper was funded by the M&T Programme, and coordinated by the author under contract to the Commission. It recognizes the problems caused by using several methods of dietary fiber analysis. A major aim of the project is to provide certified food reference materials from a range of food types for the main analytical methods that are in use. These certified materials, with supporting detailed documentation, can then be used by any laboratory for quality control and validation purposes. An important innovation is that a range of analytical methods has been used within the certification exercise. The work is not intended to recommend which method should be used for dietary fiber analysis, and it is not intended to compare the merits of the methods. It is simply intended to report the values for dietary fiber obtained by using the best technique for each method, and to certify the values on the basis of every method.

The design of the project included a management team with expertise in each of the major methods. They were from the Ministere des Affaires Economique, Brussels; the Swedish University of Agricultural Sciences, Uppsala and RHM Technology Ltd. Up to thirty-two European laboratories participated in the project from fifteen countries. They represented universities, public analysts and industrial laboratories. The background to the project was that in 1991, experts who had participated in earlier MAFF/EC collaborative trials on Englyst and AOAC methods recommended that more work should be done to improve the methods, and a wider range of reference materials should be studied with varying levels of fiber and other components. They said that it would be desirable to have more information on the polysaccharide constituents of the cell walls of the reference materials. Following these recommendations, the European Commission, M&T Programme supported a detailed study of the three main analytical methods (4). In another study (5), three reference materials based on rye flour, wheat flour and haricots verts beans were prepared and analyzed for certification purposes. Only the results by the Prosky (AOAC 985.29) method were accepted for certification, because the uncertainty of the results by the Englyst method was considered by the participants to be too high. The current project followed and built on the experience of the preceding studies. It had two parts, first, a short study of cell wall components, and second the main part of the project which was the preparation and certification of five new food reference materials.

CELL WALL STUDY

This was a qualitative study to analyze the residues from the AOAC and Englyst procedures to gather further information about their composition. The materials used were the five new food reference materials–haricot, apple, carrot, full fat soya and bran breakfast cereal. The residue was the dried material remaining after enzymic starch and protein removal steps in the two procedures, including the dimethyl sulphoxide (DMSO) dispersion step in the Englyst procedure. The AOAC residue was recovered by centrifugation to avoid contamination by the filter aid. At the TNO Nutrition and Food Research Institute, Zeist, Netherlands, the residues were analyzed directly by pyrolysis with direct chemical ionization mass spectrometry. They were also analyzed after stepwise acid hydrolysis by high performance ion exchange chromatography and by proton NMR analysis with pattern recognition. At the University of Saarlandes, Dept of Applied Physical Chemistry, the residues were analyzed after stepwise acid hydrolysis by anion exchange chromatography of the sugars followed by pulsed amperometric detection, and by capillary electrophoresis.

The results of these studies are still being analyzed. However, preliminary conclusions are that the residues can be distinguished by their pyrolysis spectra, and that residues isolated by Englyst and AOAC procedures can be differentiated. The differential rates of hydrolysis of the polysaccharides in 2M and 12M sulfuric acid can be demonstrated. The results should give some information about what the AOAC and Englyst techniques are measuring. It is anticipated that this information will become more useful as the physiologists learn more about the action of different fiber components.

MAIN STUDY

The main study was in three parts. The first was the preparation and packing of the materials and a check for homogeneity and stability. The second was the intercomparison study—optimizing the analytical methods in several laboratories, and assessing and selecting laboratories to take part in the certification study. The third part was the certification study—analyzing the new reference materials according to strict protocols in selected different laboratories, evaluating the submitted results technically and statistically, and submitting the certification report and the corresponding certificate to the advisory committee for certification of the European Commission Standards, Measurements and Testing (SM&T) Programme (formerly the Measurements and Testing, M&T, Programme).

Preparation, Packing, Homogeneity and Stability Check

The five materials were apple, bran breakfast cereal, carrot, haricot beans and full fat soya. These materials had been recommended by a previous EC/BCR meeting in 1991. They were chosen to represent a range of foods, cereal, fruit, root vegetables and legumes, and to cover a range of dietary fiber levels from approximately 10% to 30% on a dry basis. They also had different levels of other components. For instance full fat soya has a high level of fat, apple and carrot have a high level of free sugars, and bran and haricot have higher levels of starch. It was anticipated that these would be good models for a range of foods for which the materials would be used as reference materials.

In order to ensure stability and homogeneity, the foods were carefully freeze-dried to below 3 g/100 g moisture, reduced to fine powders, less than 500 μm, to ensure that there were no concentrated lumps of fiber that could cause inhomogeneity at the lowest sample mass that would be used, and they were sealed under vacuum in glass bottles with flexible seals and tamperproof screw caps. The homogeneity of the materials was checked by the Englyst 1992 procedure (6), and by the Prosky (AOAC 985.29) procedure (2). There was no significant between-bottle inhomogeneity and no significant within-bottle inhomogeneity at the 5% level using the F test. There was no significant trend due to the filling sequence and no significant trend due to the order of sampling at the 5% level using the t test. This met the European Commission M&T Programme requirements for homogeneity.

M&T Programme Requirements for Homogeneity

The coefficients of variation (CV) were all less than or equal to 4% (Table 1). These results, and particularly those using the Englyst procedure, were encouraging although they were only from single laboratories.

The values of dietary fiber measured by Englyst GC were lower than those by AOAC 985.29, except the results for full fat soya, which were similar by both procedures. This difference is in line with the findings of the COST 92 survey on dietary fiber intakes in Europe (7), where enzymatic chemical methods gave results that were approximately 18% lower than gravimetric methods. This is not surprising, because the methods measure different things. The AOAC and Uppsala methods include residual starch and lignin which are excluded in the Englyst method.

During the homogeneity tests, considerable variations in the Englyst GC results for the bran breakfast cereal were noted. The main variation was in the xylose levels. It was found that increasing the quantity of ammonia used to neu-

TABLE 1 Results of the Bottle Homogeneity Study—Dietary Fiber Levels and Coefficients of Variation of the Five New Reference Materials by the AOAC 985.29 and Englyst GC Methods

Method	Dietary fiber by AOAC 985.29 (g/100 g db)	Dietary fiber by Englyst GC (g/100 g db)	% Difference between methods	CV % by AOAC	CV % by Englyst GC
Haricot RM 514	26.1	20.7	20.6	1	2
Carrot RM 515	31.6	26.9	14.9	1	4
Apple RM 516	17.1	14.1	17.9	2	3
Soya RM 517	12.5	12.3	1.7	4	3
Bran RM 518	30.3	24.5	19.4	1	2

tralize sulfuric acid early in the derivatization step significantly increased the recovery of xylose and arabinose. The problem was probably caused by variations in the concentration of ammonia solutions. This drops when the bottles are opened frequently. The quantity of ammonia recommended in the procedure (6) was only sufficient if the solutions were the correct concentration. In the latest Englyst procedure published in 1994 (8), and subsequently used for certification analysis, the quantity of ammonia was increased. The higher level of ammonia adds tolerance to the method but it is still important to use correct concentration of ammonia.

An additional test was carried out in which extra 100% ethanol was added to the supernatant remaining after precipitation and centrifugation of the polysaccharides. This produced a further precipitate, which was analyzed by GC and found to contain significant amounts of sugars. The composition of the precipitate was not checked further. It may contain oligosaccharides. This observation has not yet been followed up.

The long term stability and possible transportation requirements of the new reference materials were checked by storage at various temperatures and analysis at intervals up to two years by Englyst GC and AOAC 985.29 methods The final analysis at two years was not complete at the time this paper was written. So far there has been no deterioration of any of the new reference materials in any storage condition.

Intercomparison Study

The aims of the intercomparison study were to optimize the methods in a wide range of laboratories, and assess the laboratories, before carrying out the certification analysis. A meeting of all the participants was held to agree the methods that should be investigated, to identify sources of error for each method and to provide suggestions for their avoidance and control. The participants in the study agreed that five methods should be used for the assessment. These were the Uppsala method (9), the AOAC Prosky method 985.29 (2), both versions of the Englyst method (gas chromatographic and colorimetric) (8) and a recent version of the AOAC method 991.43 by Lee, with MES-TRIS buffer (10).

The participants agreed that some changes or recommendations should be incorporated into the protocol of each method to optimise their performance. These were a combination of the participants' experience, some recent improvements to methods and some results from previous studies.

The changes in the Englyst procedure were all subsequently published by Englyst, Quigley and Hudson (8). They were presented to the meeting in advance of publication. The recommendations for the AOAC procedures were mainly to highlight points in the existing method that needed standardizing to avoid sources of variability. The only change to the Uppsala method was the inclusion of a factor to compensate for the difference in degradation during the hydrolysis procedure between free galacturonic acid in the standard solution and polymeric galacturonic acid in the sample. The use of this factor resulted in better agreement with other similar methods. It is now included in the published method (9).

The intercomparison study was designed to eliminate as many potential variables as possible, and some materials were supplied by the coordinator. It had originally been intended to supply the Uppsala participants with the same enzymes as the AOAC participants. However, it was found that the amyloglucosidase issued to the AOAC participants contained some unwanted hemicellulase activity. This caused losses in the Uppsala procedure, which has longer incubation stages. The Uppsala participants were therefore supplied from a purer source. This illustrates the importance of checking the activity of the enzymes in the method to be used.

Preliminary Intercomparison Analyses

Before starting the main intercomparison analysis, the participants were asked to analyze a mixture of four polysaccharide materials arabinogalactan (larch gum), fibrous cellulose, sugar free citrus pectin, and galactomannan (alcohol washed guar gum), and to obtain results within the known value ±2 SD (based on the performance in the intercomparison study). Participants who were using gas chromatography were asked, in addition, to carry out a similar exercise on a mixture of sugars. These two preliminary tests proved to be very useful, as they highlighted problems in some laboratories with the filtration step of the AOAC procedures, miscalculations, misunderstandings of the role of blanks, problems with response factors in GC, a problem with the makeup of a sugar standard and of the unknown sugar mixture, and uncovered minor errors in the protocol.

Because of this exercise, many laboratories subsequently produced very good data for the main intercomparison study by all the methods.

Table 2 shows the very low coefficients of variation between laboratories achieved with all the methods, and the good agreement between the mean values for dietary fiber. This agreement using the polysaccharide mix contrasts with the large difference in dietary fiber values found between the Englyst method and AOAC methods for many food materials and underlines its applicability for initial quality control purposes.

Main Intercomparison Analyses

The choice of suitable test materials for the study was limited. The five new reference materials could not be used because the participants must eventually carry out the analysis for certification without knowing the expected results. Alternate materials had to be found. Four dried reference materials that had already been tested for homogeneity and stability were kindly supplied by the Food Re-

TABLE 2 The Dietary Fiber Levels and Coefficients of Variation Between Laboratories Found in the Preliminary Intercomparison Test with a Mixture of Polysaccharides

Method	# of Labs	Mean TDF g/100 g db	CV(R)% (between labs)
AOAC 985.29	19	91.4	2.5
AOAC 991.43	10	92.8	1.5
Englyst GC	7	92.5	3.7
Englyst Color	9	91.0	4.0
Uppsala	5	91.2	3.3

search Institute at Norwich. They were white bread (RM 416), wholemeal bread (RM 417), a mixture of wholemeal and white bread (RM 418) and cornflakes (RM 419). These materials were analyzed by all five methods (Table 3).

The dietary fiber levels given by methods which do not exclude residual starch and lignin (Uppsala and AOAC) were higher than the values by the Englyst methods that only measure non-starch polysaccharides.

The standard deviation between laboratories was low for all methods, except the Uppsala method. This is an improvement with respect to the Englyst methods, because the uncertainty of past results was too high to permit certification. This fulfilled a major purpose of the intercomparison study which was to check that the methods, when applied by the participating laboratories, were sufficiently repeatable and reproducible to be used for certification.

The results by the AOAC 985.29 Prosky method and the AOAC 991.43

TABLE 3 Dietary Fiber Values of Four Cereal Based Reference Materials Analyzed by Five Methods During the Intercomparison Study

Reference material	# of labs	White bread	Wholemeal	Mixture	Cornflakes
AOAC 985.29	19	4.5 ± 0.7	11.8 ± 0.7	8.0 ± 0.6	3.1 ± 0.7
Englyst GC	7	3.3 ± 0.3	9.1 ± 0.7	6.3 ± 0.5	1.0 ± 0.3
Uppsala	5	5.1 ± 0.5	11.5 ± 1.7	8.2 ± 0.6	3.0 ± 1.2
AOAC 991.43	10	4.6 ± 0.4	12.1 ± 0.8	8.1 ± 0.5	3.3 ± 0.7
Englyst Color	9	3.4 ± 0.4	9.6 ± 0.6	6.8 ± 0.4	1.2 ± 0.5

Dietary fiber values, g/100 g dry basis
Mean ±1 SD

Lee method were compared statistically. The mean results for each reference material by the two methods were not significantly different ($p > 0.05$ t-test).

The participants met to discuss the results of the intercomparison study and to agree upon the criteria which would be applied to the results of each laboratory to decide which laboratories should take part in the final certification study. They also agreed upon limits that would be applied to the results of the certification study to decide whether the data was sufficiently repeatable and reproducible to be submitted for certification. They agreed upon the details to be incorporated in the instructions for the certification study to give the maximum chance of success. The project was funded on the basis of using three methods for certification and the participants agreed on the AOAC 985.29 Prosky method, the Englyst GC method and the Uppsala method. However, several laboratories had obtained very good results with the AOAC 991.43 method of Lee with MES-TRIS buffer and with the Englyst colorimetric method and they volunteered to undertake the certification analyzes without payment.

Certification Study

Structure

The certification study followed the new guidelines for the production and certification of BCR reference materials (11). The core of the study was the analysis of each of the new reference materials by each of five methods. To ensure that the methods were in control, materials with known values were tested before and at intervals during the analyzes. Certified rye flour, CRM 381 was supplied free of charge by the European Commission M&T Programme as a control for the laboratories using the AOAC 985.29 method. It was more difficult to find a suitable material for the other methods because no certified reference materials are available. The mixture of four polysaccharides was used.

For laboratories using gas chromatography, a new unknown sugar solution was prepared, and participants were required to obtain results within specified limits, for individual sugars, before continuing.

For the main analysis, three bottles of each new reference material were supplied to each laboratory, and they were analyzed in duplicate in at least two separate runs.

All the new materials, apple, bran, carrot, haricot and soya, have been analyzed by all five dietary fiber methods. Between five and nine laboratories carried out the analysis with each method. At the time of writing this paper, the certification study is almost complete. At a recent meeting of all the participants, all the data and supplementary information was discussed and evaluated to ensure that it met the Commission's rigorous standards. The data from any non-conforming laboratories is not accepted. Any results that were unusual were investigated, and discussed among the experts, to ensure that there were no technical problems or calculation errors that might explain the problem. Finally the data was technically and statistically assessed to see whether any values or data sets should be excluded. The guidelines (11) emphasize that statistically outlying data can only be excluded if there is a technical explanation because the BCR has encountered previous examples when the outlier was subsequently discovered to be the correct value. The recalculation of the data resulting from the decisions taken at the meeting, is still in progress.

During the many analyzes for intercomparison and certification, the participants have encountered and overcome several problems in carrying out the various methods. This information was collected at the meeting, and it will be added as a set of recommendations in the certification report which is sent out with the certificate and the CRM to eventual purchasers.

Results—Control Materials

The results in this paper are provisional because they have not yet been amended after evaluation at the meeting of participants. They are offered because they provided useful information for discussion at the workshop. It is anticipated that there will be few amendments, and they will tend to improve the reliability of the results. However it must be emphasized that definitive results will only be available in the final certification report.

The following results obtained with the control materials demonstrate that the methods were in control (Table 4).

The participants using the AOAC 985.29 procedure achieved excellent agreement with the certified value for the certified rye flour, CRM 381. The par-

TABLE 4 Dietary Fiber Values Obtained with the Control Standards During the Certification Analysis

Reference material	Control material	Certified value	Submitted data (mean)	Expected value 1	Submitted data (mean)
AOAC 985.29	CRM 381	8.22 ± 0.18	8.15 ± 0.18		
AOAC 991.43	P/S mixture	8.22 ± 0.18	8.15 ± 0.18	94.5 ± 2.7	93.0 ± 1.4
Englyst GC	P/S mixture	8.22 ± 0.18	8.15 ± 0.18	93.5 ± 4.6	92.9 ± 2.6
Englyst Color	P/S mixture	8.22 ± 0.18	8.15 ± 0.18	93.5 ± 4.8	93.3 ± 1.3
Uppsala	P/S mixture	8.22 ± 0.18	8.15 ± 0.18	93.5 ± 6.0	91.7 ± 3.8

Dietary fiber values g/100 g dry weight (d.w.) basis
Mean ±1 SD
Note: The expected values for the Englyst and Uppsala procedures are lower to allow for the losses of methoxyl groups during acid hydrolysis

ticipants using the other methods achieved good agreement with the expected values for the polysaccharide mix. The agreement between methods for the polysaccharide mixture was closer than in the intercomparison study—the mean values range between 91.7 and 93.3 g/100 g d.w. basis.

Results—Enzyme Testing

The enzymes used by the participants were not supplied by the coordinator, to avoid systematic bias. The enzymes were tested for activity and purity. Some participants using the AOAC methods obtained low recoveries from the substrates arabinogalactan, pectin and β-glucan when following the enzyme testing method in the AOAC procedures (985.29 and 991.43). In some cases the laboratory had not dried the substrate or allowed for the substrate's moisture content. This requirement is not clear in the AOAC methods. When allowance was made for moisture, the recovery was acceptable. However in other cases, recovery was still low after allowing for moisture, although other participants using the identical batch of enzyme obtained acceptable recoveries. One possible reason could be a loss of precipitated material through the Celite bed due to the physical nature of the precipitate and the preparation of the Celite bed. With a small quantity of pure substrate the risk of losses is probably greater. One participant commented that it was necessary to allow two hours standing time for the precipitate to develop before filtration to obtain good recoveries, rather than one hour as stated in the procedure.

Results—New Reference Material

Dietary fiber values for the five new reference materials are shown in Tables 5–8. These results are preliminary. They have yet to be amended after discussion and evaluation at the meeting of participants.

The standard deviation of the mean of means was low, enhancing the possibility of certification. The agreement with the results obtained in the previous homogeneity study was mostly good, within one standard deviation, with the exception of apple. In making this comparison, it must be remembered that the homogeneity analysis was only carried out by one laboratory per method. Agreement between the AOAC Prosky method 985.29 and the AOAC Lee method 991.43 was good for haricot, soya and Bran breakfast cereal, but outside two standard deviations for carrot and apple (Table 5).

The standard deviation of the mean of means was again low, which is an improvement on previous studies using the Englyst methods (Table 6). It is anticipated that it will be possible to certify on the basis of these results. The agreement with the homogeneity study is very good; all the results are within one standard deviation. The agreement between the gas chromatographic and colorimetric methods is good (within 1 SD), except for carrot. This may suggest that the two methods should be certified separately.

TABLE 5 Provisional Dietary Fiber Values of the Five New Reference Materials Submitted by the Participants Using the AOAC 985.29 and 991.43 Procedures

Reference material	RM 514 Haricot	RM 515 Carrot	RM 516 Apple	RM 517 Full fat soya	RM 518 Bran b'fast cereal
AOAC 985.29	25.9 ± 0.5	31.0 ± 0.6	16.4 ± 0.5	12.4 ± 0.5	30.5 ± 0.9
7 labs	(26.0 ± 0.4)	(31.6 ± 0.3)	(17.1 ± 0.3)	(12.5 ± 0.4)	(30.3 ± 0.3)
AOAC 991.43	26.1 ± 1.0	29.5 ± 0.1	14.9 ± 0.8	12.6 ± 1.0	30.5 ± 0.4
7 labs					

Dietary fiber values g/100 g dry basis
Mean of means = 1 SD (Mean ±1 SD)
Values in parentheses are from the homogeneity study

TABLE 6 Provisional Dietary Fiber Values of the Five New Reference Materials Submitted by the Participants Using the Englyst Gas Chromatographic and Colorimetric Procedures

Reference material	RM 514 Haricot	RM 515 Carrot	RM 516 Apple	RM 517 Full fat soya	RM 518 Bran b'fast cereal
Englyst GC					
6 labs	19.8 ± 0.9	27.1 ± 0.5	13.7 ± 0.5	11.9 ± 0.4	24.3 ± 0.8
Englyst Col	(20.7 ± 0.4)	(26.9 ± 1.0)	(14.1 ± 0.4)	(12.3 ± 0.3)	(24.5 ± 0.4)
6 labs	20.1 ± 0.5	25.2 ± 1.1	13.4 ± 0.4	12.3 ± 0.7	25.0 ± 1.0

Dietary fiber values g/100 g dry basis
Mean of means = 1 SD (Mean ±1 SD)
Values in parentheses are from the homogeneity study

TABLE 7 Provisional Dietary Fiber Values of the Five New Reference Materials Submitted by the Participants Using the Uppsala Procedure

Reference material	RM 514 Haricot	RM 515 Carrot	RM 516 Apple	RM 517 Full fat soya	RM 518 Bran b'fast cereal
Uppsala method	23.5 ± 0.5	29.5 ± 0.4	15.9 ± 0.5	12.8 ± 0.5	27.9 ± 1.1
4 labs					

Dietary fiber values g/100 g dry basis
Mean of means = 1 SD (Mean ±1 SD)

TABLE 8 Dietary Fiber Values Obtained on the New Reference Materials by a Variety of Analytical Methods*

Analytical method	AOAC 985.29 (Prosky)	AOAC 991.43 (Lee)	AOAC 991.43 + APP**	Englyst GC 1988	Mongeau 992.16
RM 514	23.9 ± 0.8	24.9 ± 0.3	24.6 ± 0.2	22.6 ± 0.4	20.6 ± 0.8
Haricot	(25.9)	(26.1)		(19.8)	
RM 515	30.3 ± 0.2	29.5 ± 0.2	29.4 ± 0.1	27.2 ± 0.5	25.1 ± 0.1
Carrot	(31.0)	(29.5)		(27.1)	
RM 516	16.2 ± 0.1	16.2 ± 0.2	16.2 ± 0.3	15.5 ± 0.6	14.6 ± 0.4
Apple	(16.4)	(14.9)		(13.7)	
RM 517	12.5 ± 0.1	12.8 ± 0.6	13.2 ± 0.1	14.8 ± 0.2	14.2 ± 0.2
FF Soya	(12.4)	(12.6)		(11.9)	
RM 518	30.2 ± 0.1	29.7 ± 0.2	31.0 ± 0.3	27.3 ± 0.7	29.5 ± 0.2
Bran B/C	(30.5)	(30.5)		(24.3)	

Dietary fiber values g/100 g dry basis
Mean of means = 1 SD (Mean ± 1 SD)
( ) Figures in parentheses are the results from the certification study
*Results were submitted on as-is basis. To allow comparison a dry basis figure was calculated using the mean of certification participants moisture results (max 3 g/100 g)
**APP = α-amylase from porcine pancreas

The standard deviation of the means was low. There are some differences from the values with the AOAC methods, particularly with haricot beans. The AOAC methods gave approximately 26 g/100 g and the Uppsala methods gave 23.5 g/100 g (Table 7).

Overall, the results show the expected difference between methods based on the knowledge that they measure different things.

SUPPLEMENTARY STUDY

Additional analyzes were carried out on the new reference materials by Dr. Mongeau of the Bureau of Nutritional Sciences, Ottawa, using a range of methods in his laboratory.

The following methods were used. The traditional Prosky method, AOAC 985.29 (2); the AOAC 991.43 method of Lee using MES-TRIS buffer (10) and a modification using a porcine pancreas enzyme preparation (12); the 1988 version of the Englyst gas chromatographic method (13); and the Mongeau/Brassard rapid enzymatic-gravimetric method (AOAC 992.16) that includes an initial autoclaving step (14).

The AOAC methods gave very similar values. For carrot, this contrasts with the results found by the participants in the certification study. The results by the 1988 Englyst GC method (13) are lower than the results by AOAC as expected. However they are higher than the results obtained by the participants in the certification study (shown in brackets in the table) who were using a later (1994) Englyst method (8). It is interesting to compare the Englyst GC values with the Mongeau rapid method values. Except for bran breakfast cereal, the Englyst values are higher than those obtained by the Mongeau method.

In previous studies (12) Mongeau has demonstrated that the use of porcine pancreas enzyme to replace purified enzymes in the AOAC 991.43 method with MES-TRIS buffer resulted in lower dietary fiber values with boiled legumes. This effect was not seen with the new haricot bean preparation, possibly because the material had not been boiled.

It is not the purpose of this paper to discuss the merits of the various methods or to attempt to investigate the reasons for the differences in the results obtained. What is clear is that using carefully prepared, stable, homogeneous materials, different methods of dietary fiber analysis which are under control give different results. The direction of the differences depends on the nature of the materials, and slightly different versions of the same technique can give different results depending on the nature of the reference material.

Laboratories wishing to improve and validate their dietary fiber analytical techniques must be clear about the nature of the samples they are using and the importance of following very strict protocols for carrying out the analysis.

CONCLUSIONS

The primary purpose of this study was to certify five new reference materials by a range of methods, to provide certified reference materials for laboratories that are using methods besides the AOAC 985.29 method. The work is not intended to recommend which method should be used for dietary fiber analysis, nor to compare the merits of the methods. The purpose is to report the values for dietary fiber obtained with the best technique for each method, and to certify the values on that basis. However, the results raise several interesting issues.

First, the results of dietary fiber analysis are very method dependent. This is not surprising as the methods aim to measure different things. In cereal based materials it is probable that the major differences between the Englyst and AOAC values are due to the exclusion of all residual starch and lignin in the Englyst method. However, this cannot be the explanation for the differences in carrot and apple, which contain very little starch.

The method dependency is also related to the food material being measured. The AOAC 991.43 method with MES-TRIS buffer, and the Englyst colorimetric method both give very similar results to those of their parent methods, for some materials. For other materials, there are apparent differences. This suggests that there are factors in the materials being measured which influence the results of methods apparently measuring the same components, but by different procedures.

However, for a mixture of pure polysaccharides all the methods gave remarkably similar results. This suggests that with no interfering substances, all the methods can accurately measure non-starch polysaccharides and that such materials could be used for initial quality control tests.

Some general points arose from the study. First, the laboratories in the study were all expert and competent, yet it was surprising how many minor mathematical errors crept into some calculations. Some of these significantly affected the results but were very difficult to detect. They were identified because all the submitted data was entered into computer spreadsheets which automatically carried out all the calculations in an identical way. It would appear that for this type of collaborative study, the use of spreadsheets would improve the reliability of the data. Second, moisture is a factor whose importance is often underestimated in fiber analysis. This study needed particular care because to ensure stability, the materials were dried down to below 3 g/100 g moisture, and were therefore very likely to pick up moisture from the atmosphere. The participants had to ensure that they weighed out samples for analysis at the same time as they weighed out the samples for moisture determination, so that any subsequent moisture uptake would not affect the experimental results. Precise knowledge of the moisture content of standard reagents is also vital.

Lastly, the apparently variable performance of some enzymes and the difficulties with the testing procedures suggest that further work is required in this area. It is important to carry out enzyme tests in each method that is to be used.

ACKNOWLEDGMENTS

The author wishes to thank the European Commission Measurements and Testing Programme for funding the project, the management team for their valuable assistance, and all the laboratories throughout Europe who have given their considerable skills and enthusiasm to the project.

REFERENCES

1. Council Directive on Nutrition Labelling for Foodstuffs (1990), OJ No L 276/40, European Commission, Luxembourg.
2. Official Methods of Analysis (1990) 15th Ed., AOAC, Arlington, VA, 1105–1106.
3. Lee, S. C., Prosky, L., (1995) J. AOAC Int. 78, 22–36.
4. Faulks, R. M., & Boenke, A., (1994) Dietary Fiber in Complex Food Materials, Detailed Method Study, EUR 15728 EN, European Commission, Luxembourg.
5. Hollman, P., Boenke, A., Finglas, P., & Wagstaffe, P. J. (1992) The certification of the mass fraction of major components and essential elements in rye flour, wheat

flour and lyophilized haricots verts (beans) reference materials, EUR 14553 EN, Commission of the European Communities, Luxembourg.
6. Englyst, H. N., Quigley, M. E., Hudson, G. J., & Cummings, J. H. (1992) Analyst 117, 1707–1714.
7. Dietary Fiber Intakes in Europe (1993), Cummings, J. H., & Frølich, W. (Eds), Commission of the European Communities, Luxembourg.
8. Englyst, H. N., Quigley, M. E., & Hudson, G. J. (1994) Analyst 119, 1497–1509.
9. Theander, O., Åman, P., Westerlund, E., Andersson, R., & Pettersson, D. (1995) J. AOAC Int. 78, 1030–1044.
10. Lee, S. C., Prosky, L., & DeVries, J. W. (1992) J. AOAC Int. 75, 395–416.
11. Guidelines for the production and certification of BCR Reference materials (1994), BCR/48/93, European Commission, Luxembourg.
12. Mongeau, R., & Brassard, R. (1994) J. AOAC Int. 77, 1197–1202.
13. Englyst, H. N., & Cummings, J. H. (1988) J. Assoc. Off. Anal. Chem. 71, 808–814.
14. Official Methods of Analysis (1995) 16th Ed., AOAC, Arlington, VA, sec 32.1.18.

20

High Performance Anion Exchange Chromatography with Pulsed Amperometric Detection (HPAE-PAD): A Powerful Tool for the Analysis of Dietary Fiber and Complex Carbohydrates

Alan Henshall
Dionex Corporation, Sunnyvale, California

INTRODUCTION

The quantitation of mono-, di-, and oligosaccharides from hydrolysis of non-starch polysaccharides is receiving increasing recognition as an accurate measurement of the non-lignin portion of dietary fiber. High performance liquid chromatography (HPLC) techniques based on silica bonded phase or metal-loaded cation exchange columns with RI detection have been widely used for the determination of mono-, di-, and small oligosaccharides for more than a decade. However, these techniques have proved inadequate for separating the complex mixtures of carbohydrates resulting from the hydrolysis of non-starch polysaccharides (NSP) and for separation of polysaccharides with DP >9. The more recently developed HPAE-PAD technique shows great promise for the determination of neutral sugars and uronic acid constituents derived from NSP since near-baseline separations are obtained allowing direct quantitation. The HPAE-PAD technique has also been successfully applied to the determination of sugar alcohols and the separation of polysaccharides up to DP 60. In this chapter, the basis of the HPAE-PAD technique will be reviewed along with examples of its application to the determination of dietary fiber and complex carbohydrate constituents.

The impetus to develop pulsed amperometric detection stemmed from the need for a better detection method for carbohydrates (1-3). HPLC with refractive index (RI) detection has been widely used for the detection of simple sugars in foods, however RI suffers from lack of specificity, low sensitivity, and incompatibility with gradient elution. For these reasons, conventional HPLC with RI is of limited utility for some applications due to interference resulting from inadequate resolution of sugars from sugar alcohols and organic acids coupled with the lack of detector specificity (4-8). Similarly, UV absorbance detection can only be used for detection of carbohydrates at low wavelengths (180-220 nm) where it is also nonspecific and insensitive, and interference from compounds other than the carbohydrates of interest commonly occur (8). Sodium chloride interference and the toxicity and disposal problems associated with the use of acetonitrile have also been cited as additional problems when determining carbohydrates by traditional HPLC methods (9,10).

In the case of dietary fiber analysis, traditional HPLC methods have proved inadequate for separation of the mixture of sugars released by hydrolysis of nonstarch polysaccharides (11). High performance anion exchange chromatography (also referred to as high pH anion exchange chromatography) with pulsed amperometric detection (HPAE-PAD or HPAEC-PAD) is a relatively new liquid chromatographic technique that overcomes these problems and has been successfully applied to dietary fiber and complex carbohydrate analysis. This technique is direct (no derivatization required), highly sensitive and specific, and compatible with gradient elution techniques. Sugars, sugar alcohols, oligo- and polysaccharides can be separated with high resolution in a single run and quantitated at the picomole level if necessary. HPAE-PAD is in wide use for glycoprotein research, and increasingly is being applied to a variety of routine monitoring and research applications. Recently, official methods have also been approved (12,13).

USE OF HPAE-PAD FOR DETERMINATION OF COMPLEX CARBOHYDRATES AND DIETARY FIBER

The increasing utilization of HPAE-PAD for determination of complex carbohydrates and dietary fiber constituents is illustrated by the number of publications on these topics in the last few years (11,14-23).

Englyst et al. (11,14,15) have used HPAE-PAD to determine neutral sugars, uronic acids, and hexosamines from non-starch polysaccharides. Corradini et al., have developed methods for the determination of nutritionally significant carbohydrates (16). Jane et al. have applied the technique to study debranched amylopectins (17). Coussement et al. have developed methodology for the determination of inulin and oligofructose in food products (18). Koizumi et al. have studied chain length distribution of amylopectins and oligo- and polysaccharides with DP> 50 (19,20). Fahey et al. have used HPAE-PAD to determine the neutral monosaccharide composition of various fibrous substances and have compared the HPAE-PAD method with the standard colorimetric procedure for the determination of pectic substances in fruit and vegetables (21,22). Hotchkiss et al. have applied HPAE-PAD to the analysis of pectin-derived oligogalacturonic acids with 50 or fewer residues (23).

PRINCIPLE OF PULSED AMPEROMETRIC DETECTION

Amperometric detection is based on the measurement of a change in current due to oxidation, reduction, or complex formation of an analyte at the surface of an electrode (Figure 1).

In DC amperometry the electrode is maintained at a constant potential during the determination. This technique has been applied to the determination of a number of compounds and ions e.g., catecholamines, thiols, phenols, sulfite,

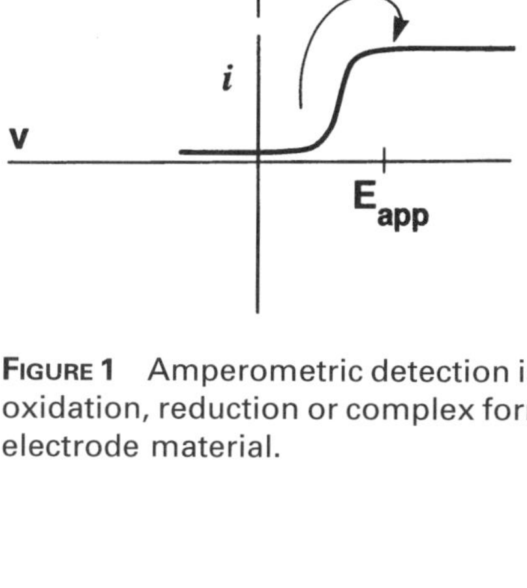

FIGURE 1 Amperometric detection is contingent on a change in current due to oxidation, reduction or complex formation at the applied potential on specific electrode material.

iodide, cyanide (24). Carbohydrates are easily oxidized on gold or platinum electrodes at high pH and are therefore good candidates for electrochemical detection. However, DC amperometry is not useful for carbohydrates since the carbohydrate oxidation products foul the electrode causing a rapidly decreasing response on subsequent determinations (Figure 2). This problem is solved by pulsed amperometry which utilizes a triple pulse sequence rather than a constant potential on the working electrode (1-3). Figure 3 illustrates the basic principle of PAD. By using a repeating sequence of high positive (E2) and negative potentials (E3) following each measurement, a clean electrode surface is maintained which ensures consistency in response. The detector signal for a particular analyte is measured at a potential which is appropriate for the particular analyte (E1) by integrating the current for a fixed length of time (typically 200 ms) and storing the resulting charge in a sample-and-hold amplifier until the next measurement.

The potential settings for a particular analyte are best determined by using cyclic voltammetry or pulsed voltammetry (25). Cyclic voltammetry plots such as the one shown in Figure 4 for glucose on a gold electrode also throw light on the mechanism of the electrochemical processes in pulsed amperometry, and the reason for the high specificity of the technique. The solid line shows the variation in current as the potential is swept from −0.8V to +0.6V and back to 0.8V for glucose in 100 mM NaOH. The dashed line shows the current as a function of

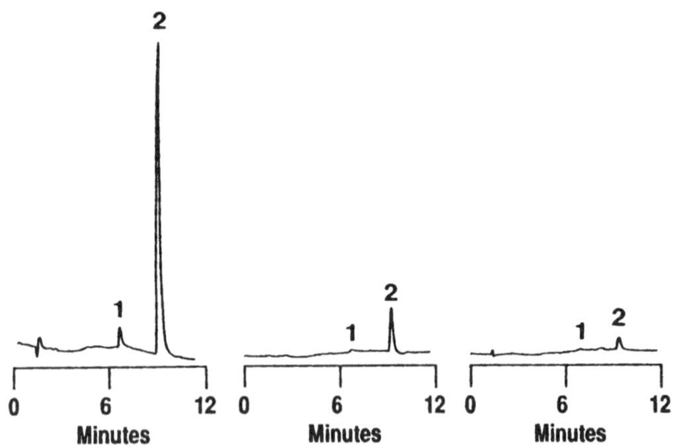

FIGURE 2 Decrease in detector response for repeat injections of a carbohydrate and an amino acid (concentration 10 μg/L in both cases) using DC amperometric detection. Peaks: (1) leucine. (2) lactose. Column: CarboPac PA1 (10 * M, 250 × 4 mm i.d.) with guard, Eluent: gradient, 15 to 150 mM NaOH in 5 min. Detection: DC amperometry, Au electrode, range 1*A, applied potential 0.15V vs. Ag/AgCL.

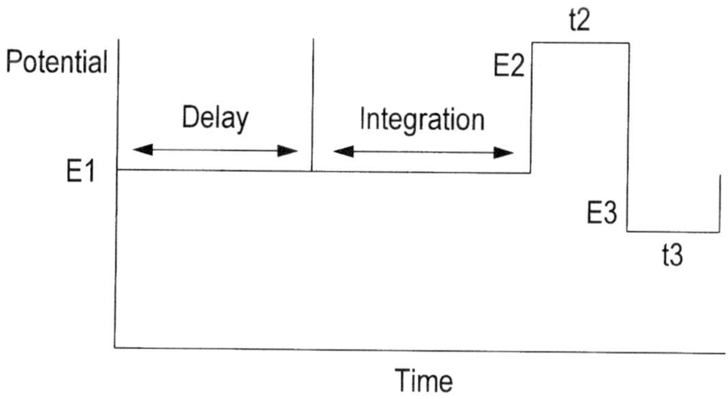

Figure 3 Triple potential sequence used in pulsed amperometry. A clean electrode surface is maintained by using a repeating sequence of a high positive followed by a negative potential after each measurement.

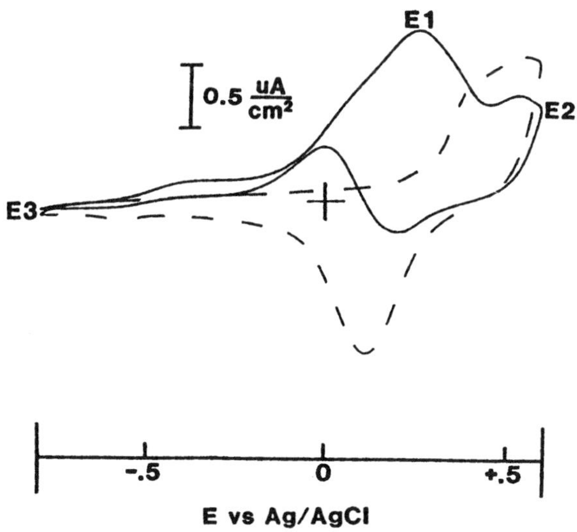

Figure 4 Cyclic voltammetry of glucose on a gold electrode. Dashed line is for 0.10 M NaOH supporting electrolyte. Solid line is for glucose + 0.10 M NaOH supporting electrolyte.

potential for the 100 mM NaOH background electrolyte in the absence of glucose. For the background electrolyte alone, the current stays fairly low and constant until a potential of approximately 0.25V is reached. At this point, onset of oxidation of the gold electrode to gold oxide occurs. The current continues to rise with further electrode oxidation until the potential sweep is reversed at 0.6V (E2). During the reverse sweep (to E3) the gold oxide on the electrode surface is reduced back to gold.

With glucose present (solid line), the current rise during the positive sweep occurs at a lower potential (−600 to -200 mV) due mainly to oxidation of the aldehyde group, and peaks at ~+0.26V due to oxidation of both the aldehyde and alcohol groups on the glucose. The current then decreases with a further increase in the potential due to the formation of gold oxide on the electrode surface which inhibits glucose oxidation. The potential at which the oxidation peak occurs is typical for carbohydrates as shown by the current vs. potential plots for several different types of carbohydrates (Figure 5) determined by pulsed voltammetry (25). The practical implication is that a single potential setting (E1)

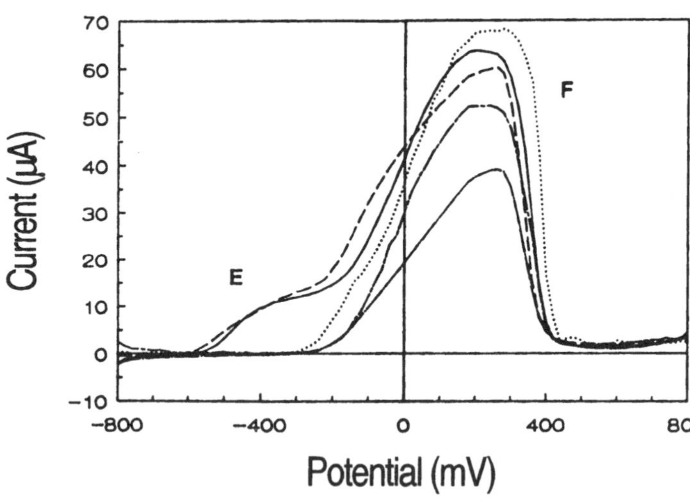

FIGURE 5 Pulsed voltammetry response for five (5) carbohydrates in 0.1 M NaOH Concentration 0.1 mM: (......) sorbitol; (—) glucose; (— —) fructose; (—•—) sucrose; (• • •) maltose. Reprinted with permission from LaCourse, W.R. and Johnson, D.C. "Optimization of waveforms for pulsed amperometric detection of carbohydrates based on pulsed voltammetry," analytical chemistry (1993) 65, 50–55. Copyright 1993 American Chemical Society.

can be used for detection of carbohydrates. In practice, a setting of 0.05V is used rather than 0.26V since this provides the best signal to noise (26). Operation at this low setting also provides higher specificity and thus freedom from interference since very few classes of organic compounds can be oxidized at this low potential. The technique of HPAE-PAD is now well established for direct detection of carbohydrates, and provides high sensitivity and specificity without the need for derivatization.

HIGH PERFORMANCE ANION EXCHANGE CHROMATOGRAPHY OF CARBOHYDRATES

In order for pulsed amperometry to have utility for the chromatographic determination of carbohydrates, a high resolution separation method is required that is also compatible with high pH. This requirement has been met by the development of column technology which allows high resolution separations of carbohydrates by anion exchange chromatography at high pH.

Carbohydrates are often thought of as neutral compounds, but in actuality they are weak acids with pKa's in the range of 12–14 (Table 1). At these pH levels, oxyanion formation occurs (Figure 6) allowing separation by ion exchange. Ion exchange separations are based on the relative affinity of the analyte ion in competition with the eluent ion for the same exchange sites (Figure 7). The greater the affinity of the ion, the longer the retention time. For carbohydrates, subtle structural differences and small differences in pKa can cause significant differences in retention characteristics.

TABLE 1 Dissociation constants of some common carbohydrates in water at 25°C

Sugar	PKa
Fructose	12.03
Mannose	12.08
Xyolse	12.15
Glucose	12.28
Galactose	12.39
Dulcitol	13.43
Sorbitol	13.60
α-Methyl glucoside	13.71

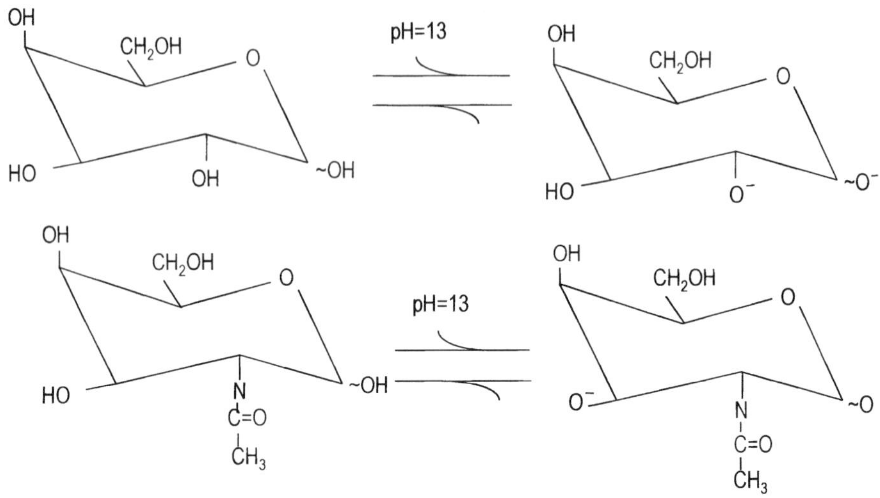

FIGURE 6 Carbohydrate oxyanion formation at high pH.

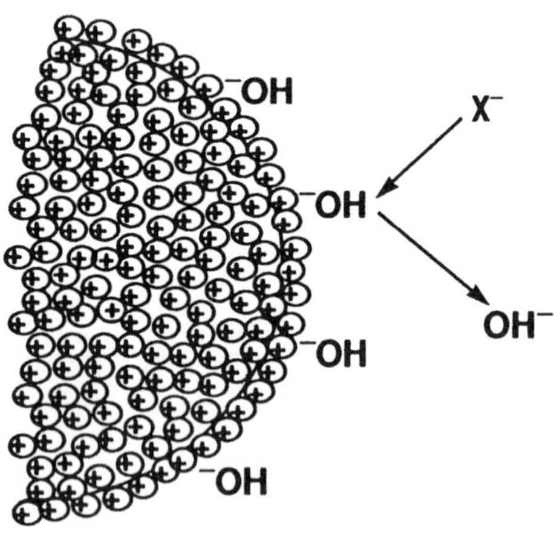

FIGURE 7 Ion exchange separations are based on the relative affinites of the analyte ions in competition with the eluent ion for the same exchange sites.

COLUMN PACKINGS FOR HIGH PH ANION EXCHANGE CHROMATOGRAPHY

The CarboPac™ series ion exchange columns developed specifically for carbohydrate separations incorporate both high selectivity characteristics with high efficiency. The basic structure of these column packings is shown in Figure 8. The core of the packing is a sulfonated, highly cross-linked and impermeable polystyrene divinylbenzene resin bead with a diameter of 10 micrometers. The core particle is covered with a pellicular layer of quaternary amine functionalized porous latex beads with a diameter of ~0.1 micrometers. This structure allows ion exchange chromatography to be carried out on a stationary phase with extremely small particle diameter yet still retaining the flow and back pressure characteristics of a conventional column packing with 10 micrometer diameter parti-

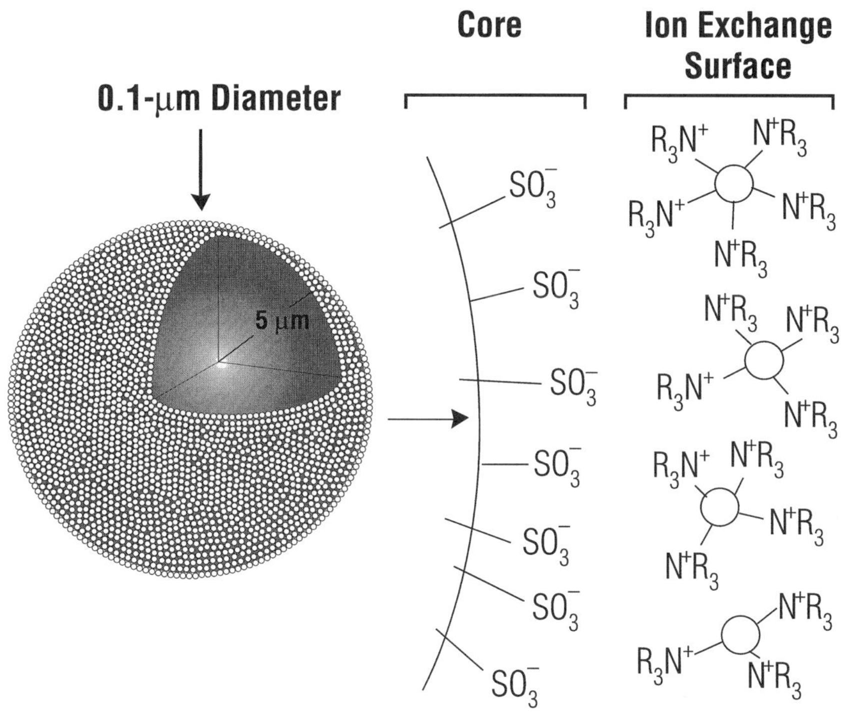

FIGURE 8 Structure of pellicular ion exchange packings for high resolution carbohydrate separations.

cles. The extremely small diameter of the pellicular beads results in excellent mass transfer characteristics and highly efficient separations. This structure also permits easy scale up from analytical columns (4 mm) to the semi-preparative scale CarboPac columns (9 mm, and 22 mm).

DETERMINATION OF SUGARS AND OLIGOSACCHARIDES

A typical isocratic separation of simple sugars is shown in Figure 9. This method was adopted in 1994 as the official method for the determination of sugars present in sugar cane molasses by the International Commission for Uniform Methods of Sugar Analysis (ICUMSA). Among the advantages cited for the new method were 1) lack of co-elution with non-sugar impurities, 2) greatly reduced possibility of overestimation of sugars due to co-eluting impurities, 3) no column heater is required. Figure 10 illustrates the use of HPAE-PAD with gradient elution to separate maltose oligomers up to DP10.

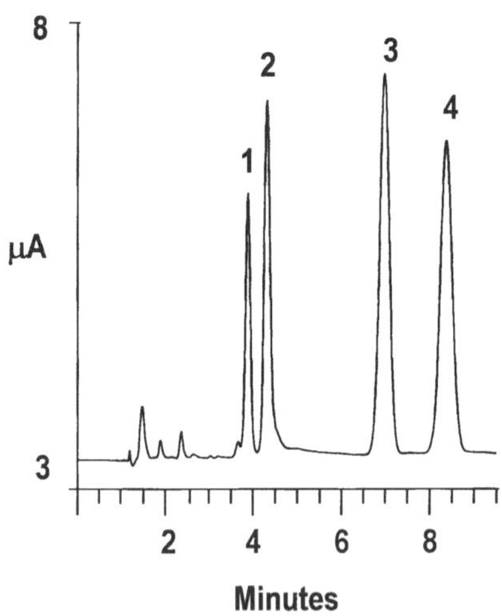

FIGURE 9 Determination of sugars in sugar cane molasses by HPAE-PAD. Column: CarboPac PA1 (10 μM, 250 × 4 mm i.d.) with guard. Eluent: 150 mM NaOH. Flowrate: 1.0 mL/min. Detection: pulsed amperometry, Au electrode. Peaks. 1 = glucose, 2 = fructose, 3 = lactose (internal standard), 4 = sucrose.

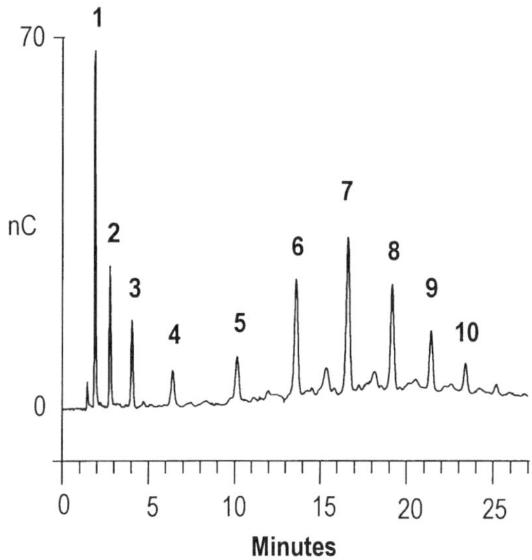

FIGURE 10 Separation of maltose oligomers by HPAE-PAD. Peak labels indicate degree of polymerization (DP). Column: CarboPac PA100 (8.5 μM, 250 × 4 mm i.d.) with guard. Eluent: NaOH/sodium acetate gradient. Flowrate: 1.0 mL/min. Detection: pulsed amperometry, Au electrode.

ANALYSIS OF STARCH AND NON-STARCH POLYSACCHARIDES

Another application of HPAE-PAD with gradient elution which is particularly relevant to the analysis of starch and dietary fiber constituents is the separation of polysaccharide mixtures. Figure 11 shows the separation of a hydrolyzed corn syrup by ion moderated partition chromatography using a typical cation exchange column. The limitation of this approach is apparent since the oligosaccharides with DP >2 are only weakly retained and the elution order is from high to low DP. Only the monosaccharide is baseline resolved from the oligosaccharides which elute as a poorly resolved envelope of peaks with the larger DP chains crowding to the front of the chromatogram, and virtually no resolution at DP >5. Figure 12 shows a separation using HPAE-PAD with sodium hydroxide gradient elution of the same hydrolyzed corn syrup. In this case the elution order is reversed as compared with the cation exchange separation, i.e. retention time increases with increase in DP. Resolution is achieved out to a DP > 20.

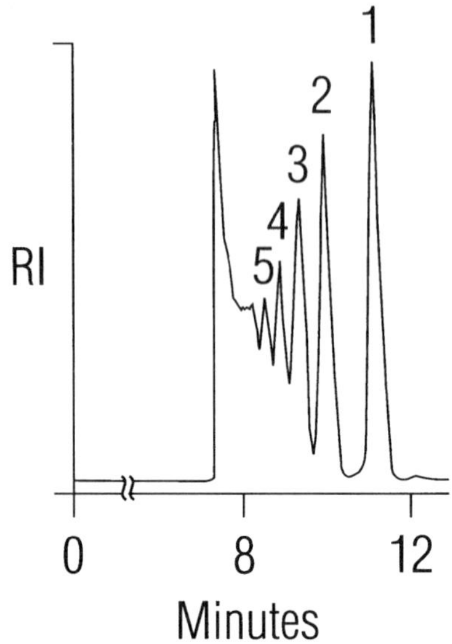

FIGURE 11 Separation of a hydrolyzed corn syrup by ion moderated partition chromatography on a cation exchange resin (calcium form). Eluent: water. Flowrate: 0.6 mL/min. Temp.: 80°C. Detector: refractive index. Peaks: 1 = DP 5, 2 = DP 4, 3 = DP 3, 4 = DP 2, 5 = glucose.

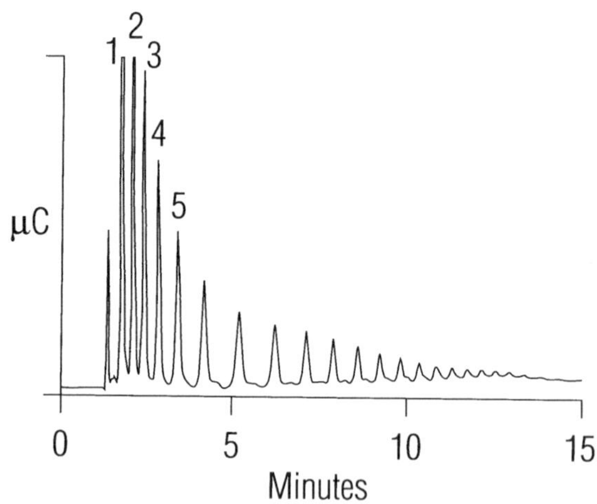

FIGURE 12 Separation of a hydrolyzed corn syrup by HPAE-PAD using gradient elution. Column: CarboPac PA1 (10 μM, 250 × 4 mm i.d.) with guard. Eluent: 150 mM sodium hydroxide with sodium acetate gradient. Flowrate: 1.0 mL min. Temp: ambient. Detector: pulsed amperometric, Au electrode. Peaks: 1 = glucose, 2 = DP 2, 3 = DP 3, 4 = DP 4, 5 = DP 5.

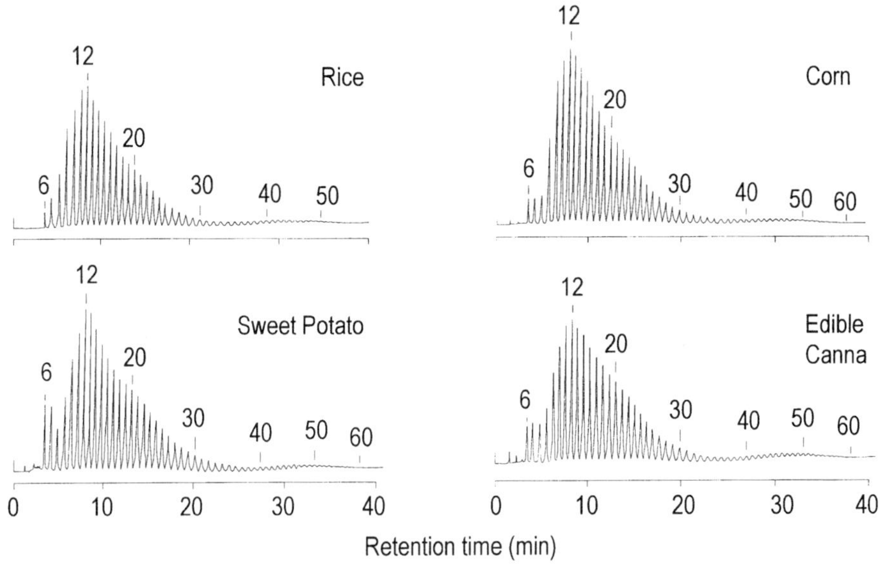

FIGURE 13 Chain length distribution of debranched amylopections from various sources determined by HPAE-PAD. column: CarboPac PA1 (10 μM, 250 × 4 mm i.d.) with guard. Eluent: A, 150 mM NaOH; B, 150 mM NaOH/500 mM sodium acetate. Gradient program: 40% B at 0 min, 50% at 2 min, 60% at 10 min, 80% at 40 min. Temp: ambient. Flowrate: 1.0 mL/min. Detector: pulsed amperometric, Au electrode, range 10 μA. Adapted with permission from Koizumi, K., Fukuda, M., Hizukuri, S., (1991), J. chrom. 585, 233–238.

STRUCTURAL STUDIES ON AMYLOPECTINS

HPAE-PAD with gradient elution has proved to be a powerful tool for structural studies on other starch-derived materials such as amylopectins since the chain length distribution is an important parameter for characterizing the molecular structure (18,19). Figure 13 shows the chain length distribution up to a DP of 55 for debranched amylopectins from various sources (19). These distributions can be used as fingerprints for the source of the amylopectin.

QUANTITATION OF POLYSACCHARIDES

For exact quantitation of each polysaccharide, the variation in PAD response over the DP range of interest is required. Relative detector response for maltose oligomers in the range DP 2 to DP 7 determined by Koizumi et al. are shown in Table 2 (20). For the maltooligomers in the range of DP 6-17, the relative

Table 2 Relative PAD responses of D-glucooligomers (DP 2 to DP 7)*

DP	# of HCOH	Relative detector response			
		(1 → 4)-α-	(1 → 2)-β-	(1 → 3)-β-	(1 → 6)-β-
2	8	1.00	1.00	1.00	1.00
3	11	1.39	1.36	1.38	1.21
4	14	1.72	1.70	1.63	1.51
5	17	2.06	2.04	2.03	1.78
6	20	2.33		2.03	1.78
7	23	2.59			

* Adapted with permission from Table II, Koizumi, K., Kubota, Y.,Tanomoto, T., Okada, Y., (1989), J. Chrom., 464, 365-373.

response factors were determined after first isolating quantities of the individual maltosaccharides (19). The data in Table 3 show that the relative response on a molar basis increases linearly for chain lengths from DP 6 to DP 15 and increments more slowly for the DP 16 and DP 17 maltosaccharides. This suggests that the differences in relative response for higher oligomers becomes smaller with increasing chain length. With the availability of semi-preparative scale (9

Table 3 Relative PAD responses of maltosaccharides (DP 6 to DP 17)*

DP	# of HCOH	RDR	RDR per HCOH unit
6	20	0.74	1.08
7	23	0.82	1.03
8	26	0.89	0.99
9	29	1.00	1.00
10	32	1.10	1.00
11	35	1.20	1.00
12	38	1.31	1.00
13	41	1.38	0.99
14	44	1.46	0.97
15	47	1.55	0.96
16	50	1.59	0.92
17	53	1.65	0.90

* Adapted with permission from Table I, Koizumi, K., Fukuda, M., Hizukuri, S., (1991), J. Chrom. 585, 233-238

mm and 22 mm i.d.) CarboPac columns, isolation of milligram quantities of individual polysaccharides in a single injection becomes feasible for any polysaccharide mixture allowing pure standards to be prepared and the relationship between DP and response factor to be accurately determined.

ANALYSIS OF PHYSIOLOGICALLY FUNCTIONAL FOOD ADDITIVES

Another class of complex carbohydrates which has been an important topic at this workshop are physiologically functional food additives such as inulin and oligosaccharide-based products. These materials are increasingly being used as fat substitutes, and for their beneficial health effects which are similar to those of dietary fiber, i.e. they are not digestible by human digestive juices, and cause an increase in the bifidobacteria population in the colon which in turn suppresses

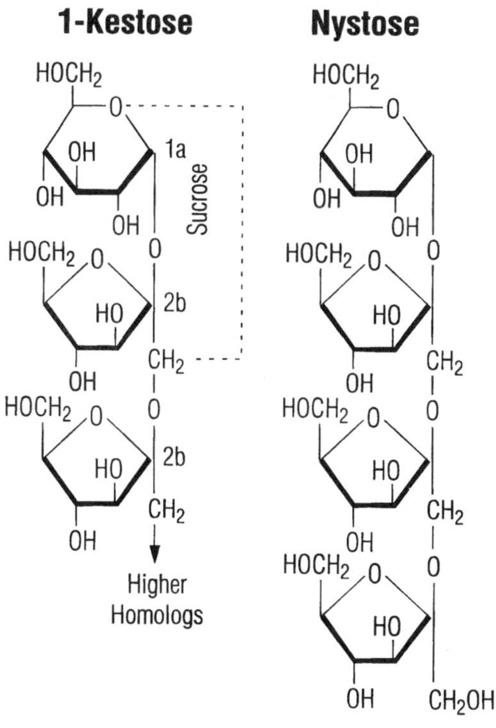

FIGURE 14 Examples of physiologically functional oligosaccharides.

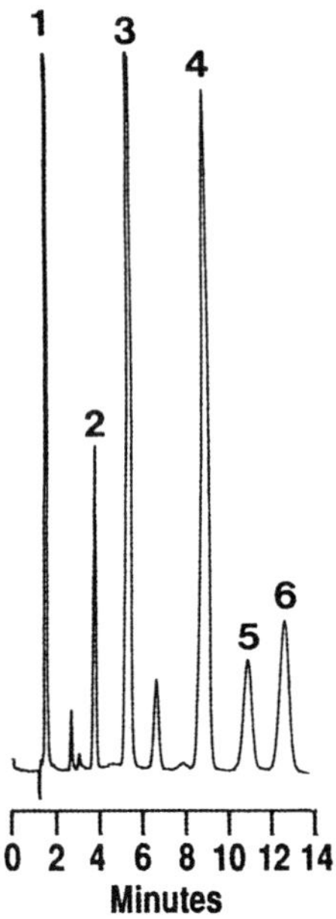

FIGURE 15 determination of ketose and related sugars by HPAE-PAD. Column: CarboPac PA1 (10 μM. 250 × 4 mm i.d.) with guard. Eluent 100 mM NaOH/20 mM sodium acetate. Flowrate: 1.0 mL/min. Temp; ambient. Detector: pulsed amperometric, Au electrode, range 1 μA. Peaks: 1 = galactinose, 2 = sucrose, 3 = 1-ketose, 4 = 6-ketose, 5 = neo-ketose, 6 = nystose.

the activity of putrefactive bacteria and reduces the formation of toxic fermentation products. In Japan, oligosaccharide additives are used in over 450 food products (27) primarily for their beneficial health effects. These products are typically mixtures of small oligosaccharides such as the fructooligosaccharides shown in Figure 14. Analysis of these types of products is straightforward using HPAE-PAD as shown in Figure 15. Oligofructose products derived from chicory inulin having DP values up to 60 can also be determined by HPAE-PAD using gradient elution as shown in Figure 16. Figure 17 shows the separation of Raftiline, a commercial inulin product from a European manufacturer in which the smaller oligofructose (Fn) chains are distinguished from the inulin (GFn) chains. Response factors have also been determined for the Fn and GFn oligomers up to DP 8. Determination of response factors for higher DP oligomers is in progress (H. Hoebregs, private communication).

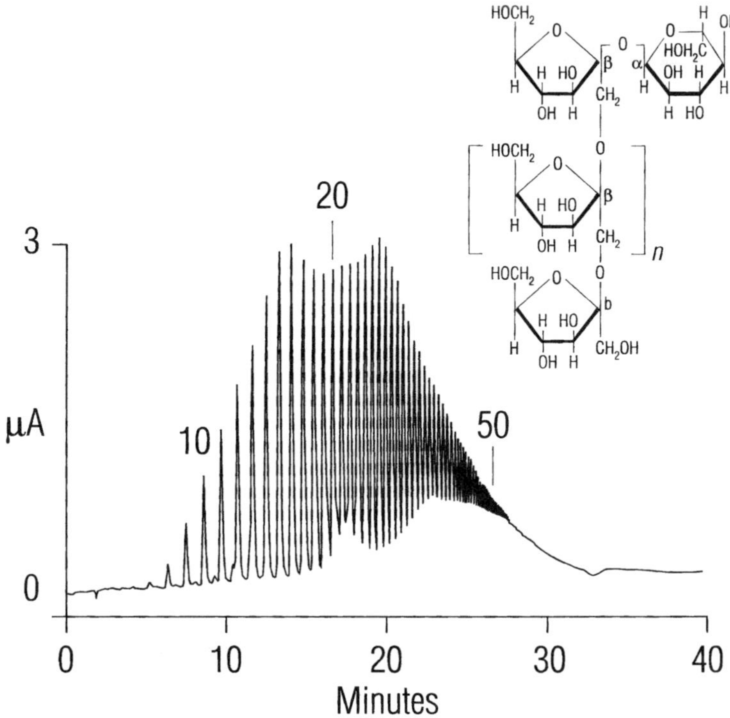

FIGURE 16 HPLC analysis of purified inulin. Column: CarboPac PA1 (10 μM, 250 × 4 mm i.d.) with guard. Eluent A, 0.1M NaOH, eluent B 0.1M NaOH/1.0M sodium acetate. Gradient 20–60% B in 40 min. Flowrate: 1.0 mL/min. Detection: pulsed amperometry, Au electrode, range 3 μA. Sample courtesy of Dr. C. Mitchell, California Natural Products, Manteca, CA.

NON-STARCH POLYSACCHARIDE ANALYSIS

The determination of non-starch polysaccharides for nutritional labeling purposes typically involves determination of the neutral sugars and uronic acid components by GC or colorimetry following hydrolysis (28). More recently, Englyst et al. have used HPAE-PAD to determine neutral sugars and uronic acids, and have demonstrated good agreement with GC and colorimetric methods (11). Uronic acids by virtue of the carboxyl group are much more strongly retained on CarboPac columns than the neutral sugars and therefore require a stronger eluent. In the Englyst procedure, uronic acids are determined separately from neutral sugars under isocratic conditions. Baseline resolution of the uronic acids is achieved

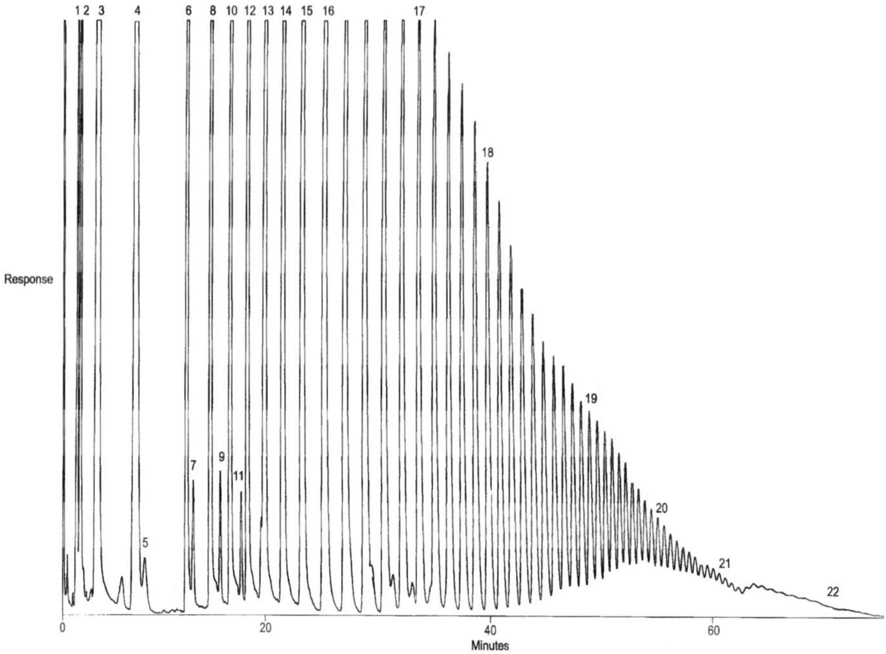

FIGURE 17 Analysis of Raftiline, a commercial inulin-based product using HPAE-PAD on a CarboPac PA1 column showing resolution of oligofructose (Fn) chains from (GFn) chains. Chromatogram and peak assignments kindly provided by H. Hoebregs, Raffinerie Tirlmontosie S.A., Tienen, Belgium. Peaks: 1 = glucose, 2 = fructose, 3 = sucrose, 4 = GF2, 5 = F3, 6 = GF3, 7 = F4, 8 = GF4, 9 = F5, 10 = GF5, 11 = F6, 12 = GF6, 13 = DP7, 14 = DP8, 15 = DP9, 16 = DP10, 17–22 = DP15, 20, 30, 40, 50, 60 respectively.

with a run time of less than 13 min. Figure 18 shows results obtained for a citrus pectin hydrolysate and a beet hydrolysate (11).

It is also possible to determine neutral sugars and uronic acids in a single run by using gradient elution (J. Prodolliet, Nestle, Lausanne, personal communication). The determination of neutral sugars and uronic acid constituents by HPAE-PAD is now accepted as an alternative method for nutritional labeling purposes in the UK (H. Englyst, personal communication).

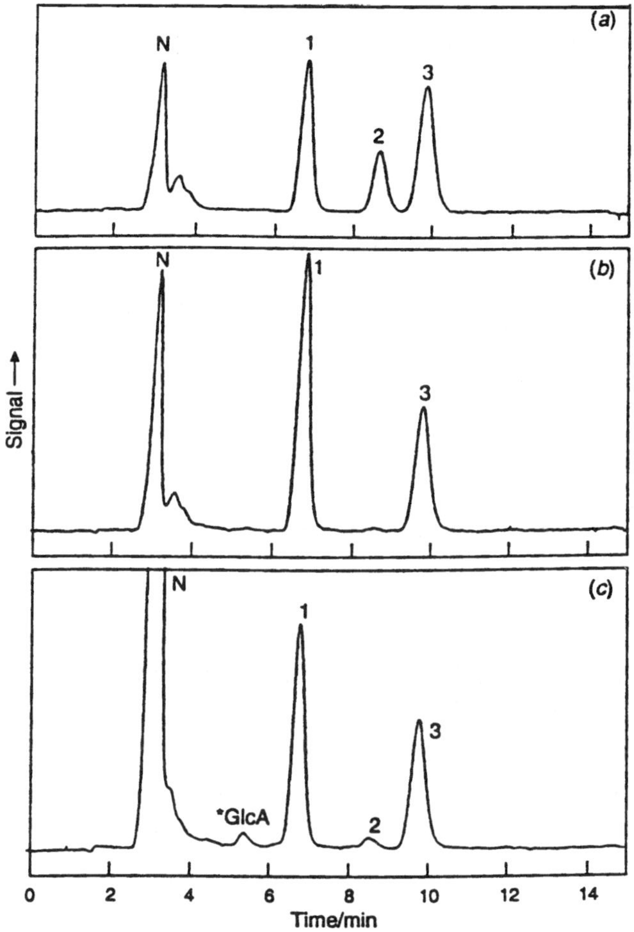

FIGURE 18 Chromatogram of (a) a standard uronic acid mixture, (b) a pectin (citrus) hydrolysate and (c) a sugar beet hydrolysate. Column: CarboPac PA1 (10 μM, 250 × 4 mm i.d.) with guard. Eluent: 25 mM NaOH/150 mM sodium acetate. Flowrate: 1.0 mL/min. Detection: pulsed amperometry, Au electrode, range 300 nA. Peaks: 1 = galacturonic acid, 2 = glucuronic acid, 3 = mannuronic acid (internal standard). The largest peak N represents the neutral sugars and the peak labeled *GlcA unidentified peak which appears to convert to glucuronic acid on further hydrolysis. Adapted with permission from Figure 1, Quigley, M. E., Englyst, H. N., (1994) Analyst, 119, 1511–1518.

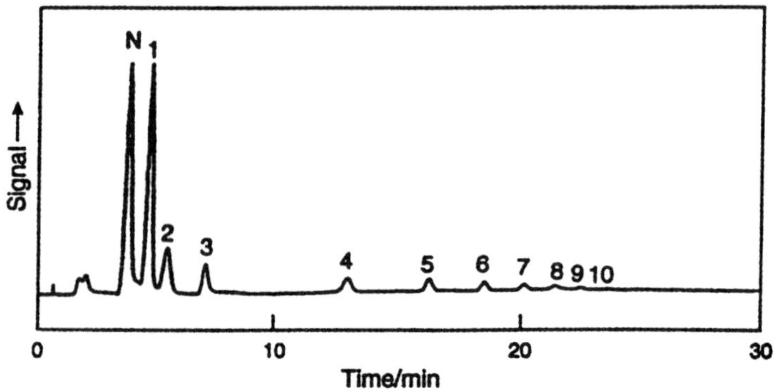

FIGURE 19 Chromatogram of a pectin hydrolysate showing incomplete conversion to free uronic acids by the hydrolysis treatment. Column: CarboPac PA1 (10 μM, 250 × 4 mm i.d.) with guard. Eluent: gradient, 100 mM NaOH/240 mM sodium acetate to 100 mM NaOH/480 mM sodium acetate in 15 min. Temp: ambient. Detection: pulsed amperometric, Au electrode, range 300 nA. Adapted with permission from Figure 1, Quigley, M. E., Englyst, H. N., (1994) Analyst, 119, 1511–1518.

USE OF HPAE-PAD IN METHOD DEVELOPMENT FOR DIETARY FIBER DETERMINATION

HPAE-PAD is proving to be valuable not only for the final determination of neutral sugars and uronic acids for nutritional labeling, but also in development of the methodology. The accuracy of dietary fiber determinations depends on the efficacy of the hydrolysis procedures used whether they be enzymatic or chemical. Fahey et al. have used HPAE-PAD to compare hydrolysis procedures for dietary fiber (21). Englyst et al. have also used HPAE-PAD to compare the relative merits of chemical and enzymatic procedures for hydrolysis of pectins (11,15). The results for a 2M sulfuric acid hydrolysis of a pectin (15) are shown in Figure 19. In addition to neutral sugars and galacturonic acid, significant peaks corresponding to uronic acid oligomers are also present indicating incomplete conversion to the free acid under these conditions.

APPLICATION OF HPAE-PAD IN PECTIN RESEARCH

Pectin is an important carbohydrate component of dietary fiber which as yet has not been fully characterized. Structural studies aimed at characterizing the complex mixture of acidic and neutral polysaccharides following partial hydrolysis of pectin have been hampered in the past due to the limitations of the chroma-

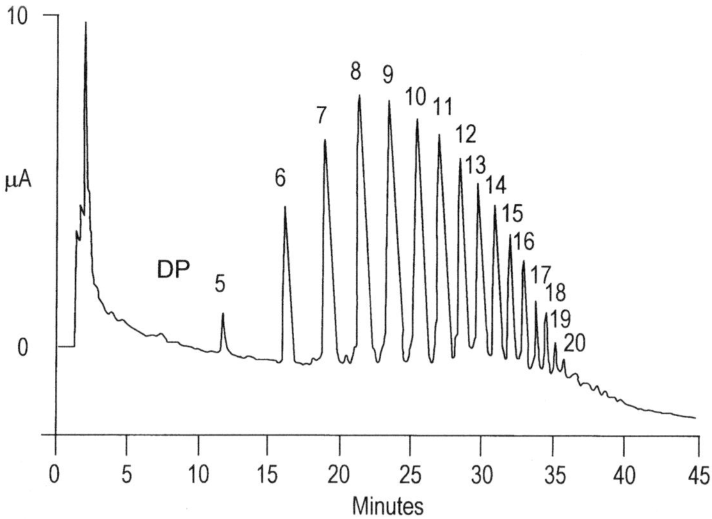

FIGURE 20 Separation of oligouronic acids in a citrus pectin hydrolysate using HPAE-PAD. Column: CarboPac PA1 (10 μM, 250 × 4 mm i.d.) with guard. Eluent: gradient from 100 mM NaOH/400 mM sodium acetate to 100 mM NaOH/900 mM sodium acetate in 45 min. Flowrate: 1.0 mL/min. Detection: pulsed amperometric, Au electrode, range 10 * A.

tographic techniques (23). Prior to the development of HPAE-PAD, the largest underivatized oligogalacturonic acid that could be separated was DP 11. Figure 20 shows a typical chromatogram of underivatized oligogalacturonic acids from a pectin hydrolysate using HPAE-PAD. Separation of oligogalacturonic acids in the range DP 2 to DP 50 have been reported by Hotchkiss et al. (23).

CONCLUSIONS

HPAE-PAD is a powerful tool both for nutritional labeling analysis and research on dietary fiber and complex carbohydrates. Accurate determination of each of the neutral sugars present in hydrolysates of complex carbohydrates and dietary fiber can be made directly without requiring derivatization. Similarly, uronic acids and oligouronic acids derived from complete or partial hydrolysis of pectin can also be determined either separately, or concurrently with the neutral sugars by using gradient elution. The compatibility of the technique with gradient elution allows chain-length distribution profiles of starch and non-starch derived oligo- and polysaccharides to be determined up to DP 60 with high resolution.

ACKNOWLEDGMENTS

The author wishes to acknowlege the contribution of the applications and research staff of Dionex Corporation who carried out the chromatographic separations shown in Figures 2, 9–12, 15,16, and 20.

REFERENCES

1. Johnson, D.C., and Polta, T.Z., (1986) Chromatogr. Forum, 1, 37.
2. Rocklin, R.D., and Pohl, C.A., (1983) J. Liquid Chromatogr., 6, 1577.
3. Johnson, D.C., LaCourse, W.R., (1990), Anal. Chem. 62(10), 589A-596A.
4. Nollet, Leo M.L. ed.; (1992) ''Food Analysis by HPLC'', Marcel Dekker, Inc., New York, p. 262.
5. Martens, D.A., Frankenberger, W.T. Jr., (1990), Chromatographia, 29, 7-12.
6. White, D.R. Jr., Widmer, W., (1990), J. Ag and Food Chem., 38 (10), 1918-1921.
7. Scott, F.W. (1992), ''Food Analysis by HPLC'', Leo M. L. Nollet ed., Marcel Dekker, Inc., New York, (a) p. 262, (b) p. 271.
8. Togami, D.W., Treat-Clemons, L.G.; Hometchko, D.J.; (1990) (June), American Lab., 15-21.
9. DeVries, J.W., and Nelson, A.L. (1994) Food Technol. 48 (7), 77.
10. Lee, S.C., DeVries, J.W., Sullivan, D.M., (1993) in Methods of Analysis for Nutrition Labeling, ADAC Int'l, Arlington, VA, p. 74.
11. Quigley, M.E., Englyst, H.N., (1992) Analyst, 117, 1715-1718.
12. Method for the Analysis of Sucrose, Glucose, and Fructose in Cane Molasses (1994) officially adopted at the 21st session of the International Commission for Uniform Methods of Sugar Analysis, Havana, Cuba. Also adopted (1995) 1st Action approval AOAC Method 996.04.
13. ISO Method 11292 :1995, Instant Coffee: Determination of Free and Total Carbohydrate-Method by High Performance Anion-Exchange Chromatography Also adopted (1995) 1st Action Approval AOAC Method 995.13.
14. Englyst, H.N., Quigley, M.E., Hudson, G.F., (1994) Analyst, 119, 1497-1509.
15. Quigley, M.E., Englyst, H.N., (1994) Analyst, 119, 1511-1518.
16. Corradini, C., Cristalli, A., Corradini, D. (1993) J. Chrom. 16(16), 3471-3485.
17. Quemener, B., Thibault, J.F., Coussement, P., (1994), Lebensm.-Wiss. u. Technol., 27, 125-132.
18. Wong, K.S., and Jane, J., (1995), J. Chrom., 18(1), 63-80.
19. Koizumi, K, Fukuda, M., Hizukuri, S. (1991), J. Chrom., 585, 233-238.
20. Koizumi, K., Kubota, Y.,Tanomoto, T., Okada, Y., (1989), J. Chrom., 464, 365-373.
21. Garleb, K.A., Bourquin, L.D., Fahey, Jr., G.C., (1991), J. Food Sci., 56(2), 423 426.
22. Garleb, K.A., Bourquin, L.D., Fahey, Jr., G.C., (1989), J. Ag. Food Chem., 37, 1287-1293.
23. Hotchkiss, Jr., A.T., Hicks, K.B., (1990), Anal. Biochem., 184, 200-206.
24. Rocklin, R.D., (1993) in A Practical Guide to HPLC Detection, Academic Press Inc., New York, NY, p. 149.

25. LaCourse, W.R., Johnson, D.C. , (1993), Anal. Chem. 65(10), 50-55.
26. Technical Note 21, Dionex Corporation, 1228 Titan Way, Sunnyvale, CA 94088
27. Tomomatsu, H., (1994) Food Technol., 48(10), 61-65.
28. Theander, O., Åman, P., Westerlund, E., Andersson, R., Petterson, D., (1995), J. AOAC, 78(4), 1030-1044.

21

NIR Analysis of Dietary Fiber

Sandra E. Kays, Franklin E. Barton II, and William R. Windham
Richard B. Russell Agricultural Research Center, Agricultural Research Service, U.S. Department of Agriculture, Athens, Georgia

INTRODUCTION

Food labeling legislation has increased the need for rapid, more efficient, and environmentally benign methods of determining the constituents of foods, particularly dietary fiber. For many agricultural products near-infrared technology has provided valuable alternatives to conventional, chemical methods of analysis. Near-infrared spectroscopy appears to provide an attractive alternative to current laboratory methods of dietary fiber determination. In this chapter, the current status of the use of near-infrared spectroscopy for the analysis of fiber in foods is reviewed. Likewise, the instrumentation and chemometrics involved in near-infrared analysis and the current applications of near-infrared spectroscopy in the food industry are critiqued. Near-infrared analysis is very rapid, requires little or no sample preparation, does not create chemical waste, and thus, has the potential to be a significant force in dietary fiber analysis in the future.

Recent United States legislation has made it necessary to seek alternative methods for the analysis of certain nutrients. The Nutrition Labeling and Education Act of 1990 requires that the amount of specific nutrients in processed and packaged foods is included on the nutrition label (1). As a result of this legislation there will be a substantial increase in the total number of analyses performed, not only in the food industry but also by monitoring agencies. Furthermore, the 1988 Resources Conservation and Recovery Act (2) advocates reduction of chemical waste generated by laboratories. Consequently there is a need for more rapid, economical methods of food analysis that do not generate chemical waste yet maintain the accuracy and repeatability of existing methods. This is particularly so for dietary fiber as the current methods of analysis (3, 4, 5, 6), although precise and repeatable for a wide variety of foods, are very time consuming, expensive, and generate waste products.

Near-infrared spectroscopy (NIRS) has been used in agriculture for many years as a rapid, accurate, non-destructive method of measuring specific constituents of grains and forages (7, 8). The technology involves measurement of sample absorptions in the electromagnetic regions of the spectrum from 750-2500 nm. Absorptions are calibrated to an analyzed component of the sample, allowing subsequent prediction of the component in new samples. Thus, NIR analysis is dependent on 1) an instrument capable of making spectral measurements with sufficient precision, 2) a reliable and accurate reference laboratory method that measures the desired quality, and 3) a mathematical model to relate the spectral data to the reference measurements. NIRS is very rapid, requiring only seconds to make a determination, needs little or no sample preparation, and does not create chemical waste. In addition to its use for agricultural crops, NIRS has been used to determine the quantity of certain constituents of foods. A small number of studies has addressed the use of NIRS to predict total dietary fiber and its constituents, soluble and insoluble fiber, in a variety of foods. The following review describes the instrumentation and model building involved in NIR analysis, gives an overview of the existing applications of NIRS for food analysis, and reviews the literature dealing with the use of NIRS for the analysis of dietary fiber in foods.

INSTRUMENTATION

The publication "Near Infrared Technology in the Agricultural and Food Industries" by Williams and Norris (1987, 7) described NIR technology as it existed in the mid-1980s. At that time there were three types of instruments in use: 1) a fixed filter instrument, which gives one data point per wavelength per filter; 2) a tilting filter instrument, which produces a segmented scan for each filter; and 3) scanning monochromators, which produce the entire spectrum. Sample presentation for these instruments consisted of a spinning cup for use with a ground product. The instruments, used to measure protein, fat, and moisture in forages, feeds, and foods (8, 9, 10), were connected to mini-computers which ran small statistical programs to develop multiple linear regression models. While adequate for simple matrices, considerable updating was required for complex systems and for use in predicting open populations. Although these systems lacked flexibility and computing power, the instruments themselves had adequate signal to noise ratios and wavelength precision.

In the late 1980s instrumentation displayed at the Pittsburgh Conferences and Eastern Analytical Symposia represented a new generation of NIR equipment. Several major analytical instrumentation manufacturers began to see NIRS as a part of their marketing scheme. Companies such as Perkin-Elmer, Boem, Nicolet, and Beckman began modifying existing optical instruments to cover the NIR. This was followed by the first dedicated FT-NIR insruments from Bran-Leubbe and Boem. In the early 1990s, sample presentation cells for unground products appeared on the market as did cells for high moisture materials and liquids, simplifying and facilitating analysis. NIRS sample presentation devices now approached those already available for mid-infrared and visible methods and could be used for finished product process control of certain products in the food industry. Over the next 2 years, instruments utilizing optic probes became available; a distinct advantage as fiber optics can be used in transmittance as well as reflectance modes. Several instruments utilized short optical fiber bundles (1–3 meters) which give excellent signal to noise ratios, while others utilized single fiber probes which could monitor samples 2–3 kilometers from the instrument. Such instruments are of use in food industries to ascertain ingredient purity and in a wide range of other industries for process control.

Coupled to advances in NIR instrumentation, there have been rapid advances in personal computers. The increased power of the personal computer and the many chemometric software packages available has been a driving force in the advancement of NIR technology. One major advance has been the ability to move data from one spectral platform and package to another. This was made possible by the hierarchy developed by instrument and software companies and by the Joint Committee on Atomic and Molecular Physical Data Protocol (JCAMP) of the American Society for Testing and Materials (11). Spectra can now be put into JCAMP format and imported into other chemometric packages, such as spread-sheets or general statistical packages, greatly expanding data analysis potential.

CHEMOMETRICS

Calibration of a NIR instrument involves: sample selection, development of a mathematical relationship between sample spectra generated by the instrument and sample values obtained from a laboratory reference method, and validation of the mathematical model developed. The choice of calibration samples determines the type of unknown samples that can be analyzed. Two important criteria in sample selection are: the calibration sample set 1) must span all significant dimensions of spectral variation, and 2) must show representative statistical distribution. Major phenomena expected to affect the spectral data of future unknown samples, (e.g. the constituent to be determined and known types of interferences) must vary independently of each other. Typical interferences include sample physical and chemical characteristics, method of sample preservation and processing, and instrument and sample environment (e.g. temperature and humidity).

If calibration samples are easily obtained and analyzed, a large number of samples can be selected, randomly, to ensure that all relevant interference phenomena are modeled. If calibration samples are difficult to obtain or expensive to analyze, then samples can be selected based on known differences. Alternatively, samples may be selected based on spectral characteristics using an algorithm (12). The algorithm identifies samples which are spectrally similar and, therefore, can be represented by one sample for the calibration.

Following sample selection, spectral data are collected for either sample reflectance or transmittance. During calibration, the spectral data pass through three conceptually different stages. The first stage is an optical correction to mathematically remove certain physical interferences (e.g. light scatter and specular reflectance). The second stage, data compression, concentrates all information in the spectra and reduces the number of NIR data points to the most important phenomena or factors that affect the spectral data. In the final stage, calibration regression, the data from data compression and the reference method values are used to build a mathematical model that predicts the constituent in question. Currently, the regression method of choice is partial least squares (PLS) regression, as it is more robust (13) and generally has lower prediction error (14) than the more classical stepwise multiple linear regression.

Multivariate calibration methods have one problem in common—determination of the optimal number of regression factors to be used for subsequent predictions. The method of predictive cross-validation is commonly used to determine the optimal number of factors and protects against overfitting. This involves temporarily removing different subsets of the calibration samples for use as validation samples. Performance statistics are accumulated for each group of removed samples. The optimal number of factors employed in the model is that which produces the minimum error between modeled and reference values (standard error of cross-validation). Two kinds of outliers may be recognized during calibration regression: 1) H statistic outliers in which the spectrum of the sample is atypical of others in the calibration set, and 2) t statistic outliers in which the reference value is significantly different from the modeled value. Outlier samples should be reanalyzed by both NIRS and the reference method.

The final step in instrument calibration is validation of the mathematical model using samples not included in the original calibration sample set but of a similar type. This step is necessary to obtain an independent measure of model accuracy, expressed as the standard error of performance (SEP). A SEP that is within 2 times the standard error of the replicated reference method is considered to be satisfactory. The slope of the modeled values plotted versus the reference method values should be close to 1, and intercept close to 0, with low scatter about the linear regression line. Unacceptable relationships between modeled and reference values are those which exhibit a bias, a change in slope, or high scatter about the linear regression line, although the intercept remains 0 and the slope 1.

After a model has been developed and validated, continual monitoring is necessary to ensure accurate results. NIR analysis can disagree with reference method values when: 1) the instrument is not working properly, 2) the sample population changes and is no longer represented by the calibration set, or 3) some aspect of the reference method changes. None of these events must take place if NIR analysis is to be accurate. A monitoring procedure has been described to distinguish between these sources of errror (15).

APPLICATIONS OF NIRS TO FOODS

Initial research in the 1960s on the application of NIRS to agricultural products was concentrated on the determination of moisture and NIR models were developed to determine moisture in a variety of ground seeds and grains (16, 17). During this time, studies were also reported on the direct determination of moisture and fat in several types of meats using their spectroscopic properties (18). In the early 1970s the technology advanced rapidly with development of several instruments for the analysis of moisture and protein in wheat (19). The Canadian Grain Commission adopted NIRS as an official method of analyzing wheat in 1975 and the United States Federal Grain Inspection Service recognized NIR analysis as an official method in 1980. The use of NIRS in the analysis of protein in wheat is, to date, one of the most important advances of NIR technology in agriculture. NIRS circumvents other time consuming methods of protein analysis and allows on-site, non-destructive determination of protein content. Currently, transmission instruments are available (such as the Infratec Whole Grain Analyzer) which allow analysis of moisture, protein, and oil in whole grains (e.g. wheat, soybeans, corn) at the elevator site. Similarly, the Infratec Meat Analyzer can be used in slaughterhouses or meat packing plants for fat monitoring and process control. In recent years the majority of food applications for NIRS have been for the determination of moisture, protein, and fat in a wide variety of products (e.g. wheat, pulses, various baked products, dough, cocoa, milk, cheese, eggs, oilseed, meat, fish, and hops) (see reviews 20, 21). Substantially fewer applications have been reported for other constituents, examples of which are: dietary fiber in cereal products (22, 23); neutral detergent fiber in breakfast cereals and snack foods (24, 25); beta-glucan in barley (26); starch in grains (27), pulses (28), and snack foods (25); starch damage in flour (29); amylose in rice (30); sucrose in chocolate (31) and wine (32); soluble solids in vegetables (33); and alcohol in beer (34) and wine (32).

MEASUREMENT OF DIETARY FIBER BY NIRS

While NIRS has been used to predict fiber in forages and grains (10, 35, 36, 37), its potential for the prediction of dietary fiber in foods has only begun to be explored. Table 1 lists the existing NIR/dietary fiber studies with calibration and validation statistics. In 1983, Baker reported the prediction of neutral detergent fiber (NDF) in a variety of ground breakfast cereals using NIR reflectance data (24). NDF (38) includes insoluble polysaccharides plus lignin and approximates insoluble dietary fiber. Using a first derivative transformation of the data and stepwise multiple linear regression, an equation was obtained utilizing 4 wavelengths for determination of NDF. The equation was used to determine NDF content of samples in the sample prediction set. The resulting standard error of prediction was 1.8% NDF and γ^2 was 0.96 (Table 1). Several samples with high fat and sugar had increased absorbance at wavelengths characteristic for fat and sugar absorbance. However, these wavelengths were avoided by the regression method, therefore, any possible interference by fat and sugar was minimized. Examples of typical reflectance spectra for dried, ground cereal products are presented in Figure 1.

Neutral detergent fiber was predicted, though less successfully, in snack

TABLE 1 Published statistics for NIR calibration and prediction of fiber foods[a,b]

Product	Fiber fraction	Calibration n	Calibration R^2	Calibration SE	Prediction n	Prediction γ^2	Prediction SE
Breakfast cereals (24)	NDF	40	0.98	1.5	50	0.96	1.8
Snack food (25)	NDF	40	0.82	1.8	49	0.83	1.4
Oat bran products (22)	IDF	45	—	—	24	0.92	1.0
	SDF	45	—	—	24	0.92	0.34
	TDF	45	—	—	24	0.97	0.85
Cereal Products (23)	TDF	90	0.99	1.6	29	0.99	1.5

[a] NDF, neutral detergent fiber; IDF, insoluble dietary fiber; SDF, soluble dietary fiber; TDF, total dietary fiber

[b] n, number of samples; R^2 and γ^2, coefficients of determination for calibration and prediction, respectively; SE, standard error

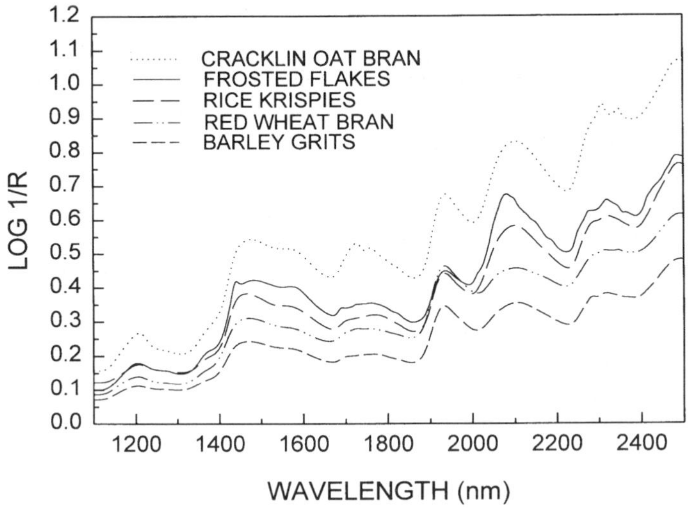

FIGURE 1 Typical NIR reflectance spectra of five cereal samples. One sample has higher fat content (Cracklin' Oat Bran) and one contains crystalline sugar (Frosted Flakes)

foods such as potato chips, pretzels, and popcorn (25). A two term, first derivative equation using 4 wavelengths was developed relating NDF to NIR reflectance spectra. The wavelengths chosen, via stepwise multiple regression analysis, were 2364, 2088, 1936, and 2342 nm and are indicative of fiber, starch, water and fat and/or protein absorbance, respectively. The poorer correlation (Table 1) was partly attributed to a skewed distribution of NDF values (62% of samples had NDF values below 2%) and partly to the inclusion of cornmeal products which, as a group, did not predict well. The authors suggested that cornmeal based products may require a separate calibration. If cornmeal samples were omitted, the standard errors for calibration and prediction are reduced to 1.4% and 1.3%, and the correlations improved to 0.91 and 0.89, respectively. Collectively the data indicate a potential relationship between insoluble fiber, as measured using the NDF method, and NIR spectra in snack foods and reiterate the importance of sample selection and a relatively normal distribution of sample values.

Williams et al. assessed the potential of analyzing total, soluble, and insoluble dietary fiber in oat bran products using NIR reflectance spectroscopy (22). Oat bran is an excellent source of soluble dietary fiber which has been associated with several health benefits. As a consequence there is interest, among manufacturers of oat based foods, in the rapid measurement of components of dietary fiber for composition assurance. Total dietary fiber and its constituents, soluble and insoluble fiber, were determined in the laboratory by the method of Mongeau and Brassard (4). Using an NIRSystems scanning monochromator for the collection of spectral data and NSAS NIR software, models were developed to predict soluble, insoluble, and total dietary fiber content of oat bran products. The accuracy of NIR prediction of the components of oat bran fiber, using PLS regression analysis, was deemed adequate for quality assurance (Table 1). A comparison between stepwise/multiple linear regression, in which specific wavelengths were selected, and PLS regression, which uses the entire NIR spectrum, indicated that the two regression methods gave very similar calibrations for soluble and insoluble dietary fiber (22). However, in the case of total dietary fiber PLS regression was the better method, having a higher γ^2 value and lower standard error of performance during verification.

Using wheat bran products only, Horvath et al. investigated relationships between NIR spectra and dietary fiber constituents (39). An enzymatic method (40) was used for water soluble and insoluble dietary fiber determination and constituents such as lignin, cellulose, hemicelluloses, and pectin were determined chemically within the dietary fiber fractions. Linear regression of a second derivative transformation of log10 1/R spectra was used to identify optimum wavelengths for predicting the soluble and insoluble dietary fiber and total dietary fiber. Correlation coefficients obtained for all constituents in this narrow population were 0.95 or greater with standard errors of calibration that were adequate for the state of the art at that time. Validation statistics were not reported.

The cereal and baking industries market products with a wide range of cereals often with multiple grains in a single product. Furthermore, regulatory agencies obtain samples from many sources, therefore, any method used in monitoring the products must be capable of assessing a broad range of samples and values. Kays et al. developed a calibration for predicting total dietary fiber in a variety of cereal products with a broad range of dietary fiber values (23). Both processed and unprocessed wheat, oats, rye, barley, amaranth, corn, and rice were included with an overall range in total dietary fiber values from <1 to 52% ($n = 90$). The samples contained $<10\%$ fat and/or $<20\%$ sugar. Higher fat/sugar samples were avoided due to difficulty in grinding and interference with the reference method. The reference method used to measure total dietary fiber was the AOAC procedure 991.43 (41), recommended for food labeling in the United States. The method includes non-starch polysaccharides, lignin, resistant starch, cutins, and plant waxes in the dietary fiber measurement. Spectral reflectance data were collected from 90 ground samples using an NIRSystems scanning monochromator and Infrasoft International software. The spectral data were transformed with standard normal variate and detrending to remove multiplicative interferences of scatter (42), and then transformed with second derivative processing. PLS was the regression method selected to relate spectral data to laboratory reference values and cross-validation was used to determine the optimal number of PLS factors for dietary fiber prediction. A NIR calibration equation was obtained for the prediction of total dietary fiber and used to determine the total dietary fiber content of samples in an independent set (Table 1, Figure 2). Linear regression of AOAC determined dietary fiber against NIRS predicted dietary fiber gave an intercept and slope not significantly different from 0.0 and 1.0, respectively.

The number of factors (nine) in the calibration developed was partly a function of the diversity of the data set. The calibration developed has broad utility for manufacturers using multiple grains and multiple grain products and for regulatory agencies monitoring products from many sources. Many companies, however, market products that contain only one or two types of grains and for these industries a simpler model may suffice. When samples containing oat and wheat only were utilized, a new calibration was obtained (n = 42) with only four factors and similar standard error of cross validation, coefficient of determination and accuracy of prediction as the model derived from the broader data set (23). Thus, calibration development and sample prediction were achieved for determination of total dietary fiber in a heterogeneous group of products and in a more homogeneous group.

Loadings express the spectral variation that corresponds to each factor of the PLS model and can provide information on the constituents exerting the greatest influence for each factor. Intensity of absorption peaks in the loading spectra

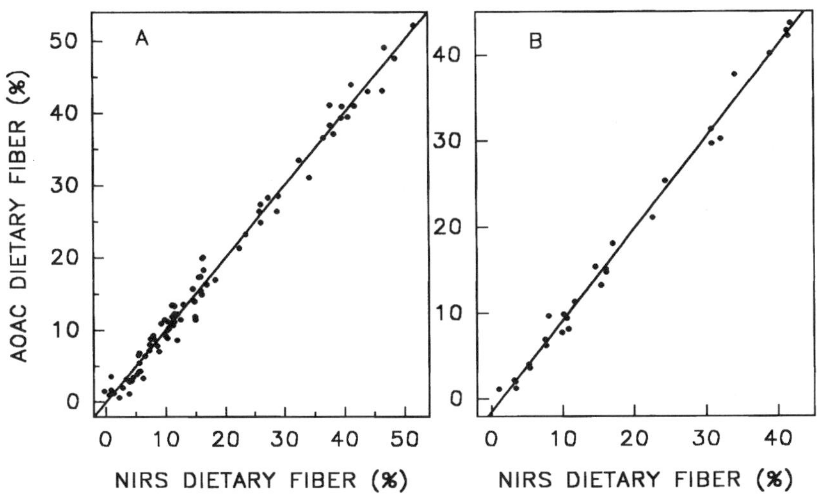

FIGURE 2 AOAC determined total dietary fiber versus NIRS predicted total dietary fiber for cereal products in the calibration (A) and validation (B) data sets (adapted from Ref. 23)

are an indication of the relative contribution of that wavelength to the model. Most software available for PLS calibrations provides a display of the loadings involved in development of the calibration model. Williams et al. found that for soluble dietary fiber in oat bran products, there were strong influences in oil and protein wavelength bands of loadings for factor one and factor two (22). This was attributed to the presence of similar amounts of soluble dietary fiber and oil in the samples and a greater concentration of protein. The third loading had strong influences from the carbohydrate wavelengths in addition to large influences in the protein wavelength bands. The loadings for NDF and total dietary fiber were similar to those for soluble dietary fiber for factors one, two, and three with the loading for factor three again having strong influences in the carbohydrate band. The influence of water on the loadings was apparent in the loadings for factor 4 for all three fiber fractions. Thus, several constituents appear to play a role in the model developed to predict dietary fiber in oat bran products.

The calibration equation developed by Kays et al. (23) for total dietary fiber prediction contained 9 factors with scores from factors 2, 3, and 4 having the highest correlation with total dietary fiber. The loading for factor 3, which was the most highly correlated to dietary fiber, showed significant intensities related to C-H absorption in the carbohydrate bands at 2262 and 2328 nm and the aliphatic C-H bands at 1722 and 2404 nm (Figure 3). Loading 3 also had

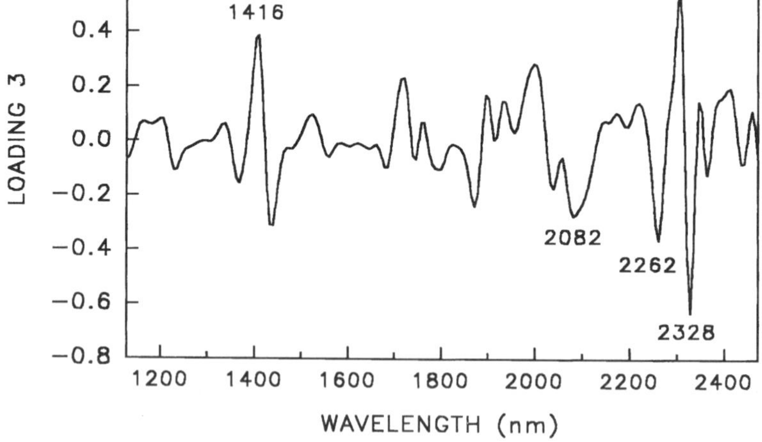

FIGURE 3 PLS loading specta for factor 3 in the total dietary fiber (reprinted in part from Ref. 23)

significant intensities related to O-H absorption in the carbohydrate band at 2082 and the water band at 1416. Factor 2 had the second highest correlation with dietary fiber and its loading was dominated by O-H absorption in the water bands at 1413 and 1920 nm. Loading 2 also had significant intensity related to C-H absorption in the carbohy-drate band at 2262 nm, the aliphatic C-H band at 2304 nm, and due to C=O absorption in the protein band at 2052. Factor 4 had the third highest correlation with dietary fiber with intensities due to C-H absorption in the carbohydrate bands at 2262 and 2328 nm and the aliphatic C-H band at 2310. Thus, for the three important loadings in the total dietary fiber prediction model, absorbance was dominated by effects due to C-H and O-H groups in the carbohydrate and water bands (23). Overall, as in the study by Williams et al. (22), absorptions by functional groups associated with several constituents (carbohydrate, water, oil, and protein) appear to contribute to the prediction model for total dietary fiber.

SUMMARY

NIR procedures have been used successfully in agriculture and on-line food processing for many years. NIR analysis has advantages over conventional laboratory techniques in that it is very rapid, requires little or no sample preparation, can be non-destructive, and does not produce chemical waste. Because of food labeling legislation, there is a need for rapid methods of dietary fiber analysis. The studies detailed in this review have demonstrated the potential of NIRS for rapid, accurate measurement of dietary fiber in processed and unprocessed cereal and snack foods. Relationships have been established between NIR spectra and total, soluble, and insoluble dietary fiber, and models developed to predict the amounts of these fiber fractions in specific data sets. Thus, NIR analysis presents an attractive alternative to current laboratory methods for dietary fiber measurement. Traditional methods, however, are still necessary to provide reference data for spectral/chemometric models. Use of the NIR and the other spectral regions is antici-pated to be a significant force in dietary fiber analysis in the future.

Reference to specific products is made for identification purposes only and does not imply endorsement by the United States Government.

REFERENCES

1. Code of Federal Regulations (1995) FDA, HHS, 21, part 101.9.
2. Resources Conservation and Recovery Act. U. S . Code 1988 Title 42, Section 6901 et seq.
3. Prosky, L., Asp, N-G., Furda, I., DeVries, J.W., Schweizer, T.F., & Harland, B.F. (1985) J. Assoc. Off. Anal. Chem. 68, 677–679.
4. Mongeau, R. & Brassard, R. (1986) J. Food Sci. 51, 1333–1336.

5. Lee, S.C., Prosky, L., & DeVries, J.W. (1992) J. AOAC Intl. 75, 395–416.
6. Englyst, H.N., Quigley, M.E., & Hudson, G.J. (1994) Analyst 119, 1497–1509.
7. Williams, P.C. & Norris, K.H., (Eds.) (1987) Near-infrared Technology in the Agricultural and Food Industries, American Association of Cereal Chemists Inc., St. Paul, MN.
8. Marten, G.C., Shenk, J.S., & Barton, F.E., II (1985) Near Infrared Reflectance Spectroscopy (NIRS): Analysis of Forage Quality, USDA Handbook No. 643, Washington, DC.
9. Williams, P.C. (1987) in Near Infrared Technology in The Agricultural and Food Industries, P.C. Williams & K.H. Norris (Eds), American Association of Cereal Chemists Inc., St. Paul, MN, pp. 107–142.
10. Barton, F.E., II & Burdick, D. (1979) J. Agric. Food Chem. 27, 1248–1252.
11. McDonald, R. S. & Wilks, P.A. Jr. (1988) Applied Spectroscopy 42, 151–162.
12. Shenk, J.S. & Westerhaus, M.O. (1991a) Crop Sci. 31, 469–47.
13. Windham, W.R. & Linn, P.C. (1992) in Near Infra-Red Spectroscopy: Bridging the Gap between Data Analysis and NIR Applications, K.I. Hildrum, T. Isaksson, T. Naes, & A. Tandberg (Eds), Ellis Horwood, London, England, pp. 459–464.
14. Shenk, J.S. & Westerhaus, M.O. (1991b) Crop Sci. 31, 1548–1555.
15. Shenk, J.S., Westerhaus, M.O., & Abrams, S.M. (1989) in Near Infrared Reflectance Spectroscopy (NIRS): Analysis of Forage Quality, G.C. Marten, J.S. Shenk, & F.E. Barton II (Eds.) USDA Handbook No. 643, Washington, DC, pp. 104–110.
16. Norris, K.H. & Hart, J.R. (1965) in Proceedings of the 1963 International Symposium on Humidity and Moisture, vol. 4, Reinhold Publishing, New York, pp. 19.
17. Ben-Gera, I. & Norris, K.H. (1968a) Israel J. Agric. Research 18, 125–132.
18. Ben-Gera, I. & Norris, K.H. (1968b) J.Food Sci. 33, 64–67.
19. Williams, P.C. (1975) Cereal Chemistry 52, 561–576.
20. Polesello, A. & Giangiacomo, R. (1983) in CRC Critical Reviews in Food Science and Nutrition 18, 203–230.
21. Osborne, B.G., Fearn, T., & Hindle, P.H. (1993) Practical NIR Spectroscopy with Applications in Food and Beverage Analysis, Longman Scientific & Technical, Harlow, England.
22. Williams, P.C., Cordeiro, H.M., & Harnden, M.F.T. (1991) Cereal Foods World 36, 571–574.
23. Kays, S.E., Windham, W.R., & Barton, F.E. II (1996) J. Agric. Food. Chem. 44, 2266–2271.
24. Baker, D. (1983) Cereal Chem. 60, 217–219.
25. Baker, D. (1985) Cereal Foods World, 30, 389–392.
26. Szczodrak, J., Czuchajowska, Z., Pomeranz, Y. (1992) Cereal Chem. 69, 419–423.
27. Kim, H-O. & Williams, P.C. (1990) J. Agric. Food Chem. 38, 682–688.
28. Davies, A.M.C., Coxon, D.T., Gavrel, G.M., & Wright, D.J. (1985) J. Sci. Food Agric. 36, 49–54.
29. Osborne, B.G. & Douglas, S. (1981) J. Sci. Food. Agric. 32, 328–332.
30. Villareal, C.P., De La Cruz, N.M. & Juliano, B.O. (1994) Cereal Chem. 71, 292–296.
31. Roberts, G. (1980) Near infrared analysis in the confectionery industry. Neotec International News Items No. 12, Pacific Scientific, Silver Spring, MD.

32. Kaffka, K.J. & Norris, K.H. (1976) Acta Alimentaria 5, 267–279.
33. Birth, G.S., Dull, G.G., Renfroe, W.T., & Kays, S.J. (1985) J. Amer. Soc. Hort. Sci. 110, 297–303.
34. Coventry, A.G. & Hunston, M.J. (1984) Cereal Foods World 29, 715–718.
35. Norris, K.H., Barnes, R.F., Moore, J.E., & Shenk, J.S. (1976) J. Animal Sci. 43, 889–897.
36. Barton, F.E., II & Windham, W.R. (1988) J. Assoc. Off. Anal. Chem. 71, 1162–1167.
37. Murray, I. (1993) in Sward Measurement Handbook (2nd Ed), A. Davies, R.D. Baker, S.A. Grant, A.S. Laidlaw (Eds), British Grassland Society, Reading, U.K., pp. 285–312.
38. Approved Methods of the AACC (1969) AACC Method 32-20, American Association of Cereal Chemists, St. Paul, MN.
39. Horvath, I., Norris, K.H., Horvath-Mosonyl, M., Rigo, J., & Hegedus-Volgyesi, E. (1984) Acta Alimenaria 13, 355–382.
40. Schweizer, T.F. & Wursch, P. (1979) J. Sci. Food Agric. 30, 613–619.
41. Official Methods of Analysis (1992) 15th Ed., 3rd Supplement, AOAC, Arlington, VA.
42. Barnes, R.J., Dhanoa, M.S ., & Lister, S.J. (1989) Appl. Spectros. 43, 772–777.

22

Definition and Analysis of Dietary Fiber

R. MONGEAU, F.W. SCOTT, AND R. BRASSARD
Food Directorate, Nutrition Research Division, Banting Research Centre, Ottawa, Ontario, Canada

INTRODUCTION

There is new evidence that the macrostructure of plant foods participates in the physiological effects of dietary fiber and this needs to be incorporated in a revised definition of dietary fiber. The first definition implied that dietary fiber is derived primarily from edible plant cell walls. The cell wall material of edible plant tissues in the diet constitutes the botanical structure of the plant foods and it is rich in micronutrients. The subsequent definitions have been either based on plant cell walls and/or on resistance to digestion, and the reference to the edible plant tissues as the origin of dietary fiber was not always mentioned. It has been shown for various edible plant tissues that the loss of structural integrity of the cell walls is associated with a significant reduction of physiological effects (regularizing colonic function, lowering peak blood glucose and insulin levels, and reducing the rate and extent of fat absorption). Relying on dietary fiber analyses alone to determine the presence of dietary fiber is problematic because (a) they cannot measure the degree of retention of the structural integrity of the cell walls and

(b) these methods cannot distinguish between dietary fiber and materials such as ruminant fiber, non-edible tissues and non-food material. Therefore, to be considered dietary fiber, a food material should meet the three following conditions: 1) originates from ''the cell walls of edible plant tissues in the traditional human diet,'' 2) retains an intact botanical structure, and 3) is measurable by current dietary fiber methods.

The term ''dietary fiber'' first appeared in 1953 and referred to hemicelluloses, cellulose and lignin (1). After observations in Africa and comparisons of dietary intakes and disease incidence with those in the United Kingdom, Burkitt and Trowell hypothesized that several western diseases were attributable to the lack of dietary fiber in the western diet. In 1972, they recommended that individuals increase dietary fiber intake to increase stool volume and softness. Trowell defined dietary fiber as that portion of food which is derived from the cell walls of plants and is digested very poorly by human beings (2–4). ''Digested very poorly'' was assumed because dietary fiber intake increases fecal volume. In the context of the 1972 definition, dietary fiber corresponds mostly to the intact or minimally processed cell wall material in edible plant tissues. The message was to avoid excessive peeling, grinding and other preparation. According to Trowell (5), dietary fiber largely corresponds to the ''skeletal framework'' of the plant as described by McCance and Lawrence (6) and refers to the structural material of the whole food.

The principal components of dietary fiber are non-starch polysaccharides (NSP). In edible cell walls, NSP is often associated with polyphenolics (e.g., lignin) and proteins. NSP is largely made up of hemicelluloses, cellulose and pectic substances. The non-carbohydrate components of cell walls are quantitatively minor constituents of most edible plant tissues but lignin and phenolic esters in lignified tissues of wheat bran, cutin and waxes in leafy vegetables, and suberin in roots and tubers have significant physiological effects (7).

The definition of 1972 (2) excluded non-cell wall material that is measured by dietary fiber methods. Although this represented a minor component of dietary fiber (7), a definition proposed in 1976 included material such as gums and some pectin (8). The latter definition was based on resistance to digestion in the upper gastrointestinal tract. For the purpose of labeling, Englyst and collaborators later proposed that dietary fiber be defined as ''nonstarch polysaccharides (NSP) and lignin in the diet that are not digested by the endogenous secretions of the human digestive tract'' in order to refer to plant cell wall and related material in the diet (9,10). In 1981, the AOAC consensus definition referred primarily to the remnants of plant cells resistant to hydrolysis by alimentary enzymes of man.

The problems with defining dietary fiber by resistance to digestion are as follows: 1) digestion by fiber methods cannot be assumed to be as efficient as by the intact gastrointestinal system (11). Resistance to digestion means resistance to acid, bile secretions, and to various enzymes with complementary simultaneous actions (e.g., amylase and protease activities). Continuous enzyme secretion and removal of the products of the reactions are characteristics of vigorous digestion in vivo that are not reproduced in vitro (12). 2) All dietary fiber fractions are assumed to reach the end of the small intestine without significant degradation but this is not necessarily the case (11,13). 3) Different materials such as ruminant fibers are resistant to digestion but are not dietary fiber. Ruminants are specially equipped to retain, grind and ferment material such as wheat straw before intestinal absorption.

Over the years, several definitions of dietary fiber have been used in various publications, with variable wording based on the concepts mentioned above. These variations in the definition were due partly to the multiplicity of concepts involved in ''dietary fiber,'' and partly to the difficulties associated with its measurement and labeling. The Canadian definition made clear that the only origin of dietary fiber is the edible part of plants in the human diet (14). It was emphasized that this definition excluded polymers made undigestible upon food processing. The Pilch definition (15) was similar and specifically excluded oligosaccharides and carbohydrate polymers of less than 50 or 60 degrees of polymerization. The latter are not recovered by dietary fiber methods.

The 1976 definition (8) did not specifically refer to the ''cell wall,'' but the notion of botanical structure has remained present since most dietary fibers have been considered to be structural cell wall components (16). Since then, evidence has accumulated on the relationship between the structural integrity of dietary fiber and its physiological effects (17).

BOTANICAL STRUCTURE AND PHYSIOLOGICAL EFFECTS

The Canadian Expert Advisory Committee on Dietary Fibre agreed that there are three specific physiological effects for different types of dietary fiber: 1) regularizing colonic function, 2) normalizing serum lipid levels, and 3) attenuating postprandial glucose response. Suppressing appetite was mentioned as a possible fourth specific effect (14). Some of the evidence supporting the position that botanical structure influences these physiological effects is reviewed below.

Colonic Function

The geometric mean particle size (MPS) affects other properties of particulate dietary fibers. Coarse wheat bran normalizes transit time (18), prevents hardening of fecal material and retains free water (19). Observations in human subjects suggested that coarse wheat bran prevents the formation of a gas phase in the colon and retains finely dispersed gas in the fiber matrix, along with free water, bacteria and other components (20). The colon has a threshold limit for the volume of gas to be absorbed and the high rates of gas production with a rapid fermentation will exceed the capacity of absorption. Effects of dietary fiber on fecal weight are apparently dependent on the type of polysaccharides and associated constituents that contribute to the architecture of the plant cell wall. Isolated polysaccharides often differ in their effects from the respective carbohydrates occurring in whole foods, probably due to a lack of intact cell wall structure (21). Although it has been recommended that volume be used rather than weight to express the concentration of colonic contents (22), few data have been generated in humans. The rat, however, is a useful model to study colonic function: rat data show that reducing the particle size of hard wheat bran affects fecal wet volume more extensively than wet weight, and they suggest that coarse bran at the 15% level in the diet has a better fecal-density lowering effect than fine bran at the 25% level (23). Rat data confirm that the coarse bran particles entrap finely dispersed gas, supporting Cummings' mechanisms of action of dietary fiber on fecal output in human (gas trapped within gut contents) (24).

Can the beneficial effect of coarse wheat bran on fecal density be obtained by a larger amount of fine bran? To answer this question, 144 rats were housed individually in Nalgene metabolic cages to permit the collection of clean feces with minimal contact with urine. They were fed one of 12 modified AIN-76 (American Institute of Nutrition) diets. With 10% oil in the diets, the nutrients in the mixed diets stuck to all bran particles and assured comparable nutrient intakes among groups. All diets except the fiber-free diet contained the same hard red wheat bran but in different amounts (0–20%) and at three MPS. Coarse bran (850 μm MPS) was provided at 4, 8, 12, 16 and 20% levels and the medium (513 μm MPS) and fine (308 μm MPS) brans were provided at the 4, 12 and 20% levels. The hard bran contained 50% dietary fiber. After 42 days on diets, fresh fecal weight, expressed per 100 g of food ingested, increased linearly ($R^2 = 0.85$) with the dietary fiber level but it was not significantly influenced by particle size. The fresh fecal volume increased with a steeper slope than the weight resulting in a reduction of density (weight/volume) well beyond that which could have been attributed to an increase in fat content. Only entrapment of finely dispersed gas could explain observed density values of £0.8. Reducing particle size affected ($P < 0.05$) the capacity of the bran to reduce fecal density, and significantly reduced the volume response. This is important considering that volume is involved in the triggering of the bowel movement. In regard to the capacity to reduce density, 20% fine bran in the diet was not as efficient as 12% medium bran or 8% coarse bran. The reduction of particle size also decreased ($P < 0.05$) the beneficial effects of wheat bran on colonic pH and fecal consistency. The reduction of particle size tended to reduce the trophic effect of wheat bran on the gastrointestinal tract, and to increase intestinal transit time, but these effects were not statistically significant.

These results show that the effect of coarse hard wheat bran on colonic function cannot be fully compensated for by larger amounts of fine hard wheat bran (same composition).

Postprandial Glucose Response

After a meal, the extent of rise of blood glucose depends on several interacting factors. At the beginning of this century, scientists assumed that the molecular size of the carbohydrate was an important determinant of its rate of digestion. Starch was thus considered to be digested and absorbed slowly whereas low-molecular-weight carbohydrates were believed to be absorbed rapidly, hence promoting high responses of plasma glucose. Studies have since shown that food properties other than molecular size influence the postprandial response and that starchy foods can have glycemic indices ranging from low to high (25–27). Any process that disrupts the physical or botanical structure of food ingredients will increase the plasma glucose and insulin responses (28).

Consumption of foods with a high glycemic index and a low dietary fiber content has been listed among the causes of insulin resistance (29). Insulin resistance occurs when high blood concentrations of insulin do not decrease hyperglycemia efficiently. The extended hyperglycemic periods continue to stimulate insulin secretion. These conditions may lead to NIDDM (non-insulin-dependent-diabetes-melitus, or type II diabetes) (29).

According to Heaton (30), dietary fiber is generally resistant to digestion but its most important characteristic is that it constitutes the physical form and texture of whole foods. This structure affects several physiological phenomena: eating time, degree of satiety, rate of digestion, and extent of digestion. The presence of dietary fiber with an intact botanical structure prevents the high insulinemic peak following mastication and ingestion of an apple, and it also prevents the resulting hypoglycemia 2h after. The homogenization of the apple in apple puree destroys its botanical structure and largely reduces the beneficial physiological effects of the whole apple, even if its composition is not affected. The food macrostructure modulates the rate of digestion by digestive enzymes; it influences the metabolic response to starchy foods (cereals, legumes) and to foods containing low-molecular-weight carbohydrates (apple, orange, carrot) (31-40).

Food structure is so important that the use of products with "as fed" food structure has been recommended when measuring their glycemic index by enzymic digestion to ensure a realistic result. Food structure must not be destroyed more than it would be by chewing (28).

Non-carbohydrate components significantly contribute to the cohesiveness of the botanical structure. Although the plant cell walls are largely made of carbohydrates, the structure has physiological effects unrelated to the carbohydrate components per se.

Fat Absorption

To alleviate the increase in fasting plasma triglyceride concentration and to improve insulin sensitivity, the diet should probably contain foods with a low glycemic index and be high in fiber (29). Few data are available on the effect of structural integrity on blood lipids. However, the amount of fat absorbed from whole (masticated) peanuts and finely ground peanuts (peanut butter) has been measured indirectly and compared to peanut oil (41). The amounts of triglycerides excreted in feces were as follows (percentage of total fat ingested): 18% for whole peanuts, 7% for creamy peanut butter, and 4.5 % for peanut oil. The whole peanut and the peanut butter had exactly the same composition. The presence of dietary fiber with an intact structure in whole, masticated peanuts limits the amount of fat that can be absorbed. By contrast, the presence of the dietary fiber components in peanut butter had little effect compared with whole peanuts and differed little from peanut oil.

DEFINITION OF DIETARY FIBER

The above examples show that we need to take into account the botanical structure of the cell walls in our foods: This structure plays an essential role in the physiological effects of dietary fiber. At this time, the notion of integrity of the botanical structure is not accounted for in the term ''complex carbohydrates'' and also, by present definitions, the term ''dietary fiber'' fails to fully acknowledge its importance. Because analysis of dietary fiber tells nothing about the origin of a sample or the integrity of its structure, clearly the methods alone cannot be used to define dietary fiber. It appears that the way to take structural integrity into account is to refer to it specifically in the definition of dietary fiber.

Therefore, in order to be included in the definition of dietary fiber, a food material should be required to meet the three following conditions:

1. It should originate from the cell walls of the edible plant tissues in the traditional human diet,
2. It should have an intact botanical structure, and
3. It should be measurable by current official dietary fiber methods (with corrections, when needed).

This definition would exclude, for example, non-edible plant tissues or organs such as apple and grape seeds that are sometimes ingested with foods, edible plant foods that have been significantly chemically or physically modified with respect to their botanical or molecular structure, non-plant sources of polysaccharide polymers such as chitin, short chain undigestible material comprising that resulting from either the breakdown of longchain nonstarch polysaccharides or synthesized from monosaccharides, and plant material available to ruminants but derived from non-edible parts of plants such as wood and straw.

Material complying with conditions 1 and 2 above would be adequately measured by the current official dietary fiber methods provided appropriate corrections are made when needed (see below). New methods would have to be evaluated according to their ability to measure such material. The material not complying with the first condition above (edible cell wall origin) but retained by current official dietary fiber methods could be classified under resistant carbohydrates.

Structural integrity (condition no. 2) of foods complying with condition no. 1 can be evaluated by such measures as particle size, and an integrity factor with an arbitrary scale based on the fact that when we cut a food into gradually smaller pieces, the surface:weight ratio increases exponentially. For example, the sugars from pieces of apple are readily released from the broken cells at their surface. This would provide a guidance to consumers for selecting foods (including processed) that comply the most with nutrient recommendations.

METHODS

An important criterion of the total dietary fiber (TDF) value determined by any method is that it should not be influenced by processing in order to be used for food labelling. If not, processing conditions favoring high values may be preferred, but this may not correspond to beneficial physiological effects.

The complete removal of starch from the dietary fiber residue has been a challenge for all dietary fiber methods (12,42–44). When present, residual starch is measured mostly as part of the insoluble fiber in gravimetric analyses and as glucose in GC analyses. In boiled legumes, the amount of starch in the residue using certain official methods can outweigh that of dietary fiber (12,43). This situation is partly due to the choice of enzymes and to the sequence of enzyme treatments. Non-mammalian (e.g., bacterial) sources of enzymes need to be purified to prevent the degradation of dietary fiber by contaminating enzymes. However, purified enzymes may have more limited activities due to loss of cofactors. A less pure mammalian enzyme has more diverse bond-breaking capacities, and multiple attacks by amylase and protease are critical (12,43). Two sequential short treatments are better than a very long one. Ideally, the fiber residue should contain only the cell wall structural protein and no other protein. Larger amounts indicate the presence of residual digestible protein and possibly an incomplete starch digestion. Starch-protein interactions are present in certain food products and the absence of a protease treatment may reduce the rate of in vitro starch hydrolysis (45). It is therefore important that proteolytic enzymes are included in the in vitro assay (28) either as a separate treatment or included with an unpurified mammalian alpha-amylase preparation (43).

Structural protein (46–47) and lignin are non-carbohydrate components of dietary fiber. One method (Englyst) overlooks lignin and only one method (Mongeau) measures the small amount of undigestible protein. Permanganate lignin and Klason lignin values are not always in agreement (43–44). Klason lignin is generally higher and more variable than permanganate lignin. Lignin is difficult to separate from some hemicelluloses and can react with protein during food processing (48). The rapid Mongeau method includes treatments that represent an appropriate preparation for measuring permanganate lignin in foods, and values are little influenced by food processing. According to Selvendran (7), the acetyl bromide method needs only a 5–10 mg sample but comparison of values has not been made. Lignin is regarded as a minor component of most plant foods but the total polyphenolic material (including lignin) represents 5–20% of the dry cell wall (7).

Food processing can solubilize some of the insoluble fiber (49). The resulting higher soluble : insoluble fiber ratio should not be interpreted as having oat-gum like physiological effects. The measurement of soluble dietary fiber increases the time and cost of analysis with some methods, and the soluble fiber values are highly method-dependent. Only the total dietary fiber values can be compared among methods, but still with certain limitations.

The Mongeau (AOAC #992.16) TDF method (42) was developed over 11 years by testing various combinations of treatments taking into account rapidity, precision and accuracy. The method uses neutral detergent but the total dietary fiber values are different from neutral detergent values. The neutral detergent method is not appropriate for measuring insoluble fiber in human foods unless it incorporates a specific preparation of alpha-amylase. The combination of neutral detergent and unpurified pancreatic amylase has a unique efficiency for digesting protein and it ensures extensive and reproducible digestion of starch. The best results with the above-mentioned TDF method are obtained when the soluble and insoluble fractions are determined sequentially in the same sample. The method provides a soluble : insoluble ratio among the highest. The solubility of dietary fiber in vivo is not well documented but it is thought to be high.

In various food samples collected throughout Canada over several years and prepared as they would have been at home, the rapid Mongeau method (y) was shown to correlate well with the integral Prosky method (x) for total dietary fiber ($y = 1.02x - 0.04$, $r = 0.993$, $n = 38$). These methods gave higher values than Englyst NSP (non-starch polysaccharides) values but the difference was partly due to the fact that lignin is not measured by the Englyst method. In a method comparison including 65 foods, the TDF values by the Mongeau method were about 1.3 times higher than Englyst NSP values. The factor remained the same when processed foods and legumes were included or excluded since both methods are not affected by processing. By contrast, when the Prosky TDF and Englyst NSP methods were compared, the factor was 1.3 when processed food and cooked dried legumes were excluded, but it reached 1.6 when they were included in the comparison (NSP × 1.6 = Prosky) (44). Thus, in spite of the close correlation mentioned above, discrepancies among dietary fiber methods can be substantial for some foods. TDF differences even between the Prosky and Lee-modified version were noticed for cooked dried legumes, but these discrepancies were attenuated when an unpurified pancreatic alpha-amylase was used in both versions of the Prosky method (12,43). On the other hand, dietary fiber values for 45 foods (fruits, vegetables, cereals and canned legumes) analyzed by the Mongeau method (y) correlate well with those published by Marlett (50) for the corresponding foods analyzed by a modified Theander method (x): $y = 0.99x + 0.06$, $r = 0.96$. Overall, the comparison of the dietary fiber value for various (>60) foods suggests a general agreement among several dietary fiber methods, and a slight modification of the Prosky and Lee methods would permit an even better agreement.

CONCLUSION

An improved definition of dietary fiber should first clarify the origin of the plant cell wall material to discriminate between human dietary fiber and ruminant fiber and other material extraneous to the human diet. Second, the relatively new information on the botanical structure should be taken into account because a significant portion of the physiological effects of dietary fiber is dependent on the structural integrity of the edible cell walls. Third, the material defined as dietary fiber should be measurable by the current dietary fiber methods. Most of these methods should be adequate, some may need corrrections.

REFERENCES

1. Hipsley, E.H. (1953) Dietary 'fibre' and pregnancy toxemia. Br. Med. J. 2, 420–422.
2. Trowell, H. (1972) Crude fibre, dietary fibre and atherosclerosis. Atherosclerosis 16, 138–140.
3. Trowell, H. (1974) Definitions of fibre. Lancet 1, 503.
4. Trowell, H. (1976) Definition of dietary fibre and hypothesis that it is a protective factor in certain diseases. Am. J. Clin. Nutr. 29, 417–427.
5. Trowell, H. (1975) Refined carbohydrate foods and disease: some implications of dietary fibre. In Refined carbohydrate foods and disease: some implications of dietary fibre, Vol 1, Academic Press, London, pp. 23–41.
6. McCance, R.A, & Lawrence, R.D. (1929) The carbohydrate content of foods. Med. Res. Coun. Spec. Rep. Ser. 135, 1–73. HM Stationary Office London.
7. Selvendran, R.R. (1987) Chemistry of plant cell walls and dietary fibre. Scand. J. Gastro. 22 (suppl 129), 33–41.

8. Trowell, H., Southgate, D.A.T., Wolever, T.M.S., Leeds, A.R., Gassull, M.A., & Jenkins, D.J.A. (1976) Dietary fibre redefined. Lancet 1, 967.
9. Englyst, H.N., Trowell, H., Southgate, D.A.T. & Cummings, J.H. (1987) Dietary fiber and resistant starch. Am. J. Clin. Nutr. 46, 873–874.
10. Englyst, H.N. & Cummings, J.H. (1988) Reply to N-G Asp et al. Am. J. Clin. Nutr. 47, 690–691.
11. Marlett, J.A. (1990) Issues in dietary fiber analysis. In New developments in dietary fiber: Physiology, physicochemical, and analytical. Advances in experimental medicine and biology, Vol 270, Plenum Press. New York, NY, pp. 183–192.
12. Mongeau, R., & Brassard, R. (1995) Importance of sample preparation and enzyme treatments in the determination of dietary fiber in dried legumes. J. AOAC Int. 78, 1444–1449.
13. Bach Knudsen, K.E., Jensen, B.B., & Hansen, I. (1993) Digestion of polysaccharides and other major components in the small and large intestine of pigs fed on diets consisting of oat fractions rich in β-D-glucan. Brit. J. Nutr. 70, 537–556.
14. Health and Welfare Canada (1985) In: Report of the expert advisory committee on dietary fibre, National Health and Welfare Canada, Ottawa, ON.
15. Pilch, S. (1987) Physiological effects and health consequences of dietary fiber. Center for Food Safety and Applied Nutrition, FDA and Life Sciences Research Office, FASEB, Bethesda.
16. McPherson, R. (1985) Classification of fibre types. In: The clinical role of dietary fibre. MES Canada Inc., Mississauga, ON., pp 13-22.
17. Asp, N.G. (1996) Dietary carbohydrates: Classification by chemistry and physiology. Food Chem. 57, 9-14.
18. Payler, D.K., Pomare, E.W., Heaton, K.W., & Harvey, R.F. (1975) The effect of wheat bran on intestinal transit. Gut 16, 209-213.
19. Eastwood, M.A. (1983) Physical properties of fibre towards bile acids, water and minerals. In Dietary Fiber, G.G. Birch & K.J. Parker (eds), Applied Science, New York, NY, pp. 149-163.
20. Brodribb, A.J.M., & Groves, C. (1978) Effect of bran particle size on stool weight. Gut 19, 60–63.
21. Wisker, E. (1994) Effect of physico-chemical properties of dietary fibre on feces. In Physico-chemical properties of dietary fibre and effects of processing on micronutrients availability. Metabolic and physiological aspects of dietary fibre in food. R. Amadó, J.-L. Barry and W. Frolich (eds). COST 92, Commission of the European Communities, pp. 75–80.
22. Lupton, J.R., & Ferrel, R.G. (1986) Using density rather than mass to express the concentration of gastrointestinal tract constituents. J. Nutr. 116, 164–168.
23. Mongeau, R., & Brassard, R. (1985) Dietary fiber and fecal characteristics in rats–effects of level and particle size of bran. J. Food Sci. 50, 654–656.
24. Cummings, J. H. (1986) The effect of dietary fiber on fecal weight and composition. In: Handbook of dietary fiber in human nutrition. G. A. Spiller (ed). CRC Press, Boca Raton, pp. 211–280.
25. Crapo, P.A., Reaven, G.M., & Olefsky, J.M. (1977) Postprandial glucose and insulin response to different complex carbohydrates. Diabetes 26, 1178–1183.
26. Hollenbeck, C.B., Coulston, A.M., Donnor, C.C., Williams, R.A., & Reaven, G.M.

(1985) The effect of variations in percent of naturally occurring complex and simple carbohydrates on plasma glucose and insulin response in individuals with non-insulin-dependent diabetes mellitus. Diabetes 34, 151–155.
27. Jenkins, D.J.A., Wolever, T.M.S., & Taylor, R.H. (1981) Glycemic index of foods: a physiological basis for carbohydrate exchange. Am. J. Clin. Nutr. 34, 184–190.
28. Björck, I., Granfeldt, Y., Liljeberg, H., Tovar, J., & Asp, N.-G. (1994) Food properties affecting the digestion and absorption of carbohydrates. Am. J. Clin. Nutr. 59(suppl), 699S–705S.
29. Smith, U. (1994) Carbohydrates, fat and insulin action. Am. J. Clin. Nutr. 59(suppl), 686S–689S.
30. Heaton, K.W. (1995) Chemical and nutritional classification of food carbohydrates. In: Recent Progress in the Analysis of Dietary Fibre, Metabolic and physiological aspects of dietary fibre in food, COST 92, Commission of the European Communities.
31. Albrink, M.J., Newman, T., & Davidson, P.C. (1979) Effect of high- and low-fiber diets on plasma lipids and insulin. Am. J. Clin. Nutr. 32, 1486–1491.
32. Bolton, R.P., Heaton, K.W., & Burroughs, L.F. (1981) The role of dietary fibre in satiety, glucose, and insulin: studies with fruit and fruit juice. Am. J. Clin. Nutr. 34, 211–217.
33. Golay, A., Coulston, A.M., & Hollenbeck, C.B. (1986) Comparison of metabolic effects of white beans processed into two different physical forms. Diabetes Care 9, 260–266.
34. Haber, G.B., Heaton, K.W., Murphy, D., & Burroughs, L. (1977) Depletion and disruption of dietary fibre. Effects on satiety, plasma-glucose, and serum-insulin. Lancet ii, 679–682.
35. O'Dea, K., Nestel, P.J., & Antonoff, L. (1980) Physical factors influencing postprandial glucose and insulin responses to starch. Am. J. Clin. Nutr. 33, 760–765.
36. Oettlé, G.J., Emmett, P. & Heaton, K.W. (1987) Glucose and insulin responses to manufactured and whole-food snacks. Am. J. Clin. Nutr. 45, 86–91.
37. Tovar, J., de Francisco, A., Björck, I., & Asp, N.-G. (1991) Relationship between microstructure and in vitro digestibility of starch in precooked leguminous seed flours. Food Structure 10, 19–26.
38. Tovar, J., Granfeldt, Y., & Björck, I. (1992) Effect of processing on blood glucose and insulin responses to legumes. J. Agric. Food Chem. 40, 1846–1851.
39. Würsch, P., Del Vedovo, S., & Koellreuter, B. (1986) Cell structure and starch nature as key determinants of the digestion rate of starch in legume. Am. J. Clin. Nutr. 43, 25–29.
40. Yoon, J.H., Thompson, L.U., & Jenkins, D.J.A. (1983) The effect of phytic acid on in vitro rate of starch digestibility and blood glucose response. Am. J. Clin. Nutr. 38, 835–842.
41. Levine, A.S., & Silvis, S.E. (1981) Absorption of peanuts (letter). N. Eng. J. Med. 304, 359–360.
42. Mongeau, R., & Brassard, R. (1993) Enzymatic-gravimetric determination in foods of dietary fiber as sum of insoluble and insoluble fiber fractions: summary of collaborative study. J. AOAC Int. 76, 923–925.
43. Mongeau, R., & Brassard, R. (1994) Comparison and assessment of the difference

in total dietary fiber in cooked dried legumes as determined by five methods. J. AOAC Int. 77, 1197–1202.

44. Mongeau, R. (1995) Experience with different official analytical methods in Canada. In: Recent Progress in the Analysis of Dietary Fibre, Metabolic and physiological aspects of dietary fibre in food, COST 92, Commission of the European Communities.
45. Tovar, J., Björck, I., & Asp, N.-G. (1990) Analytical and nutritional implications of limited enzymic availability of starch in cooked red kidney beans. J. Agric. Food Chem. 38, 488–493.
46. Dintzis, F.R. (1983) Dietary fiber analysis–Concepts and problems. Dr Lineback and GE Inglett (eds). In: Food Carbohydrates, D.R. Lineback & G.E. Inglett (eds), AVI Publishing Company, Inc. Wesport, CT, pp. 312–333.
47. Saunders, R.M., & Betschart, A.A. (1980) The significance of protein as a component of dietary fiber. Am. J. Clin. Nutr. 33, 960–961.
48. Hartley, R.D. (1978) The lignin fraction of plant cell walls. Am. J. Clin. Nutr. 31, 590–593.
49. Nyman, M., Gustafsson, K., Svanberg, M., & Asp, N.-G. (1994) Effect of processing on dietary fibre. In: Physico-chemical properties of dietary fibre and effects of processing on micronutrients availability. Metabolic and physiological aspects of dietary fibre in food. R. Amadó, J.-L. Barry & W. Frolich (eds). COST 92, Commission of the European Communities, pp. 39-45.
50. Marlett, J.A. (1992) Content and composition of dietary fiber in 117 frequently consumed foods. J. Am. Diet Assoc. 92, 175–186.

23

Estimation of Psyllium Content in Ready-to-Eat Cereals

Susan Sungsoo Cho and Mike Bussey
The Kellogg Company, Battle Creek, Michigan

INTRODUCTION

Psyllium, an acidic arabinoxylan obtained from Ispaghula husk (*Plantago ovata* Forsk), is used as a cathartic and dietary fiber ingredient to lower serum cholesterol and glycemic index. A component of the soluble dietary fiber (SDF) fraction, psyllium is determined indirectly as the xylitol acetate of the neutral polysaccharide residue by a modified capillary gas chromatographic (GC) method (994.13). Since most grains (oat, wheat, corn, and rice) utilized in cereal mixtures contain negligible amounts of xylose, its determination serves as a convenient tool for quantifying the psyllium ingredient added to ready-to-eat (RTE) cereals. Based on xylose analysis, excellent recoveries of the psyllium ingredient were obtained (76 to 109%). Repeatability (RSDs) ranging in value from 3.12 to 24.59 was consistent with the precision obtained by the official method (994.13) on which the present procedure is based.

Total dietary fiber (TDF) is composed of a diverse combination of non-starch polysaccharides (NSP) and of lignin that resist attack by digestive enzymes (1). Physiological effects of dietary fiber components seem to depend, at least in part, on their ability to form stable dispersions with water. Current official methodology (2) resolves TDF into two fractions (991.43): insoluble (IDF) and soluble (SDF). Both IDF and SDF fractions absorb water increasing fecal volume and motility (3). SDF increases satiety by retarding gastric emptying, moderates glucose absorption which reduces insulin dependence, and binds bile acids and steroids reducing serum cholesterol levels. Thus, physiological function seems to be dependent on characteristics of those constituents that compose the total dietary fiber residue.

Chemical diversity of edible plant constituents resistant to digestive enzymes remains a confounding factor in the development of inclusive analytical methodologies for dietary fiber. As Theander et al. (1) have suggested, part of the problem related to understanding the nutritional effects of dietary fiber is lack of an adequate definition upon which appropriate analytical methods depend. Present gravimetric fiber methodologies (2) involve the separation of non-fiber matrix components (primarily starches and proteins) from fiber analytes by: a) strong acid and alkali (962.09, crude fiber), b) acid detergent (973.18), or neutral detergent (4), and c) enzymatic removal (991.43, 985.29, etc., total dietary fiber).

Capillary gas chromatographic analysis (GC) has been used to quantify neutral nonstarch polysaccharides of the total dietary fiber residue as alditol acetate derivatives (5). Other residue components, uronic acids, and lignin, are determined by colorimetric and gravimetric analysis, respectively. Recently a joint AOAC/American Association of Cereal Chemists (AACC) collaborative study was completed (1) which resulted in a method for total dietary fiber (AOAC Method 994.13) based upon the Uppsala method (5).

Numerous composition tables (2,7–11) present fiber content of various fruits, vegetables and cereal products determined by methods or modifications of methods previously mentioned (2,5). With ready-to-eat (RTE) cereals that contain a variety of grains and other ingredients of plant origin, identifying and quantifying each fiber source within the mixture is often desirable.

Psyllium, an annual herb (*Plantago ovata* Forsk) grown primarily in India, southern Europe and the U.S., is cultivated principally for use as a laxative or dietary fiber ingredient (6). Recently, several clinical studies have also demonstrated the efficacy of psyllium in the reduction of serum cholesterol (12,13), glycemic index (14), and synergism with wheat bran in colon cancer prevention (15). Although the seed alone contains ample quantities of mucilage polysaccharides, the refined psyllium seed husk (PSH), commonly called Ispaghula husk, is the component most often used as a fiber source for laxatives and as a potential fiber ingredient in ready-to-eat (RTE) cereals.

Composition studies conducted by Kennedy et al. (16) demonstrated that under mild alkaline hydrolysis PSH yielded a mucilage polysaccharide fraction (85%) that contained an acidic arabinoxylan polymer with (1,4) and (1,3) linkages, as well as a non-polysaccharide (15%) component. Since PSH is composed primarily of a xylan polymer, its addition to RTE cereals increases the xylose content of the neutral polysaccharide residue substantially. With most grains (oats, wheat, corn or rice) incorporated into RTE cereals, xylose content is either negligible (oats and wheat) or absent (corn and rice). Therefore, xylose content may serve as an excellent indicator for identifying and quantifying the psyllium ingredient of the cereal mixture.

For psyllium determination, a crude SDF fraction was prepared using a modification of a TDF method (AOAC 991.43), and then subjected to acid hydrolysis. The sugars of the acid hydrolysate were neutralized, then derivatized to alditol acetates for quantification by capillary GC (1).

MATERIALS AND METHODS

Apparatus

(a) Gas chromatograph (GC).—Equipped with wide bore capillary column, [SP-2330, 30m × 0.75mm (id), 1.0m (film thickness), Supelco, Inc., Bellefonte, PA, 16823-0048, or equivalent] flame ionization detector, and integrator. Operating conditions: injector, 275°C; detector, 275°C; helium carrier gas, flow rate, 8 mL/min.
(b) Autoclave.—Capable of maintaining temperature of 121°C.
(c) Balance.—Capable of weighing to 0.1 mg.
(d) Centrifuge.—To hold 35 mL tubes; capable of operating at 1000 × *g*.
(e) Magnetic stirrer/hot plate.
(f) Mill.—Wiley type, or equivalent, capable of grinding samples to pass a 1.0 mm screen.
(g) pH meter.
(h) Pipetters.—Digital, with disposable tips, 100–300 mL and 5 mL capacity
(i) Sonicator
(j) Syringe, microliter.—Capable of delivering 1 uL
(k) Usual laboratory glassware.
(l) Vortex mixer.
(m) Water bath shakers.—(1) Capable of maintaining 100°C with automatic on-and-off timer. (2) Constant temperature, adjustable to 60°C.

Reagents

Note: Use deionized water throughout.

(a) Acetic acid, glacial.
(b) Acetic acid anhydride.
(c) Ammonium hydroxide, 12.5 M.

(d) Ammonium hydroxide/sodium borohydride solution.—Prepare by dissolving 100 g $NaBH_4$ in 1 L of 3 M NH_4OH.
(e) Amyloglucosidase solution.—Enzyme available from Sigma, St. Louis, MO, 63187, Cat. No. A9913, or equivalent. Dissolve in acetate buffer to obtain 140 u/mL. Prepare just before analysis.
(f) α-Amylase solution.—Heat-stable Termamyl, Sigma, Cat. No. A0164, or equivalent
(g) Protease solution.—Sigma, Cat. No. P3910. Prepare 50 mg/mL enzyme solution in MES-TRIS buffer fresh daily.
(h) Benzoic acid solution, saturated.—Dissolve 50 g benzoic acid in 100 mL of water (w/v).
(i) Calibration standard monosaccharide solution.—Dry monosaccharides under vacuum over SiO_2 to constant weight. Weigh 5 g each of rhamnose and xylose and dilute to volume with H_2O in separate 100 mL volumetric flasks.
(j) Internal standard sorbitol solution.—Dissolve 10 g of sorbitol in 100 mL of water.
(k) Standard sugar mixture for derivatization.—Mix 1 mL xylose and rhamnose standard solutions [B(I)] with 0.3 mL internal standard solution [B(j)] in 1 mL 2.4N sulfuric acid.
(l) Ethanol—95% (v/v).
(m) Hydrochloric acid solution.—0.561N. Add 93.5 mL 6N HCL to ca 700 mL H_2O, mix, allow to cool and dilute to 1L with H_2O.
(n) MES.—2-(N-Morpholino)ethanesulfonic acid (No. M-8250, Sigma Chemical Co., or equivalent).
(o) TRIS.—Tris(hydroxymethyl)aminomethane (No. T-1503, Sigma Chemical Co., or equivalent).
(p) EDTA.—Ethylenediaminetetraacetic acid, anhydrous (No. E-9884, Sigma Chemical Co., or equivalent).
(q) MES-TRIS buffer solution with EDTA.—pH 8.2 at 24°C, MES-0.05M, TRIS-0.05M, EDTA-0.01M. pH of buffer should be 8.2 at 24°C, 8.3 at 20°C, and ~8.1 at 27–28°C. Dissolve 19.52 g MES, 12.2 g TRIS and 5.84 EDTA, g 1.7 L H_2O. Adjust pH to 8.2 with 6N NaOH, and dilute to 2 L with H_2O.
(r) 1-Methyimidazole.
(s) pH Standards.—Buffer solutions of pH 4.0,7.0, and 10.0.
(t) Solvents.—Acetone and methylene chloride
(u) Antifoam reagent.—2-Octanol
(v) Sulfuric acid.—2.4 and 24 M.

Sample Preparation

Processed psyllium seed husks were added to ground oat, wheat, corn or rice-based RTE cereals in quantities of 0, 5, 10, and 20%. Each of the samples was mixed to achieve homogeneity. Prepared samples were stored in moisture proof containers at 4°C.

Psyllium Determination

Preparation of Soluble Dietary Fiber Residue

Weigh duplicate 0.35–0.7 g ground cereal samples into 200 mL beakers and add magnetic stirrer bar to each. Add 28 mL of MES-TRIS buffer solution with EDTA [B(o)]. Stir buffer solution at low speed while adding 140 μL Termamyl [B(f)]. Incubate in 100°C waterbath for 30 min. Cool to ca 60°C.

Insure that all materials including ring that may form above buffer solution and gelation that may occur during enzymatic hydrolysis of starches are dispersed. Add 70 μL protease solution, and continue incubation at 60°C with constant agitation for 30 min.

Adjust pH of buffer to 4.5 with 3.5 mL 0.561N HCL. Add 210 μL amyloglucosidase solution [B(e)] and incubate in waterbath at 60°C with constant agitation. Sonicate reaction mixture for 2–3 min and transfer to 50–60 mL screw-top glass tubes. Centrifuge at 1000 × *g* for 10 min to obtain supernatant containing SDF fraction. Using aspiration remove supernatant without disturbing insoluble fiber residue. Precipitate SDF by adding 4 volumes of preheated 95% ethanol (60°C) and allow to stand at ambient temperature for 1 h. Centrifuge at 2500 × *g* for 20 min; remove and discard supernatant without disturbing residue. Add 20 mL 95% ethanol to SDF residue and vortex for 5 sec. Centrifuge and remove supernatant as above. Quantitatively transfer SDF residue with 20 mL acetone to small vial and dry in oven equilibrated to <40°C.

Weigh 50 mg of residue into a 25 mL screw-cap culture tube. (Sample size may vary depending on expected xylose content.) Add 1 mL of 24N sulfuric acid and hydrolyze SDF residue at ambient temperature for 1 h; vortex for 5 sec at 15 min intervals. Adjust SDF hydrolysate to 2N sulfuric acid by adding 11 mL deionized water. Cap tube loosely with screw-cap and place in preheated autoclave at 121°C for 1 h. Remove; add 0.3 mL of internal standard sorbitol solution [B(j)] to cooled hydrolysates.

Derivatization of Psyllium-containing Sugars from SDF Fraction

(a) Reduction.—Pipet 1 mL hydrolysate or standard sugar mixture [B(k)] into glass tube. Add 256 μL 12.5M NH_4OH and vortex for 5 sec. Confirm solution alkalinity; add ca 5 μL 2-octanol and 0.1 mL of NH_4OH-$NaBH_4$ [B(d)]; vortex for 5 sec. Place tubes in 40°C water bath and incubate 1 h; remove.

(b) Acetylation.—Add 0.1 mL glacial acetic acid; vortex for 5 sec. Transfer 0.8 mL to 50 mL centrifuge tube; add 1.2 mL 1-methylimidazole [B(p)] and 8 mL acetic acid anhydride. Vortex for 5 sec and let stand at ambient temperature for 10 min. Add 15 mL deionized H_2O and vortex for 5 sec. Allow to cool; add

3 mL methylene chloride; vortex for 30–45 sec. Centrifuge at 1000 × *g* for 10 min. Transfer lower phase with Pasteur pipet to 50 mL tube. Rinsing methylene chloride phase containing alditol acetates with 15 mL of deionized H_2O; vortexing for 5 sec. Centrifuge at 1000 × *g* for 10 min. Remove upper aqueous phase by aspiration. Repeat. Evaporate lower phase containing alditol acetates to dryness under nitrogen. Redissolve dried alditol acetates in 1 mL methylene chloride; vortex for 5 sec and store in vial at −20°C, if necessary.

Determination of Xylitol and Rhamnitol Acetates

For identification and quantitation inject 1.0 μL of the alditol acetates standard solution [derivatized B(c)] onto GC widebore capillary column. Alditol acetates of the neutral sugars elute in the following order: rhamnose, xylose and sorbitol (internal standard).

Calculation

Calculate xylose content based on mean of duplicate samples. Incorporate correction factor into equation that accounts for losses sustained during hydrolysis and derivatization and that also accounts for response factor that is GC dependent:

$$\%\ \text{Xylose} = \frac{P_{spl} \times Pi_{std} \times M \times R \times S}{Pi_{spl} \times P_{std} \times G \times T} \times 100$$

where P_{spl} = peak area of xylose sample chromatogram; Pi_{std} = Peak area of sorbitol internal standard; Pi_{spl} = peak area of internal sorbitol standard from sample chromatogram; P_{std} = Peak area of xylose from standard chromatogram; M = mg internal standard added to sample (30); G = original sample weight in mg; S = SDF residue weight in mg; T = weight (mg) of residue used for acid hydrolysis step; 100 = conversion factor for percent; and R = ratio of xylose to sorbitol in calibration standard (5/3).

Compute % psyllium in product as follows:

$$\%\ \text{Psyllium} = \frac{\%\ \text{total xylose in product}}{\%\ \text{xylose in pure psyllium}} \times 100$$

or, if substantial xylose expected in product with psyllium:

$$\%\ \text{Psyllium} = \frac{\%\ \text{total xylose} - \%\ \text{xylose in product blank}}{\%\ \text{xylose in pure psyllium}} \times 100$$

RESULTS AND DISCUSSION

Grain products furnish about one-third of the total dietary fiber intake of the average North American diet (10). Thus, the addition of compatible fiber ingredients such as psyllium to cereal mixtures may provide a convenient way of increasing dietary fiber content substantially. Since most grains that are used in the manufacture of RTE cereals contain negligible quantities of xylose in their neutral sugar residues, xylose content serves as a convenient indicator of the presence and amount of psyllium ingredient added. As presented in Table 1, the SDF fractions of RTE cereals that contained no psyllium (blank values) yielded very low levels of xylose in the oat and wheat based RTE cereals (0.06 and 0.32%, respectively), whereas xylose was absent (0%) from corn and rice based products. Conversely, xylose content of the pure psyllium seed husk alone produced a mean percent of 27.86 + 4.05. Generally, as more psyllium ingredient was added to the cereal base, psyllium recoveries increased. Recoveries ranged from 76.2% for psyllium ingredient added at the 5% level in the oat-based product to 109.0%

TABLE 1 Psyllium (%) Added to RTE Cereals as Determined By GC Analysis of Xylose

Psyllium added %	(N)	Xylose (%) Mean	Xylose (%) SD	Psyllium (%) Mean	Psyllium (%) SD	RSD	Recovery (%)
RTE Cereal Base							
Oat							
Blank	(4)	0.06	0.06	0	0	—	0
5	(5)	1.06	0.08	3.81	0.27	7.09	76.2
10	(7)	2.25	0.14	8.06	0.49	5.70	80.6
20	(8)	4.82	0.55	17.30	1.97	11.39	86.5
Wheat							
Blank	(4)	0.32	0.12	0	0	—	0
5	(5)	1.27	0.24	4.55	0.86	18.90	91.0
10	(6)	2.33	0.30	8.38	1.08	12.89	83.8
15	(6)	4.28	0.64	15.35	2.30	14.98	102.3
20	(5)	5.80	0.18	20.82	0.65	3.12	104.1
Corn							
Blank	(2)	0	0	0	0	—	0
5	(6)	1.10	0.21	3.93	0.76	19.34	78.6
10	(5)	2.47	0.34	8.86	1.21	13.66	88.6
20	(7)	5.35	0.67	19.00	2.27	11.95	95.0
Rice							
Blank	(2)	0	0	0	0	—	0
5	(3)	1.20	0.30	4.31	1.06	24.59	86.2
10	(2)	3.04	0.22	10.90	0.87	7.98	109.0
20	(2)	4.64	0.67	16.64	2.41	14.48	83.2
Psyllium Ingredient							
100	(6)	27.86	4.05				

for 10% psyllium ingredient added to the rice-based product. As indicated by relative standard deviations (RSDs), variability of psyllium values with respect to amounts added did not seem to increase with increasing concentration of the psyllium ingredient. Values for RSDs ranged as low as 3.12% in the case of the wheat-based cereal containing 20% psyllium ingredient to as high as 24.59% for the rice-based cereal containing 5% added psyllium ingredient. Overall, the RSDs for most cereals varied between 6 and 19% which is consistent with the range of RSDr values obtained by Theander et al. (1) for xylose content of various plant tissues. Psyllium content of oat, wheat, corn, or rice-based RTE cereals may be determined successfully by xylose analysis of the SDF residue from the modified TDF method (994.13)

REFERENCES

1. Theander, O., Aman, P., Westerlund, E., Andersson, R. & Pettersson, D. (1995) JAOAC Int. 78, 1030–1043.
2. Official Methods of Analysis, 16th ed., AOAC International, Arlington, VA, Methods 962.09, 973.18, 985.29, & 991.43.
3. Robinson, C.H, Lawler, M.R., Chenoweth, W.L. (1990) Normal and Therapeutic Nutrition, 17th ed., Macmillan Publishing Co., New York, NY, pp 76–77.
4. Van Soest, P.J. & Wine, R.H. (1967) JAOAC 50, 50–55.
5. Theander, O. & Aman, P. (1979) Swed. J. Agric. Res. 9, 97–106.
6. The Evaluation of the Safety of Using Psyllium Seed Husk As A Food Ingredient, (1993) Federation of American Societies for Experimental Biology. Bethesda, MD, pp 3–15.
7. Pennington, J.A.T. & Church, H.N. (1989) Bowes and Church's Food Values of Portions Commonly Used, 14th ed., J.B. Lippincott Co., Philadelphia, PA.
8. Adams, C.R. (1975) Nutritive Value of American Foods. US Dept. of Agriculture Handbook No. 456.
9. Prosky, L. Asp, N.G., Schweizer, T.F., DeVries, J.W., & Furda, I.D. JAOAC (1988) 71, 1017–1023.
10. Marlatt, J.A. (1992) J. Am. Dietetic Assn. 92, 175–186.
11. Englyst, H.N. & Cummings, J.H. (1990) in CRC Handbook of Dietary Fiber in Human Nutrition, 2nd Ed., G.A. Spiller (Ed.), CRC Press, Boca Raton, FL, pp 53–71.
12. Wolever, T.M., Jenkins, D.J., Mueller, S., Boctor, D.L., Ransom, T.P., Patten. R., Chao, E.S., McMillan, K., Fulgoni, V., 3rd (1994). Method of administration influences the serum cholesterol-lowering effect of psyllium. Am. J. Clin. Nutr. 59 (5), 1055–1059.
13. Wolever, T.M., Jenkins, D.J., Mueller, S., Patten, R., Relle, L.K., Boctor, D., Ransom, T.P., Chao, E.S, McMillan, K., Fulgoni, V., 3rd (1994). Psyllium reduces blood lipids in men and women with hyperlipidemia. Am. J. Med. Sci. Apr 307 (4) 269–273.
14. Wolever, T.M., Vuksan, V., Eshuis, H., Spadafora, P., Peterson, R.D., Chao, E.S.,

Storey, M.L., Jenkins, D.J. (1991) Effect of method of administration of psyllium on glycemic response and carbohydrate digestibility. J. Am. Coll. Nutr. 10 (4) 364–371.

15. Alabaster, O; Tang, ZC; Shivapurkar, N. Dietary Fiber and the Chemopreventive Modulation of Colon Carcinogenesis. Fundamental & Molecular Mechanisms of Mutagenesis. 350:185–197.

24

Food Sources and Uses of Dietary Fiber

Mark Dreher
Nabisco, Inc., East Hanover, New Jersey

INTRODUCTION

Dietary fiber has played an important and healthful role in the history of the human food supply. Hypocrites recognized the laxative benefits of whole wheat flour over that of refined wheat flour. In the 19th century, Graham, of graham cracker fame, denounced the ''unhealthful'' effects of refined carbohydrate, and the Kellogg® and Post® cereals owe their start to increase in wheat bran consumption. The modern era of research into the health benefits of fiber began in the middle of the 20th century with the development of the ''dietary fiber hypothesis'' based on observations in Africa of distinct differences in incidence of certain chronic diseases between blacks who consumed diets rich in dietary fiber in their rural homelands and urbanized blacks and whites with low fiber diets. The people with low fiber diets had significantly more incidence of colorectal cancer, coronary heart disease, diabetes mellitus, obesity, and diverticular disease which are common in Western countries. Since the 1970s dietary fiber has become one of the most widely researched food components for both health and food technology purposes.

Today, there is strong evidence to support the positive health effects of foods rich in cereal, fruit and vegetable fiber and expanding opportunities for fiber claims in labeling. Consumer interest in fiber rich foods has had its ups and downs since the late 1980s when overexposure of oat bran claims and excessive media coverage of a contrary oat bran study confused the consumer. Despite decades of public education programs Americans still consume about half the recommended daily intake of 25–35 grams of fiber. This is in part due to challenges in developing good tasting high fiber products. However, the opportunities for fiber rich foods has growth potential because of:

1. Demographic changes with growing aging populations which can benefit from increased dietary fiber consumption
2. Changing consumer behavior towards more self-treatment to improve health
3. Economic forces focusing more attention on prevention
4. Expanded biomedical understanding and media coverage of the health benefits of dietary fiber
5. Modification of food labeling regulations giving dietary fiber more focus
6. Introduction of new grassroots avenues to communicate the health benefits of dietary fiber by the internet
7. Improved understanding of fiber food functionality which has increased the organoleptic quality of fiber rich foods

The objective of this chapter is to review the food sources and uses of dietary fiber. Dietary fiber comes from a wide variety of foods such as whole grain cereals, legumes, fruits, and vegetables or fiber-rich processed foods that are either much higher in dietary fiber, more available/convenient, or different in form than the natural sources. Organoleptic and processing challenges are frequently encountered when formulating food products high in dietary fiber. This has resulted in considerable resources devoted to better understanding dietary fiber's food functionality characteristics. Food functionality includes organoleptic, microstructural, mechanical/physical, and chemical properties. Usually the addition of high levels of dietary fiber to foods has an adverse effect on food texture and flavor, but when the functionality of fiber is understood or improved the chances of it being successfully incorporated into foods is greatly enhanced. Thus, a better awareness of food sources and uses is a good way to develop strategies that can lead to increased dietary fiber intake.

FOOD SOURCES OF DIETARY FIBER

Dietary fiber comes from a variety of sources such as vegetables, fruits, and cereal grain products. Even foods that contain small amounts of dietary fiber can make an important contribution to an individual's diet if these foods are eaten often or in large amounts.

Soluble and Insoluble Fiber

Total dietary fiber (TDF) is the analytical term for dietary fiber. It includes both insoluble dietary fiber and soluble dietary fiber. Insoluble fiber consists mainly of cell wall components such as cellulose, lignin, and hemicellulose. Soluble fiber consists of noncellulosic polysaccharides such as pectin, gums, and mucilage. About 75 percent of the dietary fiber in foods is in the form of insoluble fiber. Most fiber sources are actually mixtures of both soluble or insoluble fibers.

Insoluble Fiber

The most common form of dietary fiber is insoluble fiber which is composed of cellulose, lignin, and some hemicellulose. It promotes regularity and is being studied for its potential for reduce risk of colon/rectal cancers. Although cereal brans and whole-grain cereals are the most commonly recognized source, other good sources of insoluble fiber are dried beans, peas, vegetables, and nuts.

Soluble Fiber

Soluble fiber comprises about 25% of the dietary fiber consumed but strong evidence shows that soluble fiber as part of a low-fat, low-cholesterol diet may help lower blood cholesterol in those individuals with elevated blood cholesterol levels. It has also been shown to help control blood glucose levels in individuals with diabetes mellitus. Good sources of soluble fiber are whole-grain oats and barley, oat bran, some fruits, dried beans, and other legumes. According to current nutrition labeling regulations dietary fiber–containing food must have at least 2.5 grams fiber per reference serving to make a "good" source claims and at least 5.0 grams of fiber to make an "excellent" source claim.

Specific Food Sources

Fiber can come from a wide range of products including fresh fruits and vegetables, breakfast cereals, breads and rolls, and crackers. Recently, Rimm and coworkers (1996) demonstrated an association between doubling fiber intake from vegetables, fruit, and cereals and reduced risk of heart attacks. Table 1 lists the estimated total, insoluble, and soluble dietary fiber content of a wide variety of foods.

Table 1 Dietary fiber content of foods

Food	Moisture	Dietary fiber (g/100 g edible portion) Total	Insoluble	Soluble
Baked products				
Bagels, plain	31.6	2.1	1.5	0.6
Biscuits, baking powder	16.7	2.1	1.6	0.6
Breads:				
Boston brown	47.2	4.7	—	—
Bran	39.1	5.4	4.6	0.8
Corn	36.1	3.0	2.8	0.2
Cracked wheat	35.9	5.3	4.5	0.8
French	29.2	2.7	1.9	0.8
Italian:				
Plain	26.9	3.8	2.9	0.9
Sesame seeds	34.6	3.4	2.5	0.9
Multi-grain	38.6	5.6	4.6	1.0
Oatmeal	37.8	4.3	3.3	1.0
Pita:				
White	32.1	1.6	0.8	0.8
Whole-wheat	30.6	7.4	6.6	0.8
Pumpernickel	38.3	5.9	4.3	1.6
Reduced-calorie, high-fiber:				
Multi-grain	39.3	13.6	12.7	0.9
White	44.3	12.8	12.3	0.5
Rye (German)	36.8	8.3	6.8	1.5
Sourdough	36.4	3.0	2.0	1.0
White:	37.1	1.9	1.3	0.6
Toasted	—	2.5	—	—
Whole wheat:	39.7	8.1	7.0	1.1
Toasted	—	8.9	—	—
Bread crumbs, plain or seasoned	5.7	4.2	3.0	1.2
Bread sticks	4.6	3.0	1.8	1.2
Bread stuffing, flavored from dry mix	65.1	2.9	2.0	0.9
Cakes (prepared):				
Angel food	35.5	0.8	0.5	0.3
Chocolate	33.3	2.4	1.8	0.6
Coffee cake:				
Crumb topping	22.3	3.3	2.6	0.7
Fruit	31.7	2.5	1.5	1.0
Devil's food	30.4	2.5	1.8	0.7
Fruitcake	22.0	3.7	2.5	1.2
Yellow	26.9	1.4	1.1	0.3
Cheesecake	44.6	2.1	1.5	0.6

TABLE 1 Continued

Food	Moisture	Dietary fiber (g/100 g edible portion) Total	Insoluble	Soluble
Cookies:				
Brownies	12.8	2.5	1.7	0.8
Butter	4.7	2.4	1.6	0.8
Chocolate chip	4.1	2.6	1.9	0.7
Chocolate sandwich	2.2	2.9	2.2	0.7
Fig bar	16.7	4.6	4.0	0.6
Fortune	8.0	1.6	1.2	0.4
Ginger snaps	4.8	1.8	1.2	0.6
Oatmeal	4.9	2.6	1.5	1.1
Peanut butter	6.7	1.8	1.3	0.5
Shortbread	3.3	1.8	0.9	0.9
Sugar	3.3	1.1	0.7	0.4
Vanilla wafers	5.5	1.5	0.7	0.8
Croissants	20.4	2.3	1.4	0.9
Croutons	5.6	4.7	4.0	0.7
Doughnuts:				
Cake	19.7	1.7	1.1	0.6
Yeast, glazed	26.7	1.2	0.7	0.5
Hamburger buns	35.0	2.6	1.7	0.9
Ice cream cones:	3.0	4.6	3.4	1.2
Sugar	3.0	4.6	3.4	1.2
Wafer	5.3	4.1	3.0	1.1
Muffins:				
Blueberry	37.3	3.6	3.1	0.5
Bran-raisin	26.7	6.3	4.9	1.4
English	38.9	3.0	2.4	0.6
Oat bran	35.0	7.5	5.0	2.5
Plain	27.1	1.5	1.0	1.5
Wheat bran	23.3	3.3	2.5	0.8
Pastries:				
Plain	19.3	1.3	0.9	0.4
Fruit	27.6	1.9	1.0	0.9
Pie crust	14.9	2.3	1.8	0.5
Pies:				
Apple	44.9	1.6	1.0	0.6
Cherry	46.2	0.8	0.5	0.3
Pecan	19.8	3.5	3.0	0.5
Pumpkin	58.1	2.7	2.1	0.6

TABLE 1 Continued

Food	Moisture	Dietary fiber (g/100 g edible portion) Total	Insoluble	Soluble
Rolls:				
Brown and serve	23.5	3.0	1.9	1.1
Cinnamon	26.4	2.2	1.6	0.6
Dinner	30.4	3.8	3.0	0.8
French	30.8	3.2	2.2	1.0
Taco shells	4.2	6.3	5.4	0.9
Toaster pastries	8.9	1.0	0.6	0.4
Tortillas:				
Corn	49.0	5.1	4.4	0.7
Wheat	29.3	2.3	1.3	1.0
Waffles, frozen	45.0	2.4	1.6	0.8
Breakfast Cerals				
Bran	2.9	35.3	32.8	2.5
Bran flakes				
Plain	3.2	19.5	17.5	2.0
Raisins	7.6	13.5	15.1	2.4
Cornflakes:				
Plain	2.8	2.0	1.7	0.3
Sugar frosted	1.9	2.2	1.8	0.4
Cream of Wheat®, cooked	87.9	0.7	0.6	0.1
Crispy rice	2.4	1.9	1.4	0.5
Fruit & bran	3.0	14.8	12.0	2.8
Granola	3.3	10.5	—	—
Grapenuts®	3.1	10.4	7.3	3.1
Hominy, cooked	85.0	0.6	0.6	0.0
Muesli	5.0	12.0	—	—
Oat bran, uncooked	7.4	17.0	10.5	6.5
Oatmeal, cooked	84.2	1.9	1.2	0.7
Puffed wheat	6.9	7.5	5.1	2.4
Puffed rice	6.5	1.4	1.0	0.4
Shredded wheat	7.1	12.5	9.9	2.6
Toasted oats	3.5	7.0	4.2	2.8
Wheat flakes	2.4	11.4	9.6	1.8
Cereal Grains				
Amaranth	9.8	15.2	—	—
Amaranth flour, whole grain	10.4	10.2	—	—
Arrowroot flour	11.4	3.4	—	—
Barley	9.4	17.3	—	—
Barley, bran	3.5	70.0	67.0	3.0

TABLE 1 Continued

Food	Moisture	Dietary fiber (g/100 g edible portion)		
		Total	Insoluble	Soluble
Barley, pearled	10.1	15.6	—	—
Bulgur, dry	8.0	18.3	—	—
Corn, bran	6.5	82.4	80.4	2.0
Corn, flour, whole-grain	10.9	13.4	—	—
Cornmeal:				
Whole grain	11.0	11.0	—	—
Degermed	10.3	5.3	—	—
Cornstarch	12.0	0.9	—	—
Millet, hulled	8.2	0.9	—	—
Oat, bran	10.0	22.2	11.7	10.5
Oat, flour	7.8	9.6	—	—
Oats, rolled, or oatmeal, dry	8.8	10.3	6.5	3.8
Rice:				
Wild	8.4	5.2	—	—
Brown, long-grain:				
Raw	11.7	3.9	—	—
Cooked	73.1	1.7	—	—
Long-grain				
Dry	8.7	1.3	1.0	0.3
Cooked	77.5	0.7	0.7	0.0
Short grain	11.0	2.8	—	—
Medium grain	11.7	1.7	—	—
Parboiled rice:				
Dry	10.4	2.2	—	—
Cooked	77.0	0.5	—	—
Rice-a-roni	71.5	2.5	—	—
Rice bran	6.1	21.7	—	—
Rice flour:				
Brown	12.0	4.6	—	—
White	11.9	2.4	—	—
Semolina	12.7	3.7	—	—
Triticale	11.2	18.1	—	—
Whole grain	9.4	14.6	—	—
Wheat, bran	11.6	42.4	40.3	2.1
Wheat flour:				
White, all-purpose	11.2	2.7	1.7	1.0
Whole-grain	11.5	12.6	10.2	1.3
Wheat germ	2.9	14.0	12.9	1.1

Table 1 Continued

Food	Moisture	Dietary fiber (g/100 g edible portion)		
		Total	Insoluble	Soluble
Fruit and Fruit Products				
Apples, Red Delicious:				
Unpeeled	83.6	2.0	1.8	0.2
Peeled	84.6	1.5	1.3	0.2
Granny Smith, unpeeled	83.8	2.7	2.4	0.3
Apple juice, unsweetened	87.9	0.1	0.1	0.0
Applesauce:				
Sweetened	79.6	1.2	1.0	0.2
Unsweetened	88.4	1.5	1.3	0.2
Apricots, dried	31.1	7.8	6.0	1.8
Apricot nectar	84.9	0.6	0.5	0.1
Bananas	75.7	1.7	1.2	0.5
Blueberries:				
Fresh	85.4	2.7	2.4	0.3
Frozen	83.5	3.2	2.5	0.7
Cherries, canned	78.8	1.0	0.4	0.6
Figs, dried	28.4	9.3	—	—
Fruit cocktail	—	1.5	—	—
Grapefruit:				
Fresh	87.8	1.8	0.7	1.1
Juice	90.1	0.5	0.0	0.5
Grapes	80.6	1.2	0.7	0.5
Kiwifruit	83.0	3.4	—	—
Melons	90.1	0.7	0.4	0.3
Nectarine	89.7	1.2	0.8	0.4
Oranges:				
Fresh	86.0	1.8	0.7	1.1
Juice	89.4	0.4	0.1	0.3
Peaches:				
Fresh	87.1	1.9	1.0	0.9
Canned	83.0	1.2	0.7	0.5
Pears:				
Fresh	84.5	3.0	2.0	1.0
Canned	84.1	2.3	1.5	0.8
Pineapple, canned	84.2	0.9	0.7	0.2
Plums:				
Fresh	85.4	1.6	0.7	0.9
Canned	75.8	2.4	1.1	1.3
Prunes, dried	26.2	7.3	3.1	4.2

Table 1 Continued

Food	Moisture	Dietary fiber (g/100 g edible portion) Total	Insoluble	Soluble
Prune jucie	81.2	1.0	—	—
Raisins, seedless	12.6	3.7	2.4	1.3
Strawberries:				
Fresh	90.5	2.2	1.3	0.9
Frozen	75.0	1.6	0.9	0.7
Jam	31.8	0.9	0.7	0.2
Tangerine:				
Fresh	85.1	1.8	1.4	0.4
Canned	84.5	0.4	0.1	0.3
Watermelon	90.1	0.4	0.3	0.1
Legumes and Pulses				
Baked beans, canned:				
BBQ	—	5.8	—	—
Sweet or tomato sauce				
Plain	72.6	7.7	—	—
With franks	69.3	6.9	—	—
Black-eyed peas, canned	65.0	3.9	3.5	0.4
Lentils:				
Dried, raw	9.9	11.4	10.3	1.1
Dried, cooked	66.5	5.3	4.7	0.6
Garbanzo beans, canned	65.6	3.5	3.1	0.4
Lima beans, canned	74.5	4.2	3.8	0.4
Kidney, beans, canned	70.4	6.3	4.7	1.6
Peas, black-eyed, canned	78.6	3.1	2.7	0.4
Pinto beans:				
Dried, raw	8.2	19.5	12.1	7.4
Dried, cooked	71.2	7.0	5.8	2.2
Canned	73.3	5.2	4.0	1.2
Soybeans:				
Dry	8.0	15.0	—	—
Tofu	84.6	1.2	—	—
Nuts and seeds				
Almonds, roasted	3.3	11.2	—	—
Cashews, oil-roasted	5.4	6.0	—	—
Coconut:				
Raw	47.0	9.0	8.5	0.5
Shredded	18.5	6.6	6.2	0.4
Hazelnuts oil-roasted	1.2	6.4	—	—

Table 1 Continued

Food	Moisture	Dietary fiber (g/100 g edible portion)		
		Total	Insoluble	Soluble
Peanuts:				
Dry-roasted	1.6	8.0	7.5	0.5
Oil-roasted	2.0	8.8	8.0	0.8
Peanut butter:				
Chunky	1.1	6.6	6.0	0.6
Smooth	1.4	6.0	5.5	0.5
Pecans	4.8	6.5	—	—
Pistachio nuts	3.9	10.8	—	—
Sesame seeds:				
Dry	24.6	15.4	—	—
Roasted	5.8	11.6	—	—
Walnuts	3.5	3.8	3.7	0.1
Miscellaneous				
Avocado	77.3	3.9	2.6	1.3
Beer	92.3	0.5	—	—
Candy (caramels, vanilla)	7.6	1.2	—	—
Milk chocolate	0.8	2.8	—	—
Carob powder	1.2	32.8	—	—
Chile powder	9.1	34.2	—	—
Chocolate, baking	0.7	15.4	—	—
Cocoa, baking	1.3	29.8	—	—
Curry powder	8.7	33.2	—	—
Jelly, apple	32.3	0.6	—	—
Pancake mix	8.3	4.5	3.5	1.0
Pepper, black	9.4	25.0	—	—
Pickles	93.4	1.1	0.7	0.4
Preserves:				
Peach	32.4	0.7	—	—
Strawberry	31.7	1.2	—	—
Yeast, active, dry	6.8	31.6	—	—
Pasta				
Macaroni:				
Dry	8.5	4.3	4.1	0.2
Cooked	69.6	2.0	1.7	0.3
Noodles:				
Dry				
Spinach	8.5	6.8	—	—
Chow-mein	0.7	3.9	—	—
Egg	9.5	4.0	—	—

Table 1 Continued

Food	Moisture	Dietary fiber (g/100 g edible portion)		
		Total	Insoluble	Soluble
Cooked	67.3	1.8	1.3	0.5
Spaghetti:				
Dry:				
Regular	9.2	3.6	2.1	1.5
Whole-wheat	7.1	11.8	—	—
Spinach	8.7	10.6	—	—
Cooked	60.7	1.5	1.1	0.4
Corn chips	1.1	4.3	3.9	0.4
Corn puffs	1.5	1.0	—	—
Granola bars, crunchy:				
Chocolate chip	—	4.4	—	—
Cinnamon	—	5.0	—	—
Popcorn:				
Air-popped	—	15.1	—	—
Oil-popped	—	10.0	—	—
Potato chips	2.4	3.8	1.9	1.9
Pretzels:				
Hard	3.5	3.7	2.8	0.9
Soft	32.7	2.5	1.6	0.9
Tortilla chips	2.0	6.5	—	—
Vegetables and Vegetables Products				
Artichoke	84.4	7.6	4.4	3.2
Artichoke, globe	82.5	7.9	4.7	3.2
Asparagus:				
Fresh, cooked	90.5	2.1	1.6	0.5
Canned	93.3	1.6	1.2	0.4
Beans, green:				
Canned		2.1	1.4	0.7
Boiled		2.5	1.5	1.0
Bamboo shoots, canned	97.4	1.5	1.4	0.1
Beans sprouts	96.2	1.2	1.1	0.1
Beets, canned	92.4	1.7	1.3	0.4
Broccoli:				
Raw	88.5	3.3	3.0	0.3
Cooked	90.2	3.5	3.1	0.4
Brussels sprouts	87.2	4.1	3.6	0.6
Cabbage:				
Raw	90.9	1.8	1.1	0.7
Boiled	94.0	1.7	1.1	0.6

TABLE 1 Continued

Food	Moisture	Dietary fiber (g/100 g edible portion)		
		Total	Insoluble	Soluble
Carrots:				
Raw	88.5	2.4	1.1	1.3
Cooked	90.5	2.7	1.2	1.5
Cauliflower:				
Raw	92.6	1.8	1.1	0.7
Cooked	93.3	1.8	1.1	0.7
Celery:				
Raw	94.6	1.5	1.0	0.5
Cooked	95.2	1.4	0.9	0.5
Chives	92.0	3.2	—	—
Corn, sweet:				
Canned:				
Whole	76.7	2.1	1.8	0.3
Cream style	75.6	1.3	1.1	0.2
Fresh:				
Raw	76.0	3.2	3.0	0.2
Cooked	69.6	3.7	3.5	0.2
Frozen, whole	75.8	2.1	2.0	0.1
Cucumbers:				
Peeled	96.2	0.6	0.5	0.1
Unpeeled	95.8	0.9	0.8	0.1
Eggplant	—	6.6	5.3	1.3
Leek	90.3	2.9	2.0	0.9
Lettuce:				
Iceberg	96.0	0.7	0.5	0.2
Romaine	94.9	1.7	—	—
Mushrooms, canned	90.9	2.8	2.6	0.2
Onions, raw:				
Green	92.7	2.2	2.2	0.0
Yellow	90.3	1.7	1.6	0.1
Parsley	88.3	4.4	—	—
Peas, green:				
Canned	80.7	4.5	3.6	0.9
Boiled	76.9	6.7	5.0	1.7
Frozen, boiled	81.6	4.4	3.2	1.2
Peppers, green, raw	93.5	1.9	1.2	0.7
Potatoes:				
Baked, skin	73.3	2.5	1.9	0.6
Boiled, without skin	79.5	1.3	1.0	0.3

TABLE 1 Continued

Food	Moisture	Dietary fiber (g/100 g edible portion) Total	Insoluble	Soluble
French fried	48.6	3.0	1.5	1.5
Pumpkin, canned	90.2	2.9	2.4	0.5
Radish, red	94.2	1.4	1.3	0.1
Rutabagas:				
Raw	89.0	2.4	1.2	1.2
Boiled	92.3	2.1	1.2	0.9
Spinach:				
Raw	91.6	2.6	2.1	0.5
Cooked	93.7	2.2	1.8	0.4
Squash:				
Summer:				
Raw	93.7	1.2	—	—
Cooked	93.7	1.4	—	—
Winter:				
Raw	88.7	1.8	—	—
Cooked	89.0	2.8	—	—
Zucchini, raw	94.5	0.9	0.8	0.1
Sweet potatoes:				
Cooked	72.8	3.0	2.5	0.5
Canned	75.6	1.7	1.3	0.4
Tomatoes:				
Raw	94.5	1.2	0.8	0.4
Boiled	93.2	1.5	1.0	0.5
Canned	93.3	1.0	0.7	0.3
Sauce	90.9	1.4	0.8	0.7
Paste	74.1	4.3	—	—
Catsup	66.7	1.2	0.9	0.3
Juice	94.1	0.7	0.4	0.3
Turnip greens:				
Frozen	92.9	2.5	2.4	0.1
Cooked	93.2	3.1	2.9	0.2
Turnips	94.7	2.0	1.5	0.5
Water chestnuts	87.9	2.2	—	—

The dietary fiber contents are based on published values form the following references: American Association of Cereal Chemists, 1987; Dreher, 1987; Anderson and Bridges, 1988; Cardozo and Ettenmiller, 1988; Del Toma et al., 1988; Mongeau et al., 1989; Department of Agriculture, 1989; Toma and curtis, 1989; Ranhotra et al., 1990; Prosky and DeVries, 1992; U.S. Marlett, 1992.

Table 2 Parameters related to food functionality[a]

Parameter	Examples
Sensory	Cohesiveness Hardness Brittleness Gumminess
Mechanical/Physical	Density Expansion Shear Viscosity
Microstructural	Cellularity Crystallinity Porosity Uniformity
Functional	Water binding Emulsification Spreadability Whippability

[a] Adapted from Stanley (1986).

DIETARY FIBER SOURCES AND PROPERTIES

Composition of Dietary Fiber

The factors affecting fiber functionality are complex (Table 2). Dietary fiber is a heterogeneous mixture of materials that are the structural and some of the nonstructural components of all plants. These components are resistant to digestion by enzymes produced by humans. The components of dietary fiber include: cellulose, hemicellulose, lignins, pectins, and a variety of gums and mucilages. All except lignins are polysaccharides. The composition of dietary fiber components varies with the type and maturity of plant tissue. Effects of isolated dietary fibers are likely to be different than their effects in native foods. The heterogeneity of dietary fiber is the primary reason for the diversity of its functional properties in food systems. They include composition (e.g., hexoses, pentoses, and uronic acid), cell wall matrix characteristics, functional groups, surface area, cellulose crystallinity, surface characteristics, ionic linkages, noncovalent bonds, and structure (e.g., glycosidic linkages and degree of branching). Food uses of dietary fiber range from bulking agents to fat substitutes (Table 3).

Industry Availability

A wide variety of dietary fiber sources are available to the food industry. Since the early 1980s, the number and availability of dietary fiber sources has increased

TABLE 3 Gerneral food uses for dietary fiber

Dietary Fiber Supplements
Labeling
Calorie Control
Health Benefits
Bulking Agent
Fat Replacer
Reduced Oil Uptake during Frying
Hydrocolloid Properties
Anticaking/Antisticking
Adhesiveness

dramatically. Almost every conceivable fiber source has been considered as a potential ingredient for fiber-enriched foods. These fiber sources range from purified cellulose to sugar beet fiber, cereal brans to sunflower hulls, and guar gum to konjac flour. Not all of these sources of dietary fiber, however, have made it to the marketplace as mainstream commercial ingredients; there has been a gradual shifting out of these materials based on functionality, economics, or other reasons (Vetter, 1988).

Variations in Source Composition

Dietary fiber sources can vary widely in their composition and physicochemical properties. The TDF content is highly variable; for example, oat bran and powdered cellulose have 16 and 99 percent, respectively. The gums are completely dispersible in water, whereas powdered cellulose is completely insoluble in water and oat bran fiber is only about 50 percent water-soluble. The calorie content of dietary fiber sources reflects the TDF level; powdered cellulose is non-caloric whereas wheat bran is about 2 kilocalories per gram. Fiber comes in a wide variety of colors such as white from cellulose, cream from soy fiber and corn bran, tan/brown from apple fiber and wheat bran and off-white from guar gum. The flavor of fiber can range from bland to fruity, nutty, malty, or mild. The bulk density of fiber can range from about 12 lbs./cu. ft. to over 45 lbs./cu. ft. Additionally, particle size and water binding capacity (WBC) vary widely within sources. Fiber functionality is greatly effected by its composition and physicochemical properties.

Component Classification

Dietary fiber components are classified as either soluble or insoluble. The most common class of soluble fibers is gums (hydrocolloids). Gums have the basic properties of thickening or adding viscosity and gelling foods. They are used extensively in foods at low levels (less than 2 percent) to suspend particles, emulsify fat, inhibit ice crystallization, inhibit syneresis, form films, and mimic the properties of fat; their usage at high levels (greater than 10 percent) tends to be limited with only a few exceptions. Insoluble fibers consist of fiber sources that are rich in cell wall content such as most cereal brans (e.g., wheat and corn bran), oilseed hulls (e.g., sunflower seed and soybean hulls), and purified cellulose. Their usage in food systems is often improved by pretreatments which improve functionality. Insoluble fibers are most often used to control calories, add bulk, or provide a health benefit. Other fiber sources are a mixture of both soluble and insoluble fibers such as oat bran, legumes, and fruit fibers. The functionality of these fibers is a function of the type and level of soluble and insoluble fiber.

HYDROCOLLOIDS AS FUNCTIONAL SOLUBLE DIETARY FIBER

Basic Properties

A major class of soluble fiber ingredients are the hydrocolloids, frequently referred to as gums (Dziezak, 1991). These compounds are long-chain polymers that dissolve or disperse in water to give a thickening, gel, or viscosity. Hydrocolloids are also used for secondary effects that include stabilization of emulsions, suspensions of particulate, control of crystallization, inhibition of syneresis, encapsulation, and the formation of a film. They are classified as either food additives or ''generally recognized as safe'' (GRAS) substances by the U.S. Food and Drug Administration. Regulations of specific hydrocolloids are outlined in Title 21 of the Code of Federal Regulations in Parts 172.580-172.874 and Parts 182.1480–184.1724, respectively. Hydrocolloids are generally used at levels of less than 2 percent to achieve desired properties in food systems. They are typically used to enhance food properties rather than provide the health benefits associated with dietary fiber. Nonetheless, even at this low usage level hydrocolloids have become a large and growing business with an estimated market for nonstarch hydrocolloids approaching $1 billion.

Although using gums can sometimes be difficult, understanding several critical factors will help in their selection (Dziezak, 1991). For example, while some gums go readily into solution, others require extra care to prevent clumping such as by mixing the gum with sugar, then gradually pouring the blend into a vigorously stirred solution. In addition, there are other criteria to consider when choosing a gum that will help safeguard against making a wrong choice. Such criteria include: (a) effects of temperature, pH, and mechanical stress on solubility and dispersability, rheological characteristics, and emulsification and product stability, (b) synergism with other gums, (c) effect of the color, odor, and taste of the finished product; (d) microbiological stability, (e) regulatory status for the targeted application, and (f) cost effectiveness.

Commercial Products

Hydrocolloids usually come from: (1) plant materials such as seaweed, seeds, roots, and tree exudates, (2) microbial biosynthesis, and (3) chemical modification of natural polysaccharides. The following is a review of the important attributes of commonly used gums (Tye, 1991; Dziezak, 1991).

SEAWEED EXTRACTS

Alginates

Alginates are extracted from the class of brown seaweed known as Phaeophyceae. The principal seaweed for commercial production include *Macrocystis pyrifera, Laminaria hyperborea, Laminaria digitata*, and *Ascophyllum nodosum* which are found primarily in California, the United Kingdom, Japan, Norway, Canada, France, and Spain. They include a variety of products made up of D-mannuronic (M) acid and L-guluronic (G) acid which are arranged in regions composed solely of one unit or the other, referred to as M-blocks and G-blocks, and regions where the two units alternate. Both the ratio of mannuronic acid to guluronic acid and the structure of the polymer determine the solution properties of the alginate.

Alginates are best known for their ability to form irreversible gels in cold water when calcium ions are present. This property of gelling in cold systems distinguishes alginates from the hydrocolloids that are derived from red algae. It is possible to control both the firmness of the gel obtained and the amount of time required for gelation to occur by varying the alginate and ion system.

Alginates are used in food products for thickening, emulsion stabilization, gelation, and syneresis inhibition. For example, propylene glycol alginates incorporated into salad dressings function as emulsification and suspension of solids. Sodium alginate has been used in a cold-processed lemon pie filling to provide freeze-thaw stability. Other applications that utilize the heat stability of alginate gels include reformed red pepper strips which are stuffed into olives, structured fruit pieces that do not break down during baking, frozen jelly doughnuts, meringues, structured jelly in cake rolls, and fabricated onion rings. Some brands of fish are coated with alginates to prevent freezer burn.

Carrageenan

Carrageenans are extracted from red seaweeds (Huffman and Shah, 1995). The best known and most widely used source of carrageenan is *Chondrus crispus*, also known as Irish moss, which is typically found along the North Atlantic coasts. Carrageenans are sulfated polymers that consist of galactose and anhydrogalactose units. Three main fractions, which differ primarily in the content and distribution of sulfated ester groups, have been identified as iota-, kappa-, and lambda-carrageenan. The structure and molecular weight of the fractions determines their functional properties. Iota- and kappa-carrageenans act as gelling agents; lambda-carrageenan is non-gelling, but acts as a thickener. Iota-carrageenan gels most strongly with calcium ions to form a clear, elastic, syneresis-free gel that resets after shear. A stronger gelling agent, kappa-carrageenan forms gels in the presence of potassium ions producing a strong, rigid gel that tends toward syneresis. Both gels are thermoreversible.

Carrageenan has been used in foods because of its gelling, thickening, stabilizing, emulsifying, and suspending properties. Unique protein reactivity properties are exhibited by carrageenans useful at low levels in a number of milk-based products such as chocolate milk, ice cream, puddings, and cheese analogs. In bakery products such as pie fillings and cake icings, carrageenan has been used to replace the more expensive agar. Its reactivity with protein is useful in ham-pumping operations where kappa-carrageenan helps retain water-soluble proteins within the ham during cooking. Lambda-carrageenan can be incorporated into low-fat or fat-free salad dressings for good suspension of seasonings while providing the sensory properties of an oil-based dressing. Low sugar jams, jellies, and confections also benefit from the gelling properties of carrageenan.

SEED EXTRACTS

Locust Bean Gum

Locust bean gum is found in the endosperm of seeds from the evergreen tree, *Ceratonia siliqua*, which is native to Mediterranean countries. It has also been called carob seed gum. This hydrocolloid is a neutral polysaccharide made up of mannose and galactose in a ratio of 4:1. Locust bean gum is insoluble in cold water and must be heated to be dissolved. Maximal viscosity is obtained when the gum is heated to about 95°C, then cooled. Alone, locust bean gum will not form a gel, but it will gel when combined with xanthan gum. It interacts with kappa-carrageenan to increase gel strength, modify texture, and reduce syneresis. Further, since locust bean gum is non-ionic, it is stable over the pH range of 3.5 to 11.0.

The primary functions of locust bean gum are thickening, stabilization of emulsions, and inhibition of syneresis. This hydrocolloid is used in a number of products: canned foods, sauces, desserts, beverages, cheeses, ice cream, and processed meats. In cheese, it acts to speed up coagulation, increasing the yield of curd solids. In ice cream, locust bean gum stabilizes and binds water, which helps the ice cream withstand heat shock and melt smoothly. In meat products such as bologna and sausage, it helps to facilitate extrusion and stuffing.

Guar Gum

Guar gum is obtained from the ground endosperm of the guar plant, *Cyamopsis tetragonolobus*, an annual that is native to the arid climates of India and Pakistan. Guar has also been cultivated in Texas and Arkansas. Forming the backbone of the gum is a linear chain of mannose units with single galactose units attached as side chains in the ration of one galactose unit per every two mannose units. Since guar gum is more highly substituted than locust bean gum, it is more soluble and hydrates fully in cold water, producing high viscosity. The viscosity of guar depends on the temperature, pH, time, concentrations, degree of agitation, and particle size of the gum. Since guar gum is nonionic, it is stable from pH 4 to 10. It interacts synergistically with xanthan gum to increase solution viscosity. When mixed with either agar or kappa-carrageenan, it can increase gel strength and improve gel structure. Guar gum tends to be slightly slimy in the mouth, and is often used at low concentrations to add creaminess to foods.

Guar gum is nongelling, and it functions primarily as a viscosity builder, stabilizer, and water binder. Examples of product applications include canned foods, desserts, ice cream, soups, sauces, dressings, bakery products, and dry mixes.

ROOT FLOUR

Konjac powder from the konjac root has been traditionally used in the Far East as a food component (Tye, 1991). For over a thousand years, the Japanese have been making gels and noodles that are stable in boiling water with konjac powder. Because of its gel-forming properties and strong functional synergism with kappa-carrageenan and starches, konjac powder has been used to maintain the shape and integrity of formed foods during cooking.

Konjac powder is the dried and pulverized tuber of the perennial herb *Amorphophallus konjac* (Tye, 1991). The flour consists of fine oval whitish sacs, 100 to 500 microns in size, which swell in contact with water and rupture to release high molecular weight water-soluble aggregated glucomannans. Its molecular weight is greater than 300,000 daltons. Acetyl groups are scattered randomly along the linear glucomannan and they help promote water solubility. Konjac powder has many properties that can be useful in food formulations. Its water thickening properties are unique; when mixed with water its viscosity is a function of sac swelling which is dependent on temperature and time. Konjac sols are pseudoplastic (thin with shear and recover viscosity when the shearing stops). Konjac gels formed in the presence of mild alkali (potassium carbonate) are thermally stable. Konjac has synergism with both kappa-carrageenan and xanthan gum. Kappa-carrageenan and konjac powder solutions form an elastic, thermally reversible gel after heating and cooling. Xanthan gum and konjac flour interact to form a gel with unique viscoelastic properties. Dehydrated konjac powder dispersions can form a cohesive, tough film. Konjac powder functionally interacts with most starches to give significant increases in viscosity and gel strength.

PLANT EXUDATES

Gum Arabic

Gum arabic is the sap that is exuded from various species of acacia trees when wounded to prevent desiccation and insect infestation of the tissue beneath. Arabic is considered the oldest gum because its use can be tracked back to 2650 BC. Chemically, gum arabic is a neutral or slightly acidic salt of a complex polysaccharide containing calcium, magnesium, and potassium ions. The gum consists of six carbohydrate moieties: galactose, rhamnose, arabinopyranose, arabinofuranose, glucuronic acid, and 4-o-methylglucuronic acid. Also present in the gum is a small amount of protein. Gum arabic dissolves readily in both hot or cold water. It is the least viscous and most soluble of the hydrocolloids with possible solutions approaching a 55 percent concentration possible compared with other common hydrocolloids which are limited to levels of less than 5 percent because of their high viscosities.

Gum arabic is primarily used in the confection and soft drink industry. More than one-half of the gum arabic is used in confections where it acts to retard sugar crystallization and to promote emulsification. About one-third is incorporated in soft drinks because of its emulsifier and stabilizer properties. The remainder of the gum arabic is utilized in a variety of applications such as in the flavor industry as a fixative in spray drying applications where the gum encapsulates the flavor compound and in the beer industry where the gum promotes stabilization of foam.

Gum Karaya

Gum karaya is the dried exudate of the sterculia tree that grows in central and northern India. It consists of a main chain comprised of D-galacturonic acid, L-rhamnose, and D-galactose units with some side chains containing D-glucuronic acid. Karaya has low solubility in water and strong adhesive properties at high concentrations. It does not dissolve in water, but absorbs water and swells, producing a viscous colloidal sol. Dispersions have a greater viscosity when prepared with cold water. Boiling the dispersion increases the solubility of the gum, but it also permanently reduces its viscosity. Correspondingly, viscosity is reduced by addition of certain strong electrolytes or extremes in pH.

Gum karaya has been used in a variety of food applications. In French dressing, it functions as a stabilizer. Because of its water-binding properties, karaya has been used at low levels in ice pops and sherbets to prevent the formation of ice crystals and loss of free water. In ground meat products, such as bologna, karaya binds water and provides adhesiveness, while producing a smooth appearance.

Gum Tragacanth

Gum tragacanth is the exudate produced by certain species of the astragalus bush, a leguminous perennial that is native to Asia Minor and to the semi-desert and mountainous regions of Iran. Tragacanth is composed of a mixture of polysaccharides: tragacanthic acid, a water-insoluble component, which confers water-swelling properties to the gum; and arabinogalactan, a water-soluble polymer that gives the gum solubility. It has very high viscosity and produces viscous colloidal sols which have a texture similar to that of a soft gel. At a 1 percent concentration it can produce a viscosity of 3,600 cps. Tragacanth is cold water soluble. It is stable to heat and acid. Also, it is a good emulsifier. Despite its many functional attributes, tragacanth has not been used to its potential in the United States because of the political problems encountered with Iran, its chief exporter.

Gum tragacanth has diverse functionality in foods. It has been used in salad dressings and sauces because it imparts a creamy texture. Milk shakes made with tragacanth can contain lower levels of fat without sacrificing viscosity. In bakery fruit-based toppings and fillings, it gives the fruit a shiny, natural appearance while providing stabilization of suspended fruit pieces.

MICROBIAL GUMS

Xanthan Gum

Xanthan gum was the first gum manufactured by microbial fermentation; it is produced by culturing on a carbohydrate medium the organism *Xanthomonas campestral*. Xanthan is a high-molecular-weight polysaccharide with a cellulosic backbone that has trisaccharide branches attached to every other glucose unit in the main chain. Although xanthan is non-gelling, it can form elastic, thermoreversible gels when combined with locust bean gum. It is completely soluble in cold or hot water, and produces high viscosities at low concentrations. Xanthan gum in unaffected by enzymes and it has excellent stability to heat and pH. The viscosities of xanthan gum solutions remain unchanged across the temperature range of 0° to 100°C and over the pH range of 1 to 13. Xanthan gum solutions are pseudoplastic which helps to impart good flavor release, mouthfeel, and visual aesthetics of a food product; it also is important to the pourability of emulsions.

Xanthan is used in many food products for its thickening, suspending, and stabilizing attributes. It provides freeze-thaw stability in frozen doughs. Xanthan functions as a stabilizer in egg white substitutes made up of whey protein and gelatin. The gum is used as a stabilizer in ice cream, and it adds body to and prevents sticking in fruit gels. Tomato sauces for pizza are made with xanthan gum to attain high viscosity that keeps the sauce on the surface and inhibits absorption by the dough.

Gellan Gum

Culturing *Pseudomonas elodea* on a carbohydrate medium produces gellan gum. Its linear backbone is comprised of four saccharide units: 1,3-beta-D-glucose, 1,4-beta-D-glucuronic acid, 1,4-beta-D-glucose, and 1,4-alpha-D-rhamnose. Gellan gum is functional at very low levels with excellent gel formation at concentrations as low as 0.05 percent. Gellan needs to be heated to dissolve and requires actions to bring about gelation as the solution cools. By controlling the concentration of cations, the gel obtained can be designed to be thermoreversible or stable to retort temperatures from 65° to 120°C. Gellan gums are also stable in acid and to heat. It is approved for food use as a stabilizer and thickener in frostings, icings, glazes, non-standardized jams and jellies, and other applications.

MODIFIED CELLULOSE AND PECTIN

Cellulose Gums

Cellulose gums, which are produced by chemically modifying cellulose so that it becomes water soluble, are among the most widely used hydrocolloids. Each cellobiose unit that makes up the backbone of cellulose consists of two anhydroglucanose units, which in turn have three hydroxyl groups each. Alkaline treatment carried out under controlled conditions transforms cellulose into an ether by substituting the hydrogen on some of the hydroxyl groups with a carboxy group. The length of the cellulose ethers coupled with the nature and the number of the ether groups influence the solubility, gelling, and thickening properties of the derivative. Chemically modified celluloses include carboxymethylcellulose, methylcellulose, and hydroxypropylmethylcellulose.

Sodium carboxymethylcellulose, which is commonly called cellulose gum, is available in a variety of types based on particle size, degree of substitution, viscosity, and hydration abilities. Solutions of these gums are pseudoplastic. Their viscosities decrease with an increase in temperature and they are stable over the pH range of 4 to 10. Cellulose gum is used to thicken, suspend, stabilize, gel, and modify flow characteristics of aqueous solutions or suspensions. It is used in a wide range of food products as a bulking agent in low-calorie foods, as a water binder in starch-based pie fillings, and in association with soybean protein and caseinate it acts as a stabilizer to prevent precipitation at their isoelectric points.

Methylcellulose and hydroxypropylmethylcellulose come in a range of viscosities. They are the only gums that gel when heated and return to their original liquid state when cooled. This attribute makes these gums well suited for use in fried foods in which they improve the adhesion of batter and create a barrier to oil absorption. It is important that these gums be solubilized at cool temperatures in order to thermally gel. In bakery products, these gums improve batter consistency via emulsification and strengthen cell walls of gas bubbles formed during baking. They can also improve the viscosity of creamed soups and sauces and pie and pastry fillings.

Pectin

Pectins are commercially extracted from citrus peels or apple pomace. Pectin functions as a gelling agent, thickener, and suspending agent in a number of products. It consists of repeated D-galacturonic acid units which have side chains made up of L-arabinose and D-galactose. Methyl groups esterified to a portion of the carboxyl group on the main chain determine the gelling time, setting conditions, and gel strength of the pectin. The degree of methylation (DM) is the criterion which classifies pectins into low-methoxyl (LM) or high-methoxyl (HM) types, depending on whether the DM is less than or greater than 50 percent.

The selection of the pectin type depends on the requirements of the particular application. LM pectin requires only a controlled amount of calcium ions to form gels. Gelation can take place across the pH range of 2.9 to 5.5 and soluble solids content from 10 to 80 percent. The resulting gels are thermoreversible and are softer and more elastic than those from HM pectins. Alternatively, HM pectins are dependent upon acidic conditions (pH 2.0 to 3.5) and a soluble solid level of 55 percent or greater for gelation. Commercially, HM pectins are further classified as slow-, medium-, or rapid-set, referring to the relative speed of gelation. Rapid-set pectins have a DM of around 75 percent while slow-set pectins have a DM of about 60 percent. Generally, slow-set pectins are used in confections, and rapid-set pectins in specialized applications such as in ensuring a uniform distribution of fruit particles in jams.

Pectins are used in a variety of food applications. Pectins are frequently used in jams, preserves, confections, barbecue sauces, processed tomato products, carbonated beverages, and fruit toppings. Small amounts of LM pectin improve the texture of yogurt. HM pectins are used in fruit drink concentrates and powder to stabilize oil emulsions, suspend fruit particles, and to provide a natural mouthfeel.

SELECTED HYDROCOLLOID APPLICATIONS

Dietary Fiber Supplements in Beverages

Hydrocolloids with relatively low viscosities such as gum arabic and low viscosity grades of methylcellulose have application as dietary fiber supplements in beverages and soups. In contrast, moderate to high viscosity gums, which in cludes most gums, will thicken or gel and insoluble fibers such as brans will settle out or, if suspended, add an undesirable grittiness. Low viscosity hydrocolloids can become fully integrated into beverage or soup formulations in significant levels with only a small increase in viscosity. Gum arabic is especially suited for use as a direct fiber additive to liquid foods. Even at a 10 percent level, gum arabic does not increase viscosity above 20 cps. Beverages containing up to 3 grams gum arabic per 8 fluid ounce serving were equivalent to control beverages in taste and texture (Andon, 1987).

Reduced-Fat Foods

Today's consumers are more aware of the nutritional value of the foods they eat. Although Americans have a growing preference for less fat in their food, they do not want to compromise organoleptic properties such as mouthfeel or taste. Hydrocolloids are ideally suited for the production of fine emulsions and fat-like systems. Moderate levels of hydrocolloids sequester larger amounts of water while maintaining fat-like texture in some fat-containing foods such as salad dressings, ground meat, processed cheese, and frozen desserts. For example, the use of gums to reduce the fat content in processed cheese spreads has been extensively studied (Brummel and Lee, 1990). Aqueous dispersions of gums have been shown to replace up to 50 percent of the fat, relative to the control cheese spread containing 25 percent fat, by increasing the moisture proportionally. Additionally, the addition of hydrocolloids to the formulation of fried snacks may help repel oil uptake during frying.

BAKERY PRODUCT APPLICATIONS

Structure Enhancer in Bread Products

Methylcellulose has an ability to improve the structure of bakery products which makes it a gluten replacer or enhancer (Bell, 1990). Methylcellulose results in improved dough strength and loaf volume, softness, and exterior and interior appearance scores of whole wheat bread and roll formulations. It gives bread formulations several unique properties including enhanced interfacial activity within the dough system and increased dough viscosity during baking. During dough proofing, the improved interfacial activity provides stability to the gas cells during expansion during fermentation. This translates into dough better able to sustain mechanical abuses caused by conveyors and more able to resist other stresses, like changing temperatures and humidity, caused by the dynamic environmental conditions of automated baking processing lines. During baking, as the temperature of the dough rises in the oven, a point is reached where the polymer molecules no longer bond directly to water and instead interact with one another to form a temporary network (thermal gelation). This network serves to increase viscosity and strengthens the boundaries of the expanding cells in the dough, reducing gas loss, and protecting the dough from losing volume. This thermal gel reverts to its previous form upon cooling after baking. The optimal results in whole wheat bread are obtained with at least 2 percent methylcellulose (based on flour weight).

Bread Staling

Wheat bread supplemented with soluble pentosans has a reduced rate of staling. Bread slices containing 1.5 to 3.0 percent soluble pentosans isolated from rye and stored for 6 days at 20°C have less staling than controls as measured by compression analysis. Bread staling is correlated with increasing force necessary to reach crumb depression; breads supplemented with 1.5 to 3.0 percent soluble pentosans have reduced crumb depression. The soluble pentosans appear to reduce the rate of starch retrogradation (staling). Breads with soluble pentosans maintain their freshness and good sensory properties much better than breads without these pentosans.

COMMON DIETARY FIBER COMPONENTS AND SOURCES

Numerous sources of dietary fibers are commercially available as supplements for use in foods such as bakery goods. Unfortunately, many of these sources result in gritty textures and degradation in functional properties when they are added to foods. One of the reasons for these functional problems is that these fiber sources tend to hydrate more completely on the particle surface than the particle interior, reducing the extent to which the particle can soften and swell in food systems such as dough and cake mixes. However, many of these functional problems can be overcome by modifying the source with chemical or physical treatments, selecting the appropriate source for a specific application, using the isolated fiber components, or blending different sources. Care must be taken to balance product functionality with potential health benefit. For example, oat hulls can be added to foods at high levels to add bulk and reduce calories but oat hulls contain no soluble beta-glucan that is needed to reduce the risk of coronary heart disease.

Cellulose

Powdered Cellulose

Cellulose is the most abundant source of complex carbohydrate in the world. Powdered cellulose is a beta-1,4-glucan (not to be confused with alpha-1,4-glucan, which is common starch) (Ang and Miller, 1991). Where starch is digestible in the human digestive tract, powdered cellulose, which is over 99 percent total dietary fiber, is considered to be non-caloric. Powdered cellulose is ''generally recognized as safe'' (GRAS) by the FDA. Since cellulose is a fiber, its physical dimensions are commonly expressed as fiber lengths. Although it has an approximate diameter of 17 microns its length is dependent upon the manufacturing process. Commercial forms of powdered cellulose for food applications are readily available in a variety of fiber lengths, ranging from about 22 to 290 microns. The bulk volumes for this ingredient vary from about 2 to 6 cm^3/gram.

Powdered cellulose is widely used as a non-caloric bulking agent in reduced calorie foods (Ang and Miller, 1991). Since water and oil also play important roles in these products, the physicochemical properties of powdered cellulose and their relationship to these components have been extensively studied. The water binding capacity (WBC) of powdered cellulose is directly related to its average fiber length: WBC increases as the fiber length increases. Depending on fiber length powdered cellulose can retain about 3.5 to 10 times its weight in water. The WBC of cellulose with fiber lengths greater than 100 microns does not vary as much as those with fiber lengths between 35 and 100 microns. Below 35 microns WBC is found to be less dependent on fiber length. The WBC of powdered cellulose is similar to that of wheat bran. For most practical purposes pH and temperature do not significantly alter the WBC of powdered cellulose. A similar pattern is obtained when vegetable oil is substituted for water. However, the retention capacities for the oil are generally slightly lower than that of water. Powdered cellulose with fiber lengths between 22 to 290 microns retained 2.5 to 85 times its weight of vegetable oil. With the exception of cellulose fibers greater in length than 110 microns, powdered cellulose does not possess thickening properties when suspended in water. It is generally observed that upon sitting without agitation, powdered cellulose fibers settle out of suspension. It is also observed that the use of other stabilizers is needed to hold these fibers in suspension for any length of time. The average cellulose fiber length has a significant impact on food application. Cellulose fibers with relatively short lengths of about 50 microns or less have good functionality as bulking agents or dietary fiber supplements. The smallest cellulose fibers with a length of 22 microns are used as anti-caking agents. Larger cellulose fibers of 120 microns or more are used to prevent the separation of fat and water in canned meat products.

Powdered cellulose has been shown to improve the functionality of cakes (Ang and Miller, 1991). One use of powdered cellulose has been to improve specific cake volume. In most cake batters, foams are formed by dispersion of air by mixing. However, the foams are thermodynamically unstable. Foam stability can be enhanced by increasing the viscosity of the batter or by introducing fine particulate mater. Cellulose fibers of 110 microns can function in both these ways. The addition of cellulose fiber to yellow layer, devil's food and angel food cakes has been shown to increase cake volume. Although 1 percent cellulose did not affect the volume of devil's food cake, additions of higher levels up to 4 percent increased cake volume significantly. It has been demonstrated that the shrinkage commonly experienced when cakes cool after the baking process is minimized in cakes with cellulose, suggesting that powdered cellulose may impart dimensional stability to baked products. Another use for powdered cellulose, particularly the 110 micron material, has been to improve cake texture. Compression force, a measure of firmness, increases with the addition of cellulose. Cellulose supplemented cakes (at the 2 to 4 percent level) tend to be stronger structurally, making them spongier and more highly rated by taste testers compared to controls. A possible explanation of the increased strength is possibly related to the formation of a network of cellulose fibers within the cake interior. This may be advantageous to the baking industry because of better handling properties, less loss from breakage, and improved product appearance.

Powdered cellulose can help reduce the fat absorption of some fried foods (Ang and Miller, 1991). When powdered cellulose is added to batter or breading coatings at the 1 percent level, the fat content of these batters is significantly ($P < 0.05$) lower after frying compared to controls. At the same time their moisture contents are increased. These observations are independent of the frying medium used, the batter formulation, or the type of food. Additionally, powdered cellulose has been shown to reduce the fat content of cake-type doughnuts. The data indicates that the level of cellulose added to the doughnut formulation is inversely related to the fat content. For example, 1 to 3 percent cellulose added to doughnuts results in a 10 to 21 percent decrease in fat content. As with the batters, the moisture content of the doughnuts is increased by 3 to 12 percent. Doughnuts with cellulose also appear to have improvement in appearance, more volume, and better pliability (less breakage during handling) than those without cellulose. The color is more uniform and lighter because powdered cellulose does not undergo nonenzymic browning. Sensory evaluations with untrained taste panels could not detect any significant differences from the control in the eating qualities of doughnuts containing 1 and 2 percent cellulose; the panelists tended to prefer the cellulose doughnuts because of their lighter color and reduced oiliness.

Microcrystalline Cellulose

Microcrystalline cellulose is acid hydrolyzed cellulose (Dreher, 1987; McGinley, 1991). It is purified, partially depolymerized cellulose prepared by treating alpha-cellulose, obtained as a pulp from fibrous plant materials, with mineral acids. Microcrystalline cellulose occurs as a fine, white, odorless, soft, crystalline powder which is insoluble in water and most organic solvents. It is the nonfibrous form of cellulose with particles typically ranging in size from 0.2 to 25 microns.

Microcrystalline cellulose is ''generally recognized as safe'' (GRAS) by experts in accordance with Food and Drug regulations and it can be labeled as cellulose gel.

The powdered microcrystalline cellulose products are usually spray-dried to create particles that are aggregates of microcrystals with unique physical properties (FMC Corporation, 1985; Dreher, 1987). The spray-dried particles tend to be very porous, deformable, and compressible. Cellulose gels have smaller fiber particle size (100 microns or less) than most powdered celluloses (300 microns or less). Particle size appears to have little effect on the density, specific volume, or WBC within the range of 20 to 50 microns. Some cellulose gels are spherical in shape that may provide better organoleptic acceptance when added to products at high levels compared to powered cellulose. The customary applications of powdered MCC is foods are as anti-caking agents, extrusion aids, bulking agents, non-nutritive sources of dietary fiber, and flavor carriers. They have a wide range of food applications (Brys and Zabik, 1976; Ferguson and Malick, 1983; Dreher, 1987).

Colloidal microcrystalline cellulose is a mixture of powdered microcrystalline cellulose (cellulose gel) and sodium carboxymethylcellulose (cellulose gum) (FMC Corporation, 1985). Cellulose gum is usually between 8.5 to 15 percent (w/w) of the colloidal microcrystalline cellulose. The colloidal material can be dispersed in water to form a suspendable, insoluble network of cellulose crystallites with highly functional properties. The bulk-dried grades required homogenization to disperse the microcrystals and, therefore, are generally used in whipped toppings and frozen desserts. The spray-dried grades require shear from a high-speed mixer for proper dispersion. These grades of cellulose are useful in a variety of food systems such as: fat-reduced foods, calorie-controlled foods, microwaved foods, bakery products, batters, breadings, beverages, canned foods, confections, dairy products, dry mixes, formed foods, frozen desserts, salad dressings, sauces, and whipped toppings.

When colloidal cellulose gel products are properly dispersed, the cellulose crystallites set up a network with particles less than 0.2 microns. These cellulose networks are responsible for the unique functional properties because they can be dispersed in water to form an aqueous hydrocolloid. The network is held together by weak hydrogen bonds which continue to form over time. Viscosity continues to increase over a 24-hour period. An aqueous hydrocolloid of cellulose gel differs from a gum solution because it binds water to a much lesser extent; the primary mechanism for controlling moisture flow is the cellulose network acting as a physical barrier. The gel network has a variety of important functional properties: (1) its thixotropic, viscosity decreases with shear and once the shear is removed the gel reforms with minimal loss in viscosity; (2) it is stable over a wide range of temperatures and pH—temperature and pH changes have little effect on functionality and viscosity of dispersions; (3) it thickens with clean mouthfeel that is non-greasy, non-stringy with some lubricity, and it does not mask flavors; and (4) it is noncaloric and provides dietary fiber.

Colloidal cellulose gel products have many functions in foods (FMC Corporation, 1985). First, they are premier foam stabilizers because the gel network acts as a physical barrier to hold air cells in suspension and thicken the water phase between air bubbles. This is effective in frozen desserts and whipped toppings to stabilize foam and improve overrun control. Second, they increase the viscosity of sugar solutions at concentrations of less than 1 percent. Reduced calorie, pourable syrups are developed by the use of this property. Third, they are used to extend and improve the properties of starch. A blend of 3 to 4 parts starch to 1 part colloidal cellulose can reduce the amount of starch thickener required by up to 25 percent. Fourth, they control ice crystal growth in frozen foods because the gel network provides a flexible stabilizing system that allows for the reabsorption of water and redispersion of components during the thaw cycle. Finally, they have the ability to improve the clingability (flow control) of starch sauces.

Colloidal cellulose gel products can be used as fat mimetics (McGinley, 1991; Penichter and McGinley, 1991). Cellulose gels simulate many of the rheological properties of oil-in-water emulsions without contributing calories. Typical use levels are from 0.75 to 2.5 percent in ice cream/frozen desserts, salad dressings, whipped toppings, icings, and puddings. A basic emulsion containing 60 percent soybean oil has similar rheological properties and stability characteristics as a 20 percent soybean oil emulsion containing 1 percent colloidal gel. They can reduce the fat and calorie content of extruded snacks such as cheese flavored puffed corn (Mottur and Glass, 1985).

Hemicellulose

Hemicellulose (sometimes called pentosans) consists of a diverse variety of polymers, varying in composition from a simple sugar such as is found in beta-glucans to polymers that may contain pentoses, hexoses, side chains, proteins, and phenolics (Hoseney, 1986; Dreher, 1987). Sugars that are often reported to be constituents of hemicelluloses include D-galactose, L-arabinose, D-xylose, D-glucose, D-glucuronic acid, and 4-O-methyl-D-glucuronic acids. Taken together they encompass the noncellulosic polysaccharides. They are widely distributed in plants and are generally thought to make up part of the cell wall and the cementing materials that holds cells together. Hemicelluloses are usually insoluble, but they can also be soluble. Purified hemicelluloses are not presently readily available for commercial food uses. Refined dry milled corn bran is, however, a very concentrated source of hemicellulose; this bran contains about 90 percent total dietary fiber and as much as 70 percent of that can be hemicellulose.

Insoluble hemicellulose is associated with a positive effect on cake and cookie functional properties. Jeltema and Zabik (1979) used fiber components to partially predict the following parameters of cake quality: tenderness, volume, cell size, cell wall thickness, and grain. Hemicelluloses have the largest effect on cake quality; insoluble hemicellulose is directly related to good cake quality whereas soluble hemicellulose is associated with poor cake quality. Jeltema and coworkers (1983) used fiber components to partially predict the following parameters of cookie quality: toughness, top grain, moisture, shape, cell distribution, cell size and spread. Insoluble hemicellulose is associated with improvements in cookie quality attributes such as reduced toughness and increased moistness. Further, insoluble hemicelluloses restrict cookie spread whereas soluble hemicellulose enhances cookie spread.

The role of pentosans in the formation and properties of dough has been the subject of many investigations (D'Appolonia and Gilles, 1971; Kim and D'Appolonia, 1977; Hoseney, 1984; Amado and Neukom, 1985; Meuser and Suckow, 1986; Kuhn and Grosch, 1989; Michniewicz et al., 1991). Because of their high water binding capacity, pentosans strongly influence the breadmaking properties of cereal flours. The water-insoluble pentosans make up about 2.4 percent of the wheat endosperm. The functional effect of pentosans on wheat dough and bread seems to depend on the properties of the base flour (Jelaca and Hlynka, 1972; and Michniewicz et al., 1991). One study shows that the addition of 2% insoluble endosperm pentosans to relatively weak Belgian wheat bread formulations can increase the loaf volume by 30 to 45 percent. However, the additions of insoluble pentosans to flours typically used in the United States do not tend to be as effective. Insoluble pentosans may also improve bread shelf life (Kim and D'Appolonia, 1977). Pentosans have been shown to reduce bread staling rate; insoluble pentosans are more effective than soluble pentosans.

Beta-Glucan

Beta-glucan is a cell wall polysaccharide which is present in oats and barley in much greater concentration than in other grains (Marlett, 1993). The typical range of beta-glucan in oat bran is from 5.5 to 9.0 percent and in barley bran from 4.0 to 8.5 percent; however, cultivars with higher beta-glucan are in development. Newman and coworkers (1990) found that up to about two-thirds of the barley beta-glucan is water-soluble. Marlett (1991) found that processing barley bran flour into cereal increased beta-glucan solubility to 90 percent. Beta-glucans consist of linear, unbranched polysaccharides composed of 1,4-beta-glucan units and 1,3-beta-glucan units found in endosperm cell walls. The beta-glucan molecule consists of 1,4 linkages occurring in groups of 2 to 4 units linked by single 1,3 linkages. The resulting structure consists mainly of beta-1,3-linked cellotriosyl and cellotetraosyl units. Oat and barley beta-glucans are generally categorized as structurally similar (Wood, 1991; Wood, 1993). Thus, oat and barley beta-glucan tend to produce similar high viscous aqueous solution.

Fibercel® was developed by Alpha-Beta Technology, Inc., in Worcester, Massachusetts as a concentrated source of beta-glucan (Ostroff et al., 1990). Fibercel® is a highly purified, beta-glucan fiber prepared from food-grade yeast, such as brewer's or baker's yeast. Beta-glucan is a major structural component of the yeast cell wall. Fibercel® consists of 86 percent beta-glucan, which is over 10 times more beta-glucan than is found in oat bran. Fibercel® is formulated by a patented process (US patent number 4,962,094) as discrete, 2–5 micron beta-glucan microspheres which readily disperse in liquids and do not gel. Due to their size and spherical morphology, they impart a smooth, creamy mouthfeel normally associated with fat. Fibercel® can be manufactured with a range of hydrodynamic properties to optimize its functionality for specific food uses. In low viscosity liquid systems, such as beverages, 10 grams of Fibercel-M®, with a low hydrodynamic volume (4 g/dl), can be added without any significant changes in viscosity. Fibercel-B®, however, with its higher hydrodynamic volume, is recommended for semi-liquid formulations such as ice cream, frostings, and puddings. Fibercel® is stable over a wide range of temperatures (−80°C to 120°C), unlike microparticulate protein preparations.

Lignin

Lignin is an amorphous, high molecular weight, aromatic polymer composed of phenylpropane residues which are formed in a matrix type arrangement by the condensation of three primary phenolic alcohols—coniferyl, sinapyl, and p-coumaryl alcohols (Dreher, 1987). Lignin is usually associated with mature plant cells or it is concentrated in plant tissues that have specialized support functions. Dietary fiber sources vary widely in lignin content; for example, cereal and oilseed fibers usually have only a few percent lignin, but rice and sunflower hulls may contain as high as 25 percent lignin.

Lignin is usually not considered to be a functional ingredient. However, it has been shown to exhibit antioxidant properties in the presence of vegetable oil (Catignani and Carter, 1982). Experimental evidence indicates that both lignin and tocopherol have a similar ability to reduce the rate of oxidation as measured by peroxide value. The chemical structure of lignin precursors is similar to that of many commonly used antioxidants. The phenolic moiety is believed to interrupt the free-radical chain of oxidative reactions by contributing hydrogen from the phenolic hydroxyl groups, themselves forming stable free radicals which do not initiate or propagate further oxidation of lipids (free-radical terminators) (IFT, 1986).

Resistant Starch

Resistant starch (RS) is known to develop in starchy foods after heating and during the cooling period. The amount depends mainly on the content of amylose and water (Rabe, 1994). Cooking and cooling of high amylose corn starch several times can result in as much as 60 percent RS. Since bakery products cannot undergo repeated heating and cooling in a high moisture environment without excessive texture and flavor problems, the best way to increase RS in bread and other baked goods is to enrich them with preprocessed high amylose starch. The RS amount for pasta has been shown to increase from 1.8 percent to 5.0 percent for cooked pasta (Rabe, 1994). The physiological properties of RS tend to act like dietary fiber. Commercial concentrated sources of resistant starch are available with 30 percent total dietary fiber (National Starch and Chemical Company).

Cereal Brans

Cereal brans are one of the most commonly used ingredients for increasing the dietary fiber content of processed foods. The main reasons for their widespread usage is: (1) low cost, (2) availability, (3) familiarity, (4) functionality, and (5) acceptable organoleptic characteristics. The dietary fiber content ranges from about 16 percent for oat bran to 90 percent for corn bran.

Cereals are the fruits of cultivated grasses belonging to the genus *Gramineae* (Fisher, 1985). The main cereals grown for human food are wheat, corn, rice, barley, oats, rye, sorghum, and millet. Cereal grains have similar structures which include a hull (husks) and a kernel (caryopsis). Grains of wheat, rye, corn, and sorghum are without hulls because the kernel and the hull separate readily during threshing whereas the grains of oats, rice, and mulch barley retain hulls after threshing (Fincher and Stone, 1986). The kernel consists of three basic components—bran, germ, and endosperm.

Wheat Bran

Wheat bran is the coarse outer layer of the wheat kernel (Vetter and Ranhotra, 1990). It is separated from cleaned and scoured wheat during milling. All wheat brans are not alike. Bran can be processed from red or white, hard or soft, and durum wheat. Besides the obvious color difference the bran from white wheat has a milder flavor than the bran from red wheat. The bran to be used in a specific application depends on the flavor, color, and appearance desired. The breakfast cereal industry uses both red and white wheat brans, but the bakery industry primarily uses red wheat bran. White bran has excellent potential for use in flour tortillas and pizza doughs.

Saunders (1980) and Posner (1991) have reviewed the morphology and composition of wheat bran and its milling fractions. The commercial end products of milling are not pure anatomical parts of the wheat kernel. Each consists of a mixture of endosperm and the outer fibrous layers of the kernel because when wheat is milled a break occurs in the endosperm. There are three main bran-containing fractions: bran, shorts, and red dog. The bran consists mostly of the nuclear epidermis, seed coat, pericarp, and a small amount of endosperm. It contains about 11 percent of the wheat kernel with an average particle size of over 900 microns. The shorts include the fibrous parts of the bran, endosperm, and germ. About 12 percent of the wheat kernels end up in the short fraction, with an average particle size of 500-900 microns. Red dog is actually low-grade flour, a mixture of endosperm and bran powder taken from the tail of the mill. It accounts for about 3 percent of the kernel with a particle size of 100–300 microns. The compositions of white and red wheat bran are summarized in Table 4. The wheat bran dietary fiber content may also be concentrated by further processing. A concentrated wheat bran between 60 and 80% dietary fiber can be produced by air classification (Posner, 1991) and/or enzyme-hydrolysis.

Grinding of wheat bran reduced the average particle size and increases the surface area which has a significant impact on its food functionality and its usefulness as a laxative. The main property affected is water binding capacity (WBC). Particle reduction causes the collapse of the fiber matrix of wheat bran which changes the WBC of wheat bran. In coarse wheat bran, water entrapped in the fiber matrix has an important influence on WBC. The finely ground wheat bran is less porous and unable to absorb as much water as the course bran which results in a lower WBC (Mongeau and Brassard, 1982).

Wheat bran has been shown to be detrimental to bread loaf volume (Pomeranz, 1977; Pomeranz et al., 1977; Shogren et al., 1981; Rogers and Hoseney, 1982; Finney et al., 1985; Lai et al., 1989). There are reports that wheat bran particle size affects bread quality. Finer wheat bran tends to be associated with better loaf volume and this appears to be related to dough water absorption properties. The detrimental effects of wheat bran on bread volume can be partially overcome by the addition of water and certain ingredients (Lai et al., 1989). The reduction in loaf volume due to the addition of wheat bran can be partially reversed by adding more water to the formulation or by soaking the bran in water

TABLE 4 AACC Certified Wheat Bran

	Soft White	Hard Red
Moisture	6.4%	9.7%
Protein (N × 6.31)	16.4%	16.0%
Fat	6.8%	5.9%
Ash	6.5%	6.1%
Total Dietary Fiber	44.5%	42.7%
Lignin	—	2.0%
Pectin	2.3%	1.6%
Pentosans	—	23.9%
Cellulose	—	15.2%
Starch	11.1%	16.2%
Water Binding Capacity	1.1 g/g	4.5 g/g

prior to use. Other ingredients are also useful in improving loaf volume. The addition of shortening and/or surfactants (e.g., sodium stearoyl lactylate) helps to increase the loaf volume of bran supplemented breads.

Corn Bran

There are two types of corn milling processes (Hoseney, 1986). Dry milling primarily separates the anatomical parts of the corn: bran, germ, and endosperm. Wet milling separates corn into its chemical constituents: starch, protein, oil, and fiber. Although most corn is processed by wet milling, dry milling is typically used for the production of corn bran for human consumption (Burge and Duensing, 1989). Because of density differences between germ and bran, raw corn bran can be aspirated from the bran/germ stream for further refining, concentrating, and sizing. This results in a very high fiber corn bran product with about 85 percent or more dietary fiber which is about 65 percent hemicellulose and 20 percent cellulose. Its calorie content is low at about 0.5 kcal/g. Corn bran exhibits a water binding capacity of about 2.4 to 3.7 g/g depending on the particle size and dietary fiber content. This product comes in various particle sizes, from fine to coarse, as needed for a variety of specific food applications.

Rice Bran

Rice is in the form of paddy (where the kernel is fully enveloped by the rice hull) when harvested from the field (Saunders, 1990). After being dried, the first stage in milling is removal of the hull, yielding brown rice. In the second state, the outer brown layer is removed from the brown rice kernel by abrasive milling operation to yield the familiar white rice. The separated brown layer is designated rice bran, which includes the germ in the United States. Under normal milling conditions, when brown rice is milled to white rice, the oil in the bran and a potent lipase also in the bran come into contact, resulting in rapid degradation of the oil. The bran thus produced is unpalatable and only fit as a feedstuff. However, if the bran is subjected to a short-term high temperature heat treatment the lipase activity is destroyed and a stabilized bran is produced. The compositions of rice brans are summarized in Table 5.

Rice bran has a number of unique properties (Saunders, 1990). Rice bran protein is of relatively high nutritional value. Protein efficiency ratio values reported for bran generally range from 1.6 to 1.9 compared to casein value of 2.5. Digestibility of protein in rice bran is about 75 percent. The bran usually contains 16–22 percent oil, although this value is higher in parboiled bran due to the absence of broken starch fragments. The three major fatty acids in rice bran are palmitic, oleic, and linoleic and they make up more than 90 percent of the total fatty acids. Rice bran oils contain 3–4 percent waxes and about 4 percent unsaponifiable lipids. Rice bran oil has a higher content of unsaponifiable material

TABLE 5 Typical composition of rice bran

Atribute	Stabilized Rice Bran	Parboiled Rice Bran
Moisture	8–12%	7–9%
Protein	12–16%	14–20%
Fat	16–22%	23–32%
Ash	7–10%	8–13%
Total Dietary Fiber	20–25%	31–33%
Soluble Dietary Fiber	2–3%	2–3%
Calories/g	3.2	3.5

From Saunders (1990).

than other vegetable oils. The unsaponifiable fraction consists of compounds such as oryzanols, beta-sitosterol, and tocopherols, which may have cholesterol-lowering activity. The major carbohydrates in commercial rice bran are cellulose, hemicellulose, and starch. Starch is not present in the outer pericarp layers, but because of endosperm breakage during milling it appears in the bran. The quantity varies according to the amount of breakage and degree of milling, but values of 10–20 percent are typical. Hemicellulose and cellulose have been reported to comprise 8.7–11.4 percent and 9.6–12.8 percent of the bran. Beta-glucans in the bran are present at levels of less than 1 percent.

The functional properties of rice bran are compatible with a wide variety of food uses (Barber and Benedito de Barber, 1980; Saunders, 1990). The water and oil absorption capacities are 2.0 and 1.5 g/g, respectively. Bran from parboiled food-grade rice bran is normally finely granulated, light tan in color, and possesses a relatively bland flavor with a nutty, toasted overtone. Its applications include use in baked goods, breads, cookies, breakfast cereals, granola-type bars, snacks, muffins, many other product. Parboiled rice bran appears to be a good dietary fiber supplement for bakery products (Skurray et al., 1986).

Barley Bran

Most barley, like rice and oats, is usually harvested with the hull intact, but some hull-less varieties are also available. Barley bran from hull varieties is obtained by pearling, which is the process of cutting away the outer layers of the barley with an abrasive surface. Barley bran from hull-less varieties is obtained by traditional milling techniques. Most commercially available barley bran flour is produced from brewers' grain by drying, milling, and fractionation procedures to produce flours that are tan, bland, and have a mild roasted grain flavor. The physical properties of barley bran are suitable for a number of food uses. Breads with barley bran flour have significantly increased dietary fiber and reduced calories with little change in loaf volume, texture and flavor according to Chaudhary and Weber (1990).

Barley, like oats, has much greater concentrations of betaglucan in the cell wall than other cereal grains (Marlett, 1993). Barley flour contains between 3.7 and 8.2 percent beta-glucan. Newman and coworkers (1990) found that 55 to 63 percent of the beta-glucan in typical barley cultivars is soluble. Henry (1985) shows that barley contains more soluble beta-glucan than oats. Hull-less barley cultivars can have up to 16 percent beta-glucan (Newman et al., 1989).

Oat Bran

Oat bran is produced by grinding clean oat groats or rolled oats and separating the resulting oat flour by sieving, bolting, and/or other suitable means into fractions such as the oat bran fraction, which should not be more than 50 percent of the starting material (Committee on Oat Bran, 1989). Oat bran has a total dietary fiber content of at least 16.0 percent and at least one-third of the fiber consists of the soluble fiber beta-glucan. Oat bran must contain at least 5.5 percent total beta-glucan. Beta-glucans of the oat cell walls are composed of linear polysaccharides chains (Inglett, 1991). Their structural components are glucose units connected with beta-(1-3) and beta-(1-4) linkages. It has been reported that the oat beta-glucan consists of about 70 percent of (1-4)-linked and about 30 percent of the (1-3)-linked beta-D-glucosyl residues.

Water binding capacity (WBC) of oat bran is an important determinant of its functionality in foods. The processing of oat groats differs from the processing of other cereals (Cadden, 1987). Oat groats must first be steam-treated and kiln-dried to inactivate the lipase enzymes present in the bran layers of the groat. Layers of the plant cell wall matrix of commercial oat brans are usually collapsed making absorption (taking water through pores) ineffective. This makes adsorption (surface binding of water) more important. The effect of oat bran particle size on WBC is demonstrated in Table 6. Since oat bran has a collapsed fiber

TABLE 6 Effect of bran particle size on physical properties and water binding capacity (WBC)[a]

Bran Source		Particle Size (microns)	Specific Volume (cc/g)	WBC (ml/g)
Oat Bran	Coarse	624	0.77	2.1
	Fine	256	0.77	3.3
Wheat Bran	Coarse	804	0.70	4.0
	Fine	308	0.66	2.4

[a] Adapted from Cadden (1987)

matrix, the grinding of oat bran, which increases surface area, has a major impact on increasing WBC. The effect of oat bran particle size on bread loaf volume has been studied by Krishnan et al. (1987). The finer the oat bran particle size the lower the bread volume. This effect appears to be related to WBC.

Krishnan and coworkers (1987) studied the impact of oat bran on bread properties. The effect of oat bran (at 10–15 percent and several granulations) on dough properties and bread quality were examined. The oat bran doughs had increased absorption as bran levels were increased and particle size was reduced. Breads with 10 percent substitution of the bran had better loaf volume, grain, and texture than the 15 percent bran bread. Other baked products such as cookies and muffins also show excellent potential for inclusion of oat bran as an ingredient (Seibert, 1987). Further, finely grounded oat bran shows potential as a carrier and dispersant, such as in seasoning mixes.

Oatrim is produced by a process that involves the conversion of starch in oat flour or bran to maltodextrins using alpha-amylase for starch liquefaction (Inglett, 1991). After starch liquefaction is complete, the enzyme is inactivated and the soluble materials containing the maltodextrin and beta-glucan are separated from the insoluble components by centrifugation. Oatrim has functional properties that make it uniquely suitable as a fat substitute. Oatrim containing maltodextrins with a low dextrose equivalent has the most suitable fat substitute properties. Oatrim can be made with various beta-glucan contents from 1 to 15 percent depending upon the functional and nutritional requirements. Oatrim comes in three forms: Oatrim-1, -5, and -10. The number after the Oatrim refers to the percent of beta-glucan present on a dry weight basis (Oatrim-1, Oatrim-5, Oatrim-10 are prepared from debranned oat flour, whole oat flour, and oat bran, respectively). Dr. George Inglett, USDA Agricultural Research Service, developed Oatrim. This technology was licensed by two corporations, ConAgra and Rhone-Poulene, in 1990.

TREATMENTS TO IMPROVE FIBER FUNCTIONALITY AND UNIQUE FIBER SOURCES

Alkaline Hydrogen Peroxide (AHP) Treatment

Partial delignification of lignocellulose by alkaline hydrogen peroxide treatment produces highly water absorbent, swellable, cellulosic products that can be used at high levels in food products such as bakery goods (Gould, 1987; Gould and Dexter, 1988). This treatment solubilizes a portion of the lignin present in the lignocellulosic matrix, leaving a cell wall material with higher water absorbency and improved softening and swelling characteristics.

Lignocellulosic materials suspended in an alkaline hydrogen peroxide aqueous solution have a special ability to solubilize lignin and conserve other fiber components such as hemicellulose. Typically between 40 and 60 percent of the original lignin content of the fiber is removed and solubilized. Upon completion of the reaction, the partially delignified fiber can be recovered by certrifugation, washed, and dried. As compared with the original substrate, the processed material exhibits a significant increase in water absorbency. The degree of water absorbency depends on the processing conditions. This suggests two possible mechanisms.

1. The selective removal of only a portion of the lignin by this process produces a highly porous cell wall matrix that allows increased hydration of the polysaccharides normally shielded by lignin. Complete delignification, which occurs in the production of cellulose, allows for the increased association of cellulose chains into highly crystalline structures that are resistant to internal hydration. In other words, if a little delignification is good, more is not better.
2. In the AHP-treated material, there is a decreased in the proportion of total crystalline cellulose. It is interesting to note that this reduction in cellulose crystallinity is irreversible and does not change after drying. This process appears to disrupt the hydrogen bonding pattern between the chains which maintains a highly open structure and allows the free hydroxyl groups to become moe available for binding to water molecules.

Regardless of the mechanism or combination of mechanisms, the increased internal hydration of these fibers produces a less gritty particle with enhanced interactions between the fiber polysaccharides and starch/gluten.

These AHP-treated fibers have been used as a high-fiber non-caloric flour substitute for use in baked goods (Jasberg et al., 1987). Mixograph peak heights for bread doughs increased when AHP-treated fibers replaced up to 30 percent of the flour, whereas untreated materials and purified cellulose decreased peak height. Loaf volumes at the 30 percent replacement level, without added gluten, were comparable to the controls. AHP-treated fibers could replace up to 40 percent of the flour in cakes without reducing baked volume or introducing gritty texture or off-flavors.

Extrusion Modification

Bran is subjected to a high temperature, high shear extrusion in a counter-rotating twin screw extruder, which modifies the structure of the bran ot make it more readily millable (Fulgar and Bradbury, 1985). additionally, the invention allows the naturally present starch to coat the lignocellulosic bran material during the extrusion process. After milling, the modified bran has an acceptable mouthfeel with an absence of grittiness, higher water binding capacity, and textural properties that are compatible with a wide variety of food products.

Encapsulation

Hutchinson and Swanson (1985) coated cellulose powder with soluble fiber to produce a low calorie base foold ingredient. The gum coating imparts to the fibrous cellulose particles a smooth texture that is more pleasant to the mouth and easier to chew and swallow than the unmodified cellulose. The gum coating greatly reduces the dry and gritty surface testure usually associated with powdered cellulose. Specifically, the powdered cellulose, wwith an average particle lenght of less than 75 microns, needs to be coated with between 2 and 15 percent soluble fiber for this to be effective (4 percent glycerol is required for optimal fiber characteristics).

Morley and Sharma (1986) coated ceral bran with soluble fiber to produce an improved low calorie food ingredient. The process works best with refined bran that has been chemically and/or enzymatically purified to provide a concentrated source of insoluble fiber. This refined fiber is then coated with 1.5 to 8.0 percent soluble fiber (dry weight basis) to provide a smooth, non-fibrous texture and mouthfeel.

Enzymatic Modification

Enzymatic modification of dietary fiber may improve sensory properites due to a change in chemical composition and physical properties (Caprez et al., 1987). Enzymatic treatments lead to an increase in soluble fiber content. The modified fiber sources show reduced wter binding capacity, which is advantageous for technology purposes. Also, the enzymatically treated fibers have a softer texture, which facilitates their use in food products.

Extrusion processing conditions have been shown to increase the dietary fiber content of wheat flour (Theander, 1987). During the extrusion process there tends to be an increse in both soluble and insoluble glucans and soluble pentosans. A portion of the insoluble glucans might be ''resistant starch,'' but the soluble glucans probably represent chemically modified starch. klason lignin increased directly with increased extrusion temperature.

CONCLUSIONS

The comsumer interest in fiber rich foods is expected to grow because of its increased visibility on food labels an s association with reduced chronic disease risk and enhanced weight maintenance. Dietary fiber is found in a wide array of foods such as vegetables, fruits, and cereal grains which should help increase the level of American comsumption which is about half the recommended intake for optimal health.

REFERENCES

Amado, R., and Neukom, H. 1985. Minor constituents of wheat flour: the pentosans.
American Association of Cereal Cheimists. 1987. Dietary fiber guide. Cereal Foods World. 32(8): 555–570.
Anderson, J. W. and Bridges, S. R. 1988. Dietary fiber content of selected foods. Am. J. Clinl. Nutr. 47:440–447.
Andon, S. A. 1987. Application of soluble fiber. Food Technology. 41(1);74–75.
Ang, J. F. and Miller, W. B. 1991. Multiple functions of powdered cellulose as a food ingredient. Cereal Foods World. 36(7): 558 -564.
R. D. Hill and L. Munck, Eds. 1985. Approaches to Research on Cereal Carbohydrates. Elsevier Science Publishers. Amsterdam. p. 249.
Barber, S. and benedito De Barber, C. 1980. Rice bran: chemistry and technology. Rice: Production & Utilization. B.S. Luh (Ed). AVI Publishing Company, Inc., Westport, Connecticut. pp. 809–817.
Becker, A. J., Egan, J. E., and Medri, M. 1987. Snack food product with high dietary fiber content and process for producing the same. Warner-Lambert Co., U.S. Patent 4,673,578.
Bell, D. A. 1990. Methylcellulose as a structure enhancer in bread baking. Cereal Foods World. 35(10):1001–1006.
Brummel, S. E. and Lee, K. 1990. Soluble hydrocolloids enable fat reduction in process cheese spreads. J. Food Sci. 55(5):1290–1292, 1307.
Brys, K. D. and Zabik, M. E. 1976. Microcrystalline cellulose replacement in cakes and biscuits. Journal of the American Dietetic Association. 69:50–55.
Burge, R. M. and Duensing, W. J. 1989. Processing and dietary fiber ingredient applications of corn bran. Cereal Foods World. 34(7):535–538.
Bushuk, W. 1966. Distribution of water in dough and bread. Bakers Digest. 40(5):38.
Cadden, A. M. 1987. Comparative effects of particle size reduction on physical structure and water binding properties of several plant fibers. J. Food Sci. 52(6):1595–1599.
Cadden, A. M., Sosulski, F. W., and Olson, J. P. 1983. Physiological responses of rats to high fiber bread diets containing several sources of hulls or bran. J. Food Sci. 48: 1151–1156.
Caprez, A., Arrigoni, E., Neukom, H., and Amado, R. 1987. Improvement of the sensory properties of two different dietary fiber sources through enzymatic modification. Lebensm.-Wiss.U.-Technol. 20:245–250.
Cardozo, M. S. and Ettenmiller, R. R. 1988. Total dietary fiber analysis of selected baked and cereal products. Cereal Foods World. 33(5): 414-418.
Catignani, G. L. and Carter, M. E. 1982. Antioxidant properties of lignin. J. Food Sci. 47:1745,1748.

Chaudhary, V. K. and Weber, F. E. 1990. Barley bran flour evaluated as dietary fiber ingredient in wheat bread. Cereal Foods World. 35(6):560–562.

D'Appolonia, B. L. and Gilles, K. A. 1971. Pentosans associated with gluten. Cereal Chem. 7:427.

DeFouw, C., Zabik, M. E., Uebersax, M. A., Aguilera, J. M., and Lusas, E. 1982. Effects of heat treatment and level of navy bean hulls in sugar-snap cookies. Cereal Chemistry. 59(4):245–248.

Del Toma, E., Clementi, A., Marcelli, M., Cappelloni, M., and Lintas, C. 1988. Food fiber choices for diabetic diets. Am. J. Clin. Nutr. 47:243–246.

Dreher, M. L., 1987. Dietary fiber content of food sources. Handbook of Dietary Fiber: An Applied Approach. Marcel Dekker, Inc., New York.

Duvall, L. F. 1982. Corn bran expanded cereal. The Quaker Oats Co. U.S. Patent 4,350,714.

Dziezak, J. D. 1991. A focus on gums. Food Technology. 45(3):116–132.

Editors. 1987. Dietary fiber guide. Cereal Foods World. 32(8):555–570.

English, C., Ross, J. K., Schlenker, E. D., and Perlmutter, C. A. 1987. Fiber content and cost of selected vegetable and fruits. Home Economics Research Journal. 16(2):96–102.

Ferguson, A. M. and Malick, H. M. 1983. Processing of mushrooms with reduced weight loss. U.S. Patent 4,407,832.

Fincher, G. B. and Stone, B. A. 1986. Cell walls and their components in cereal grain technology. Advances in Cereal Science and Technology. Volume VIII. Y. Pomeranz (Ed.). American Association of Cereal Chemists, Inc., St. Paul, MN. pp. 207–295.

Finney, P. L., Henrey, S., and Jeffers, H. 1985. Effects of wheat variety, flour grind, and egg yolk on whole wheat bread quality. Cereal Chem. 62:170.

Fisher, N. 1985. Cereals, milling and fibre. Dietary Fibre, Fibre-Depleted Foods and Disease. H. Trowell, D. Burkitt, and K. Heaton (Eds.) Chapter 25. Academic Press. Londong. pp. 377–390.

FMC Corporation. 1985. Avicel Bulleting G-34. Philadelphia, Pa.

Fulgar, C. V. and Bradbury, A. G. 1985. Modification of bran by extrusion. General Foods Corp., U.S. Patent 4,500,558.

Glicksman, M. 1982. Food applications of gum. Food Carbohydrates. AVI Publishing Co., Inc., Westport, CT. pp. 270–295.

Gould, J. M. 1987. Alkaline peroxide treatment of non-woody lignocellulosics. U.S. Patent No. 4,649,113.

Gould, J. M. and Dexter, L. B. 1988. Modified plant fiber additive for food formulations. U.S. Patent 4,774,098.

Henry, R. J. 1985. A comparison of non-starch carbohydrate in cereal grains. J. Sci. Food Agric. 36: 1243–1253.

Hoseney, R. C. 1984. Functional properties of pentosans in baked foods. Food Technology. 38(1):114–117.

Hoseney, R. C. 1986. Principles of Cereal Science and Technology. American Association of Cereal Chemist, Inc., St. Paul, MN.

Huffman, F. G. and Shah, Z. C. 1995. Carrageenans uses in foods and other industries. Nutrition Today. 30(6):246–253.

Hutchinson, B. R. and Swanson, A. M. 1985. Coated fibrous cellulose product and process. Maxfibe, Inc. U.S. Patent 4,565,702.

IFT. 1986. Preservatives: antioxidants. Food Technology. 40(9):94–102.

Inglett, G. E. 1991. Oatrim-a new fat substitute. Cholesterol Reduced Foods Technologies and Ingredients Conference. International Business Communications. Second Annual Industry Forum. Atlanta, Georgia. March 14–16.

International Food Information Council. 1991. How Americans are making food choices. Washington, D.C.

Jasberg, B. K., Gould, J. M., and Warner, K. 1987. High-fiber, non-calorie flour substitute for use in baked foods. Agricultural and Food Chemistry. ACS Abstract.

Jelaca, S. L. and Hlynka, I. 1972. Effect of wheat-flour pentosans in dough, gluten, and bread. Cereal Chem. 49:489.

Jeltema, M. S. and Zabik, M. E. 1979. Fiber components–quantification and relationship to cake quality. J. Food Science. 44:1732–1735.

Jeltema, M. A., Zabik, M. E., and Thiel, L. J. 1983. Prediction of cookie quality from dietary fiber components. Cereal Chemistry. 60(3):227–230.

Johnson, C. D., Berry, M. F., and Weaver, C. M. 1985. Soybean hulls as an iron source for bread enrichment. J. Food Science. 50:1275–1277.

Kim, S. K. and D'Appolonia, B. L. 1977. Bread staling studies. III. Effect of pentosans on dough, bread, and bread staling rate. Cereal Chemistry. 54:225.

Krishnan, P. G., Chang, K. C., and Brown, G. 1987. Effects of commercial oat bran on the characteristics and composition of bread. Cereal Chem. 64(1):55–58.

Kuhn, M. C. and Grosch, W. 1989. Baking functionality of reconstituted rye flours having different nonstarch polysaccharides and starch contents. Cereal Chem. 66:149.

Kuiper, A. and Schroder, K. 1982. Process for extruding a dietary fiber snack product. Meggie Milchindustrie GmbH & Co., KG. U.S. Patent 4,315,954.

Labuza, T. P. 1989. Fiber addition to foods. Cereal Foods World. 34(6):489.

Lai, C. S., Hoseney, R. C., and Davis, A. B. 1989. Effects of wheat bran in bread making. Cereal Chem. 66(3):217–219.

Lanza, E., Jones, Y., Block, G., and Kessler, L. 1987. Dietary fiber intake in the U.S. population. Am. J. Clin. Nutr. 46:790–797.

Marlett, J. A. 1991. Dietary fiber content and effect of processing on two barley varieties. Cereal Foods World. 36(7):576–578.

Marlett, J. A. 1992. Content and composition of dietary fiber in 177 frequently consumed foods. J. Am. Diet. Assoc. 92:175–186.

Marlett, J. A. 1993. Comparisons of dietary fiber and selected nutrient composition of oat and other grain fractions. Oat Bran. P. J. Wood, Ed. American Association of Cereal Chemists, Inc., St. Paul, MN. pp. 49–82.

McGinley, E. J. 1991. Functionality of collodial cellulose in low fat processed foods. Cholesterol Reduced Foods Technologies and Ingredients Conference. International Business Communications. Second Annual Industry Forum. Atlanta, Georgia. March 14–16.

Meuser, F. and Suckow, P. 1986. Non-starch polysaccharides. Chemistry and Physics of Baking. J. M. V. Blanshard, P. J. Fraizer, and T. Galliard, Eds. Royal Society of Chemistry. London. pp. 42–61.

Michniewicz, J., Biliaderis, C. G., and Bushuk, W. 1991. Effect of added pentosans on some physical and technological characteristic of dough and gluten. Cereal Chem. 68: 252–258.

Mongeau, R. and Brassard, R. 1982. Insoluble dietary fiber from breakfast cereals and brans: bile salt binding and water-holding capacity in relation to particle size. Cereal Chemistry. 59(5):413–417.

Mongeau, R., Brassard, R., and Verdier, P. 1989. Measurement of dietary fiber in a total diet study. Journal Food Composition and Analysis. 2:317–326.

Morley, R. C. and Sharma, S. C. 1986. Dietary fiber products and method of manufacture. Warner-Lambert Co., U.S. Patent 4,565,702.

Mottur, G. P. and Glass, R. W. 1985. Reduced calorie puffed snack food products. Frito-Lay, Inc., U.S. Patent 4,500,558.

Newman, R K, Newman C W, and Graham, H. 1989. The hypocholesterolemic function of barley beta-glucans. Cereal Foods World. 34:883-886.

Newman, R K, McGuire, C F, and Newman, C W. 1990. Composition and muffin-baking characteristics of flours from barley cultivars. Cereal Food World. 35(6):563–566.

Ostroff, G. R., James, S., and Easson, D. D. 1990. A new microspherical fiber with fat-mimetic properties. Alpha-Beta Technology, Inc., Worcester, MA.

Parrott, M. E. and Thrall, B. E. 1978. Functional properties of various fibers: physical properties. 43:759–763.

Penichter, K. A. and McGinley, E. J. 1991. Cellulose gel for fat-free food applications. Food Technology. 45(6):105.

Pilot, S. M. 1987. Physiological Effects of Health Consequences of Dietary Fiber. Life Sciences Research Office. Federation of American Societies for Experimental Biology. Beheads, Maryland. Contract Number FDA 223-84-2059, pp. 162, 163.

Pomeranz, Y. 1977. Fiber in breadmaking: a review of recent studies. Baker's Digest. 51(10):94.

Pomeranz, Y., Shogren, M. D., Finney, K. F., and Bechtel, D. B. 1977. Fiber in breadmaking–effects on functional properties. Cereal Chemistry. 54(1):25–41.

Posner, E. S. 1991. Mechanical separation of a high dietary fiber fraction from wheat bran. Cereal Foods World. 36(7):553–556.

Proctor & Gamble 1990. Your Guide to a High-Fiber Diet. Cincinnati, Ohio.

Prosky, L. and DeVries, J. 1992. Controlling Dietary Fiber in Food Products. Van Nostrand Reinhold, New York.

Rabe, E. 1994. Affecting the RS-content by household cooking. Proceedings of the concluding plenary meeting of EURESTA. Asp, N-G, Van Amelsvoor, JMM and Hautvast, JG. pp. 146–148.

Ranhotra, G. S., Gelroth, J. A., and Astroth, K. 1990. Total and soluble fiber in selected bakery and other cereal products. Cereal Chem. 67(5):499–501.

Rimm, E. B., Ascherio, A., Giovannucci, E., Spiegelman, D., Stampfer, M. J. and Willett, W. C. 1996. Vegetable, fruit, and cereal fiber intake and risk of coronary heart disease among men. JAMA. 275(6):447–451.

Rogers, D. and Hoseney, R. C. 1982. Problems associated with producing whole wheat bread. Cereal Foods World. 27:451.

Rogols, S. 1986. Technical services report. Grain Processing Corp.

Satin, M., McKeown, B., and Findlay, C. 1978. Design of a commercial natural fiber white bread. Cereal Foods World. 23(11):676–680.
Saunders, R. M. 1990. The properties of rice bran as a foodstuff. Cereal Foods World. 35(7):632–636.
Saunders, R. M. 1980. Wheat bran as dietary fiber. Cereals for Food and Beverages Recent Progress in Cereal Chemistry and Technology. G.E. Inglett and L. Munck (Eds.) Academic Press. New York. pp. 137–153.
Seibert, S. E. 1987. Oat bran as a source of soluble dietary fiber. Cereal Foods World. 32(8):552–553.
Shogren, M. D., Pomeranz, Y., and Finney, K. F. 1981. Counteracting the effects of fiber in breadmaking. Cereal Chem. 58:142.
Skurray, G. R., Woolbridge, D. A., and Nguyen, M. 1986. Rice bran a source of dietary fibre in bread. J. Food Tech. 21:727–730.
Slavin, J. L. 1987. Dietary fiber: classification, chemical analysis, and food sources. J. Am. Diet. Assoc. 87(9):1164–1171.
Stanley, D. W. 1986. Chemical and structural determinations of texture of fabricated foods. Food Technology. March: 65–76.
Theander, O. 1987. Chemistry of dietary fibre components. Scandinavian Journal of Gastroenterology. 22 (129):21–28.
TIC Gums. 1987. Water soluble gums booklet.
Toma, R. B. and Curtis, D. J. 1989. Ready-to-eat cereals: role in a balanced diet. Cereal Foods World. 34(5):387–390.
Toma, R. B., Orr, P. H., D'Appolonia, B., Dintzis, F. R., and Tabekhia, M. M. 1979. Physical and chemical properties of potato peel as a source of dietary fiber in bread. J. Food Science. 44(5):1403–1407, 1417.
Tye, R. J. 1991. Konjac flour: properties and applications. Food Technol. 45(3), 82, 84, 86, 88, 90, 92.
U.S. Department of Agriculture 1989. Composition of Foods: Cereal Grains and Pasta. Agricultural Handbook No. 8–20.
Vetter, J. L. 1988. Commercial available fiber ingredients and bulking agents. AIB Technical Bulletin. X(5):1–5.
Vetter, J. L. and Ranhotra, G. S. 1990. Wheat bran: functional, physiological, and dietary application. AACC Short Course on Fiber in Food: Biochemistry, Physiology, and Technology. October 11–13. Dallas, TX.
Weber, F. E. and Chaudhary, V. K. 1987. Recovery and nutritional evaluation of dietary fiber ingredients from a barley by-product. Cereal Foods World. 32(8):548–550.
Wolever, T. M. S., Vuksan, V., Eshuis, H., Spadafora, P., Peterson, D., Chao, E. S. M., Storey, M. L., and Jenkins, D.J.A. 1991. Effect of method of administration of psyllium on glycemic response and carbohydrate digestibility. J. Am. Coll. Nutr. 10(4): 364–371.
Wood, P. J. 1991. Oat beta-glucan physicochemical properties and physiological effects. Trends in Food Science & Technology. December. pp. 311–314.
Wood, P. J. 1993. Physicochemical characteristics and physiological properties of oat beta-D-glucan. Oat Bran. P. J. Wood, Ed., American Association of Cereal Chemists, Inc. St. Paul, MN. pp. 83–112.

Wrick, K. L., Robertson, J. B., Van Soest, P. J., Lewis, B. A., Rivers, J. M., Roe, D. A., and Hackler, L. R. 1983. The influence of dietary fiber source on human intestinal transit and stool output. J. Nutr. 113:1464–1479.

Wright, H. S., Guthrie, H. A., Wang, M. Q., and Bernardo, V. 1991. The 1987–88 nationwide food consumption survey: an update on the nutrient intake of respondents. Nutrition Today. May/June: 21–27.

Zabik, M. E., Shafer, M. A. M., and Kukorowski, B. W. 1977. Dietary fiber source for baked products. J. Food Science. 42(6):1428–1431

25

Chemical and Physical Modifications of Dietary Fiber

Mary Ellen Camire
University of Maine, Orono, Maine

INTRODUCTION

The importance of dietary fiber to human nutrition and food processing is well-known, but less is understood of the effects of common food processing techniques on the properties of fiber molecules. Removal of native lipids, proteins and starches from a fiber-rich food changes hydration characteristics. Milling modifies surface properties, with important nutritional implications. Processes involving moist heat may leach soluble fiber; canning produces the most severe changes. Extrusion cooking fragments carbohydrates into smaller molecules that may recombine in unique ways. New food processing methods may have yet other effects on dietary fiber molecules.

For many years the complex of compounds known as dietary fiber was considered to be roughage: of little importance to humans except for laxative effects. Since the 1970s the value of cellulose, hemicelluloses, pectins, gums and lignin to human health has become apparent. Numerous studies have examined the effects of fiber on the prevention of cancer (1,2), heart disease (3,4), and other disorders. Some studies have had contradictory findings. While some of the disagreement may be attributable to differences in definitions of dietary fiber, changes in the chemical and physical structure of fiber constituents due to processing may have had profound influences on nutritional properties (5). Epidemiological studies often fail to consider food preparation techniques in the analysis of data. Stir-frying used in Asia should have less severe effects on the fiber in vegetables than would boiling, which is used extensively in Europe and the United States to cook vegetables. Nutrient content data such as the United States Department of Agriculture's Handbook 8 contain limited information on the differences in fiber due to common food preparation techniques. This chapter will summarize information on reported changes to the molecular structure of fiber and subsequent nutritional and functional changes.

INDUSTRIAL PROCESSING

Manufacturers process fiber-rich materials into concentrated forms of fiber often as a by-product of some other food operation. Cereal brans, soy fiber (bran and cotyledon), apple fiber, and many other products were once part of the wastestream from food processing operations. Isolated, concentrated fiber has different physical and nutritional properties from the parent material. Vitamins, minerals and phytochemicals are removed along with protein, lipid, and starch, depending upon the process used. Rice bran, for example, may contain tocotrienols that are beneficial for cardiovascular health. Defatted rice bran may have substantial amounts of these compounds removed, thereby altering potential health benefits. Removal of other macromolecules could alter water-binding properties. Psyllium gum supplements proved hazardous when not ingested with sufficient liquid, since an insoluble mass formed, preventing passage through the gastrointestinal tract. Purified fiber supplements also exhibited different in vitro fermentabilities (6). Fermentation of pectin, tragacanth gum, psyllium, guar gum, soy fiber (type not available) produced significantly greater amounts of short-chain fatty acids and methane than did cellulose fermentation. Hydrogen production in the study was variable.

Fiber Separation Techniques

Removal of the fiber-rich component from the rest of the food material significantly changes the dietary fiber content of the materials. Brans typically are richer in cellulose and lignin, while cereal endosperm and legume cotyledon tissue contain a greater proportion of water-soluble molecules, principally hemicelluloses. Milling grain removes bran from endosperm, resulting in a product with less insoluble fiber and possibly total fiber. This physical treatment is not expected to modify the fiber molecules in each co-product (bran and flour). Table 1 shows the dietary fiber composition of common wheat products. All-purpose and cake flours have substantial amounts of fiber removed during milling.

Oat gum extracted from oat bran with aqueous sodium carbonate (pH 10) at 40°C had different properties depending upon the concentration procedure used (7). Dialysis of the extract produced gums with greater viscosity than did ultrafiltration or ethanol precipitation methods. Alcohol precipitation had the highest yields, however. Inactivation of enzymes by 75% ethanol at 80°C also resulted in gums of higher viscosity but much of the β-glucanase present in the original bran had been reduced by a prior steaming by the supplier.

Alkali extractions were also effective in removing soluble fiber from defatted rice bran. Extracts obtained with either sodium hydroxide or calcium hydroxide at pH 12 significantly lowered serum cholesterol in rats fed a cholesterol-enriched diet (8). The $Ca(OH)_2$ method was preferred because it produced a lighter colored-product. NaOH had a better yield, however, of 8 g per 100 g rice bran versus 5 g for the calcium salt.

Removal of starch, protein and other water-soluble compounds by various treatments affected wheat bran composition, water-holding capacity, and bread-baking properties (9) (Figure 1). Amylase treatments produced the highest neutral fiber contents; protease with amylase yielded more fiber, but that fiber was not suitable for baking. Rinsing following chemical or enzyme treatment may have removed too much soluble material.

Microwave heating has been proposed as a pretreatment for fruit waste to enhance pectin extraction. A ten-minute treatment at 2450 MHz and 0.5 kW improved pectin yields from orange and lemon peels and apple pressings without affecting the amount of anhydrouronic acid content or degree of esterification (10). Microwave heating, whether or not followed by drying, increased pectin gel strength compared to pectin extracted directly from fresh fruit or from dried

TABLE 1 Total dietary fiber content of wheat milling products

Wheat Product	TDF (%)[a]
Whole wheat flour	12.2
All-purpose flour	2.7
Cake flour	1.7
Wheat bran	42.8
Wheat germ	13.2

[a] Percent total dietary fiber, as is basis.
Adapted from the USDA Nutrient Database.

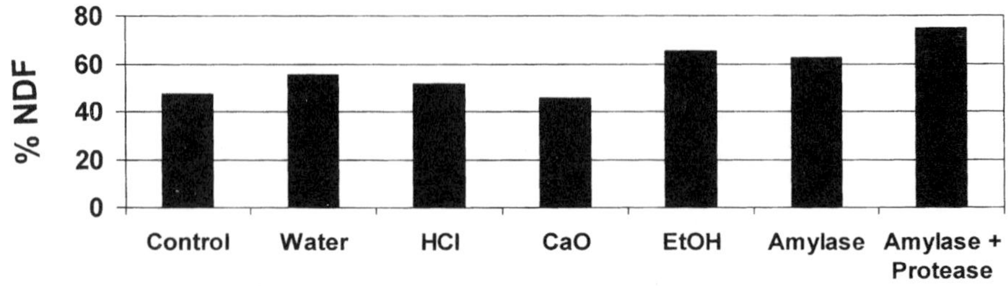

Figure 1 Neutral detergent fiber of treated wheat bran.

material. The beneficial effects of microwave pretreatment may be due to inactivation of pectin enzymes and simultaneous collapse of cell structure.

Particle Size Reduction

Milling may be taken for granted since most consumers are familiar with foods containing flour or bran. Intact foods such as kernel corn and sesame seeds can pass completely through the gut with little apparent change; clearly particle size determines many factors in vivo. Particle size reduction increases surface area, and presumably accessibility to enzymes and water. The water holding capacity (WHC) of a fiber source is believed to be especially important for stool bulk, but in vitro measurements of WHC cannot predict in vivo effects (11). Grinding or milling influences water binding properties according to the composition and prior processing history of the fiber. Grinding reduced water binding by wheat bran because the cell matrix was disrupted, yet ground oat bran exhibited higher binding (12). Since the oats were subjected to steam, then dried to inactivate enzymes, the cell structure was modified prior to grinding.

"Harder" portions of a food, probably rich in lignin and cellulose, are more resistant to grinding, while softer portions may contain more starch and water-soluble nonstarch polysaccharides. These fractions have different hydration properties, thus fractions collected according to particle size after milling are expected to have different hydration properties. Smaller particles of hammer-milled wheat bran, sugar beet fiber, and citrus fiber had reduced water holding and swelling capacities, while water holding capacity was higher for smaller pea hull particles (13). Grinding may have increased pore size for the pea hulls. In that same study, magnetic stirring increased the water binding capacity of sugar beet fiber over time.

The type of mill used also influences particle size. A Wiley mill produced a greater percentage of coarse food particles than did a Cyclotec mill (14). Wheat and potato samples ground in the Cyclotec mill had higher soluble fiber recoveries, suggesting the some previously insoluble material was made more soluble by reducing particle size.

Chemical Treatments

Chemical Modifications

Carboxymethylcellulose, methylcellulose and hydroxymethylcellulose products are available for controlling viscosity and oil use or absorption in foods (5,15). Although these cellulose derivatives are considered fiber molecules, they have some solubility in aqueous ethanol solutions, thus they may not be detected by analytical procedures that employ an ethanol precipitation step.

Bleaching

Brans, fruits, and other dark or highly colored products may be difficult to use in those foods where lightness in color is important. Bleaching may be used to lighten fiber materials, but chlorine-based bleaching agents should be avoided. Hydrogen peroxide treatment of wheat bran resulted in lighter, less red, and more yellow product (9). Wheat straw bleached with hydrogen peroxide could be incorporated into cakes without affecting flavor or producing gritty mouthfeel (16). Rats fed bleached oat hulls showed no abnormalities (17).

Peroxide bleaching frees carbohydrates bound to lignin. Bleaching increased soluble fiber neutral sugars in oat hulls by over 3%, while lignin decreased over 6% compared to non-bleached hulls (18). Health benefits due to phenolic compounds and other phytochemicals associated with fiber in foods may be lost during bleaching (19). As more consumers appreciate the importance of fiber in their diets, there may be less need to bleach fiber-rich materials to enhance marketability.

Enzymes

Oat beta-glucans and guar gum have been enzymatically hydrolyzed to improve functionality. The primary change after enzyme treatment is a reduction in molecular weight, which in turn leads to lower viscosities when the gums are dispersed in water. While a fiber-enriched mineral water may appeal to some consumers, there may not be a nutritional advantage to such supplementation. Bile acid binding and delayed glycemic response (20) are two health benefits that are dependent upon the viscous gels formed in the intestine. Further study is needed on the changes this procedure has on physiological effects.

Enzymes naturally present in fiber-rich materials can reduce food quality. Lipase inactivation is necessary for rice bran use. Although most processors employ some type of thermal treatment to destroy the enzyme, USDA researchers have found solvent extractions to be effective as well. Ethanol at room temperature and hexane at 68°C inhibited lipid hydrolysis in rice kernels and flour during storage while producing slightly higher total dietary fiber contents (21).

Food Processing

Food processors utilize a variety of methods. Foods in microwavable frozen dinners may have been subjected to boiling, steaming, chemical peeling, baking, dehydration, or extrusion in addition to freezing and microwaving. Knowledge of the effects of these methods on fiber composition and properties is limited. Changes in fiber analytical methodology have made older reports less useful since many reported only total fiber or soluble plus insoluble fiber.

Wet Heat Treatments

Autoclaving

Solubilization of sugarbeet fiber was temperature- and pressure-dependent (22). No changes were observed at 10-minute intervals when sugarbeet pulp was autoclaved at 50° or 100°C and atmospheric pressure; soluble fiber content doubled after 10 minutes at 121°C and 1.2 bar.

Boiling

Cooking foods in an excess volume of water leads to loss of water-soluble materials into the cooking water. Despite the potential nutrition impairment, this method of cooking remains common in households and institutions. Seaweed boiled for one hour lost up to 40% of insoluble fiber (23). Soaked and boiled chickpeas and kidney beans retained more dietary fiber than when soaked and pressure-cooked, presumably due to losses of soluble fiber into the cooking water (24).

Canning

The combination of time and temperature required to produce commercially sterile foods can severely affect fiber composition. Retorted (121°C, 60 minutes) green bean and carrot purees lost significant amounts of pectic material (25). No changes were found in the neutral sugar fractions of the vegetables. Since this type of processing is used to prepare fruits and vegetables for infants and elderly persons, the health implications of such changes warrant further study. However, the vegetables in this study were subjected to many processes (freezing, freeze-drying, milling) prior to analysis. Fiber changes at each step were not evaluated.

Although blanching produced minor changes in carrot fiber compared to a frozen standard, boiling, microwaving and canning carrots caused increases in soluble fiber molecules (26). Canning also resulted in larger changes in molecular weight distribution of nonstarch polysaccharides in green beans, Brussels sprouts, and green peas compared with boiling and microwaving (27).

Steaming

More fiber should be retained in steamed vegetables since the food is not immersed in the cooking medium and leaching is minimized. Steam-cooking wheat bran increased IDF, but boiling and autoclaving increased SDF (28). Oil absorption, but not water-binding capacity, was increased by steaming and autoclaving; boiling significantly increased both properties. The processed brans also exhibited different farinogram effects when mixed with flour. These changes were attributed to physical, not chemical, modifications of fiber during processing.

Microwaving

Vegetables vary in their changes due to microwave cooking. Green beans and Brussels sprouts showed little change in molecular weight of fiber molecules, but green peas showed significant loss of higher molecular weight compounds (MW > 40000) with increased recovery of middle-sized polymers (MW 10000–40000) (27). Microwaved (previously blanched and frozen) carrots elicited higher postprandial glucose values in volunteers fed a mixed meal than did raw carrots (29). Total dietary fiber was lower in raw carrots during the first year of the study, and a significantly higher satiety score was obtained for raw carrots that year.

Dry Heat Treatments

Baking

Breads and other baked grain products are popular world-wide, yet relatively little is known about the effects of baking on dietary fiber composition. Baking for one hour at 135°C had no effect on the dietary fiber composition or hydration capacity of cornmeal or oatmeal, but for baked potato peels, insoluble nonstarch polysaccharides increased and hydration capacity decreased (30). Baking bread transforms wheat starch into resistant starch that is digested and fermented like dietary fiber (31). More resistant starch was formed in the crumb than in the crust. These chemical changes are difficult to predict. Estimation of fiber content after baking from the total dietary fiber content of ingredients was inadequate (32). Formation of Klason lignin during baking cannot be predicted reliably, but content of other fiber components correlated well with predicted values. Some baked foods have increased soluble fiber and prediction of this change in solubility was also limited.

Roasting

Several commodities such as nuts are heated at high temperatures (>170°C) to produce characteristic colors and flavors via Maillard reactions. Roasting/toasting significantly increased the lignin content of wheat bran (25) and cocoa beans (33). Although total fiber values were unaffected, both neutral sugars and uronic acids decreased in the insoluble fiber fraction of cocoa beans after roasting. The involvement of these carbohydrates in the formation of Maillard polymers is most likely responsible for the higher apparent lignin formation.

Extrusion

Many foods and feeds are now processed by extrusion cooking. This unique process performs several unit operations simultaneously. Foods are subjected to heat and shear during transportation along the extruder barrel. Fiber-rich materials may be extrusion-cooked to modify functional properties. Extruded bran mills into smaller pieces with reduced grittiness and improved water absorption (34). Increased screw speed during extrusion increased soluble fiber and enzyme-susceptible starch contents for whole wheat and wheat bran (35).

Branched molecules are more susceptible to shear during extrusion than is cellulose. Extrusion significantly increased the water solubility of sugar beet pulp fiber by decreasing the molecular weight of pectin and hemicelluloses molecules (36). No difference in X-ray diffraction patterns was found after extrusion of corn fiber–corn starch blends, suggesting than semi-crystalline cellulose is more resistant to degradation under typical extrusion conditions (37).

Prior processing can influence fiber changes during extrusion. Both acid and alkaline treatments increased soluble fiber somewhat in corn bran (38). Although grinding doubled the soluble fiber of pea hulls to 8% (dry basis), all extruded hulls contained over 10% soluble fiber (39). Total fiber content after extrusion was lower, perhaps due to losses of smaller molecular weight compounds formed from fiber during the process.

Soluble fiber created during extrusion is chemically different from naturally soluble fiber compounds such as pectin and gums, and thus should be expected to have different nutritional properties. The soluble fiber content of potato peels was about doubled by extrusion, and barrel temperature significantly increased in vitro binding of cholic acid and deoxycholic acid (40). Those findings agreed with a rat feeding study. Total serum and liver cholesterol levels were lower in young rats fed extruded oats, barley or wheat than in rats fed a control diet or feeds containing unextruded grains (41). Soluble fiber was higher in all extruded feeds, and soluble β-glucans increased slightly in extruded oats and barley. Higher viscosities of aqueous suspensions of extruded grains were also found.

Extruded citrus peels had higher levels of soluble fiber and increased in vitro viscosity (42). Starch digestion and glucose diffusion were not different from those of non-extruded products, however. Additional research could lead to extruded products with improved glycemic properties designed for diabetic consumers.

Extrusion-induced molecular changes could influence the ability of fiber to bind carcinogens. Few studies have been published on this subject. Extrusion conditions, with one exception (110°C, 30% feed moisture), did not affect the ability of potato peels to bind benzo[a]pyrene, a polycyclic aromatic hydrocarbon (43). Ready-to-eat breakfast cereals are often produced by extrusion. Sixteen commercial cereals bound at least 40% of the benzo[a]pyrene added during in vitro digestion, but carcinogen binding was not correlated with a specific dietary fiber fraction (44).

Non-Thermal Treatments

Freezing

Many vegetables are blanched prior to freezing to inactivate enzymes, and this brief treatment may produce slight fiber solubilization (45). Fruits are generally not blanched to maintain texture and prevent juice loss. Pectinase activity is only slowed at freezer temperatures. Pectin solubilization and degradation may occur during frozen storage since consumers may keep frozen items for a year or more. Starch retrogradation may also occur in frozen foods; the formation of resistant starch by this mechanism is possible.

Fermentation

Insoluble dietary fiber increased after fermentation in three legumes (Bengal gram, cow pea, and green gram) (46). Since many microorganisms can use soluble fiber as an energy source, the increase in insoluble fiber was probably due to removal of soluble molecules.

Malting/Sprouting

Germination produced slight increases in legume IDF (46). Rolled flakes made from malted barley contained only 1.2% soluble beta-glucans, compared with 2.9% in flakes made from untreated barley (47). Total dietary fiber was also lower in the malted flakes.

SUMMARY

Common processing methods can produce important changes in food dietary fiber composition. These changes are summarized in Table 2. Although calculation of nutrient content of processed foods from ingredient content is an accepted procedure in the United States, dietary fiber composition will most likely be incorrect. New sterilization methods such as ohmic heating and magnetic field processing may also affect fiber. As new methods are developed, care should be taken to analyze the fractions of fiber, not simply total fiber. Processing-induced changes in fiber molecules may significantly alter health benefits, leading to public health and food labeling issues.

TABLE 2 Changes in dietary fiber composition due to processing

Food Processing Method	↓ Soluble Fiber		↑ Soluble Fiber		↑ Insoluble Fiber	
	Cooking Losses	Soluble Fiber	Cell Wall Release	Insoluble Fiber Splitting	↑ Resistant Starch	↑ Klason Lignin
Boiling	*					
Canning	*	*				
Microwaving	*	*	*			
Baking					*	*
Roasting						*
Extrusion				*	*	*
Freezing		*	*	*		

ACKNOWLEDGMENTS

Maine Agricultural and Forest Experiment Station publication #2068. The author appreciates the assistance of Michael Dougherty in the preparation of this manuscript.

REFERENCES

1. Kritchevsky, D. (1991) Evaluation of Publicly Available Scientific Evidence Regarding Certain Nutrient-Disease Relationships: 5. Dietary Fiber and Cancer, Federation of American Societies for Experimental Biology, Bethesda, MD.
2. Harris, P.J., & Ferguson, L.R. (1993) Mutation Res. 290, 97–110.
3. Anderson, J.W., Deakins, D. A., Floore, T. L., Smith, B.M., & Whitis, S. E. (1990) Crit. Rev. Food Sci. Nutr. 29, 95–147.
4. Kritchevsky, D. (1991) Evaluation of Publicly Available Scientific Evidence Regarding Certain Nutrient-Disease Relationships: 6. Dietary Fiber and Cardiovascular Disease, Federation of American Societies for Experimental Biology, Bethesda, MD.
5. Dreher, M. L. (1987) Handbook of Dietary Fiber, Marcel Dekker, Inc., New York, NY.
6. McBurney, M. I., & Thompson, L.U. (1989) J. Food Sci., 54, 347–350.
7. Beer, M.U., Arrigoni, E., & Amado, R. (1996) Cereal Chem. 73, 58–62.
8. Aoe, S., Oda, T., Tatsumi, K., Yamauchi, M., & Ayano, Y. (1993) Cereal Chem. 70, 423–425.
9. Rasco, B. A., Borhan, M., Yegge, J.M., Lee, M.H., Siffing, K, & Bruinsma, B. (1991) Cereal Chem. 68, 295–299.
10. Kratchanova, M., Panchev, E., & Shtereva, L. (1994) Carbohydrate Polymers 25, 141–144.

11. Robertson, J. A., & Eastwood, M. A. (1981) Brit. J. Nutr. 45, 83–89, Roehrig, K.L. (1988) Food Hydrocolloids 2, 1–18.
12. Cadden, A.-M. (1987) J. Food Sci. 52, 1595–1599, 1631.
13. Auffret, A., Ralet, M.-C., Guillon, F., Barry, J.-L., & Thibault, J.-F. (1994) Lebensm.-Wiss. u.-Technol. 27, 166–172.
14. Mullin, W.J., & Wolynetz, M. S. (1995) J. AOAC Intl. 78, 83–87.
15. Whistler, R.L., & BeMiller, Miller, J.N. (1997) Carbohydrate Chemistry for Food Scientists, Am. Assoc. Cereal Chem., St. Paul, MN.
16. Jasberg, B.K., Gould, J.M., & Warner, K.. (1989) Cereal Chem. 66, 209–213.
17. Kehoe, D.F., Kong, L.L., Tisdel, P.J., MacKenzie, K.H., Hall, T. L., Field, W. E., & Rao, C. S. (1990) Cereal Foods World 35, 1026–1029.
18. Lopez-Guisa, J.M., Harned, M.C., Dubielzig, R., Rao, S.C., & Marlett, J. A. (1988) J. Nutr. 118, 953–962.
19. Ranum, P.M., & DeStephanis, V. A. (1989) Cereal Foods World 34, 984–988.
20. Wood, P.J. (1994) Carbohydr. Polym. 61, 331–336.
21. Champagne, E. T., Hron, R. J., & Abraham, G. (1991) Cereal Chem. 68, 267–271.
22. Quaglia, G. B., & Carletti, G. (1993) La Rivista di Sci. dell'Alimentazione 22, 109–114.
23. Suzuki, T., Nakai, K., Yoshie, Y., Shirai, T., & Hirano, T. (1993) Nippon Suisan Gakkaishi 59, 1371–1375.
24. Vidal-Valverde, C., & Frias, J. (1991) J. Food Sci. 56, 1350–1352.
25. Anderson, N.E., & Clydesdale, F. M. (1980) J. Food Sci. 45, 1533–1537.
26. Nyman, M., Nylander, T., & Asp, N.G. (1993) Food Chem. 47, 169–176.
27. Nyman, E.M., Svanberg, S.J.M., & Asp, N.-G. (1994) J. Sci. Food Agric. 66, 83–91.
28. Caprez, A., Arrigoni, E., Amadó, R., & Neukom, H. (1986) J. Cereal Sci. 4, 233–239.
29. Gustafsson, K., Asp, N.-G., Hagander, B., Nyman, M., & Schweizer, T. (1995) Intl. J. Food Sci. Nutr. 46, 3–12.
30. Camire, M.E., & Flint, S.I. (1991) Cereal Chem. 68, 645–647.
31. Bjorck, I., Nyman, M., Pederson, B., Siljestrom, M., Asp, N.G., & Eggum, B. O. (1986) J. Cereal Sci. 4, 1–11.
32. Vollendorf, N. W., & Marlett, J. A. (1994) Cereal Chem. 71, 99–105.
33. Valiente, C., Esteban, R.M., Molla, E., & Lopez-Andreau, F.J. (1994) J. Food Sci. 59, 123–124, 141.
34. Fulger, C.V., & Bradbury, A.G. (1985) Modification of bran by extrusion, U.S. Patent 4,500,558.
35. Wang, W.-M., Klopfenstein, C.F., & Ponte, J.G. (1993) Cereal Chem. 70, 707–711.
36. Ralet, M.-C., Della Valle, G., & Thibault, J.-F. (1991) Lebensm.-Wiss. u.-Technol. 24, 107–112.
37. Artz, W.E., Warren, C.C., & Villota, R. (1990) J. Food Sci. 55, 746–750, 754.
38. Ning, L., Villota, R., & Artz, W.E. (1991) Cereal Chem. 68, 632–636.
39. Ralet, M.-C., Della Valle, G., & Thibault, J.-F. (1993) Carbohydrate Polymers 20, 17–23.
40. Camire, M.E., Zhao, J., & Violette, D. A. (1994) J. Agric. Food Chem. 41, 2391–2394.

41. Wang, W.-M., & Klopfenstein, C.F. (1993) Cereal Chem. 70, 712–715.
42. Gourgue, C., Champ, M., Guillon, F., & Delort-Laval, J. (1994) J. Sci. Food Agric. 64, 493–499.
43. Camire, M.E., Zhao, J., Dougherty, M.P., & Bushway, R. J. (1995) J. Agric. Food Chem. 43, 970–973.
44. Camire, M.E., Zhao, J., Dougherty, M.P., & Bushway, R. J. (1995) Cereal Foods World 40, 447–450.
45. Nyman, M. (1995) Eur. J. Clin. Nutr. 49, S215-S218.
46. Veena, A., Urooj, A., & Puttaraj, S. (1995) Die Nahrung 39, 132–138.
47. Sundberg, B., Abrahamsson, L., & Aman, P. (1994) Plant Foods Human Nutr. 45, 145–154.

26

Production of Resistant Starch

PIERRE WÜRSCH
Nestlé Research Centre, Vers-chez-les-Blanc, Switzerland

INTRODUCTION

Resistant starch (RS) is defined as the sum of starch and of the product of starch degradation not absorbed in the small intestine of healthy individuals. Most of the RS is formed in food during normal processing and much is known about how to promote its formation. Highest yields are achieved with potato and legumes (7% and 11% of total starch, respectively) due to the special nature of their starch. The main source of starch in the diet is cereal, in which only limited amounts of RS are produced by the usual processing, namely baking and extrusion cooking (2–6% of total starch). RS is constituted mainly of retrograded amylose, which consists of an association of the linear chains. Yields as high as 45% RS have been obtained with 70% amylose which is gelatinized and cooled under controlled conditions (concentration, temperature, storage time). The yield can be increased by subsequent hydrolysis of the unretrograded starch with enzymes. RS can be easily incorporated in food without altering the texture and appearance, partly due to its white color, bland taste, and microparticulate structure. It can thus be used as fat mimetic or to increase the dietary fiber content of food.

Resistant starch was identified in the early 1980s and for years remained just an analytical curiosity: Was it a starch or a fiber? How does one analyze it? How was it produced, and had it any physiological role? All these questions were systematically studied by a few groups (1–4) and in the early 1990s by Euresta (5). The first task was to define resistant starch (RS): ''the sum of starch and products of starch degradation not absorbed in the small intestine of healthy individuals'' (6). The RS population has been identified and quantified in vivo in a few studies. It appears to be composed of roughly two physically and/or chemically different groups of glucosidic polymers: digestible starch and dextrins, and retrograded starch (7–10). However, retrograded starch itself is composed of ordered structures of portions of double helical amylose chains which crystallize generally in B-type and amorphous portions which are not accessible to the pancreatic α-amylase (11,12). This is the fraction that has been defined as RS using the pancreatic α-amylase digestion method (13–15). The amorphous portion of RS seems to be hydrolyzed by thermally stable enzymes such as α-amylase from *Bacillus licheniformis* (Termamyl L) used in the analysis of the dietary fiber by the AOAC method (16,17), and in part by amyloglucosidase from *Aspergillus niger* (personal communication). Resistant starch recovered from extensive pancreatic α-amylase digestion had a chain length distribution between 15 and 80 glucose units (12,17), but this decreased to 15–65 glucose units when subsequently digested by Termamyl at 80°C. The fraction digested represented 35% of the RS (17). Consequently, the residual starch found in the dietary fiber fraction, sometimes defined as RS (4,9), represents only part of the starch resistant to digestive enzymes, which in turn is a significant fraction of the RS as defined above.

The RS measured in food using the simulation of digestion gives generally similar RS values as the in vivo measurements using ileostomy subjects (14,18–20). However, in some cases underestimation was found due to residual starch, dextrin, and sugars that are not accounted for in the in vitro method. In the case of white bean flakes, 3.4% of total starch was recovered in the dietary fiber residue (9), 11.5% was measured using pancreatic α-amylase (= RS) (5), and 16.5% was recovered in ileostomy effluents (9). Recovery of starch (including RS, residual starch, dextrin, and sugars) in ileostomy effluent, from cooked and cooled potato was as high as 12.2%, although the RS part of starch was 3.4% (8).

A simpler classification of RS has been proposed based on its physical nature: RS1, physically inaccessible starch; RS2, resistant native starch granules; and RS3, retrograded starch (13). These classes are described in more detail by Champ et al. (21). The measurement of RS following various methods creates a lot of confusion especially when the method applied is not stated. The data collected in this review are based on various methods; to avoid any misunderstanding, the method using pancreatic α-amylase will be referred to as method A and the one measuring starch in the dietary fiber residue as method B.

RESISTANT STARCH IN FOODS

Resistant starch is found in a few raw starchy foods, namely raw potato starch, green banana starch, and amylomaize starch (RS2). However, they become partially to totally digestible by hydrothermal treatment (cooking). Analysis of many processed food products indicates RS content is generally below 5% of the dry matter (Table 1), but a high amount of RS1 can be found in cereals which are cooked and eaten and in grains such as pearled barley, buckwheat or puffed wheat. RS in legumes is generally very high due to encapsulation of starch in the cells and its rather high amylose content (23).

Resistant starch in common foods can be increased by storing the wet cooked food in the cold, by heating and cooling, or by freezing. This is especially the case for potato and beans. Although instant mashed potato has negligible amounts of RS, deep-fat frying or storing cooked potato in the cold converts up to 12.2% of its starch into RS (7,24).

In the case of cooked cereal products (rice, pasta, bread), RS content does not seem to increase during storage or freezing. The best example is bread that has a rather stable resistant starch content, although amylopectin retrogradation occurs during storage (2,25). Retrogradation of amylopectin consists in the reassociation of external chains of the macromolecules, which have an average chain length of 13–16 glucose units in cereal starch. They are completely digested, but at a slower rate (26). Some endogenous or added lipids, although present in low quantity, reduce the RS yield. These lipids (monoglycerides, phospholipids) form enzyme-digestible inclusion complexes with amylose; less amylose is then available to form RS (27–29). The RS yield of autoclaved, non-defatted starch is 5.6%, and increased to 7.3% after lipid extraction, but was almost nil after addition of 3% SDS (28).

TABLE 1 Resistant Starch (Method A) Content in Common Foods

Food	% of total starch
Bread	2.2–4.3
Special breads	7.2–9.5
Breakfast cereals	0.0–9.0
Wholegrain cereals	1.7–12.3
Potato	0.6–9.0
Pasta	1.3–4.2
Pulses	12–20

PRODUCTION OF RESISTANT STARCH

Resistant starch is produced during processing and storage of starchy food, although the amount formed is quite limited. Processing involves the application of heat (cooking) and cooling. The starch is gelatinized in an excess of water, which leads to melting of the A- and B-crystalline forms and swelling by absorption of water at 50–80°C. Amylose re-adopts a helical structure upon cooling, reassociates, and progressively crystallizes into B-type crystals. However, RS also includes an amorphous portion of amylose, which is not hydrolyzed by α-amylase (12).

Crystallization derives from an amorphous matrix. It consists of three steps: 1. nucleation (i.e. formation of critical nuclei); 2. propagation (i.e. growth of crystals from the nuclei formed); 3. maturation (i.e. crystal perfection and/or continuing slow growth). The extent to which these processes occur is clearly dependent on the temperature and time. The nucleation rate is nil at the melting temperature of the crystal (130–150°) and increases with decreasing temperature. At the temperature below the glass transition temperature (ca. −5°) the nucleation rate is negligible and the system is frozen (30). The propagation rate is reversed. It increases with increased temperature. Thus, the conditions for fastest rate of RS formation must be found between these two temperatures. A compromise can be found by inducing nucleation at low temperature followed by propagation at a higher temperature.

Yield and quality of RS in a mixture of amylose and amylopectin thus greatly depends on the storage temperature. At 100°C for several days, 10% RS with an A-type crystalline structure is produced, and at between 0 and 70°C, 3–4% RS (method A) with a B-type structure (31).

Sievert and Würsch (29) studied the effect of heating and cooling of different starches in water. Melting transitions occurred at 140–160°C. On cooling, the chains of amylose reassociated between 60 and 40°C. Reassociation is, however, inhibited by fast cooling rates (>10°C/min), but when the linear chains were small, e.g. DP 65, reassociation occurred even at a very fast cooling rate, due to a much higher mobility of the chains.

The highest yield of RS is obtained by controlled retrogradation of amylose, high amylose starch, or debranched amylopectin and amylose after autoclaving. For pure pea amylose the optimum concentration is equal or higher than 10% and yields of up to 50% RS (method A) were obtained after one day of storage at room temperature (12). In starch, reassociation of amylose chains during retrogradation is lower since amylopectin apparently restricts the extent of conformational ordering of amylose chain (32). However, the RS content after extended storage time at subzero temperature was proportional to the amylose content (Figure 1). Furthermore, RS can be purified by enzymatic or acid hydrolysis to remove the amorphous regions of the starch molecule.

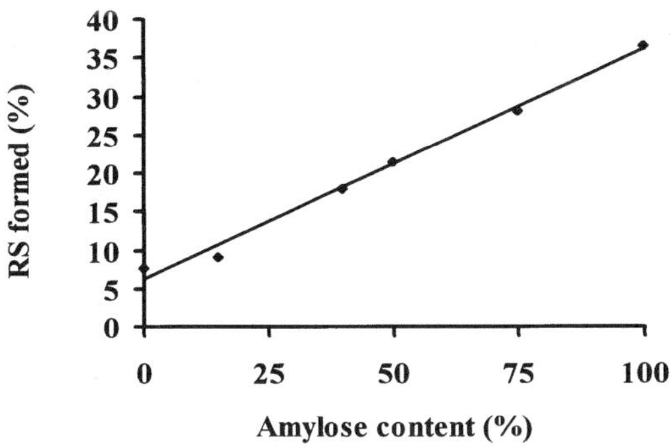

FIGURE 1 RS yield obtained after autoclaving and retrogradation of mixtures of amylose and amylopectin (method A).

Several patents have been filed over the last six years for the production of RS for use in food as bulking agent, dietary fiber, or fat mimetic (34–40). Generally starch is heated in water at more than 100°C to hydrate and gelatinize starch and then cooled for a sufficient time to cause starch retrogradation and formation of RS fractions. The yield of RS depends on the amylose content, and consequently the preferred sources are starches having 70% or more amylose content (amylomaize with 70 or 85% amylose, high amylose pea starch and high amylose barley starch). Starch is mixed in 3 to 10 volumes of water, but the highest RS yield is achieved with greater starch concentration (4,34–37). The suspension is heated in an autoclave at a temperature above 100°C to ensure starch gelatinization and complete disruption of the granules. High temperatures are particularly necessary for the high amylose starches (120–150°C). In one of the proposed processes (4,34), the mixture is then cooled to below room temperature to allow amylose retro-gradation to take place and the heating-cooling process is repeated up to three times (Table 2). The yield of RS is systematically much lower with method B used for RS determination compared with the milder pancreatic α-amylase assay shown in the last column. Storage at 4°C for periods of 2–24 hours is recommended to complete amylose reordering. RS contents increased when heating from 121 to 134°C, and decreased again at 148°C (4). The yield of RS shown in Figure 1 is inversely related to the amylose content.

RS3 has been produced by extrusion cooking of amylomaize starch in a double screw extruder with one volume of water added, followed by two days storage at 4°C, oven-dried and milled. The in vitro RS content was 30% (Table 3), but reached 49% in ileostomy subjects (19). This partially retrograded starch was used as the reference sample in the Euresta project. By autoclaving at 145°C

TABLE 2 Yield of RS after retrogradation and enrichment by enzymatic treatment with termamyl at 70–100°C

Starch	Amylose (%)	RS (%) Method B (4)	RS-enriched (%) Method B (34)	RS (%) Method A (3)
Amylomaize VII	70%	21.3	70.8	28.5
Amylomaize V	53	17.8		26.2
Pea starch	33	10.5	66	
Wheat starch	25	7.8	63.1	4.0
Maize	26	7	59.6	
Potato	20	4.4	48.6	
Waxy maize	<1	2.5		0.5

Starch:water ratio 1:3.5 for amylomaize VII and 1:2 for the others. Autoclaving temp. 134°C. Autoclaving time: 1h.

for 45 minutes, followed by freeze-drying, the in vitro and in vivo RS were comparable at 40% (40).

Alternatively 70% amylose starch was autoclaved at 150°C and retrogradation took place at room temperature for 20 hours (35). The retrograded amylose was then treated with acid for several hours at 70°C. The insoluble fraction was isolated by microfiltration of the slurry at around 95°C, and consists in a single domain that peaked at 120°C (RS3).

After autoclaving at >120°C for 8 hours, the slurry was maintained at 120°C for 8 hours, then 24°C for 16 hours and 8°C for 48 hours and hydrolyzed with a thermostable α-amylase. High yields were obtained with the enzyme from

TABLE 3 In vitro and in vivo RS content in starches (% starch)

Food Source	In vitro RS Method A (Ref.)	In vivo RS (Ref.)
Raw potato starch	65 (13)	84 (19)
Raw green banana starch	74 (13)	76 (19)
Amylomaize 85% amylose (in bread)	26 (46)	33 (46)
Raw amylomaize 70% amylose	69 (13)	51 (19)
Amylomaize 70% amylose (in bread)	38 (45)	ND
Autoclaved, retrograded high amylose starch	40 (40)	43 (40)
Extruded retrograded high amylose starch	30 (13)	49 (19)

Bacillus licheniformis at 70–100°C for about one hour. Up to 70% RS was found in the recovered residue (method B) (34,36). These ingredients have very low water holding capacity and a small particle size (<50 mm), making them advantageous as an insoluble bulking agent in extruded products and baked products (37).

The yield of RS thus can be increased by varying various processing steps and conditions as shown in Figure 2 (37). High amylose starch, after high temperature gelatinization (>150°C), contained 9.4% RS (method B), and 14.3% RS when followed by extrusion cooking. The RS was increased to 27% by enzymatic debranching of the gelatinized starch and fractionation. Extrusion cooking of the debranched high amylose starch yielded 30% RS. The highest yield was achieved by holding the debranched amylomaize slurry in a high salt solution at 95°C for 24 hours. The ethanol-water 1 : 1 insoluble fraction contained 44% RS.

RS has also been produced by mild heat-moisture treatment of amylomaize, but in this process no granule disruption occurred. A 15% aqueous slurry of maize starch containing 70% amylose was heated at 95°C and maintained at that temperature for 15–30 minutes under gentle mixing, cooled slowly to 30°C, reheated to 60°C, then finally cooled and spray-dried. The RS yield reached 42% (method A) (42). In a similar approach, 85% amylose starch was heated at 85°C for one hour followed by debranching with pullulanase. The RS content in the insoluble starch was 30% (method B)(43). The enzymatic hydrolysis with Termamyl during the heat treatment increased the concentration of RS. The enzyme produced only exoerosion and pits.

Up to 60% RS yield (method A) has been obtained by debranching with isoamylase, an aqueous slurry of at least 20% of a partially hydrolyzed starch (dextrose equivalent of 2–3) containing less than 40% amylose (44). However, native high amylose starch, which contains a very high amount of RS2, is a

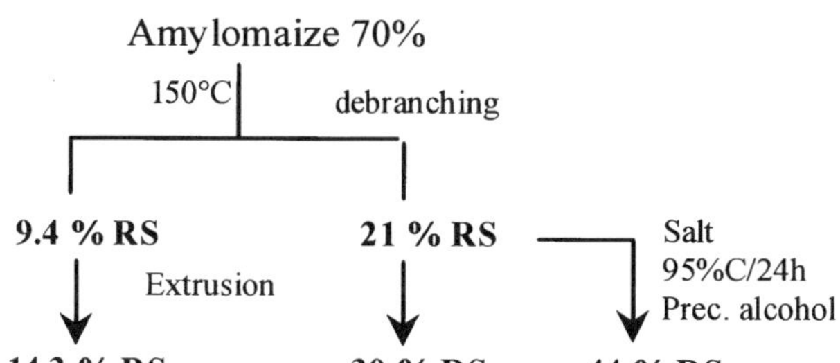

FIGURE 2 Yield in RS (method B) from amylomaize treated in different ways (method B).

readily available source of RS, or dietary fiber. Breads and breakfast cereals enriched with Hi-maize are already on the market in Australia (39,40). Bread has been enriched up to 11% RS (based on DM, method A) by replacing part of the flour by retrograded amylomaize (70% amylose) or native amylomaize and gluten without altering the texture and taste of the product (45). These application studies show that RS content in amylomaize is markedly lower, around 30–40%, after the processing of the food (Table 3).

Chemical modification of starch (CMS) can be another way to significantly reduce its digestibility. Chemically modified starches are widely used in the food industry as texture agent. Chemical modification such as substitution and cross-linking confers to the starch heat and shear resistance, and/or improved pH and freeze-thaw stability. The in vitro digestibility of acetylated and cross-linked gelatinized starches was nearly equal to native gelatinized starches (47), whereas etherification with hydroxypropyl groups significantly reduced the digestibility (47, 48). Increasing molar substitution (MS) decreased the in vitro and in vivo digestibility to around 42% for a MS of 0.16 (49). The undigested fraction was metabolized in rats only to a very limited extent due to the very high MS of this residue (DS = 0.6) (49). These studies and others indicate that only substitution with ether groups decreases the digestibility of gelatinized starch, but the resulting resistant starch is not metabolized by the intestinal microflora.

CONCLUSIONS

Resistant starch has been known for 15 years, and its chemical and physical natures have been well defined. The increase in RS in everyday food by processing adaptation is quite limited, thus the attention has been concentrated on high-amylose starch, particularly from corn, which is itself in great part resistant to digestion. Starches with 50% RS or more when the starch was purified can be produced, and they withstand heat treatment. These starches can be easily incorporated in food to increase the fermentable polysaccharide content without altering the sensory properties. RS is slowly fermented in the large intestine by the colonic flora. The metabolites formed include volatile fatty acids (acetic, propionic and butyric acids), resulting in a decrease in the pH of the feces (49,50). RS seems to yield more butyrate than some highly fermentable soluble fibers, which is of special interest regarding the prevention of colonic cancer (51).

REFERENCES

1. Englyst, H., Wiggins, H.S. & Cummings, J.H. (1982) Analyst 107, 307–318.
2. Siljestrom, M. & Asp, N.G. (1985) Z. Lebensm. Unters forsch. 148, 4–8.
3. Berry, C.S.J. (1986) Cereal Sci. 4, 301–314.
4. Sievert, D. & Pomeranz, Y. (1989) Cereal Chem. 66, 342–347.

5. Champ, M. (1992) Eur. J. Clin. Nutr. 46(Suppl.2), S51–S62.
6. Asp, N.-J. (1992) Eur. J. Clin. Nutr. 46(Suppl.2), S1.
7. Englyst, H.N. & Cummings, J.H. (1987) Am J Clin Nutr. 45, 423–431.
8. Englyst, H.N. & Cummings, J.H. (1985) Am. J. Clin. Nutr. 42, 778–787.
9. Schweizer, T.F., Andersson. H., Langkilde, A.M., Reimann, S. & Torsdottir, I. (1990) Eur. J. Clin. Nutr. 44, 567–575.
10. Faisant, N., Champ, M., Colonna, P., Buleon, A., Molis, C., Langkilde, A.-M., Schweizer, T., Flourié, B. & Galmiche, J.-P. (1993) Eur. J. Clin. Nutr. 47, 285–296.
11. Leloup, V.M., Colonna, P. & Ring, S.G. (1992) J. Cereal Sci. 16, 253–266.
12. Cairns, P., Sun, L., Morris, V.J. & Ring, S.G. (1995) J. Cereal Sci. 21, 37–47.
13. Englyst, H.N., Kingman, S.M. & Cummings, J.H. (1992) Eur. J. Clin. Nutr. 46 (Suppl.2), S33–S50.
14. Muir, J.G. & O'Dea, K. (1993) J. Am. Clin. Nutr. 57, 540–546.
15. Goni, I., Garcia-Diz, L., Manas, E. & Saura-Calixto, F. (1996) Food Chem. 56, 445–449.
16. Prosky, L., Asp, N.G., Schweizer, T.F., De Vries, J.W. & Furda, I. (1988) J. Assoc. Off. Analyt. Chem. 71, 1017–1023.
17. Würsch, P. & Koellreutter, B. (1992) Eur. J. Clin. Nutr. 46 (Suppl.2), S113–S116.
18. Muir, J.G., Birkett, A., Brown, I., Jones, G. & O'Dea, K. (1995) J. Am. Clin. Nutr. 61, 82–89.
19. Langkilde, A.M. & Andersson, H. (1994) in Proceeding of the concluding plenary meeting of Euresta, N.-G. Asp, J.M.M. van Amelsvoort & J.G.A.J. Hautvast (Eds.), Flair Food-linked Agroindustrial Research. pp. 31–32.
20. Silvester, K.R., Englyst, H.N. & Cummings, J.H. (1995) Am. J. Clin. Nutr. 62, 403–411.
21. Champ, M., Noah, L., Loizeau, G. & Kozlowski, F. (1998), Chap. 13, pp. 151–163.
22. Englyst, H.N. & Hudson, G.J. (1996) Food Chem. 57, 15–21.
23. Würsch, P., Del Vedovo, S. and Koellreutter, B. (1986) Am. J. Clin. Nutr. 43, 25–29.
24. Thed, S.T. & Phillips, R. D. (1995) Food Chem. 52, 301–304.
25. Rabe, E. & Sievert, D. (1992) Eur. J. Clin. Nutr. 46(Suppl.2), S105–S107.
26. Eerlingen, R.C., Jacobs, H. & Delcour, J. A. (1994) Cereal Chem. 71, 351–355.
27. Molis, C., Champ, M., Flourié, B., Pellier, P., Bornet, F., Colonna, P., Kozlowski, F., Rambaud, J.-C. & Galmiche, J.P. (1992) Eur. J. Clin. Nutr. 46 (Suppl.2), S131–S132.
28. Eerlingen, R.C., Cillen, G. & Delcour, J. A. (1994) Cereal Chem. 71, 170–177.
29. Sievert, D. & Würsch, P. (1993) Cereal Chem. 70, 333–338.
30. Levine, H. & Slade, L. (1984) in Dough Rheology and Baked Product Texture. H. Faridi & J.M. Faubion (Eds): Van Nostrand Reinhold, NY.
31. Eerlingen, R.C. & Crombez, M., Delcour, J. A. (1993) Cereal Chem. 70, 339–344.
32. Sievert, D. & Würsch, P. (1993) J. Food Sci. 58, 1332–1334.
33. Escarpa, A., Gonzalez, M.C., Manas, E., Garcia-Diz, L., Saura-Calixto, F. (1996) J. Agric. Food Chem. 44, 924–928.

34. Pomeranz, Y. & Sievert, D. Purified resistant starch products and their preparation. WO 90/15147.
35. Harris, D.W., Little, J.A., Stanley, K.D. Method of preparing reduced fat foods. WO-A-94/09645.
36. Iyengar, R., Zaks, A., Gross, A. A starch-derived, food grade, insoluble bulking agent. WO 91/07106.
37. Kevin, K. (1995) Food Processing 56, 65–67.
38. Chiu, C.-W., Matthew, H., Altieri, P. Process for making amylase resistant starch from high amylose starch. US Patent 5,281,276.
39. Brown, I.L., McNaught, K.J. & Moloney, E. (1995) Food Australia 47, 272–275.
40. McNaught, K.J, Maloney, E., and Knight, A.T. High amylose starch and resistant starch fractions. WO 94/03049.
41. Ekwall, H.R., Langkilde, A.M., Asp, N.-G., Björck, M.E. & Andersson, H. (1995) Scand. J. Nutr. 39, 145–150.
42. Baench, J., Gumy, D., Sievert, D. & Würsch, P. WO-A-96/03057.
43. Brown, I., Mc Naught, K.J., Ganly, R., Conway, P.L., Evans, A.J. & Topping, D.L. WO 9608261A1.
44. Anger, H., Kettlitz, B., Moorthamer, E. & Stoof, G. EP 688872.
45. Eerlingen, R.C., Van Haesendonck, L. P., De Paepe, G. & Delcour, J.A (1994) Cereal Chem. 71, 165–170.
46. Muir, J.G., Birkett, A., Brown, I., Jones, G. P. & O'Dea, K. (1995) Am. J. Clin. Nutr. 61, 82–89.
47. Oestergard, K., Björck, I. & Gunnarsson, A. (1988) Straerke 40, 58–66.
48. Mohd. Azemi, B.M.N. & Wootton, M., (1984) Staerke 36, 273–275.
49. Björck, I., Gunnarsson, A. & Oestergard, K. (1989) Staerke 41, 128–134.
50. van Munster, I.P, Tangerman, A. & Nagengast, K.N. (1994) Dig. Dis. Sci 39, 834–842.
51. Würsch, P. (1995) Lebensm.-Technol. 28, 434–440.
52. Cummings, J.H. & Macfarlane, G.T. (1991) J. Appl. Bacteriol. 70, 443–59.

27

Effect of Processing on Dietary Fiber in Foods

ECKHARD RABE
Federal Center for Cereal, Potato and Lipid Research, Detmold, Germany

INTRODUCTION

Thermal treatments such as baking, roasting, drying, microwaving, and extrusion-cooking can affect the amount and composition of dietary fiber. The making of bread is not accompanied by great changes in TDF during the different stages of preparation such as dough processing or baking. The content of insoluble hemicelluloses decreases as the content of the soluble hemicellulose increases. The RS content starting from the dough-making step results in higher dietary fiber values at the time of cooling. There is an elevated lignin content, especially in the crust, which increases with baking time. Baking of rye bread with sour dough or with lactic and acetic acid enhances the DF content by formation of RS and diminishes the non-starch polysaccharide fraction; the loss in the insoluble hemicelluloses starts with dough making. The cellulose is not degraded. The repeated heating of starch-rich foods like pasta, potatoes or rice shows the possibility of accumulation of RS. Cooking increases the DF content of potato by formation of RS. In vegetables and fruit the amount of pectic substances decreases with boiling. The greatest changes in the DF content is with extrusion cooking. The total amount of DF is nearly the same, as with most products. The content of soluble fiber increases with increased severity of treatment.

POSSIBLE CHANGES BY PROCESSING

Dietary fiber (DF) is defined as the material surviving digestion with human enzymes, but the different components, which form the DF complex, can be degraded or modified by other enzymes, e.g. microbial, by acids and bases or by temperature and pressure. While this either reduces the DF content or modifies it, new components, determined as DF, can be increased, too. During production of cereal foods and baked products, different treatments such as grinding, fermentation, cooking, baking, deep-fat frying, extrusion cooking, popping, or steam flaking are possible. This means conditions of temperature, pressure, heat treatment and shear force, electrolytes, and pH can change or be extreme and, therefore, alter DF values.

Heat treatment of starch-containing food may result in chemical modification and fragmentation of the starch. Changes in chemical characteristics may also alter physiological properties of the fiber. In this chapter, alterations in the DF content by physical adjustment or by making a product edible will not be considered. (Milling reduces the particle size, changing the DF content drastically. This reduction is due to the removal of the outer layer of the cereal grain, which contains the highest concentrations of DF. The peeling of fruit and tubers has the same effect.) Most plant food is consumed only after a mechanical and/or thermal treatment. Most fruits rich in pectins are consumed raw, while DF from cereals contain high amounts of hemicelluloses. Vegetables, on the other hand, are normally eaten after cooking in water. During cooking, hemicelluloses and pectins are leached into the water. These polymers can partly be disintegrated. Pectins are depolymerized by heat and cannot be found in the cooking water.

It is worth mentioning that even the preparation of samples for the analyses can partly enhance the DF content: drying and grinding of bread crumb, made only from wheat starch, was accompanied by an increase in the insoluble DF (IDF) content from 2.5 to 3.6% d.m. This was found with bread from normal flour, too. The reason is the building of enzyme-resistant starch (1).

The effect of fiber particle size on functionality has been addressed, and evidence was found that particle size is highly influential on the functionality and nutritional value of dietary fiber containing raw material. For instance, the bile salt-binding capacity decreases with decreased particle size (2). The susceptibility to fermentation in the colon of human subjects is inversely proportional to the size of bran particles (3). The moisture content in feces is significantly higher in humans given a coarse bran diet than in humans given a fine bran diet (4,5). The Englyst definition (6) of DF as non-starch polysaccharidic (NSP) cell-wall material has the benefit of not being effected by processing. So the NSP values for white, brown and wholemeal bread are very similar to the values for the corresponding flours from which they are made; total NSP in the crumb is also similar to NSP values for the breads. Arabinose content in the crust is slightly lower with a higher proportion of xylose residues being measured in the soluble fraction than in the crumb (7). On the other hand, if enzyme-resistant starch (RS) is unfermentable by human enzymes and only is degraded by the colonic microflora in the large intestine, it should be included in the DF value. This part of DF is not accounted for in the Englyst method.

There are different possibilities of changing the DF content by processing (Table 1). These may lead to increased solubility of the fiber, decreased dietary fiber content (if low molecular fragments are formed), and loss of physiological properties of the fiber.

Resistant starch (RS), which is retrograded amylose, is known to develop in starchy food after heating during the cooling period, the amount depending mainly on the content of amylose or the amylose/amylopectin ratio, respectively, and water. However, other important factors are the processing temperature, the physical form, degree of gelatinization, and cooling and storage conditions (1, 8–11). Raw and processed foods contain appreciable amounts of RS, depending on the botanical source of the starch and the type of processing. In the case of waxy maize starch (normally zero amylose content), yields of RS were extremely low at all temperatures in contrast to Hylon VII (nominal 70% amylose), for which yields were high (approximately 34%) (11). By autoclaving and cooling high-amylose corn starch several times, the amount of RS can be increased up to about 60%. DF determined by the AOAC method is known to contain the RS as part of the complex. Today RS is accepted as part of the DF complex (9,10).

Discrepancies in the declaration of the RS content of foods occur because RS was initially defined as that starch which was determined after solubilization

TABLE 1 Possible changes in DF content by processing

Leaching of SDF, like pectins or fragments of hemicelluloses, into the process water
Decomposition of SDF or IDF into fragments, not determined as DF
Decomposition of insoluble to soluble DF (accompanied with a relatively constant DF content)
Decrease of degradable products like starch or protein, which means an indirect DF enrichment
Formation of enzyme-resistant starch
Formation of acid-insoluble material Maillard products (“lignins”)
Increase of enzyme-resistant compounds such as Maillard products (“lignins”) and RS

with 2 M KOH or DMSO. RS was the starch solubilized in the DF residue or the difference in starch content with and without added DMSO. Different methods for starch determination were used, too. In products with a high starch to fiber ratio, formation of enzyme-resistant starch during processing may contribute significantly to the DF content of the product. RS has been identified in cooked and baked foods such as bread, boiled potatoes, pasta, legumes, porridge, and corn flakes at levels of 1–4 g/100 g d.m. Cooked, dried, and ground legume seeds, such as beans, which are rich in amylose, showed an RS content of 3–6%, which is considerably higher than that formed during baking of bread. As the raw beans showed 0.8% RS it may be that these products have a high content of RS2 (12,13), which is resistant starch like raw potato starch.

Although Englyst (14) proposed a method for the determination of different kinds of RS, which was accepted initially, there is still the need for a quick and reliable method, mainly for the determination of RS3, the retrograded amylose. The true RS content of foods may be higher than that recorded for RS3 in fiber residues since only a fraction of retrograded starch remains in the residues. The continuing development of new methods (15) shows there still is demand for it. Although interesting from a scientific point of view, the physically inaccessible kinds of RS are not of great importance, as most food is consumed after heating. To take this to the extreme, it means RS2 from potatoes should not be considered, because when they are consumed, there is only RS3. On the other hand, in eating raw cereals like muesli, there really is a greater consumption of RS2, physically trapped starch, but only a small part of the population consumes it.

The repeated heating of starch-rich foods (Table 2), measured by the IDF fraction, shows the possibility of accumulation of RS. Potatoes (variety ''Hansa'') were cooked in water, drained, cooled to room temperature, and stored in a refrigerator for 18 h (overnight). Heating of the cooked potatoes, the cooked polished rice, and the pasta (100% durum wheat) in the microwave oven was done without additional water.

It can be seen from Table 2 that the content of IDF, or of RS, respectively, is greater in products heated with excess water in a normal cooking pot than in products heated without water, e.g. in a microwave oven, as expected. On the other hand, in heating in the microwave oven, there was an increase, too. The highest amount of RS, compared to the original but low value for the uncooked food, was formed in rice heated in a normal cooking pot or a microwave oven. In pasta, too, there was a great increase, but only about half that in rice. The reason was that these foods are rich in amylose and underwent complete starch gelatinization during cooking. The least amount was formed in potatoes, independent of the method of heating. The decrease in RS in rice during heating in the normal pot results from the fact that in this case, there was a great amount of insoluble material poured away with the cooking water, which was opaque from it (16).

TABLE 2 RS formation in reheated foods as seen by IDF (% d.m.)

Food	Normal Cooking pot	Microwave oven	Pressure cooker
Potatoes, uncooked:	5.0%	—	5.8%
Cookng time: 15 min	7.2%	—	6.2% (6 min)
+ 2 min	8.3%	6.1%	8.6%
+ 2 min	8.9%	8.1%	9.8%
Rice, uncooked	1.0%		
Cooking time: 10 min	4.6%		
+ 2 min	7.9%	5.4%	
+ 2 min	5.1%	7.2%	
Pasta, uncooked	1.8%		
Cooking time: 12 min	4.0%		
+ 3 min	5.0%	4.4%	
+ 3 min	5.8%	4.8%	

As can be seen from these results, the reheating of already cooked pasta, (salad-) potatoes, and rice is a way to increase the RS or DF content, respectively, in normal starchy food without adding other material. In order to reach a higher intake of RS, consumers can be told to prepare a greater amount than is actually needed, refrigerate the surplus, and reheat as needed. This heating is best done with additional water and in a normal cooking pot or in a pressure cooker. The increase in the absolute amounts is relatively small after repeated heating/cooling cycles compared to the first heating (16).

EFFECTS OF PROCESSING ON DIFFERENT FOODS

Thermal treatments of wheat bran such as toasting, roasting, drum drying, autoclaving and drum drying, microwaving and drum drying, and extrusion do not significantly affect total DF content of wheat bran. Increased Klason lignin content of wheat bran is generally observed following thermal processing (17). Effect of dry heat on wheat bran was that toasting for 30 min and 60 min at 177°C resulted first in a decrease from 44.1% to 42.6% after 30 min and an increase to 51.3% after 60 min. The largest change was in the lignin fraction from 2.9% at time 0 to 4.3% after 30 min and 12.0% after 60 min of processing. Visually, the samples were significantly brown after 30 min and dark brown after 60 min of toasting. There was no significant difference in the hemicellulose content with processing; however, there was a small decrease in the cellulose content. Boiling wheat bran for 30 min had relatively little effect on the DF constituents. There was no significant difference in the hemicellulose or cellulose fraction; only a small but significant increase in the lignin fraction was realized. The major effects appear to have been a dramatic decrease in the pectic substances: wet heat tends to first solubilize the pectins and then destroy them. This effect was also found in boiling pureed carrots, but there was no significant difference in the lignin fraction of carrots (18).

Wheat and rye bran, extruded with or without addition of lactic acid, showed a significant loss of cellulose on one hand, and on the other an increase of ''lignins'' by Maillard products. As the reaction time is very short (about 40 seconds) compared to the baking time of pumpernickel bread (at least 16 hours), the changes are not that great. Extrusion with lactic acid results in an increase of the SDF as a disintegration of the IDF without changing the TDF content. Extrusion of wheat or rye flour under normal conditions does not result in production of high amounts of RS. This might be due to starch gelatinization, disintegration of the starch granule or even destruction of amylolytic enzymes. Another reason is the low water content ($< 20\%$), so that no gelatinization and no reorganization of the amylose molecules is possible (19). While under extreme extrusion conditions it was found that the amount of soluble fiber increased. Conversely, corn fiber, extruded at pH 3 to 11, showed statistically no change in their soluble and insoluble fiber content (20). An increase in SDF is expected to improve the nutritional value of fiber sources such as corn or soy bean hulls.

Cooking increases the DF content of potato. Wet heat processing, such as boiling, tends to first solubilize and then destroy the pectin substances by degrading galacturonan chains. Pectin molecules are depolymerized by chain splitting via β-elimination. Once the chain length of the degraded parts is small enough and the molecules are no longer bound in the framework of the cell wall gel by cations, pectic galacturonan is partly solubilized. Ions accelerate this breakdown. Calcium ions retard the solubilization of pectin in comparison with potassium. Calcium-binding anions (citrate, phytate and malate) favor the solubilization of pectin (21). The SDF of instant mashed potatoes and of French fries remain unchanged during domestic cooking. The major SDF constituents of potato have been identified as pectin and hemicellulose. Boiling and microwave-heating appear to increase the IDF of instant mashed potatoes. In French fries, deep-fat frying significantly increases the IDF while baking causes only a minor additional change in IDF fraction. The formation of lignin-like substances and enzyme-resistant starch is also responsible for the increased IDF. Since the SDF content in processed potato remains constant during cooking, any increase in TDF can therefore be attributed to the elevated IDF level. In French fries, baking does not alter the starch composition but deep-fat frying reduces digestible starch and significantly increases the amount of RS (22).

The amount of TDF [non-cellulosic polysaccharides (NCP) + cellulose] in untreated potato was 6.8% of dry matter. All treatments increased total DF, most changes being statistically significant. The maximum value was 10.9% (130°C, pH 4.2). Total DF in untreated, mashed tomatoes was 23.2%. Autoclaving without added water reduced it further to a minimum of 18.6% (130°C, pH 4.2). Baking in an oven increased the total DF in tomato to 26.0% d.m., while microwave treatment did not cause significant changes. Potato cellulose increased very significantly in all treatments, and most in the excessive autoclaving at 130°C. Lignin and cellulose contents of autoclaved tomato samples were smaller than those of untreated tomato. Baking increased the quantities of all constituents. Microwave treatment also significantly increased the NCP values of tomato. Acidification of the cooking water of potato or the tomato slurry did not have a clear effect on DF, but it tended to reduce the NCP values. Uronic acid concentration of tomato and potato was lowest in the samples autoclaved at 130°C. DF was increased more by boiling and pressure cooking than by baking or microwave treatment. The increment in the total DF was due to the increases in both water insoluble NCP and cellulose, and was evidently caused by retrograded starch. The total DF of tomato was lowered by all autoclave treatments, but only the changes at 130°C were statistically significant. Baking increased TDF significantly. This treatment caused considerable drying and scorching of the product, increasing not only the lignin, but also all other fractions (23). Cooking increases solubility of pectic substances while decreasing the water insoluble fraction. There is essentially no difference in the total insoluble pectic substances due to the method of cooking.

The DF contents in drum-dried wheat flour products are not significantly different from those of the unprocessed flours. Extruded flours, on the other hand, have a significantly lower content of insoluble fiber regardless of processing conditions. Extrusion cooking, autoclaving, steam flaking and, in particular, popping of wheat results in a redistribution of insoluble to soluble DF. The influence of the various processes on the TDF are small, but a slight solubilization of fiber components is observed for all processes, except drum-drying, when severe conditions were used (24).

The SDF fraction isolated from rye DF showed interesting properties. Partly hydrolyzed and marketed in dried form, they can be incorporated in rolls with a remarkable enrichment of the SDF of up to 150% related to the flour DF. A 10% enrichment of the rye SDF in mashed strawberries or raspberries, which means a consumption of 5.6 g SDF per day, were accepted by patients. In type II diabetics the DF showed a leveling effect to the course in the blood glucose (25).

The baking of bread (extraction flour or wholemeal) is not accompanied by great influences on DF during the different stages like dough processing, baking, storage, drying (freeze-drying or drying with normal pressure), freezing or thawing. Only the RS content, starting from the dough-making, growing during the baking process and resulting in the greatest differences during the time of cooling is the reason for higher DF values (26).

Because of the long and intensive influence of heat, the DF content of the crust differs from that of the crumb: on a dry matter basis the insoluble fiber content is lower. This is because of a lower content of RS, caused by the reduced availability of water. On the other hand, insoluble hemicelluloses become soluble. Dextrination can cause breaking of α-1,4-glucosidic bonds of starch. The arabinoxylans are more influenced by heat than the xylose chains. The cleaved xylose molecules are not determined as DF any more.

In relation to the used wholemeal wheat flour, the insoluble hemicelluloses are diminished by 1.1% d.m. in the crust after a baking time of 55 min compared to the corresponding wheat flour. After a baking time of 80 min there is a decrease of 2.1% d.m. Only small amounts of these show up as SDF. The cellulose is not affected by the heat (Table 3) (27). The rising of the lignin and protein content in the IDF residues is taken as a marker for condensation and polymerization reactions taking place in the crust, yielding nitrogen-containing substances, not degraded by the enzymes for DF determination. At the moment it is not clear if part of the insoluble DF is becoming soluble, and part of the soluble hemicellulose is hydrolyzed, or if a part of the insoluble hemicellulose is hydrolyzed directly to molecules not determined as DF. At low moisture levels, intramolecular rupture of α-1,4-linkages in starch produces oligosaccharides and more high-molecular fragments containing 1,6-anhydropyranose end-units. These anhydro units are

TABLE 3 Dietary fiber and components in bread and corresponding flour, %DM

	Components of IDF (29)				Components of TDF (27)		
	Hemicellulose	Cellulose	Lignin	RS	IDF	SDF	TDF
Wholemeal flour	5.5	1.5	0.8	< 0.1	8.2	2.6	10.8
Dough, freeze dried	5.5	1.8	0.7	< 0.1	8.1	2.5	10.6
Bread, whole, fresh baked 55 min	5.3	1.9	1.1	0.4	8.7	2.7	11.4
Crumb, fresh	5.4	1.8	0.9	0.4	8.5	2.6	11.1
Crumb, dried	5.5	1.8	1.0	0.6	8.9	2.5	11.4
Crust, baked 55 min	4.4	1.8	1.4	0.2	7.8	3.2	11.0
Crust, baked 80 min	3.4	1.7	2.7	0.1	7.9	2.7	10.6

Adapted from Refs. 27,29

able to react either with water, thus forming maltodextrins, or with hydroxyl groups on starch or other polysaccharides, to form new branched structures. Such new linkages are not degradable with amylolytic enzymes and represent an irreversible chemical modification (28).

Fermentation can also result in changes of the DF content. Total DF in natto and tempeh decreased slightly during fermentation. Pectic substances in natto increased 14% versus the control. Among component sugars, the relative amounts of arabinose, galactose, and galacturonic acid increased during the fermentation because of the growing of the bacteria, while no significant change was observed in the amount of DF. The hemicellulose fraction decreased in the case of tempeh during fermentation (30). During sourdough fermentation there is a decrease of the insoluble hemicelluloses by 2.7%, and even the soluble hemicelluloses are diminished by 0.9%; the xylose and arabinose are not determined as DF anymore (31).

Baking of rye bread with sour dough containing acetic and lactic acid enhances the DF content by formation of RS during cooling, too; on the other side, the non-starch polysaccharide (NSP) fraction is diminished. The same results are gained by addition of the acid itself or with wheat bread, baked with wheat-sourdough. The loss in the insoluble hemicelluloses starts with dough making, mainly by destruction of the xylose side chains, and mannose- and galactose-containing polymers, which does not result in a greater rising of the amount of soluble hemicelluloses; most are not determined as DF anymore. There is a greater influence of the acids on fine particles in flour than on coarse particles as DF is not protected by intact cell structures and there is more destruction during the baking process. During baking there is a further reduction of the insoluble hemicelluloses, accompanied by a rising of the soluble part, without a change in the arabinose/xylose ratio. In the crust there again is a reduction of the IDF accompanied by a higher SDF and an increase of the lignin fraction. Baking of pumpernickel bread, which has a long baking time (up to 24 hours), accompanied by lower baking temperatures (12°C) results in a continuing reduction of insoluble hemicelluloses, which in the end is about 2.4% lower than in the corresponding whole grain flour. Parallel to this is a modest rising in the soluble hemicelluloses and a continuous rise of the lignin and the RS content, so that in the end the DF in this process remains nearly constant (31).

It was shown (8) that low-temperature, extended (20 h at 120°C) baked wholemeal breads contain higher amounts of RS than a corresponding ordinary baked bread (40 min at 200°C): 3.0% or 5.4% (starch basis), respectively. With added lactic acid (10.5 g lactic acid, 90 wt%, with 650 g flour, pH 4.3) or lactic acid in combination with malt the RS formation was even more pronounced: 6.6% and 6.7% (starch basis), respectively. Addition of acetic acid on an equivalent molar basis did not exert this effect, nor did malt or malt in combination with acetic acid (8). With lactic acid added to bread baked under ordinary conditions, there was no increase in RS formation, which means the baking process is the important part in RS formation. Sourdough-baking is an old traditionally used process in Europe. Bread baked from flour containing a high amylose content, e.g. wholemeal high-amylose barley flour, with the low-temperature, extended process showed 7.7% RS (starch basis). This shows the formation of RS is strongly related to the amylose content.

The baking process increases the content of Klason lignin. Since phenolic propane lignin cannot be formed by baking, the increase is probably due to formation of highly resistant products such as Maillard products. Staling of bread affects neither the content nor the composition of DF. The formation of RS takes place within hours after gelatinization of starch. It involves recrystallization of the amylose fraction (linear-(1,4)-α-D-glucose) whereas staling involves retrogradation of amylopectin (branched (1,4),(1,6)-α-D-glucose). The slow retrogradation of amylopectin is due to difficulties with which bulky molecules crystallize. On the other hand, linear amylose molecules associate very easily and therefore retrograde easily (32).

Fiber enrichment in cereal products like bread or rolls is possible without difficulties with material such as bran. Changes of theses products by processing are very small compared to their DF content. As bakery products cannot further be heated and cooled again without changing their appearance by browning products dramatically, the best way to get more RS into bread is by enrichment of bread and fine baked goods with RS-rich material from high-amylose corn starch. This can be done without problems by minimal changes in the production process adjusting the water absorption; the bakery products show a whiter color than with wheat bran. The incorporated RS remains practically unchanged. Dried and ground crumb of wheat bread was added in concentrations of 5 and 10% to normal flour and bread baked from it. The IDF content raised from 1.4% to 1.5–1.6% with addition of 5% and to 1.7–1.8% with the addition of 10%. This small increase is because the RS is a minor component in the dried bread, too. But it shows RS is not affected by mixing, fermenting or baking. RS physiologically shows functions similar to DF, but technologically it shows the same properties as insoluble DF. Addition of 10% autoclaved wheat starch, high in RS, gives breads with RS contents that are three times that of normal breads. Because the production of RS is a costly procedure, especially if the product contains as much RS as possible (which means a further treatment with α-amylase), the RS enrichment in bread might be useful only in few cases, especially today where there is a growing interest in food prepared without ''additives.''

Eerlingen et al. replaced 24% of wheat flour with 4% vital gluten and 20% extruded, retrograded high-amylose starch. They produced breads with 8.4% RS d.m. and 6.1% d.m. DF and with an excellent taste and shelf life. But the RS level of the bread was lower than could be predicted from the analytical data of the starting material, which they thought might be due to some RS destruction in the bread making process. They found that the RS content in breads increased significantly after seven days of storage (about 3% d.m.), while the DF content remained unchanged. This indicates the observed increase could not be ascribed to the formation of resistant retrograded amylose, but it seems possible that retrogradation of amylopectin increased the resistance to hydrolysis of the starch. This was confirmed by DSC analysis (33).

Enrichment of cakes with fiber isolated from different seed hulls or waste pulp of pineapple resulted in cakes with TDF up to 8% d.m. with no altered sensory characteristics and volume. It was found that, although rich in insoluble fraction, the incorporated fibers did not reflect a proportionate increase in the insoluble fiber content of the products. This could possibly be due to heat processing, which is often known to reduce the IDF components followed by a release of SDF (34).

When the brown seaweed hijiki (*Hizikia fusiformis*) was steamed for 6 h or the brown seaweed kombu (*Laminaria ochotensis*) and the red seaweed nori (*Porphyra* spp.) were boiled for 2 h (these treatments simulate conventional processing of the seaweed), the SDF of all three seaweeds increased during heat processing. Molecular weight of the soluble fraction decreased during heat treatment, the decrease being greatest in nori (boiling for 1 h decreased Molecular weight to 15% of the value in non-heated samples). IDF content decreased during heating, the decrease being greatest for kombu (boiling for 1 h reduced the value to approx. 40% of the IDF content of raw samples). Molecular weights of the main leached-out fractions were comparable to those of the SDF (35).

Total DF in 15 kinds of fresh and cooked vegetables commercially available was 1.1 to 6.2 g/100 g fresh weight, and the ratio of insoluble to soluble DF was from 90:10 to 58:42 according to the kind of sample. TDF in normally cooked vegetables was 1.4 to 5.6 g/100 g weight, and the ratio of insoluble to soluble DF was from 86:14 to 57:43. Changes in TDF contents during normal heat treatment occurred in edible burdock, green peas with pod, garland chrysanthemum, Japanese radish, eggplant, Chinese cabbage, spinach and sweet pepper. The changes were within 6 to 17%. Turnip, cauliflower, cabbage, onion, Chinese chives, carrot, and broccoli showed little or no change in content during normal heat treatment. DF was further decreased by boiling for up to 22.5 min in turnip, cauliflower, edible burdock, Japanese radish, eggplant, carrot, Chinese cabbage, and sweet pepper, whereas the content did not change in other vegetables (36).

EFFECTS OF DIFFERENT PROCESSES

Temperature changes in extrusion-cooking are less important than those observed for mechanical energy. Solubilization results from mechanical transformation rather than from thermal effects. The total amounts of DF are similar (50.4–

52.2%) for most of the extruded products (Table 4) (37). A remarkable fact is that the content of soluble fiber increases from 8 to 16% with increased severity of treatment. The xylose to arabinose ratio in the SDF increased after extrusion-cooking indicating preferential solubilization of slightly branched arabinoxylans. Phenolic acids, mainly ferulic acid, which are ester-linked to the arabinoxylans, are also solubilized. Water absorption capacity, as measured by the Baumann method, increases from 270 for untreated bran to 375% for the products processed under low severity treatments (6).

The influence of various processes on the TDF content is small. The most significant changes are found when autoclaving or popping under severe conditions. These processes decrease the TDF content by 0.7% and 2.0-3.2% d.m., respectively. The effect of autoclaving is mainly seen as a loss of arabinoxylans. These components are known to be sensitive to thermal degradation under the weakly acidic conditions commonly prevailing in foods. Processing under severe conditions produces a redistribution of DF from insoluble to soluble, most pronounced in the case of popping (24).

Deep fat frying does not change the DF content very much, because the water content of the products is nearly the same as in the dough (loss about 10%) and the frying time is not very long. The same processes take place in the crust of bread, i.e., changing from insoluble to soluble hemicelluloses and building of "lignins"; the temperatures are not that high (about 180°C) (26). During the production of normal pasta, the changing DF content is only affected by RS. After cold extrusion of the pasta dough, the RS content of the fresh pasta is about 0.8% d.m., changing to negligible amounts (0.1%) after drying for 12 hours. The explanation is this RS might be formed during the hydrolysis for the DF determination. Only small amounts of hemicellulosic material are leached into the water during cooking of pasta in plenty of water. On the other hand, non-

TABLE 4 Insoluble, soluble, and total DF content (%DM) of wheat bran after different conditions of extrusion cooking

Screw speed (rev/min)	Water added (% of dry matter)	Product temperature (°C)	Spec. mechanical. energy (KWh/t)	Dietary fiber		
				Insol.	Sol.	Total
250	17.5	120	232	41.4	10.8	52.2
250	8.7	126	301	38.3	12.0	50.3
240	11.3	113	316	37.3	13.9	51.4
240	6.1	105	386	30.7	16.0	46.7

Adapted from Ref. 37

DF-material is extracted into the water, too, resulting in higher DF values. This is also found with cooked vegetables. On the other hand, RS is built in large amounts (about 1% d.m.), because during cooking, the starch is completely gelatinized. During cooling more amylose can recrystallize than in bread, where the available water is limiting this process. Corresponding to this, more RS is found in bread that was baked with higher amounts of dough water (38).

HTST (high-temperature, short-time) extrusion-cooking causes a redistribution of insoluble to soluble DF with a constant TDF content. Thus in raw wheat flour 40% of total fiber is soluble versus 50-75% in the extruded products. Even in the products processed under mild conditions (screw speed 150 rpm, mass temperature 161°C), the redistribution is statistically significant. In raw whole grain wheat flour, 15% of the total fiber is soluble, versus about 20% after processing. Extrusion cooking of pure wheat starch does not affect its digestibility. However, extrusion cooking of wheat flour increases the fermentability. No such effect is obtained with extruded whole grain wheat flour. Extrusion cooking primarily affects the fermentability of the smaller fiber fraction connected with the endosperm. In extruded wheat flour, the solubilization of fiber might be a factor in increasing the availability to microorganisms. In general, soluble fiber is more easily fermented than insoluble fiber (19,39).

Considering the different components of IDF, i.e., cellulose, lignins, and insoluble hemicelluloses, it is the hemicelluloses that are broken down during processing. Cellulose and lignins are resistant to the attack of acids in concentrations used in food processing. Enzymes like cellulase, which can degrade cellulose and lignins, but which are proteins, are inactivated soon after the beginning of the heating. That means these enzymes can only act during the period before baking, proofing, or fermentation. Heating, on the other hand, induces the building of new structures as temperature and time chemical reactions start. These reactions become evident with the appearance of browning products by the Maillard reaction. As the resulting products can be quite complex, they show the same attributes as lignins, e.g. insoluble and undegradable. In SDF, it is mainly the pectins and soluble hemicelluloses that are degraded. If there is enough water, as in cooking fruit and vegetables, hemicelluloses and pectins are leached into the water. Wet heat first solubilizes the pectins and then destroys them by degrading the galacturonan chains. In products rich in starch or amylose, there is the building of the enzyme-resistant starch fraction in cooling after the heating-process. Generally, the level of water soluble fraction increases with severity of processing conditions, the water soluble fraction coming mainly from hemicellulose (18). Extrusion most significantly modifies the properties of DF.

Altogether, processing under normal conditions has little effect on the amount of TDF content when expressed on an "as is" basis. Results on dry matter basis are more affected. Additionally, other, indirect effects can also be seen: cooking can cause a small but significant increase in DF due to loss of non-fiber components, resulting in an ''enrichment'' of the fiber. Deep-fat frying, on the other hand, results in a dilution of the DF due to the incorporation of fat in the baked goods. Different methods of DF and RS determinations might be the reason for conflicting results. Considering the small amount of dietary fiber in and consumed from vegetables and fruits, the changes in DF by processing may not be of physiological significance. Physically modified high-fiber products such as wheat bran with an altered relation of soluble and insoluble dietary fiber may be of interest in the future as the physiological effects with the components of the fiber.

REFERENCES

1. Sievert, D., Seibel, W., Rabe, E. & Pfeilsticker, K. (1987) Getreide Mehl Brot 41, 172–177
2. Mongeau, R. & Brassard, R. (1982) Cereal Chem. 59, 413–417
3. Brodribb, A.J.M. & Groves, C. (1978) Gut 19, 60–65
4. Wyman, J.B., Heaton, K.W, Manning, A. P. & Wicks, A.C.B. (1976) Am. J. Clin. Nutr. 29, 1474–1479
5. Björck, I., Nyman, M. & Asp, N.-G. (1984) Cereal Chem. 61, 174–179
6. Englyst, H.N., Quigley, M.E. & Hudson, G.J. (1995) European J. Clin. Nutr. 49, Suppl.3, S48–S62
7. Englyst, H.N., Anderson, V. & Cummings, J.H. (1983) J. Sci. Food Agric. 34, 1434–1440
8. Liljeberg, H., Akerberg, A. & Björck, I. (1996) Food Chem. 56, 389–394
9. Delcour, J. A. & Eerlingen, R.C. (1996) Cereal Foods World 41, 85–86
10. Eerlingen, R.C. & Delcour, J.A. (1995) J. Cer. Sci. 22, 129–138
11. Berry, C.S. (1986) J. Cereal Sci. 4, 301–314
12. Tovar, J., Björck, I. M. & Asp, A.-G. (1990) J. Agric. Food Chem. 38, 488–493
13. Tovar, J., Björck, I. M. & Asp, A.-G. (1980) J. Agric. Food Chem. 38, 1818–1823
14. Englyst, H. N., Kingman, S. M. & Cummings, J. H. (1992) European J. Clin. Nutr. 46, Suppl.2, S33–S50
15. Goni, I., Garcia-Diz, L., Manas, E. & Saura-Calixto, F. (1996) Food Chem. 56, 445–449
16. Rabe, E. (1994) in: Asp, N.-G., van Amelsvoort, J.M.M. & and Hautvast, J.G.A.J. (Ed.) Proceedings of the concluding plenary meeting of EURESTA–Wageningen: EURESTA, 146–148
17. Jae-Kwan, H., Chong-Tai, K., Sung-Ja, C. & Chul-Jin, K. (1995) Korean J. Food Sci. Technol. 27, 394–403; from English summary
18. Anderson, N.E. & Clydesdale, F. M. (1980) J. Food Sci 45, 1533–1537
19. Seibel, W. Sievert, D. & Seiler, K. (1988) Mühle + Mischfuttertechn. 125, 487–489
20. Artz, W.E., Warren, C. &Villota, R. (1990) J. Food Sci. 55, 746–750,754
21. Keijbets, M.J.H., Pilnik, W. & Vaal, J.F.A. (1976) Potato Res. 19, 289–303
22. Thed, S.T. & Phillips, R. D. (1995) Food Chem. 52, 301–304

23. Varo, P., Veijalainen, K. & Koivistoinen, P. (1984) J. Food Technol. 19, 485–492
24. Siljeström, M., Westerlund, E., Björck, I., Holm, J., Asp, N.-G. & Theander, O. (1986) J. Cereal Sci. 4, 315–323
25. Gebhardt, E. (1996) Ernähr./Nutr. 20, 397–405
26. Sievert, D., Seibel, W., Rabe, E. & Pfeilsticker, K. (1988) Getreide Mehl Brot 42, 48–152
27. Sievert, D., Seibel, W., Rabe, E. & Pfeilsticker, K. (1989) Ernähr./Nutr. 13, 75–81
28. Siljestöm, M., Björck, I. and Westerlund, E. (1989) Starch/Stärke 41, 95–100
29. Meuser, F., P. Suckow and W. Kulikowski (1985) Z. Lebensm. Unters. Forsch. 181, 101–106
30. Taguchi, K., Kawabata, M., Ohtsuki, K. & Tanaka, Y. (1986) J. Japan. Soc. Nutr. Food Sci. 39, 203–208; from English summary
31. Sievert, D., Seibel, W. Rabe, E. & Pfeilsticker, K. (1988) Getreide Mehl Brot 42, 172–176
32. Hansen, H. B., Östergaard, K. & Bach Knudsen, K.E. (1988) J. Cereal Sci. 7, 135–144
33. Eerlingen, R. C., van Hesendonc, I. P. dePaepe, G. & Delcour, J.A. (1994) Cereal Chem. 71, 165–170
34. Sreenath, H.K., Sudarshanakrishna, K.R., Prassad, N.N., and Santhanam, K. (1996) Starch/Stärke 48, 72–76
35. Suzuki, T., Nakai, K., Yoshie, Y., Shirai, T., & Hirano, T. (1993) Bul. Japan. Soc. Sci Fisheries 59, 1371–1375; from English summary
36. Takahishi, R., Ogawa, H., Satoh, E. & Mori, B. (1989) Japan. J. Nutr. 47, 189197; from English summary
37. Ralet, M.-C., Thibault, J.-F. & Della Valle, G. (1990) J Cereal Sci. 11, 249–259
38. Sievert, D., Seibel, W., Rabe, E. & Pfeilsticker, K. (1988) Getreide Mehl Brot 42, 259–264
39. Björck, I., M. Nyman and N.-G. Asp (1984) Cereal Chem. 61, 174–179

28

Application of Complex Carbohydrates to Food Product Fat Mimetics

SUSAN SUNGSOO CHO
The Kellogg Company, Battle Creek, Michigan
LEON PROSKY
Prosky Associates, Rockville, Maryland

INTRODUCTION

Except in cases of obesity, where the energy consumed had to be reduced in order to lose weight, fat in the diet and its effect on the overall health of the consumer was hardly considered to be of importance until the 1980s. Reduced-calorie foods shared a small portion of the market, which was directed toward persons with obesity or persons deciding to maintain their body weight through calorie restriction. For the most part, calorie reduction was sought through the reduction in the intake of carbohydrates even though carbohydrate restriction resulted in smaller calorie reductions compared to fats.

Consumers are growing increasingly aware of the link between fat intake and excess weight and heart disease. Dietary recommendations are to reduce the current fat intake at 37% of calories to no more than 30% (1). Unfortunately, this task is made more difficult by the presence of hidden saturated fat present in processed foods, particularly packaged dry goods (2). Nevertheless, over the past 15 years, low-fat food products incorporating fat substitutes or replacers have risen exponentially to meet consumer demand. The major classes of fat replacers are carbohydrates, proteins, emulsifiers, reduced-calorie fats, and synthetic fats. The focus of this chapter will be on carbohydrate-based replacers and their functions in low-fat products. But first, some of the reasons for the shift towards consuming less fat will be discussed.

FAT INTAKE AND DISEASE

There is a growing body of evidence that suggests high fat intake may specifically contribute to overeating and obesity, more so than other dietary energy sources like carbohydrates. Although fat is energy dense, it appears to have a weak effect on satiety (3). In contrast to the carbohydrates, fat oxidation seems to be is largely unrelated to fat intake, and dietary fats are more efficiently used and more readily converted to body fat (3). In fact, recent evidence suggests that carbohydrates may not make a significant contribution to body fat in humans under normal feeding conditions in humans (3). Finally, there is longitudinal data that point to a causal relationship between fat intake and weight gain over time in certain individuals (3).

Official recommendations are based on the evidence that reduced fat, particularly saturated fat, leads to a reduction in serum cholesterol, a known risk factor for coronary heart disease. Some investigators have also postulated that a reduction in fat intake may decrease mortality from breast, colon, and prostate cancers (4–6). Browner and colleagues have estimated that if the population were to follow the current dietary recommendations for fat intake, coronary heart disease mortality rates could decrease as much as 20% depending on age (7). Based on their assumptions of the relationship between fat intake and heart disease and cancer, they have also estimated that 42,000 of the 2.3 million adult deaths occurring in the U.S. each year could be deferred (7).

The general consensus is that both the quantity and type of dietary fat are important in preventing certain chronic diseases such as coronary heart disease. The Eskimos, for example, ingest mainly a high fat diet of fish, and experience less coronary heart disease and thrombosis than persons eating the high fat diets that contain mostly saturated fats (9). The major mechanism would seem to be the effects of the fats on the proportion of serum cholesterol associated with the high-density lipoproteins (HDL) as compared with the serum cholesterol associated with the low-density lipoproteins (LDL). That is, the diets that have a higher proportion of polyunsaturated fats, such as those diets that contain fish and certain vegetable sources or the monounsaturated (e.g. olive oil) fats, tend to reduce the risk from CHD. Conversely, diets rich in saturated fats increase the ratio of LDL-cholesterol to HDL-cholesterol increasing the risk of a coronary heart disease incident (9,10). However, it is not quite as simple as it seems because different saturated fats and dietary sources of saturated fat have different influences on the level of LDL-cholesterol (11). For example, dairy products which are high in myristic acid (14:0) appear to increase levels of LDL-cholesterol whereas beef fat, containing palmitic (16:0) and stearic (18:0) acids, do so to a lesser extent and cocoa butter, with a high proportion of stearic acid, increases LDL-cholesterol only slightly. This would strongly indicate that other dietary constituents are interacting and playing a vital role in this process.

DEVELOPMENT OF THE FAT REPLACER MARKET

In the 1980s, significant changes in the official nutritional recommendations were made when the relationship of carbohydrates and of fats to diet and health were better understood. Reports of the National Advisory Committee on Nutrition Education (NACNE) and the Committee on Medical Aspects of Food Policy (COMA) in the United Kingdom indicated that fat intake should be reduced from 42%, at the time, to 34% or 35% of total food energy in the diet (12,13). Further recommendations were to reduce the intake of saturated fat to 10% (NACNE) or 15% (COMA) of the food energy, to decrease salt intake, and to increase in the consumption of complex carbohydrates and dietary fiber (12,13).

Similar developments took place in the United States. The U.S. Surgeon General published a major review on nutrition and health proposing that the dietary energy from fat be reduced to 30% (1). A further review carried out by the National Academy of Sciences (14) resulted in the U.S. government report "Nutrition and Your Health: Dietary Guidelines for Americans" (15). Recent data from the Third National Health and Nutrition Examination Survey (NHANES III, 1989–91) showed that Americans are currently consuming approximately 34% of their total calories as fat (16), but this is still considerably higher than the goal.

Nevertheless, there is an increasing trend to reduce dietary fat intake by consuming low-fat and reduced-fat foods (17). The production of low-fat, high-fiber products came to the forefront with the U.S. Food and Drug Administration (FDA) final rule published in the Federal Register. The ruling stated that the grams of total dietary fiber could be subtracted from the grams of carbohydrate of the food before using the Atwater conversion factor (4 kcal/g) to determine the caloric content of the food (18). This provided a mechanism for calorie reduction through the ingestion of more fruits, cereal grains, and vegetables, all containing high dietary fiber, and manufacturing of foods supplemented with dietary fiber fractions. At the present time, only the insoluble dietary fiber may be subtracted from the carbohydrate content before calculating the calorie content of the food (19).

However, the major reduction in calories could only be obtained when along with the higher content of dietary fiber, the fat in the product could be replaced by a fat substitute. Because of consumer demand for low-fat and low-cholesterol products, reduced-calorie and low-fat or fat-free food products represent the fastest-growing segments of the food industry (20). It has been estimated that the total retail sales of all products using fat substitutes would reach $6.2 billion in 1996 (20).

In order to be a successful reducer of fat content of a food, the fat replacer or substitute must impart certain characteristics to the food product. Among these are flavor, mouthfeel, texture, structure, process performance, shelf life and appearance. The sensation of a fatty mouthfeel is formed by a combination of several inadequately defined and quantified parameters including viscosity, absorption, cohesiveness, and waxiness (21). The food industry has also found that instead of trying to match particular products, it may be better to create something different. Many times a familiar brand name may at first attract persons to the product, but it also gives them a standard frame of reference. Sometimes the process must be dramatically altered to accommodate the new formulation and yet yield a product similar to full-fat product.

The real potential for growth of low-fat foods and therefore fat replacers depends upon the quality of the low-fat product, technology to further improve quality, marketing to widen the range of low-fat foods, and consumer willingness to accept low-fat foods as an essential part of their diet (21). The taste and texture of low-fat foods must be equivalent to that of standard products for consumer acceptance. Consumers will not trade off product quality even if the product is perceived to have healthy aspects which are important to the consumer (17). Many of the lightly processed low-fat cheeses, biscuits, and mayonnaise produced to date have failed in this regard. Sauces and dressings have been more successful because the strong flavor systems are largely independent of fat content (21).

CARBOHYDRATE-BASED FAT REPLACERS

The major carbohydrate-based fat substitutes include starches, maltodextrins, polydextrose, altered sugars, pectin, gums, and other dietary fibers. By stabilizing substantial quantities of water in a gel-like matrix, this group of fat replacers mimics some of the textural and functional characteristics of fat. The functionalities of the different carbohydrate-based fat replacers are described below. Most of the carbohydrate-based ingredients are "label-friendly" and have GRAS (Generally Recognized As Safe) status by the U.S. FDA. However, certain carbohydrate-based fat substitutes (e.g. polydextrose, xanthan gum, and gellan gum) are approved for use only in specific applications (22,23). An extensive listing of companies that have produced carbohydrate-based products to reduce, extend, or replace fat in low-fat products are listed in a chapter by Jones (25). The leading manufacturers and their products are shown in Table 1.

Polydextrose

Polydextrose is prepared by vacuum thermal polymerization of glucose, using sorbitol as a plasticizer and citric acid as a catalyst (25). Although 1–6 glycosidic bonds predominate (both alpha and beta), polydextrose is composed almost entirely of randomly cross-linked glucose polymers. The energy value of polydextrose is only 1 kcal/g because the random bonding renders it relatively resistant to digestive enzymes, with a large proportion excreted unchanged in the feces (26). Because of the low digestibility of polydextrose, laxative effects have been observed above the threshold value of 90 g/d (26). No deleterious effects of polydextrose have been observed in animal testing, and it does not appear to interfere with the absorption and utilization of essential vitamins, minerals, or amino acids (27).

Polydextrose exists in five forms, all of which are highly stable (28). The original polydextrose powder is available in coarse (Pfizer, Inc.) and fine (A. E. Staley) granulations and has a tart/bitter aftertaste (pH of 2.5 to 3.5). Type N polydextrose is a 70% solution neutralized with potassium hydroxide to a pH of 5.0 to 6.0 and has been described as being slightly sweet-salty-bitter (26–28). Type K polydextrose is a powder buffered to the same pH as type N with potassium bicarbonate. In solution, polydextrose type K has a slightly sweet-sour-bitter taste (30). The fourth form, type F (Litesse®, Pfizer, Inc.), is an improved polydextrose powder with reduced titratable acidity and a bland/neutral taste. The recently developed Litesse II® (Pfizer, Inc.) has tenfold lower titratable acidity than Litesse and has been described as having a clean, mildly sweet taste. With lower acidity levels, Litesse II can be used at much higher concentrations than previous versions of polydextrose and has negligible sucrose inversion and minimal effects on fat rancidity (26).

As a low-calorie bulking agent, polydextrose reduces the calories of full-sugar foods while maintaining body and texture. Polydextrose can also contribute to the mouthfeel and creaminess of fat-reduced formulations because of its high viscosity in solution (26). Because polydextrose slows moisture changes in foods, its use in dry mixes improves flowability, assures uniform dispersion, and prevents lumping (28). The essentially bland taste of polydextrose renders it applicable to both sweet and savory applications. However, certain sweet products, such as confectionary, usually require the addition of a high intensity sweetener like aspartame, acesulfame-K, or alitame (26). An example of a low-fat confectionary product containing polydextrose is Lo, launched in 1991 by the Leaf Group in Finland. Thus, polydextrose has been used in the preparation of bakery goods

TABLE 1 Carbohydrate-based fat replacers and their manufacturers

Trade Name	Manufacturer/Developer	Product Components
AF Fiber®	ITD Corp.	Almond hemicelluloses
Amalean I™, Amalean II™	American Maize Products Co.	Modified high amylose maize starch
Avicel®	FMC Corp.	Microcrystalline cellulose + carboxymethylcellulose gel
Avicel® RCN-30	FMC Corp.	Cellulose + maltodextrin + xanthan gum
Avicel® RCN-15, Avicel® RCN-10	FMC Corp.	Cellulose + guar gum
CentuTex	Woodstone Foods	Golden pea fiber
C*Pur 01906	Cerestar	Potato maltodextrin
Fibercel	Alpha-Beta Technology	β-Glucan from yeast
Fibrex®	Delta Fibre Foods	Sugarbeet fiber
Fibrim®	Protein Technologies International	Soy hemicelluloses
Fibruline	Cosucra	Inulin
Frutafit	Suiker Unie	Inulin
Kelcogel	Kelco	Carrageenan
Kelcogel BF	Kelco	Gellan gum
Kel-Lite	Kelco	Xanthan/Guar gum blend
Litesse®, Litesse® II	Pfizer Food Science	Polydextrose
Natureal	Alko	Oat starch, oat fiber
N-Lite™	National Starch and Chemical Co.	Starch
Novagel™ NC 200	FMC Corp.	Microcrystalline cellulose + carageenan
Nutricol®	FMC Corp.	Konjac flour gel
Paselli Excel	Avebe	Maltodextrin
Pretested Colloid No Fat 102	TIC Gums	Gum arabic, modified starch, and alginate blend
Raftiline®	Orafti	Inulin
Raftincreaming®	Tiense Suikkerraffinaderij Services	Inulin
Slendid™	Hercules	Pectin gel
Solka Floc®	James River Corp.	β-1,4-Glucan polymer
Stellar™	Amylum	Maize starch
TrimChoice (Oatrim)	A. E. Staley Manufacturing Co. (ConAgra Specialty Grain Products)	β-Glucans (dextrins) from oat flour
Vitacel	J. Rettenmaier and Sohne	Microfibrillated wheat fibers + maltodextrin

and baking mixtures, in confectionery products to partially replace either sugar (including corn syrup) or fat, in frozen desserts and dairy products to replace sugar and butter fat, and in fruit jellies (29). In contrast to other high-weight polysaccharides, polydextrose can achieve a 90% or greater calorie reduction in gelatin-type desserts. Polydextrose has also been shown to provide mouthfeel, viscosity, and bulk to low-fat spoonable and pourable dressings (26).

Maltodextrins

The success of starchy products in reducing the fat content in food formulations is partially dependent upon having particle sizes small enough to simulate fat emulsions. Small particle native starches from certain grass and cereal seeds exist, but their use is uneconomical due to the production costs involved in their preparation (17). For this reason, enzymatic degradation of starch polysaccharides has been employed to produce maltodextrins as fat replacers. Typical starch sources are corn, potato, tapioca, and rice. With dextrose equivalents (DE, an indication of the extent of starch hydrolysis) below 20, maltodextrins are highly digestible (supplying 4 kcal/g), are easy to blend with other dry ingredients, are readily dissolved, and have low viscosity in solution (30). Low-DE maltodextrin gels (consisting of 1 part maltodextrin and 3 parts water) only have 1 kcal/g.

The most useful characteristic of maltodextrins in fat replacement is their ability to form thermoreversible gels that melt upon heating and reset to comparable gel strength when cooled (31). The main function of the soft and spreadable maltodextrin gels is to provide texture and mouthfeel simulation of fats in food products. Maltodextrins may also act as bulking agents. However, like native starches, maltodextrins have the tendency to retrograde slowly in food products during storage (31). Low-DE (i.e. DE < 5) maltodextrins can also exhibit variable freeze-thaw stability, unreliable heat and acid stability, and an undesirable starchy flavor to delicate foods if used at high concentrations (38). Many stable food starches used as fat replacers are chemically modified to be resistant to temperature, shear, and low pH levels encountered in processing (17,28) (Table 1).

Low-DE maltodextrins derived from potato starch have advantages over those produced from other starch sources. Potato starch is thought to retrograde less readily than other starches because of its longer chain amylose molecules, reducing the tendency for turbidity and undesirable texture (30). In addition to being thermoreversible, the potato-based maltodextrin gels are pH stable (pH 3–7), can withstand shearing and heating effects, and have a unique plastic, spreadable, shorthening-like texture (30). Commercial maltodextrins derived from potato starch include C*Pur 01906 (Cerestar), Paselli SA2 (Avebe), and Lycadex® 100 (Roquette).

Maltodextrins can be used in a variety of products. The shortening-like texture of potato maltodextrins makes them ideal as fat replacers in baked products such as cakes, muffins, and cookies by increasing dough viscosity and improving aeration (30). Low-DE maltodextrins promote water-in-oil emulsions and have thus been used in low-fat cheese products, spreads, sauces, soups, and salad dressings (29,39,40). Because Cerestar's C*Pur 01906 has a minimum gelling concentration of 12% (vs. 18% of other maltodextrins), lower levels are required in low-fat spread formulations and the unpleasant starchy flavor associated with high maltodextrins levels can be avoided. C*Pur 01906 has also been shown to provide better flavor release in low-fat spreads due to its ability to lose 50% of its gel structure at oral temperatures (31). In addition to being a fat replacer, maltodextrins can stabilize and enhance the body and viscosity of ice cream and other dairy products (32,33). There have also been recommendations for maltodextrin use as fat replacers in meat products such as frankfurters and hamburgers (31).

CELLULOSE DERIVATIVES

Microcrystalline Cellulose

Microcrystalline cellulose powder (Avicel®, FMC Corp.) is a nonfibrous form of cellulose produced by acid hydrolysis of the cellulose pulp (34). Intense shear forces (i.e. wet mechanical disintegration) are used to form the colloidal variant of microcrystalline cellulose. To prevent reaggregation of the colloidal crystalline aggregates during drying, soluble hydrocolloids such as carboxymethylcellulose (Avicel® RC/CL), xanthan gum (Avicel® RCN30), or alginate (Avicel® AC815) are introduced (42). Powdered forms of microcrystalline cellulose are commonly used as an inert fiber source and non-caloric bulking agent. Colloidal microcrystalline cellulose is physically and structurally similar to an oil-in-water emulsion and imparts the fat-like mouthfeel of full-fat products (34). In addition to being a general stabilizer in food formulations, colloidal Avicel® products are used as fat replacers in salad dressings, bakery products, dairy products, ice cream and frozen desserts, cheese, spreads, and processed meats. In frozen foods, colloidal microcrystalline cellulose prevents ice crystal formation during freeze-thaw cycles (42).

The Novagel® (FMC Corp.) range of fat mimetics, developed in the late 1980s, are cellulose microcrystals co-processed with 10–15% guar gum (Novagel® RCN 10, Novagel® RCN 15) which forms pliable, spherical particles in solution (34). In food formulations, these particles impart a creamy mouthfeel, body, opacity, and fat-like consistency to products. Novagel® and Avicel® products have similar food applications. In reduced fat cheese products, Novagel® breaks and lubricates the elastic protein structure formed in the absence of fat, improving both melting and eating properties (43). Recent ''light'' processed cheese formulations with Novagel® NC 200 have employed carageenan gum (extracted from red seaweed) to interact directly with casein micelles from the milk-based ingredients, resulting in textures resembling the full-fat control (35). Often, the whey and water separation is the most difficult process operation to control when making reduced-fat cheeses that contain fat substitutes (35).

Methylcellulose Gums

Methylcellulose (MC) and hydroxypropyl methylcellulose (HPMC) are gums derived from chemical modification of cellulose (Methocel®, Dow Chemical Co.). In forming MC, cellulose is treated with alkali (e.g. sodium hydroxide) followed by methyl chloride. For the production of HPMC, propylene oxide is added to the reaction mixture (36). The degree of substitution (amount of substituent groups up to a maximum of three on the anhydroglucose units of cellulose) and the molar substitution (average number of molecules of substituent per anhydroglucose molecule; used for HPMC only) affects the physicochemical properties of MC and HPMC (37). Such properties include water retention, electrolyte sensitivity, dissolution temperature, gelation characteristics, and solubility in nonaqueous systems.

Both MC and HPMC gel at high temperatures, which is opposite to that observed with plant-derived gums. This unique property reduces fat uptake in fried foods and provides a barrier to moisture loss during baking and cooling. MC and HPMC provide controlled pourability and mouthfeel characteristics to low-calorie sauces and salad dressings. HPMC stabilizes fat droplets and air cells in reduced-fat frozen desserts, and both MC and HPMC inhibit ice-crystal formation during freeze-thaw cycles. Foam stability characteristics of MC and HPMC, as well as fat-like mouthfeel, have led to their incorporation in low-fat whipped toppings as well (36).

Bacterial Cellulose

A new form of cellulose called bacterial cellulose has been produced by the action of *Acetobacter aceti*. At 97% water by weight, bacterial cellulose is paste-like and comprised of flocks of microfibrils which swell and disperse homogeneously at a level of 3% in solution. The viscosity of the suspension is low compared to common thickeners. This cellulose has the highest water-holding capacity among commercial cellulose products and is considered as a low-calorie material and fat substitute (38). In food formulations, bacterial cellulose functions as a heat-stable suspending agent and as a filler to reinforce the body of fragile food hydrogels. Bacterial cellulose improves the quality of pastry products by reducing their stickiness. It also can be added to meat products as a fat substitute and to jam as a non-caloric bulking agent (39).

Pectin

Pectin is a soluble dietary fiber obtained by mildly acidic aqueous extraction of plant material, the main sources being citrus peel and apple pomace (40). Slendid® products (Hercules Inc.) are fat replacers based on pectin fiber. Pectins have different degrees of esterification (the percentage of methyl-esterified galacturonic acid units). Low-ester pectins (Slendid® 100 and 110) typically range from 20–40% whereas high-ester pectins (Slendid® 200) are between 55 and 75% (40). To function as a fat replacers, Slendid® is dissolved in water, gelled with calcium ions, and sheared into small particles to mimic the physical and sensory characteristics of emulsified fats (41). In contrast, Slendid® 200 does not gel or dissolve in water but swells and instantaneously forms soft and flexible particles with an average size greater than 200 μm. The original size of these soft particles is significantly reduced with food processing (40,41). The Slendid® line of products are stable to heat, pH, shear, and salt, have a neutral taste, and are almost calorie-free (40).

Slendid® may be used to partially or fully replace fat in a wide range of products: spreads, mayonnaises, salad dressings, processed meats, ice cream, processed cheeses, soups and sauces, desserts, and bakery products. The use of Slendid® in spreads and mayonnaise can reduce the fat content from 80% in the full-fat version to 20% and 3%, respectively (40). Slendid® 200 was developed for use in low-fat spreads and emulsified meat products to eliminate the water homogenization step (41). In soups and sauces, Slendid® 100 and 110 (the 110 type being more viscous) are preferentially used because of their superior heat stability to Slendid® 200 (40).

GUMS

Gums, due to their high water-holding capacity, are used as thickeners and viscosity enhancers in food applications. Gums provide texture and gloss and often add a fat-like mouthfeel to food products. The type of gum used for a particular food application is dependent upon many factors. Temperature and shear affects the solubility and dispersibility of gums. Time, pH, temperature, and concentration can also affect viscosity formation as well as gel-forming characteristics of gums (22). Gums used in food applications, some of which are described below, include agar, alginate, gum arabic, carrageenan, curdlan, konjac, guar gum, gellan gum, locust bean gum, pectin, and xanthan gum.

Galactomannan Gums

The main galactomannan gums used in commercial applications are guar gum and locust bean gum. Both gums are composed of a linear chain of α-1,4 linked

D-mannose with single α-D-galactose units linked 1,6 with the main mannan chain (42). Because of its lower mannose:galactose ratio, guar gum solubilizes at lower temperatures than locust bean gum. Thus guar gum is cold water soluble and produces highly viscous, pseudoplastic solutions (43). In contrast, locust bean gum must be heated (80°C) for complete hydration and viscosity development.

The main function of galactomannans in low-fat foods is not as a fat-replacer per se but to imbibe water and control viscosity (28). This becomes increasingly important as the fat level in foods is reduced. Both locust bean gum and guar gum have been used as stabilizers in ice cream and other frozen desserts to control ice and sugar crystal growth (42). The stabilizing properties of galactomannan gums have made them useful in low-fat cheese products, bakery goods, and sauces and dressings.

Xanthan Gum

Unlike galactomannans, xanthan is produced from the microorganism *Xanthamonas campestris* under anaerobic fermentation conditions. The main polymer chain consists of β-1,4 linked D-glucose units as in cellulose but with alternate residues substituted with a charged trisaccharide group (mannose-glucuronic acid-mannose) linked 1,3 with the main chain (42). Solutions of xanthan gum, which is readily soluble in hot or cold water, are highly pseudoplastic, resulting in extremely high viscosities when not under the influence of shear. These properties persist even at very low (0.1%) concentrations of xanthan which contributes to its effectiveness as a stabilizer in low-fat foods (42).

Xanthan gums are generally used as stabilizers in dressing, sauces, and mayonnaises to exploit its weak-gel, pseudoplastic properties. In pourable dressings, the resting gel structure suspends particulate matter, making the dressing visually attractive. The small shear forces produced by the act of pouring are enough to break down this structure and allow the dressing to pour from the bottle. The dressing clings to the food instead of draining off because the gel structure rapidly reforms (52). Xanthan gums also have good flavor release characteristic due to its highly pseudoplastic nature. Kelco has a line of products (Keltrol, Keltrol BT, and Keltrol RD) made from xanthan gum. Keltrol BT (brine tolerant), with improved hydration over regular Keltrol in high salt systems, is suitable for use in chili sauces, marinades, barbecue sauces, thickened soy sauce, and relishes. Keltrol RD, a readily dispersible xanthan gum, requires mimimal mixing and eliminates dust problems during processing (24).

Other Gums

The three types of carrageenan gums (κ-, ι-, and λ-carrageenan), extracted from red seaweed, differ in the content and distribution of sulfate ester groups (53,54). ι-Carrageenan forms thermoreversible gels that are clear, elastic and syneresis-free in the presence of calcium ions (53,54). κ-Carrageenan forms strong, rigid gels, and its tendency toward syneresis is controlled by blending with ι-carrageenan (53,54). λ-Carrageenan acts as a thickener but has no gel-forming properties (54). Of the three types of carrageenans, the ι-type has the greatest freeze-thaw stability (53,54). Carrageenans bind water, improve the texture and slicing properties of processed meats, and reduce cooking losses (49). Carrageenans have been used in the production of low-fat cheese products, gelled milk desserts, milk drinks, and low sugar jams and jellies (43,49). A commercial brand of carrageenan is Kelcogel by Kelco.

Kelco has recently developed the biosynthetic gellan gum (Kelcogel BF) which was approved for non-standardized food use by the U.S. Food and Drug Administration (FDA) in November 1992 (24). Kelcogel BF produces strong gels, which have excellent clarity and are stable to heat and a wide range of pH levels. Highly versatile, Kelcogel BF has created new textural variations for confections, dessert gels, dairy products, frostings, icings and glazes, puddings, jams and jellies, and structured foods (24).

Konjac flour gel is the basis of the Nutricol® product from FMC Corp. Like other hydrocolloid gums, Nutricol provides viscosity and simulates the sensory properties of fats. The incorporation of the konjac flour gel at 10–20% in low-fat prerigor pork sausage resulted in a product with similar shear force and sensory textural attributes to the full-fat control. The cooked low-fat sausage with konjac flour gel was less than 15% whereas the full-fat control sausage fat levels were over 40% (55).

Hydrocolloid Gum Blends

Gelatin is a well-established product that has an important use as a fat replacer in low-fat spreads, yogurt, sauces, dressings, desserts, and ice cream (56). The introduction of combinations of gelatin with various hydrocolloids has resulted in new plastic textures that closely mimic the mouthfeel of fats. Slimgel® (PB Gelatins), launched in 1992, is a family of blends consisting of gelatin and guar or locust bean gum (Slimgel® 100 and 200, respectively) (56). With gelatin, both galactomannan gums exhibit thermodynamic incompatibility with phase separation. That is, when dissolved at an appropriate concentration in water and allowed to set with cooling, the gelatin is dispersed as discrete beads of gel in a continuous viscous galactomannan matrix. Although gelatin melts in the mouth much like solid triglycerides, the galactomannan keeps the melted products sufficiently viscous to provide proper flavor release and mouthfeel (56).

A Slimgel® dispersion in water exhibits similar rheology to solutions of xanthan gum where it is gel-like when at rest and liquifies with low levels of shear. Slimgel® 100/i, composed of gelatin, guar gum, pectin, and maltodextrin, is less gel-like, but has more viscous character than Slimgel® 100 or 200 (56).

Slimgel® 100/i also has higher stability to a variety of food processing conditions (56). Slimgel® products are used in meat products (Slimgel® 100), spreads (usually Slimgel® 200), dairy products and desserts, dressings and sauces, and baked products (56). Slimgel® 100/i is preferably used in frozen desserts, dressings, and sauces because of its cold solubility, ease of use, and improved mouthfeel due to slower melting (56).

Blends of galactomannans and xanthan are often used in food applications because they have been found to have functionalities that were at least the same or better than either gum alone at a reduced cost. When locust bean gum and xanthan gum are heated together, the resulting solution has a much higher viscosity than would be obtained with either gum alone. At high enough concentrations, locust bean/xanthan gum blends form thermoreversible gels with a melting temperature between 50 and 55°C (57). Guar gum/xanthan gum blends have a synergistic increase in viscosity but without gel formation (58). Kel-Lite CM (Kelco) is a xanthan/guar gum blend used to eliminate shortening in baked goods through its stabilizing and emulsifying properties (24).

Galactomannans are also used with certain types of carrageenans. Guar gum with low concentrations of λ-carageenan produce an increase in viscosity whereas high carageenan concentrations increase gel strength. Locust bean gum and κ-carageenan enhances gel strength and a range of textures from brittle to elastic. Locust bean gum/carageenan also lessens the degree of syneresis (23).

FIBERS

A number of fat replacers have been based on fiber from a variety of sources such as soy beans, oats, sugar beets, almonds, peas, and wheat (Table 1). In addition to replacing fat, products containing β-glucan and inulin have been reported to reduce serum cholesterol (59,60). The fat replacer products Oatrim, Z-trim, Vitacel, and inulin are described in more detail below.

Oatrim

In 1991, the U.S. Department of Agriculture (USDA) developed an oat-based fat substitute called Oatrim. (α-Amylase enzymes were used to break down the amylose and amylopectin chains in the oat flour or bran to maltodextrins. The enzyme treatment conditions were selected so that the β-glucan bound to the cellular matrix was liberated, ranging in levels from 1–10%. The blend of β-glucan and low-DE maltodextrin produced a product with improved functional properties and fat-like mouthfeel in comparison with other maltodextrin gels. An added benefit of the β-glucan is its reported lowering effects on blood cholesterol and triglycerides (50). ConAgra Specialty Grain Products and Rhone-Poulenc/Quaker Oats Companies are currently producing Oatrim under a licensing agreement with the USDA. Oatrim is presently marketed by A. E. Staley under the name of TrimChoice.

Z-trim

Z-trim is another product recently developed by the USDA as a calorie-free, high fiber fat replacer (54). In a two-fold shearing process, the fiber structure of hulls of oats, soybeans, peas, and rice, or bran from corn or wheat are reduced to microscopic sizes with the aid of peroxide and alkali. Z-trim has zero calories, no taste, smooth texture, large water-holding capacity, and high viscosity. Z-trim provides moistness, density and smoothness to foods such as reduced-calorie cheese products, hamburger, and baked goods. Replacement of 100 g fat with Z-trim reduces the caloric content of the food by 900 calories and adds 10 g of fiber.

Vitacel

Microfibrillation of wheat fibers with enrichment of a special grade of maltodextrin has produced the product Vitacel by Rettenmaier (55). Vitacel is composed of 70% wheat fibers and 30% maltodextrin. This wheat fiber gel has many functional properties that make it ideal as a fat replacer: viscosity, creamy mouthfeel, body, and substance. This product can thus be used instead of hydrocolloids for many applications. Vitacel can be used as a thickener and binder and for stabilization of emulsions, foams, and liquid media. Its freeze-thaw stability allows for applications in frozen foods (55).

Inulin

Inulin is a polymer of up to 35 fructose units terminating with a sucrose molecule (56) with a sweetening power of 30–65% that of sucrose (28). The main sources of inulin are Jerusalem artichokes and chicory tubers (28). Like the altered sugars isomalt (an equimolar mixture of α-D-glucopyranosyl-1,6-D-sorbitol and α-D-glucopyranosyl-1,1-D-mannitol) and alternan (α-D-glucansucrase, i.e. a polymer of the enzymatically hydrolyzed glucose of sucrose), inulin can be considered as a sucrose replacer because it can provide some sweetness as well as other functional properties of sucrose. Inulin can also be thought of as a fiber and will be under consideration as such by the U.S. FDA now that the methodology for determining inulin in foods has been approved by AOAC International. In addition to replacing sugar in foods, inulin has been used in ice cream to replace both butterfat and sugar, providing a product, sweetened with aspartame, with a 16% dietary fiber content and 52% fewer calories than conventional ice cream (56). Inulin has also been suggested for use in confectionary and bakery products. Fat replacers based on inulin are Fibruline by Cosucra, Fruitafit by Suiker Unie,

Raftiline® by Orafti, and Raftincreaming® by Tiense Suikkerraffinaderij Services.

APPLICABILITY OF CARBOHYDRATE-BASED FAT MIMETICS IN DIFFERENT LOW-FAT PRODUCTS

Presently, xanthan gum, guar gum, carrageenan, and cellulose gel are the most widely used carbohydrate-based fat substitutes. Nevertheless, the market remains highly fragmented because an ingredient that works well in one product may not be suited for another (20). In addition, the flavor profiles can vary widely depending on the type of fat mimetic used. Previous limitations to the use of these fat mimetics have been overcome such as applicability in fried foods (e.g. MC and HPMC) and better control in water activity changes in foods (e.g. polydextrose), increasing product shelf life.

The highest level of penetration of carbohydrate-based replacers has been in the dairy sector. Polydextrose, cellulose-based products, and gums have greatly improved the quality of ice cream and other frozen desserts because of their freeze-thaw stability. In contrast, consumer acceptance of low-fat cheese products has been typically low because of inadequacies in texture, consistency and flavor. However, the development of reduced-fat cheese foods with microcrystalline cellulose in conjunction with gums like carrageenan are making some progress in this area (35).

The use of carbohydrate-replacers in bakery products, especially cookies, biscuits, and crackers, has met with some difficulty because of their low moisture content. The fat in baked goods is important for tenderness and mechanical handling. Some of the problems that have been encountered—loss of viscosity and moisture, poor aeration, poor heat transfer, poor flavor release, and reduced shelf life—have been reduced with improved forms of polydextrose (Litesse II), potato maltodextrins (C*Pur 01906), cellulose gums (MC and HPMC), and fiber-derived products like Z-trim. Nevertheless, emulsifiers (fatty-acid derived compounds) are usually needed to provide the texture and cohesiveness found in regular fats (57). Experiments using carbohydrate-based fat substitutes (Litesse®, N-Flate, RiceTrin, Stellar or TrimChoice) and emulsifiers [diacetyl-tartaric esters of monoglycerides (DATEN), glycerol monostearate (GMS), or sodium stearoyl-2-lactylate (SSL)] had breaking force and toughness values similar to traditional full-fat cookies with fat-substitute level of 35% (58). Thus, it is possible to achieve 15-20% reductions in fat content by making certain modifications to conventional bakery formulations. Nutricia (Nutricia, Netherlands), an 89% fat-free Maderia Cake, was such a product launched in 1994 and is based on xanthan and other gums (22).

The most difficult sector with relatively low activity in new product development is confectionary. Low-fat products are less likely to succeed in such "indulgence" products. With chocolate confectionary, compositional requirements such as the presence of cocoa butter or cocoa butter equivalent make the development of low-fat chocolate an onerous task (21). Total fat reductions can be at most 20–25% with the current technology and regulatory systems if quality is to be maintained (22). Of the few low fat confectionary products available, polydextrose has been the basis for "Lo" launched by the Leaf Group in Finland in 1991.

SUMMARY AND CONCLUSIONS

With the mounting scientific evidence of the role of dietary fats, especially saturated fats, in coronary heart disease, more consumers will see the need to have low-fat foods as a regular part of their diet. Clear labeling of the hidden saturated fat contents in foods would allow the consumer to make a more informed choice (2). Carbohydrate-based fat replacers play an important role in the growing industry of low-fat and reduced-fat foods. Technological advances in this group of fat mimetics have led to applications previously not believed to be possible. However, no single fat replacer has all the properties suitable for different food applications. The food chemist and manufacturer must consider the processing conditions as well as the rheological and functional capabilities of the fat replacer. Despite the health benefits of consuming low-fat foods, deficits in taste, texture, and other sensory qualities limit its success. With successful marketing and improvements in technology and quality, low-fat products will have a considerable impact upon most sectors of the food industry.

REFERENCES

1. U.S. Department of Health and Human Services (DHHS), Public Health Service (PHS), (1988) The Surgeon General's Report on Nutrition and Health, Washington, DC, DHHS (PHS) Publication No. 88-50210, U.S.Government Printing Office.
2. Black, D. M. and Knauer, S. L. (1991) The legal implications of dietary fats: risks of cardiovascular disease and the duty of food manufacturers. J. Nutr. 121, 578–582.
3. Mela, D.J. (1996) Implications of fat replacement for food choice and energy balance. Chemistry and Industry, Vol 9, 329–332.
4. Committee on Diet, Nutrition, and Cancer, National Academy of Sciences. (1992) In: Diet, Nutrition, and Cancer. Washington, DC, National Academy Press.
5. Anon. (1984) Nutrition and Cancer: Cause and Prevention: Special Report. New York, NY, American Cancer Society.
6. National Cancer Institute. Cancer Prevention. Washington, DC, U.S. Department of Health and Human Services, (1984) NIH publication 84-2671.

7. Browner, W. S., Westenhouse, J., Tice, J. A. (1991) What if Americans ate less fat? A quantitative estimate of the effect on mortality. JAMA, 265 (24), 3285–3291.
8. Dyerberg, J. and Bang, H. O. (1979) Haemostatic function and platelet polyunsaturated fatty acid in Eskimos. Lancet 2, 433.
9. Dyerberg, J., Bang, H. O., Stoffersent, E., Moncada, S., and Vane, J. R. (1978) Eicopentoenoic acid and prevention of thrombosis and atherosclerosis? Lancet 2, 117.
10. Grundy, S. M. (1994) Lipids and cardiovascular disease, in Nutrition and Disease Update, Heart Disease. Kritchevsky, D. and Carroll, K.K. (Eds.), American Oil Chemists Society Press, Champaign, Illinois, p. 211.
11. Richardson, D. P. (1995) The food industry response to the health of the Nation White Paper, Br. Food J. 93, 3.
12. National Advisory Committee on Nutrition Education (NACE). (1983) A discussion paper on proposals for nutritional guidelines for health education in Britain, prepared for the National Advisory Committee on Nutrition Education by an ad hoc working party under the Chairmanship of Professor W.P.T. James. Health Education Council, London.
13. Department of Health and Social Security (1984) Diet and cardiovascular disease. Committee on Medical Aspects of Food Policy (COMA). HMSO, London.
14. Committee on Diet and Health, Food and Nutrition Board, Commission on Life Sciences, National Academy of Sciences, National Research Council. (1989) Diet and Health: Implication for reducing chronic disease risk, National Academy Press, Washington, DC.
15. USDA and DHHS. (1990) Nutrition and your health, dietary guidelines for Americans, Home and Garden Bulletin No. 232, 3rd ed., U.S. Government Printing Office, Washington, DC.
16. USDHHS (1994) Energy and macronutrient intakes of persons ages 2 months and over in the United States: Third National Health and Nutrition Examination Survey, Phase I, 1988–1991.
17. Anon. (1993) Simply Starch. Food Manufacture 51–56.
18. U.S. Food and Drug Administration. (1987) Nutrition labeling of food: Calorie content. Final rule. Federal Register 52 (148), p. 28690-28691.
19. U.S. Food and Drug Administration. (1993) Food Labeling. Federal Register. 58 (3) 2175, 2302–2941.
20. Anon. (1993) Heavy demand drives market for fat substitutes to over $3 billion. Frozen Food Digest, 2, 36.
21. Anon. (1996) Innovation in food ingredients. Datamonitor, 72–96.
22. Lucca, P. A. and Tepper, B. J. (1994) Fat replacers and the functionality of fat in foods. Trends Food Sci Tech, 5, 12–19.
23. Anon. (1993) A world of gum solutions. Food Industries of South Africa, p. 23.
24. Jones, S. A. (1996) Classified list of fat replacers and their applications. p. 275-305, In Handbook of fat replacers. Sibel Roller and S.A. Jones, (Eds.). C.R.C. Press, Inc., Boca Raton, NY, London, Tokyo, pp 275–305.
25. Craig, S. A. S., Holden, J. F., Troup, J. P. Auerbach, M. H. and Frier, H. L. (1998) Polydextrose as soluble fiber and complex carbohydrate. Chap. 18, this volume.
26. Mitchell, H. L. (1996) The role of the bulking agent polydextrose in fat replacement.

In: Handbook of Fat Replacers. S. Roller and S. A. Jones (eds.). CRC Press, Boca Raton; pp. 235–249.
27. Anon. (1981) Fat replacer cuts fatty-foods' calories. Food Engineering International 6 (9), 70.
28. Setser, C. S., and Racette, W. L. (1992) Macromolecule replacers in foods. Crit. Rev. Food Sci. Nutr. 32, 275–297.
29. Spector, S. (1998) The effect of surcose and milkfat substitition on sensory textural and physical propertries in a frozen dessert system. M.S. Thesis, Kansas State University, Manhattan.
30. Harkema, J. (1996) Starch-derived fat memetics from potato. In: Handbook of Fat Replacers. S. Roller and S. A. Jones (eds.) CRC Press, Boca Raton; pp 119–129.
31. Roller, S. (1996) Starch-derived fat mimetics: maltodextrins. In: Handbook of Fat Replacers. S. Roller and S. A. Jones (eds.). CRC Press, Boca Raton; pp. 99–118.
32. Nonaka, H. H. (1997) Plant carbohydrates-derived products as fat replacers and calorie reducers. Cereal Foods World 42, 377–378.
33. Vom Dorp, M. (1996) Carbohydrates as fat replacers in ice cream. Food Marketing and Technology, 20–22.
34. Humphreys, W. M. (1996) Fiber-based fat mimetics: microcrystalline cellulose. In: Handbook of Fat Replacers. S. Roller and S. A. Jones (eds.). CRC Press, Boca Raton; pp. 132–144.
35. Bullens, C. B., Krawczyk, G., and Geithman, L. (1994) Reduced-fat cheese products using carrageenan and microcrystalline cellulose. Food Technol. 79–81.
36. De Mariscal, P. and Bell, D. A. (1996) Fiber-based fat mimetics: methylcellulose gums. In: Handbook of Fat Replacers. S. Roller and S. A. Jones (eds.). CRC Press, Boca Raton; pp. 145–159.
37. Grover, J. A. (1981) Methylcellulose (MC) and hydroxypropylcellulose (HPMC) gums. In: Food Hydrocolloids, 2nd ed., Vol 3. M. Glicksman (ed.). CRC Press, Boca Raton; pp. 121–154.
38. Okiyama, A., Motoki, M. and Yamanaka, S. (1993) Bacterial cellulose III. Development of a new form of cellulose. Food Hydrocolloids 6, 493–501.
39. Okiyama, A., Motoki, M. and Yamanaka, S. (1993) Bacterial cellulose IV. Application to processed foods. Food Hydrocolloids 6, 503–511.
40. Nielsen, B. U. (1996) Fiber-based fat mimetics: pectin. In: Handbook of Fat Replacers. S. Roller and S. A. Jones (eds.). CRC Press, Boca Raton; pp. 161–173.
41. Anon. (1994) Gum, set, and match. Food Manufacture, July.
42. Clegg, S. M. (1996) The use of hydrocolloid gums as fat mimetics. In: Handbook of Fat Replacers. S. Roller and S. A. Jones (eds.). CRC Press, Boca Raton; pp. 191–211.
43. Herald, C. T. Guar gum. (1986) In: Food Hydrocolloids, Vol. 3, M. Glicksman (ed.). CRC Press, Boca Raton; pp. 171–184.
44. Morris, E. R. (1991) Pourable Gels, IFI NR, 1, 32.
45. Glicksman, M. (1983) In: Food Hydrocolloids. M. Glicksman (ed.). CRC Press, Boca Raton; pp. 73–113.
46. Osburn, W. E. and Keeton, J. T. (1994) Konjac flour gel as fat substitute in low-fat prerigor fresh sausage. J. Food. Sci. 59, 484–489.
47. Muyldermans, G. (1996) The use of blends as fat mimetics: gelatin/hydrocolloid

combinations. In; Handbook of Fat Replacers. S. Roller and S. A. Jones (eds.). CRC Press, Boca Raton; pp. 251–263.
48. Pettit, D. J. (1982) In: Food Hydrocolloids. M. Glicksman (ed.). CRC Press, Boca Raton; pp. 127–149.
49. Morris, E. R. (1990) Mixed polymer gels. In: Food Gels. P. Harris (ed.). Elsevier Science, London; pp. 291.
50. Duxbury, D. D. (1990) Oatrim: Rat reducer, cholesterol fighter. Fed. Proc. 51 (8), 48.
51. Jamas, S., Easson, D. D., Jr., and Bistrian, B. R. (1990) Glucan dietary additives, U.S. Patent 388572.
52. Duxbury, D. D. (1993) Fat substitute with fiber now commercialized. Food Processing, March, p. 82.
53. Inglett, G. E. (1997) Developmemt of a dietary fiber gel for calorie reduced foods. Cereal Foods World 42, 382–385.
54. Bollinger H. (1995) Wheat fiber gel in the food industry. Food Marketing and Technology, October 4–6.
55. Anon. (1991) Showcase: Bulking agents. Prep. Foods. 160 (12), 91.
56. Orthoefer, F. and McCaskill, D. (1992) Emulsifiers and their role in low-fat and no-fat processed foods. INFORM, 3(12), 1270–1282.
57. Sanchez, C., Klopfenstein, C. F., and Walker, C. E. (1995) Use of carbohydrate-based fat substitutes and emulsifying agents in reduced-fat shortbread cookies. Cereal Chemistry 72, 25–29.

29

Patent Literature Review on Complex Carbohydrates as Fat Mimetics

Susan Sungsoo Cho
The Kellogg Company, Battle Creek, Michigan

INTRODUCTION

As demonstrated in the previous chapter there is a multifactorial need and desire for complex carbohydrates to be used as fat replacers. The detriment that is caused by consuming a diet that is high in saturated fat has been well documented with regard to several disease states, particularly coronary heart disease. Fat intake and the preponderance of obesity in the United States is another indication of the need to reduce the overall fat intake in the diet. Due to this unprecedented demand and the unlimited potential to develop products that emulate the characteristics of fat, a deluge of related patents has been filed.

There are several different types of complex carbohydrates used as fat mimetics. Starch based fat mimetics are predominantly maltodextrins. Hydrocolloid fat mimetics include carboxylmethyl cellulose (CMC), carrageenan and xanthan gum. Conventional fiber based mimetics include products such as Oatrim, Z-trim, and Vitacel. Oligosaccharides or low molecular weight polysaccharides based fat mimetics include polydextrose and inulin. The range of applications of these fat replacers include products such as: beverages, desserts, baked goods, dairy products (milk, ice cream), thickening agents, emulsifiers, suspending agents, salad dressing, meat products (sausages, hamburger), as well as fruit and vegetable products.

The patents included in this chapter are evidence of the growing market of low-fat foods and more specifically those using complex carbohydrate fat mimetics. The potential for food companies who implement these new ideas is enormous.

STARCH-BASED FAT SUBSTITUTES

Starch—General 1

Fat-free mimetic economical use compsn. useful for prepd. foodstuffs—comprises starch, cellulose, protein, gum and flavouring, useful for easy to use bakery fillings, ice-cream, cheese or baked goods.

Patent Assignee: GRIFFITH LAB WORLDWIDE INC (GRIF-N)
Inventor: TANG P S
Number of Countries: 001 Number of Patents: 001
Patent No Kind Date Applicat No Kind Date Main IPC Week
US 5589215 A 19961231 US 93128602 A 19930929 A21D-002/00 199707 B
Abstract (Basic): US 5589215 A

Fat-free compsn. comprises:

(a) 10–85 wt.% starch (I);
(b) 2–25 wt.% of cellulose (II);
(c) 4–70 wt.% protein (III);
(d) 0–4 wt.% gum; and
(e) 0–8.2 wt.% flavouring (IV).

Also claimed are:

(i) a reduced fat biscuit;
(ii) a reduced fat cream soup;
(iii) a reduced fat cheese sauce;
(iv) a reduced fat cream sauce;
(v) a reduced fat chicken gravy;
(vi) a method for preparing a foodstuff comprising replacing at least a portion of the fat in the foodstuff with a fat-free mimetic comprising dry components;
(vii) a foodstuff made by the above process; and
(viii) a method (I) for preparing a foodstuff; and
(ix) a foodstuff made by the above method (I).

USE—The compsn. is a fat mimetic useful in a range of prepd.

foodstuffs including soup, sauce, gravy, salad dressing, bakery fillings, ice-cream, cheese, and baked goods, etc.

ADVANTAGE—The compsn. is partic. economical and easy to use.

Starch—General 2

Starch-based texturising agent derived from high amylose starch—by pre-gelatinising to disrupt starch granules with or without retrograding the starch.

Patent Assignee: OPTA FOOD INGREDIENTS INC (OPTA-N)
Inventor: FINOCCHIARO E T
Number of Countries: 001 Number of Patents: 001
Patent No Kind Date Applicat No Kind Date Main IPC Week
US 5584937 A 19961217 US 92900899 A 19920618 C08B-030/12 199705 B
US 93138541 A 19931015 WO 94US11654 A 19941014 US 95460223 A 19950602
Abstract (Basic): US 5584937 A

A food formulation (I) contains a starch-based texturising agent (IIa), (IIb) or (II) derived from high amylose starch (III). (IIa) is essentially crystalline. It is derived by pre-gelatinising the starch under aq. conditions at temp., pressure and time to disrupt the granules and cause the starch to retrograde. (IIc) is essentially non-crystalline. It is derived by pre-gelatinising the starch to disrupt the granules without retrograding. (IIb) is partially crystalline. It is derived by pre-gelatinising the starch to disrupt the granules and cause partial degradation.

USE—Claimed foods are mayonnaise, salad dressing, cheesecake, mousse, no-fat sour cream, meat products, yogurt, cottage cheese dressing, ice cream, frozen dessert, cream cheese, processed cheese, topping, whipped cream, sauces, cake frosting, peanut butter spread, confection, non-dairy creamer, cheese-based sauce, cultured dairy product, baked or cold processed food, cream based sauces, savory sauces and non-cultured dairy products.

ADVANTAGE—(II) can fully or partially replace fats in a food product, to obtain a reduced fat or fat-free formulation. It provides fat-like attributes e.g., structure, viscosity, smoothness and opacity. It can also stabilise full fat food.

Starch—General 3

Low fat meat prods. or meat analogues—contg. thermo-irreversible starch gel, esp. potato starch gel, as fat substitute.

Patent Assignee: SWIFT-ECKRICH INC (SWIF-N)
Inventor: LAI D
Number of Countries: 016 Number of Patents: 001

Patent No Kind Date Applicat No Kind Date Main IPC Week
WO 9615685 A1 19960530 WO 95US15132 A 19951121 A23L-001/314 199627 B
Abstract (Basic): WO 9615685 A

Low fat meat foods comprise meat and thermo-irreversible starch gel. Low fat meat analogues comprise plant protein and the gel.

Prods. also contain vegetables, pastry, breading, gravy or seasonings. The gel is 1 tapioca, corn, wheat, rice or, esp. potato starch gel, which are pre-gelled. The gel is at 5–50 (10–40) (30) wt.% w.r.t. meat. The gel has average particle size 0.1–3 times that of the meat. It is at most 5 wt.% of the prods. The meat is beef, poultry, pork or mutton, esp. ground beef, turkey, or a mixt. of turkey and beef. In the analogues, the plant protein is soya bean protein.

USE—Prod. have reduced total fat, satd. fat, cholesterol and calories, giving sausages, salami, meatballs, etc. of good mouthfeel and flavour.

Starch—General 4

Thermally stabilised swelling-resistant non-crystalline particles of high amylose starch—for use as non-chemically modified fat replacers and/or food whiteners.

Patent Assignee: SOC PROD NESTLE SA (NEST)
Inventor: BAENSCH J; GUMY D; SIEVERT D; WURSCH P; WUERSCH P
Number of Countries: 022 Number of Patents: 004
Patent No Kind Date Applicat No Kind Date Main IPC Week
WO 9603057 A1 19960208 WO 95IB556 A 19950713 A23L-001/0522 199612 B
AU 9528058 A 19960222 AU 9528058 A 19950713 A23L-001/0522 199621
NZ 288729 A 19970424 NZ 288729 A 19950713 A23L-001/0522 199723
WO 95IB556 A 19950713
EP 773723 A1 19970521 EP 95923521 A 19950713 A23L-001/0522 199725
WO 95IB556 A 19950713
Abstract (Basic): WO 9603057 A

Novel food grade texture agents (I) are in the form of thermally stabilised swelling-resistant non-crystalline particles of high amylose starch. They present a gelled soft structure in which the amylose content of the starch is 40–70% and in which 90% of particles have dia. 5–30 μm.

USE—(I) are used as fat replacers (claimed) and/or as whitening agents.

ADVANTAGE—(I) are non-chemically modified and are therefore more acceptable to the consumer. They have a good combination of taste and mouthfeel, and are prepd. easily and inexpensively.

Starch—General 5

Thickened foodstuff—comprises foodstuff, water and as essential thickening agent a starch extracted from plant having sugary-2 starch genotype.

Patent Assignee: AMERICAN MAIZE PROD CO (AMEM); AMERICAN MAIZE TECHNOLOGY INC (AMEM)
Inventor: FRIEDMAN R; HAUBER R; KATZ F
Number of Countries: 022 Number of Patents: 007
Patent No Kind Date Applicat No Kind Date Main IPC Week
WO 9526642 A1 19951012 WO 95US4182 A 19950404 A23L-001/0522 199551 B
AU 9522394 A 19951023 AU 9522394 A 19950404 A23L-001/0522 199605
US 5476674 A 19951219 US 94223518 A 19940405 A23L-001/0522 199605
FI 9505863 A 19951205 WO 95US4182 A 19950404 A23L-000/00 199609
FI 955863 A 19951205
EP 701405 A1 19960320 EP 95915547 A 19950404 A23L-001/0522 199616
WO 95US4182 A 19950404
EP 701405 A4 19960703 EP 95915547 A 19950000 A23L-001/0522 199644
AU 677904 B 19970508 AU 9522394 A 19950404 A23L-001/0522 199727
Abstract (Basic): WO 9526642 A

A thickened foodstuff comprises of a foodstuff, water, and an essential thickening ingredient—a starch extracted from a starch bearing plant having a sugary-2 (su2) starch genotype. The starch thickens the food at a rate faster than conventional starch and provides the foodstuff with a paste that has a stronger gel strength than a paste made from a conventional starch.

Also claimed is a method for making a thickened foodstuff, the starch used in granular form, a process for replacing high amylose starch with the starch extracted from the plant of su2 genotype, a thickened foodstuff for canning, a process for making the foodstuff and a batter mix for breaded deep fat fried foods comprising the starch.

USE—The su2 starch is ideal ingredient for use as a thickening agent in foodstuffs such as pie fillings, starch jelly candies, soups, sauces, breadings, batters, and snack foods, and as replacement for conventional high amylose starches, and as thin-thick canning starch. The starch can also be used in the manufacture of gum-type candies, and as fat mimetics.

ADVANTAGE—The su2 genotype starch produces a gel having a higher strength and a faster set than conventional starches and has lower gelatinisation temp. Because of lower temps. necessary to cook and absence of special equipment cost savings result.

Starch—General 6

Prepn. of non-separable starch-oil compsn.—used as food coating, lipid replacement, seed coating, thickener, etc.

Patent Assignee: US SEC OF AGRIC (USDA)
Inventor: ESKINS K; FANTA G F; ESKINS K L
Number of Countries: 018 Number of Patents: 003
Patent No Kind Date Applicat No Kind Date Main IPC Week
WO 9528849 A1 19951102 WO 95US4909 A 19950421 A23D-009/02 199549 B
AU 9524259 A 19951116 AU 9524259 A 19950421 A23D-009/02 199608
EP 758198 A1 19970219 EP 95918272 A 19950421 A23D-009/02 199713
WO 95US4909 A 19950421
Abstract (Basic): WO 9528849 A

Preparing a compsn. having a uniform and stable distribution of lipid in a continuous starch phase comprises: (a) cooking an aq. dispersion of starch to solubilise the starch to form an aq. soln.; (b) maintaining in a non-retrograded state while combining with lipid under sufficient turbulence to produce an emulsion comprising droplets of the lipid uniformly dispersed through the soln.; and (c) recovering the emulsion under conditions which stabilise the distribution of lipid.

USE—The formulation is opt. used as a coating on a food prod. pref. on nuts, legumes, cereals (pref. popcorn), fruit and vegetables or is used to partially or wholly replace a lipid component which is normally present in a food prod. pref. in sour cream, yogurt, ice cream, cheese, cheese spread, cake mix, cookie dough mix, salad dressing, meat, margarine, powdered shortening, instant gravy or confectionary. Alternatively, the formulation is a carrier or vehicle for active agents in health care prods. such as hand lotion, hand cream, body lotion, body cream, bath oil, shampoo, hair conditioner, suntan lotion, lipstick, eye shadow, dusting powder, foot powder, medicinal oil, vitamin, antibiotic or antifungal agent. The formulation may also be used as a thickener in paint, ink, polish, paint remover, lubricant, toner and drilling mud. It may also be used as a fat substitute and seed coating.

ADVANTAGE—The compsns. have a non-greasy, yet slippery texture. They form soft gels which can be easily converted to pourable fluids by application of heat.

Starch—General 7

Prepn. of starch-based texturing agent—comprises heating a slurry of amylose starch, filtering and reducing temp. to allow starch to retrograde.

Patent Assignee: OPTA FOOD INGREDIENTS INC (OPTA-N)
Inventor: FINOCCHIARO E T; MALLEE F M; STONE J A
Number of Countries: 060 Number of Patents: 004
Patent No Kind Date Applicat No Kind Date Main IPC Week
WO 9510196 A1 19950420 WO 94US11654 A 19941014 A23L-001/0522 199521 B
AU 9480170 A 19950504 AU 9480170 A 19941014 199536
US 5470391 A 19951128 US 92900899 A 19920618 C13K-001/06 199602
US 93138541 A 19931015
EP 723403 A1 19960731 EP 94931364 A 19941014 199635
WO 94US11654 A 19941014

Abstract (Basic): WO 9510196 A

Method for preparing. a starch-based texturising agent, comprises:

a) heating a slurry of high amylose starch in an aq. medium for a temp. and time sufficient to disrupt starch granules to produce a solubilised starch soln.;
b) filtering the resultant soln. to remove impurities; and
c) reducing the temp. of the resultant soln. to a temp. and for a period of time sufficient for the starch to retrograde.

Texturising agent derived from high amylose starch which is non-degraded, retrograde and crystalline or non-crystalline in structure, is also claimed.

Methods of removing the off-flavour and off-colour from a high amylose starch; producing a high amylose starch-based texturising agent; and making a reduced fat or non-fat food formulation; are also claimed.

USE—The starch-based texturising agent provides several fat-like attributes such as structure, viscosity, smoothness and opacity to reduce and/or replace the fat content in foods. The texturising agent can also be used in full fat foods as a stabiliser, and be incorporated into drug and cosmetic formulations.

ADVANTAGE—The texturising agent provides a safe and cost effective product for use in foods, drugs or cosmetics. The functionality of the agent as a fat replacer and stabiliser is achieved without chemical modification of the starch polymer, does not necessitate the use of numerous adjunct ingredients, and prod. is stable for use in a variety of food processing schemes.

In full fat products, the texturising agent provides improved mouthfeel, body and stability. Food formulations contg. the texturising agents exhibit excellent freeze/thaw and frozen storage stability, shelf stability and resistance to shear and thermal abuse.

Starch—General 8

Fat substitute compsns. for use in foods—comprising starch and protein obtd. from seeds by solvent extraction of lipids.
Patent Assignee: NURTURE INC (NURT-N)
Inventor: BIXBY S H; TARR B D
Number of Countries: 003 Number of Patents: 006
Patent No Kind Date Applicat No Kind Date Main IPC Week
WO 9423587 A1 19941027 WO 94US4119 A 19940414 A23L-001/05 199442 B
AU 9466344 A 19941108 AU 9466344 A 19940414 A23L-001/05 199507
US 5393550 A 19950228 US 9347846 A 19930415 A23L-001/0522 199514
EP 693883 A1 19960131 EP 94914172 A 19940414 A23L-001/05 199609
WO 94US4119 A 19940414
AU 673435 B 19961107 AU 9466344 A 19940414 A23L-001/05 199701
JP 8509126 W 19961001 JP 94523453 A 19940414 A23L-001/05 199705
WO 94US4119 A 19940414
Abstract (Basic): WO 9423587 A

Fat substitute compsns. (I) for use in foods comprise a microparticulate, starch/protein material obtd. by solvent extraction of lipids from seeds. (I) contain at least 60% starch (by dry wt.) and are gelled by heating with an aq. material. Low fat or fat-free foods are prepd. by combining (I) with other animals or vegetable food ingredients.

The seeds are canola, beans, rape, soya, oats, barley. The size of the microparticles are 0.5–20 μm before gelling. The ratio of starch: protein is 60:40–95:5, esp. 85:15.

The material is obtd. from oats by milling, solvent extraction and physical sepn. of the particles. It is free from denaturation due to alkaline extraction

USE—(I) allow low fat foods to be prepd. that do not inhibit assimilation of fat-soluble vitamins and other nutrients. They are esp. dairy prods. or their substitutes (claimed).

Starch—General 9

Prepn. of compsn. for replacing fat and/or oil in food—by gelatinising starch contg. amylose and amylopectin, membrane separation, pptn. of amylose, recrystallising and fragmenting to form particle gel.
Patent Assignee: STALEY MFG CO A E (STAL)
Inventor: HARRIS D W; LITTLE J A
Number of Countries: 018 Number of Patents: 002
Patent Family:
Patent No Kind Date Applicat No Kind Date Main IPC Week
WO 9418849 A1 19940901 WO 94US697 A 19940118 A23L-001/05 199436 B

US 5374442 A 19941220 US 90483208 A 19900220 199505
US 90578994 A 19900906 US 91746381 A 19910816
US 91798291 A 19911126 US 92908728 A 19920706
US 92918862 A 19920730 US 9319162 A 19930216

Abstract (Basic): WO 9418849 A

Prepn. of compsn. of matter useful in replacing fat and/or oil in food formulation comprises: (a) gelatinising starch having amylose and amylopectin components to form aq. mixt.; (b) exposing mixt. to membrane that will only allow aq. soln. of pure amylose to pass through, but no amylopectin; (c) sepg. amylopectin by passing through membrane with less than 15 wt.% of dry solid through membrane being amylopectin; (d) precipitating amylose from aq. soln.; (e) successively heating and cooling pptd. amylose in contact with major amt. of an aq. liquid to recrystallise at least a portion of pptd. amylose; and (f) fragmenting minor amt. of prod. in major amt. of aq. liquid to form a particle gel of the compsn.

USE—The recrystallised and fragmented amylose ppte. allows for the replacement of a portion (10–100 wt.%) of the fat and/or oil in foods, with little or no effect on the organoleptic desirability of the food. Typical foods in which fat and/or oil can be replaced include frostings, creme fillings, frozen desserts, dressings, meat prods. margarine, fruit butters, puddings, sauces, topping, etc. Thus lower calorie and lower cholesterol prods. can be prepd. The processed amylose can also be used as a thickener, etc.

Starch—General 10

New pullulanase from Bacillus deramificans—for starch saccharification etc., with good stability over wide temp. and pH ranges, also related DNA vectors, transformed cells etc.

Patent Assignee: SOLVAY SA (SOLV); SOLVAY & CIE (SOLV)
Inventor: AMORY A; DEWEER P
Number of Countries: 006 Number of Patents: 009
Patent No Kind Date Applicat No Kind Date Main IPC Week
EP 605040 A1 19940706 EP 93203593 A 19931220 C12N-015/56 199426 B
AU 9352759 A 19940707 AU 9352759 A 19931230 C12N-009/44 199431
FI 9305900 A 19940629 FI 935900 A 19931228 C12N-009/44 199433
CA 2112028 A 19940629 CA 2112028 A 19931229 C12N-015/56 199434
JP 6217770 A 19940809 JP 93337202 A 19931228 C12N-009/44 199436
BE 1006483 A3 19940913 BE 921156 A 19921228 C12N-000/00 199439
BE 1007313 A3 19950516 BE 93744 A 19930715 C12N-000/00 199526
BE 1007723 A6 19951010 BE 931278 A 19931119 C12N-000/00 199546
CN 1090325 A 19940803 CN 93121736 A 19931228 C12N-009/44 199713

Abstract (Basic): EP 605040 A

Pullulanase (I) produced by a strain of Bacillus deramificans (or its derivs. or mutants) is new. Also new are (1) DNA (II, sequence of 27846p reproduced) coding for (I); (2) expression or chromosomal integration vectors contg. (II); (3) transformed strains of B. licheniformis contg. (II) or such vectors; (4) recombinant (I) produced by these strains and (5) isolated and pure cultures of B. deramificans.

USE/ADVANTAGE—(I) hydrolyses the alpha 1-6 glycosidic bonds of both amylopectin and pullulan. It is useful (together with glucoamylase) for saccharification of starch in the food, pharmaceutical and chemical industries. Typical applications are as anti-staling additives in bread making and brewing (prodn. of low calorie beer); in prepn. of low calorie foods where amylose replaces fats; in prodn. of oligosaccharides from amylopectin; prodn. of tetraholosides by condensation of maltose; to condense mono/oligo-saccharides with 1-6 bond formation, and to clarify fruit juices.

(I) has better stability than known pullulanases over a wide temp. and pH range (partic. at about 60°C and pH 4.5, where half-life is about 55 hr). It may allow a redn. in the amt. of glucoamylase used (opt.) thus of byproducts formed) without adverse effect on glucose yield. Also it can be used in concn. solns. (high content of liquefied starch) so costs of evapn. are reduced.

Starch—General 11

Compsns. used as fat replacements in e.g., baking—comprise viscous liq., liq. humectant, starch and fibre.

Patent Assignee: ORCHID ISLAND TECHNOLOGIES INC (ORCH-N)
Inventor: VANDERVEER F
Number of Countries: 044 Number of Patents: 002
Patent No Kind Date Applicat No Kind Date Main IPC Week
WO 9412054 A1 19940609 WO 93US11646 A 19931201 A23L-001/0522 199424 B
AU 9456838 A 19940622 AU 9456838 A 19931201 A23L-001/0522 199436
Abstract (Basic): WO 9412054 A

Reduced fat food prods. are prepd. using a compsn. of an edible viscous liq. (I), a liq. humectant (II), a starch (III) and a fibre (IV).

Pref., (I) is corn syrup. (II) is glycerine. (III) is arrowroot, corn, high amylose, pea, potato, rice, tapioca, waxy maize and/or wheat. (IV) is amaranth bran, apple, barley, cellulose, citrus, cocoa bran, corn bran, fruit, multigrain, mustard, oat bran, pea bran, peanut bran, pear, psyllium, rice bran, soy bran, sugar beet, sunflower, tomato, vegetable and/or wheat bran. Compsns. also contain an emulsifier (V), esp. acetylated.

USE/ADVANTAGE—For pastries, biscuits, icings, sweets and sweet fillings, fillers, meats, salad dressings, yoghurt and ice-cream can be made using the compsns. Reduced fat prods. have acceptable taste, texture and consistency and do not increase water activity.

Starch—General 12

Low-calorie food used as fat substitute—contains polysaccharide and branched dextrin.
Patent Assignee: DAINIPPON PHARM CO LTD (DAIN)
Number of Countries: 001 Number of Patents: 001
Patent No Kind Date Applicat No Kind Date Main IPC Week
JP 5276898 A 19931026 JP 92112136 A 19920403 A23L-001/307 199347 B
Abstract (Basic): JP 5276898 A

Food contains polysaccharide(s), opt. xanthan, carageenan, alginates or cellulose and branched dextrin, e.g., enzymatically decomposed or acidified starch comprising amylopectin.

USE—Low-calorie food having reduced fat content is used as a substitute for fats.

Starch—General 13

Starch hydrolysates as fat replacements—prepd. by heating granular starch in aq. acid-solvent mixt., to cleave some amylose gps but not gelatinise.
Patent Assignee: EASTMAN J E (EAST-I)
Inventor: EASTMAN J E
Number of Countries: 002 Number of Patents: 002
Patent No Kind Date Applicat No Kind Date Main IPC Week
US 5275837 A 19940104 US 92884693 A 19920518 A23L-001/05 199402 B
CA 2095875 A 19931119 CA 2095875 A 19930510 A23L-001/052 199406
Abstract (Basic): US 5275837 A

The amt. of fat in food is reduced by using as at least partial fat replacement a starch hydrolysate (D.P. 20–200; D.E. 0.5–5) prepd. as follows: (a) a granular starch (I) slurry comprising at least 20 wt.% amylopectin (II), H_2O, an H_2O-miscible organic solvent, and acid (to 0.1-2N) is heated to effect cleavage of at least 20% of the terminal amylose gps. from (II) without gelatinising (I); and (b) the resulting granular starch hydrolysates are sepd. from the liq.

USE/ADVANTAGE—The hydrolysates are prepd. in a single-step, high yield process that rapidly goes to completion, and readily sepd. from the liq., while biological contamination is no problem. The hydrolysates are useful as fat replacements over a very broad range of solids (1–75 wt.%), and in a wide variety of goods, including salad dressings, frostings, glazings, ice creams, margarines, yogurts, breads, cakes and pastries etc. The hydrolysates are also useful in other food applications (replacements for caseinates in cheeses) and non-food uses (pharmaceuticals), etc.

Starch—General 14

Low-fat and non-fat bakery dough—comprises wheat flour, fat substitute e.g., potato flour, non-fat dry milk solids, emulsifying binder, fat-like sensory additive and leavening agent.

Patent Assignee: JEWELL A M (JEWE-I)
Inventor: JEWELL A M; SEAMAN T
Number of Countries: 002 Number of Patents: 002
Patent No Kind Date Applicat No Kind Date Main IPC Week
CA 2087318 A 19930716 CA 2087318 A 19930114 A21D-008/02 199340 B
US 5344663 A 19940906 US 92821735 A 19920115 A23L-001/10 199435
Abstract (Basic): CA 2087318 A

A fat substd. shortened bakery dough comprises wheat flour, 8–62% potato flour (all percentages are based on the wt. of the wheat flour), as a fat substitute. A bakery prod. produced from the bakery dough contains less than 15% fat, 1.1–12% of a caseinate protein source, 7–60 wt.% of an ovalbumin emulsifying binder source, 15–93% of a fat-like sensory additive, a leavening agent; and 7–28% of a liq. whereby a bakery prod. produced from the bakery dough has a moisture content less than 15% and has a coarse crumb grain structure.

Also claimed, a process for preparing a fat substitute bakery dough, comprises mixing a wheat flour, 8–62% of potato flour as a fat substitute, from 1.1–12% of a water absorbing binder, from 7–60% of an emulsifying binder, 11–93% of a fat-like sensory additive and a leavening agent, where all percentages are based on the wt. of wheat flour.

USE/ADVANTAGE—The fat substitute dough produces a baked prod. with satisfactory colour (browning), flavour and texture qualities combined with a desirable open, coarse crumb grain structure (not cake-like). The dough produces cookies with a high moisture content, yet does not require preservatives to avoid microbial contamination. The dough has improved freeze-thaw and storage stability. Also, the dough and its baked prods. are relatively cheap to produce compared to those produced from enzyme- or acid-modified starches used as fat substitutes or synethetic fat substitutes.

Starch—General 15

Fat substitute useful in foods esp. in non-fat coffee whitener—prepd. by heating mixt. of starch, corn syrup solids, malto-dextrin non-fat dry milk, etc. to specified temp. and drying the prod.

Patent Assignee: BORDEN INC (BORD)
Inventor: BIBEAU L S; KELLER D J; MCKENNA R J
Number of Countries: 001 Number of Patents: 001
Patent No Kind Date Applicat No Kind Date Main IPC Week
CA 2047266 A 19921121 CA 2047266 A 19910717 A23C-011/02 199312 B
Abstract (Basic): CA 2047266 A

A process for producing a fat substitute useful in foods comprises: (a) combining starch, corn syrup solids, malto-dextrin and non-fat dry milk, dipotassium phosphate, Na-hexametaphosphate, Na-citrate, water, and glycine; (b) heating the soln. of step (a) to a temp. above 150°C for a time sufficient to form a viscous gel and (c) drying the prod. from step (b) to produce a powder prod. Also claimed is the fat substitute compsn. produced and coffee whitener, cheese prod., frozen dessert, yoghurt prod, cottage cheese prod., imitation sour cream and a hot beverage prod., each contg. the fat substitute compsn.

USE/ADVANTAGE—The fat substitute is derived primarily from potato starch, corn syrup solids and non-fat dry milk. The non-fat coffee whitener contg. the substitute exhibits at least 18 months non-refrigerated shelf life.

Starch—General 16

Powdery edible material in aq. suspension—comprises cellulose material regenerated from edible polysaccharide in suspension, for use as edible fat substitute.

Patent Assignee: ASAHI CHEM IND CO LTD (ASAH)
Number of Countries: 001 Number of Patents: 001
Patent No Kind Date Applicat No Kind Date Main IPC Week
JP 5023119 A 19930202 JP 91198232 A 19910715 A23L-001/0534 199310 B
Abstract (Basic): JP 5023119 A

The material comprises cellulose regenerated from aq. alkali metal hydroxide and edible polysaccharide, homogeneous mixt. of both ingredients being at least 10% in the continuous form and its particle size of 50% of accumulated vol. being 50 microns or less. Water suspension contains the material in an amt. of 3 to 40 wt.%.

Pref. the edible polysaccharide comprises gum arabicum, alginic acid, carrageenan, pectin, pluran, mannan, starch, etc. The polysaccharide is 10% or more in the material. The cellulose is dissolved in alkaline soln. and then polysaccharide followed by mixing and kneading, to give dope. The dope is extruded in water to coagulate, and it is washed and dried.

USE/ADVANTAGE—Material has good touch and feeling and bitter taste is reduced, used as substitute for edible fat material, etc.

Starch—General 17

Foodstuffs with reduced fat content—have fat or oil content replaced with fragmented enzyme de-branched amylopectin starch.
Patent Assignee: STALEY MFG CO A E (STAL)
Inventor: HARRIS D W; LITTLE J A
Number of Countries: 017 Number of Patents: 001
Patent No Kind Date Applicat No Kind Date Main IPC Week
EP 529894 A1 19930303 EP 92307461 A 19920814 A23L-001/09 199309 B
Abstract (Basic): EP 529894 A

A foodstuff having a reduced content of fat and/or oil, comprising a mixt. of a foodstuff and a fragmented, debranched amylopectin starch ppte. being capable of forming a particle gel in aq. dispersion.

The debranched amylopectin starch is pref. derived from a starch consisting essentially of amylopectin, esp. waxy maize starch, and is composed of more than 80 wt.% short chain amylose and essentially free of amylopectin having a mol. wt. of greater than 20,000 g/mol.

USE/ADVANTAGE—Amylopectin starches which have been subjected to enzymatic debranching followed by pptn. and then mechanical disintegration of the ppte. into fragments, can be used to replace at least a substantial portion of the fat and/or oil content of foodstuffs such as salad dressings, icings, cream filling, ice cream, margarine, meat prods. such as sausages, processed meats etc., cheese prods. such as cheese spreads, puddings such as mousse desserts, candies such as chocolates, nougat etc., sauces, toppings, etc. The prods. are esp. useful to replace part of the shortening used in making layered pastry articles, in which layers of dough are assembled with a roll-in contg. a shortening placed between the layers and the assembly is then baked.

Starch—General 18

Foodstuffs with reduced fat content—has fat or oil content replaced with enzyme-de-branched amylopectin starch.
Patent Assignee: STALEY MFG CO A E (STAL)
Inventor: HARRIS D W; LITTLE J A
Number of Countries: 017 Number of Patents: 001
Patent No Kind Date Applicat No Kind Date Main IPC Week
EP 529893 A1 19930303 EP 92307460 A 19920814 A23L-001/09 199309 B
Abstract (Basic): EP 529893 A

A foodstuff having a reduced content of fat and/or oil, comprising a mixt. of a foodstuff and a particle gel comprising a minor amt. of debranched amylopectin starch particles dispersed in a major amt. of an aq. liq. as replacement for at least a substantial portion of the fat and/or oil of the foodstuff.

Pref. the particle gel exhibits a transition in dynamic elastic modules versus shear strain from substantially constant dynamic elastic modulus to decreasing dynamic elastic modulus, the transition being exhibited at a shear strain of less than ca. 50 millistrain. The debranched amylopectin starch is pref. derived from a starch consisting essentially of amylopectin, esp. waxy maize starch, and is composed or more than 80 wt.% short chain amylose and essentially free of amylopectin having a mol.wt. of greater than 20,000 g/mol.

USE/ADVANTAGE—Amylopectin starches have been subjected to enzymatic debranching following by dissolution in an aq. liq. and then particle formation to form a particle gel, can be used to replace at least a substantial part of the fat and/or oil content of foodstuffs such as salad dressings, icing, cream fillings, ice cream, margarine, meat prods. such as sausages, processed meats, etc., cheese prods. such as cheese spreads, puddings such as mousse desserts, candies such as chocolates, nougat, etc., sauces, toppings, etc. The prods. are esp. useful to replace part of the shortening used in making layered pastry articles, in which layers of dough are assembled with a roll-in contg. a shortening placed between the layers, and the assembly is then baked.

Starch—General 19

Prodn. of amylodextrin prods. for food use—by fractionation of starch hydrolysate(s) or soluble components from amylase treatment of milled cereal, oil seed or vegetable fibre substrates.

Patent Assignee: US SEC OF AGRIC (USDA)
Inventor: INGLETT G E
Number of Countries: 001 Number of Patents: 001
Patent No Kind Date Applicat No Kind Date Main IPC Week
US 5225219 A 19930706 US 92815996 A 19920102 A23L-001/105 199328 B
Abstract (Basic): US 5225219 A

Prodn. comprise (A) treating an aq. dispersion of a milled cereal, oil seed or vegetable fibre substrate with an alpha-amylase (I) to hydrolyse the substrate and liberate soluble fibre; sepg. the resulting water-soluble and water-insol. fractions; and fractionating the water-soluble fraction; or (B) preparing an aq. soln. of a starch hydrolysate with a DE below 10; and fractionating the soln.

In (A), the substrate is pref. an oat, barley, rice or wheat flour, a corresp. bran flour, a soya, pea or psyllium husk flour, or sugar beet fibre. (I) is a thermostable alpha-amylase and the substrate is gelatinised concurrently with hydrolysis. The fractions are sepd. by filtration or centrifugation. In (B), the starch hydrolysate is selected from corn, potato, tapioca and wheat dextrins and maltodextrins. Fractionation is effected by pptn. of amylodextrins with a water-miscible organic solvent, pref. isopropanol, acetone or esp. ethanol.

USE/ADVANTAGE—The prods. are useful as functional and nutritional components of foods such as dairy prods., meats, bakery prods., frozen foods, yoghurt, snacks, confectioneries, coatings, beverages and breakfast foods. They have higher gel strengths and a blander taste than the corresp. unfractionated prods. (cf US4996063) and can be used as aq. gels to replace fat in ice-cream, whipped cream, cheese.

Starch—General 20

Starch hydrolysates formed with strong acid—used in foodstuffs partic. as substitute for fats and/or oils.

Patent Assignee: STALEY MFG CO A E (STAL)
Inventor: ANDERSON K F; BROWN C C; CHIOU R G; COONTZ H D; HAMDEN C J; HARRIS D W; LEHNHARDT W F; LITTLE J A; SCHANEFELT R V; SLOWINSKI L A; STANLEY K D; WITCZAK Z J; WOLF-RUEFF J A; YOUNG A H; ANDERSON K R; HAMDAN C J; BROWN C S; CHIOU R
Number of Countries: 027 Number of Patents: 013
Patent No Kind Date Applicat No Kind Date Main IPC Week
EP 443844 A 19910828 EP 91301368 A 19910220 199135 B
WO 9112728 A 19910905 199138
CA 2036490 A 19910821 199145
AU 9173337 A 19910918 199150
CS 9102191 A2 19920513 CS 912191 A 19910715 C08B-030/14 199247
FI 9203749 A 19920820 WO 91US1029 A 19910215 A23L-000/00 199247
FI 923749 A 19920820
NO 9203259 A 19921019 WO 91US1029 A 19910215 A23L-001/307 199305
NO 923259 A 19920819
JP 5506776 W 19931007 JP 91505572 A 19910215 A23G-003/00 199345
WO 91US1029 A 19910215
AU 652743 B 19940908 AU 9173337 A 19910215 A23L-001/09 199437
US 5378286 A 19950103 US 90483208 A 19900220 C13K-001/06 199507
US 90578994 A 19900906
US 92857532 A 19920421
HU 67293 T 19950328 WO 91US1029 A 19910215 A23G-003/00 199518
HU 922707 A 19910215
EP 443844 B1 19960619 EP 91301368 A 19910220 A23L-001/09 199629

DE 69120314 E 19960725 DE 620314 A 19910220 A23L-001/09 199635
EP 91301368 A 19910220
Abstract (Basic): EP 443844 A

The following are claimed (A) use as for the prepn. of a foodstuffs material of a granular starch hydrolysate which in aq. dispersion is organoleptically fat-like, (B) use as for the prepn. of a foodstuffs material of a fragmented granular starch hydrolysate which in aq. dispersion is organoleptically fat-like; (C) a process for prepg. a starch hydrolysate, (D) a process for prepg. an insol. starch hydrolysate and EtOH, (E) processes for sepg. a granular starch hydrolysate residue from a liquid phase, the granulates of the granular starch hydrolysate residue being susceptible to physical fragmentation, (F) a dry granular starch hydrolysate compsn., (G) a starch hydrolysate compsn. and (H) an aq. fragmented starch hydrolysate dispersion.

USE—The starch hydrolysates are used in foodstuffs partic. as at least partial substitutes for fats and/or oils.

Starch—General 21

New partially esterified polysaccharide(s)—useful as non-absorbed, non-hydrolysed fat substitutes having good organoleptic prop.
Patent Assignee: ARCO CHEM TECHNOLOGY INC (ATLF)
Inventor: WHITE J F
Number of Countries: 007 Number of Patents: 002
Patent No Kind Date Applicat No Kind Date Main IPC Week
US 4959466 A 19900925 US 88147806 A 19880125 199041 B
EP 463245 A 19920102 EP 90306871 A 19900622 199202 N
Abstract (Basic): US 4959466 A

Partially esterified polysaccharides (PEPs) of the formula (P-O(R)x)n having the structure (I) are new: where P is a polysaccharide; n has average value 3-50; R is H or 2-28C acyl; and x is deg. of esterification (1–80%; to render the PEPs resistant to digestive tract hydrolysis and absorption, and to be oils, fats or greases).

Pref. polysaccharides have the polysaccharide as an oligosaccharide where n = 3-10, the acyl gps. are one or more 8-24C acyl (same or different), and y = 1 or 2 (n, x, y, R selected to impart lipase hydrolysis rate less than 20% as compared with olive oil); esp. prefd. oligosaccharides are xanthan gum, guar gum, gum arabic, alginates, cellulose or starch hydrolysis prods., hydroxypropylcellulose, casein, Karaya gum, pectin, or mixts.

USE/ADVANTAGE—The partially esterified polysaccharides (PEPs) have substantial resistance to intestinal absorption and do not appreciably hydrolyse in the digestive tract, have good organoleptic props., and (as well as any hydrolysis prods.) are non-toxic. The PEPs have characteristics similar to vegetable oils and fats, and are useful in a range of low calorie food prods.

Starch—General 22

Starch hydrolysate for use in reduced fat foods as fat replacement—prepd. by maintaining a strongly acidic aq. slurry of the starch at specified temp.

Patent Assignee: STALEY MFG CO A E (STAL)
Inventor: HARRIS D W; STANLY K D
Number of Countries: 017 Number of Patents: 001
Patent No Kind Date Applicat No Kind Date Main IPC Week
EP 529891 A1 19930303 EP 92307458 A 19920814 A23L-001/09 199309 B
Abstract (Basic): EP 529891 A

Preparing a starch hydrolysate comprises maintaining a strongly acidic aq. slurry comprises of a granular amylose starch at greater than 70°C and below both (i) the gelatinisation temp. of the granular starch in the slurry and (ii) the atmos. b.pt. of the slurry, to hydrolyse a substantial portion of the starch and retain a starch hydrolysate residue insoluble in the aq. slurry.

Also claimed is the aq. dispersion of the starch hydrolysate, a method of preparing a starch hydrolyate comprising maintaining a strongly acidic aq. slurry of granular amylose starch at up to 70°C or gelatinisation temp. of the starch, a method of pasteurising a foodstuff, a method of formulating a food having a reduced fat and/or oil, the food formulation produced and an edible compsn. contg. a mixt. of food or foodstuff with a fragmented, granular amylose starch hydrolysate.

USE/ADVANTAGE—The fragmented, granular, amylose starch hydrolysate allows for the replacement of a substantialy portion (10–100 wt.%) of the fat and/or oil in a food formulation. In a French-style salad dressing all the oil component can be replaced. In other foods such as frostings, icings, cream fillings etc. 50–80% of fat and/or oil can be replaced. The replacements do not result in any loss of organoleptic qualities of food. The hydrolysates can also be used as a thickener, bodying agent, etc. The food formulation include flavours, thickeners, nutrients, antioxidants, antimicrobial agents, non-fat milk solids, acidulants, etc.

Starch—General 23

Fat-like carbohydrate contg. short chain amylose—for use as fat replacement in foods, made by enzymatic de-branching of starch.

Patent Assignee: NAT STARCH & CHEM INVESTMENT (NATT)
Inventor: CHIU C W; MASON W; CHIU C
Number of Countries: 015 Number of Patents: 007

Patent No Kind Date Applicat No Kind Date Main IPC Week
EP 486936 A1 19920527 EP 91119368 A 19911113 A23L-001/09 199222 B
AU 9187811 A 19920521 AU 9187811 A 19911112 A23L-001/09 199229
CA 2055856 A 19920520 CA 2055856 A 19911119 C08B-030/20 199232
JP 4351601 A 19921207 JP 91303376 A 19911119 C08B-030/20 199303
EP 486936 B1 19940810 EP 91119368 A 19911113 A23L-001/09 199431
DE 69103383 E 19940915 DE 603383 A 19911113 A23L-001/09 199436
EP 91119368 A 19911113
JP 2597058 B2 19970402 JP 91303376 A 19911119 A23L-001/307 199718
Abstract (Basic): EP 486936 A
Fat-like carbohydrate (A) contains 12–100 wt.% short-chain amylose (I) and is used to replace up to 100% of one or more fats in foods. Also new are foods contg. (A) as a fat replacement to provide comparable functional and organoleptic qualities.

More specifically, (A) are made by debranching starch, using an enzyme which specifically degrades the alpha-1,6-D-glucoside linkages. It is used in foods as a 20–30 wt.% aq. dispersion or in powdered form.

USE/ADVANTAGE—(A) is useful as a fat replacement in dairy prods., salad dressings, baked goods, puddings, coffee whiteners, etc. Aq. dispersions of (A) have a variety of fat-like textures (oily, creamy or waxy) and produce high-strength or thermoreversible gels.

Abstract (Equivalent): EP 486936 B

Use of a fat-like carbohydrate, comprising 12 to 100% by weight, short chain amylose in foods in an amount effective to function as a replacement for up to 100%, by weight of one or more fat(s) contained in the foods.

Starch—General 24

Prodn. of reduced fat foodstuff—comprises replacing fat and/or oil with water and high amylose starch hydrolysate with DE 5-15., pref. made from corn starch.

Patent Assignee: AMERICAN MAIZE PROD CO (AMEM)
Inventor: FARON E J; FURCSIK S L; KORNACKI L; MAURO D J; OWEN R; TURNAK F L; TURNAK F
Number of Countries: 016 Number of Patents: 007
Patent No Kind Date Applicat No Kind Date Main IPC Week
WO 9101091 A 19910207 199108 B
AU 9060630 A 19910222 199120
US 5094872 A 19920310 US 90617405 A 19901121 199213
EP 482094 A 19920429 EP 90911792 A 19900717 199218
EP 482094 B1 19940907 EP 90911792 A 19900717 A23L-001/0522 199434
WO 90US4013 A 19900717

DE 69012331 E 19941013 DE 612331 A 19900717 A23L-001/0522 199440
EP 90911792 A 19900717
WO 90US4013 A 19900717
EP 482094 A4 19920513 EP 90911792 A 19900000 199522
Abstract (Basic): WO 9101091 A

A method of preparing a reduced fat foodstuff comprises replacing at least part of the fat and/or oil with water and a high amylose starch hydrolysate which has a DE of 5-15 and a peak average molecular weight of less than 10,000, and is made from a base starch with an apparent amylose content of greater than 40%, esp. 60%.

The high amylose starch hydrolysate is an aq. dispersion, esp. as a paste, with a solids content of 5–50 wt.%. The foodstuff is a salad dressing, frozen novelty, ice cream, whipping topping, icing, cookie or sauce. A high amylose corn starch is the pref. starch base. Up to 90% of the fat and/or oil is replaced.

ADVANTAGE—An aq. dispersion of the high amylose starch hydrolysate possesses good gel strength (greater than 25g, esp. 500–1100g). The gels are smooth, creamy and white, and have no starchy or roasted flavour. A caloric decrease of greater than 90% is obtained by replacing all of the fat and/or oil.

Starch—General 25

Edible fat substitute material—comprising carbohydrate particle cores with covalently bonded hydrophobic shell material.
Patent Assignee: SERES LAB INC (SERE-N)
Inventor: JENNINGS R A; STEARNS J F
Number of Countries: 013 Number of Patents: 001
Patent No Kind Date Applicat No Kind Date Main IPC Week
EP 388572 A 19900926 EP 89710019 A 19890323 199039 B
Abstract (Basic): EP 388572 A

Composite particles comprise solid core material (I) with shell components (II) bonded to its surfaces. (I) has particle size 0.1–20.0 microns, comprises naturally-occurring polysaccharides and has surface OH gps. for bonding covalently with (II). (II) is of formula -X′-Y-Z, where X′ is derived from any functional gp., X, which can bond covalently with (I), and Y and Z together form a gp. which makes the particles hydrophobic.

The polysaccharides are microcrystalline cellulose, cellulose pulp, colloidal cellulose, starch, flow and/or inulin. X is an acid chloride which esterifies with the surface of (I). Y is an opt. branched 1-30C hydrocarbonyl with up to 5 double bonds. Z is ester gp(s)., esp. a phosphatidyl chlorine residue. Edible food prods comprise staple food prods. with the particles dispersed therein. The staple food is butter, oil, salad dressing, ice cream, milk, cheese, margarine, mayonnaise or shortening. The covalent bond is stable w.r.t. human digestive tract enzymes.

USE/ADVANTAGE—Particles are edible fat substitutes, as they resemble and are used in the same way as conventional triglyceride fats, but reduces caloric and cholesterol intake without decreasing absorption of oil-soluble vitamins or causing diarrhea.

Starch—General 26

Carbohydrate based fat or cream substitute—using hydrated macro-colloidal spherical particles of given size distribution.

Patent Assignee: NUTRASWEET CO (NUTR-N)
Inventor: CHANG H; DUNN J M; SINGER N S; TANG P
Number of Countries: 028 Number of Patents: 029
Patent No Kind Date Applicat No Kind Date Main IPC Week
WO 8912403 A 19891228 WO 89US726 A 19890621 199003 B
PT 90968 A 19891229 199004 AU 8938323 A 19900112 199013
US 4911946 A 19900327 US 88211494 A 19880624 199018
FI 9000926 A 19900223 199022 NO 9000879 A 19900423 19000489
A 19900223 199025 EP 380614 A 19900808
EP 89907903 A 19890621 199032 CN 1040311 A 19900314 199050
EP 403696 A 19901227 EP 89121654 A 19891123 199101
HU 53796 T 19901228 199107 ES 2019574 A 19910701 199131
DD 288748 A 19910411 199136
JP 3505666 W 19911212 JP 89507401 A 19890621 199205
US 5153020 A 19921006 US 88211494 A 19880624 A23L-001/307 199243
US 89367322 A 19890620 US 91678897 A 19910328
IL 90739 A 19921115 IL 90739 A 19890623 A23L-001/19 199250
CZ 8903820 A3 19930414 CS 893820 A 19890623 A23L-001/30 199331
CZ 277987 B6 19930714 CS 893820 A 19890623 A23L-001/30 199340
NO 173361 B 19930830 WO 89US2726 A 19890621 A23L-001/19 199340
NO 90879 A 19900223
AU 642852 B 19931104 AU 8938323 A 19890621 A23L-001/29 199351
EP 403696 B1 19940119 EP 89121654 A 19891123 A23L-001/10 199403
ES 2019574 T3 19940316 EP 89121654 A 19891123 A23L-001/10 199415
EP 380614 B1 19941012 EP 89907903 A 19890621 A23L-001/10 199439
WO 89US2726 A 19890621
DE 68918838 E 19941117 DE 618838 A 19890621 A23L-001/10 199445
EP 89907903 A 19890621
WO 89US2726 A 19890621
CA 1333019 C 19941115 CA 603772 A 19890623 A23L-001/052 199501

JP 95032685 B2 19950412 JP 89507401 A 19890621 A23L-001/19 199519
WO 89US2726 A 19890621
CN 1023759 C 19940216 CN 89106568 A 19890624 A23L-001/19 199520
RU 2039449 C1 19950720 SU 4614610 A 19890629 A23C-023/00 199614
FI 98600 B 19970415 WO 89US2726 A 19890621 A23L-001/19 199721
FI 90926 A 19900223

Abstract (Basic): WO 8912403 A

Water-dispersible macrocolloids comprise hydrated macrocolloidal particles of carbohydrate. These are spherical and have such a particle size distribution as to give the smooth organoleptic character of an oil-in-water emulsion.

USE/ADVANTAGE—Ice cream, frozen desserts, salad dressing, mayonnaise, cheese, cream cheese, sour cream, yoghurt, milk, cream, icing, spread, whipped topping, sauce all use these microcolloids as fat substitute. Unlike sucrose polyester fat substitutes, the macrocolloids are stable over a wide temp. range, do not cause anal leakage and do not leach vitamins from the gut. The particles are non-aggregated. The mean particle size ranges from 0.1–4 microns with less than 2% of particles over 5 microns. The particles are of starch, dextran, gum, konjak and/or cellulose, esp. starch. They are of cross-linked quinoa starch, cross-linked dextran, konjak or Ca alginate. Use of the macrocolloid simulates the mouth feed of fat and/or cream.

Starch—General 27

Oil replacement compsn. for foodstuffs—comprising complexed hydrated protein and cellulose gum, swelled gelatinised modified starch and air bubbles.

Patent Assignee: GENERAL FOODS CORP (GENO)
Inventor: GIULIANO C; HO A S; RISPOLI J M; SABHLOK J P; SCHERER B G
Number of Countries: 006 Number of Patents: 008
Patent No Kind Date Applicat No Kind Date Main IPC Week
GB 2078483 A 19820113 GB 8118592 A 19810617 198202 B
US 4308294 A 19811229 198203 FR 2484793 A 19811224 198205
DE 3123775 A 19820616 198225 CA 1151943 A 19830816 198337
GB 2078483 B 19840411 198415 IT 1171294 B 19870610 199004
DE 3123775 C 19900613 199024

Abstract (Basic): GB 2078483 A

Compsn. comprises a complex of hydrated protein and a hydrated cellulose gum which coats swelled gelatinised modified starch units at pH 3–6; and has air bubbles incorporated in it.

The use of egg, soy or whey protein or casein; and hydroxypropyl, hydroxymethyl, microcrystalline or carboxymethyl cellulose is claimed.

The compsn. has the texture, mouthfeel and lubricity of an oil. It can be used to replace, at least partially, an oil in a food compsn. such as dessert, margarine or salad dressing

Starch—General 28

Microcrystalline starch useful as fat substitute—is prepd. by disintegration of microporous starch granules produced by hydrolysis of granular starch.

Patent Assignee: WHISTLER R L (WHIS-I)
Inventor: WHISTLER R L
Number of Countries: 001 Number of Patents: 003
Patent No Kind Date Applicat No Kind Date Main IPC Week
WO 9221703 A1 19921210 WO 92US4740 A 19920528 C08B-030/00 199252 B
US 5445678 A 19950829 US 91706894 A 19910529 C08B-030/12 199540
US 9386227 A 19930701
US 5580390 A 19961203 US 91706894 A 19910529 C08B-030/12 199703
US 9386227 A 19930701
US 95455425 A 19950531
Abstract (Basic): WO 9221703 A

A method for preparing a microcrystalline starch compsn, useful as a fat substitute in reduced calorie foods, comprises partially hydrolysing granular starch to form a microporous granular starch and disintegrating the prod. into crystalline starch particles. Also claimed is the microcrystalline starch compsn. produced.

Pref. the microporous granular starch is formed by action of an amylase enzyme on granular starch and the microporous granular starch is mechanically or chemically disintegrated to form the starch compsn.

USE/ADVANTAGE—The compsn. can be opt. treated with starch reactive cross-linking agents and/or other surface modifying agents to optimise its rheological properties and organoleptic qualities of processed foods contg. the compsn. The compsn. imparts the sensory perception of fattiness with less calorie content and without compromising other organoleptic qualities of the food prod.

Starch—General 29

Starch-derived, food-grade, insol bulking agent—for total or partial replacement of sugar, flour and/or fat in foods to reduce calorie or fat content.

Patent Assignee: OPTA FOOD INGREDIENTS INC (OPTA-N); ENZYTECH INC (ENZY-N); OPTA FOOD INGREDIEN (OPTA-N)
Inventor: GROSS A; IYENGAR R; ZAKS A
Number of Countries: 017 Number of Patents: 006
Patent No Kind Date Applicat No Kind Date Main IPC Week
WO 9107106 A 19910530 199124 B
US 5051271 A 19910924 US 89440585 A 19891122 199141
EP 502102 A1 19920909 WO 90US6865 A 19901121 A23L-001/308 199237
EP 91900500 A 19901121
JP 5506564 W 19930930 WO 90US6865 A 19901121 A23L-001/308 199344
JP 91501093 A 19901121
EP 502102 B1 19940713 WO 90US6865 A 19901121 A23L-001/308 199427
EP 91900500 A 19901121
DE 69010694 E 19940818 DE 610694 A 19901121 A23L-001/308 199432
WO 90US6865 A 19901121
EP 91900500 A 19901121
Abstract (Basic): WO 9107106 A

The calorie content of food is reduced by replacing all or some of the sugar and/or flour with a food-grade insol. bulking agent. The agent is a retrograded starch having a crystalline structure free of amorphous starch (I). Fat content can be reduced by replacing all or some of the fat by (I). The starch is amylose, amylopectin, dextran, glycogen, galactomannan, or corn, wheat, oat or potato starch. (I) is made by (a) incubating a polysaccharide dispersion under retrogradation conditions, (b) incubating the dispersion formed with a catalyst under hydrolysis conditions and (c) washing to remove the catalyst and water-soluble by-prods. The catalyst is an acid, esp. HCl, H_2SO_4 or TFA. Before (a) the polysaccharide is pretreated with a glycosidase. Step (b) is opt. omitted.

USE/ADVANTAGE—margarine, biscuits, frosting, brownies, fudge, chocolate syrup or frozen desserts. (I) can be easily modified.

Starch—Meat Product 1

Redn. of animal fat content of meat prods.—by addn. of a triglyceride- and ester-free animal fat replacement prod. comprising maltodextrin cpds., and a matrix structure forming agent.

Patent Assignee: LIFEWISE INGREDIENTS INC (LIFE-N)
Inventor: BROZ R T; SHARE R A
Number of Countries: 001 Number of Patents: 001
Patent No Kind Date Applicat No Kind Date Main IPC Week
US 5603976 A 19970218 US 93163983 A 19931207 A23L-001/314 199720 B
US 95418784 A 19950407

Abstract (Basic): US 5603976 A

Redn. of the animal fat content of a meat prod. comprises replacing at least a portion of the animal fat with a triglyceride- and ester-free animal fat replacement prod. consisting of an aq. gel of (a) at least one maltodextrin having a dextrose equiv. = 1–20, or (b) at least one such maltodextrin and starch having a dextrose equiv. = 0, entrained in a matrix formed by at least one matrix structure forming agent selected from an alginate, gum tragacanth, pectin and konjac flour. The fat replacement prod. contains (a) 10–30 wt.% maltodextrins and 0.1–5.0 wt.% matrix structure forming agent or (b) 5–30 wt.% maltodextrins, 0.5–12.0 wt.% starch and 0.1–5.0 wt.% matrix structure forming agent.

USE—The fat substitute is used as a total or partial replacement for animal fat in the prepn. of low fat meats and meat prods. from cattle, buffalo, sheep, swine, goat, chicken, turkey, duck, quail or ostrich. It possibly may be used as a meat extender.

ADVANTAGE—The fat replacement prod. is inexpensive, has few or no calories, is an odourless white solid and can be incorporated into meat just like an animal fat. It can be used without adverse organoleptic effects. It provides excellent lubricity and juiciness and undergoes rendering on heating. It behaves quite similarly to animal fat. It is an excellent vehicle for incorporation of other agents often added to meat.

Starch—Meat Product 2

Fat mimetic compsns. that do not cause off-flavours—comprise starch, cellulose, protein, gum and flavouring.

Patent Assignee: GRIFFITH LAB WORLDWIDE INC (GRIF-N)
Inventor: TANG P S
Number of Countries: 018 Number of Patents: 001
Patent No Kind Date Applicat No Kind Date Main IPC Week
WO 9611587 A1 19960425 WO 94US11794 A 19941017 A23L-001/05 199622 B

Abstract (Basic): WO 9611587 A

Fat mimetic compsns. comprise 10–85 wt.% starch, 2–25% cellulose, 4–70% protein, 0–4% gum and 0–8.2% flavouring.

Also claimed is the prepn. of a foodstuff by replacing at least part of the fat in the foodstuff with the fat mimetic compsn.

Starch is present in an amt. 24–84 wt.%. It is esp. (modified) corn, potato, rice, wheat or tapioca starch or (modified) tapioca (malto)dextrin, esp. tapioca dextrin or modified corn starch.

Cellulose is in powder form with particle size 5-100 (pref. 20) μm and is esp. cellulose, cellulose gel or cellulose ether. Protein is present at 6.9–62.4

wt.% and is whey, whey protein concentrate, milk, non fat dried milk, casein, rice protein, pea protein, soya, egg albumin or gelatin.

Gum is present in an amt. 1–2% and is esp. guar, carrageenan, arabic, xanthan, alginate, methocel or curet gum. The flavouring is cream, butter, cheese, chicken or beef flavour. Compsns. include sufficient water to give a smooth and creamy consistency.

USE—The fat mimetic compsn. is used to replace normal fat in reduced fat biscuits, cream soup, cheese sauce, cream sauce and chicken gravy, as well as salad dressing, icing and bakery fillings, mayonnaise, ice-cream, cakes, cookies and processed meats e.g., hot dogs and sausages.

ADVANTAGE—The compsns. reduce satd. and unsatd. fat and cholesterol whilst maintaining the same flavour and other organoleptic properties as their full-fat counterparts. The compsns. do not cause off-flavours or undesirable appearance or mouthfeel.

Starch—Meat Product 3

Hydrolysed starch blends with fruit concentrates—to provide nutritive sweetening and fat substitution in foods or beverages, esp. baked goods.

Patent Assignee: GREENLAND F A (GREE-I); LYNCH R J (LYNC-I); MITCHELL C R (MITC-I); MITCHELL P R (MITC-I); MYERS T R (MYER-I)

Inventor: GREENLAND F A; LYNCH R J; MITCHELL C R; MITCHELL P R; MYERS T R

Number of Countries: 001 Number of Patents: 001

Patent No Kind Date Applicat No Kind Date Main IPC Week

US 5492715 A 19960220 US 94222291 A 19940331 A23L-001/222 199613 B

Abstract (Basic): US 5492715 A

Fruit concentrate compsns. are a blend of hydrolysed starch (I) of dextrose equiv. (DE) 40 and a fruit concentrate (II) contg. no insolubles and at least as sweet as sucrose. (II) contains 77% soluble solids with 70% simple carbohydrates and 3–20% complex carbohydrates. (I) provides at most 60% of the simple carbohydrates.

USE—Compsns. are used in foods or beverages, esp. in baked goods.

ADVANTAGE—The dual functionality in food formulations achieves both nutritive sweetening and fat substitution.

Starch—Meat Product 4

Reduced fat processed meat—with fragmented aq. dispersion of granular starch hydrolysate as fat substitute.

Patent Assignee: STALEY MFG CO A E (STAL)

Inventor: SCHANEFELT R V; SMICK C

Number of Countries: 001 Number of Patents: 001
Patent No Kind Date Applicat No Kind Date Main IPC Week
US 5368878 A 19941129 US 90483208 A 19900220 A23L-001/317 199502 B
US 90578994 A 19900906 US 92896096 A 19920610
US 9390570 A 19930706
Abstract (Basic): US 5368878 A

Processed meat with reduced fat comprises ground meat contg. a minor amount of a fragmented granular starch hydrolysate. Most of the hydrolysate, but not all, is insoluble in cold water.

The carbohydrate replaces fat and/or oil in the meat, giving calorie-reduced and low cholesterol products.

Starch—Meat Product 5

Cereal hydrolysate contg. compsn. for use as fat mimetic in foods—comprises cereal hydrolysate comprising water-soluble dietary fibre prepd. by hydrolysing aq. dispersion of substrate with enzyme, isolating fibre and adding hydrocolloid gum.

Patent Assignee: RHONE POULENC INC (RHON); RHONE POULENC SPECIALTIES CHEM CO (RHON)
Inventor: JENKINS R K; WILD J L
Number of Countries: 008 Number of Patents: 014
Patent No Kind Date Applicat No Kind Date Main IPC Week
EP 577294 A2 19940105 EP 93304705 A 19930616 A23L-001/308 199402 B
BR 9302393 A 19940111 BR 932393 A 19930617 A23J-001/12 199406
AU 9341349 A 19931223 AU 9341349 A 19930618 A23L-001/10 199407
NO 9302262 A 19931220 NO 932262 A 19930618 A23L-001/308 199407
CA 2098552 A 19931220 CA 2098552 A 19930616 A23L-001/308 199410
US 5294456 A 19940315 US 92901331 A 19920619 A23L-001/105 199411
US 5294457 A 19940315 US 92901464 A 19920619 A23L-001/103 199411
JP 6098704 A 19940412 JP 93149041 A 19930621 A23L-001/10 199419
ZA 9304328 A 19940831 ZA 934328 A 19930617 A23L-000/00 199435
US 5380542 A 19950110 US 92901331 A 19920619 A23L-001/0522 199508
US 92901464 A 19920619 US 9373358 A 19930611
NZ 247925 A 19950328 NZ 247925 A 19930618 A23L-001/05 199519
EP 577294 A3 19940907 EP 93304705 A 19930616 A23L-001/308 199532
AU 663957 B 19951026 AU 9341349 A 19930618 A23L-001/10 199550
US 5585131 A 19961217 US 92901331 A 19920619 A23L-001/314 199705
US 92901464 A 19920619 US 9373358 A 19930611
US 94212076 A 19940314
Abstract (Basic): EP 577294 A

A cereal hydrolysate contg. compsn. for use as a fat mimetic in foods comprises: (A) a cereal hydrolysate comprising water soluble dietary fibre material prepd. by hydrolysing an aq. dispersion of a cereal substrate with an enzyme under conditions which will hydrolyze substrate starch without appreciable solubilization of substrate protein to yield water soluble and insoluble fractions. The water soluble dietary fibre material is isolated from the water soluble fraction; and (B) a hydrocolloid gum effective and in an amt. sufficient to form a thermo-irreversible gel with water-soluble dietary fibre material.

Also claimed is a food compsn. contg. the fat mimetic and a food compsn. comprising the dietary fibre prod.

USE/ADVANTAGE—The hydrolysate compsn. is useful as a fat mimetic in preparing low fat comminuted meat prods. such as sausages. The compsn. is obtd. in good yield and has good water holding capacity and provides a fat reduced prod. with the visual, taste and mouthfeel properties characteristic of a full fat meat prod. The gels can withstand the heating and cooking needed to provide a prod. with the visual, taste and mouthfeel characteristics desired in a fat mimetic particle of meat prods.

Starch—Meat Product 6

Foodstuff comprising native granular starch—is encapsulated in continuous amorphous starch, used as substitute for fats in butchery and biscuit prodn.

Patent Assignee: TIPIAK SA (TIPI-N)
Inventor: GROULT P; SIGONNEY L
Number of Countries: 001 Number of Patents: 001
Patent No Kind Date Applicat No Kind Date Main IPC Week
FR 2661317 A 19911031 FR 905444 A 19900427 199203 B
Abstract (Basic): FR 2661317 A

Starch based foodstuff is produced by: (i) preparing a paste of starch and water from native starch grains; (ii) fragmenting the paste; (iii) cooking the fragments while effecting cooking differences between the starch grains; (iv) drying the obtd. prod. and (v) grinding and sieving.

The obtd. prod. comprises granular starch associated (i.e., encapsulated) with starch in a continuous amorphous state.

USE/ADVANTAGE—The prod. is used as a substitute for fatty materials in food prods., partic. in pork butchery and biscuit prodn. The prod. is easily dispersible in water (cold or hot). It is slightly soluble in cold water, the solubility increasing rapidly at 60–70°C, but, unlike native starch, this solubility is not complete at high temp., a large fraction of the prod. remaining in the state of insoluble particles even after intensive heat and mechanical treatment. The prod. also has a high water retention capacity; the particles are very hydrophilic and their swelling capacity in water at 95°C is higher than 50 g water/g starch.

Starch—Meat Product 7

Foodstuff having reduced level of fat and/or oil—consists of particle gel comprising water and material prepd. by precipitating amylose and treating ppte. with alpha-amylase.

Patent Assignee: STALEY MFG CO A E (STAL)
Inventor: HARRIS D W; LITTLE J A
Number of Countries: 017 Number of Patents: 001
Patent No Kind Date Applicat No Kind Date Main IPC Week
EP 529892 A1 19930303 EP 92307459 A 19920814 A23L-001/09 199309 B
Abstract (Basic): EP 529892 A

A foodstuff having a reduced level of fat and/or oil comprises a mixt. of foodstuffs and a particle gel as a replacement for at least a portion of the fat and/or oil of the foodstuff. The particle gel comprises a minor amt. of hydrolysed amylose precipitate regenerates by alpha-amylase and a major amt. of an aq. liquid.

Also claimed is a method of formulating the foodstuffs contg. the fat and/or oil ingredient replaced with the particle gel, an aq. dispersion useful as a replacement for fats and/or oils contg. the particle gel, an edible compsn. contg. the particle gel and an edible fat and/or oil replacement compsn. contg. water and the particle gel.

Starch—Meat Product 8

Microcrystalline starch useful as fat substitute—is prepd. by disintegration of microporous starch granules produced by hydrolysis of granular starch.

Patent Assignee: WHISTLER R L (WHIS-I)
Inventor: WHISTLER R L
Number of Countries: 001 Number of Patents: 003
Patent Family:
Patent No Kind Date Applicat No Kind Date Main IPC Week
WO 9221703 A1 19921210 WO 92US4740 A 19920528 C08B-030/00 199252 B
US 5445678 A 19950829 US 91706894 A 19910529 C08B-030/12 199540
US 9386227 A 19930701 US 5580390 A 19961203
US 91706894 A 19910529 C08B-030/12 199703
US 9386227 A 19930701 US 95455425 A 19950531
Abstract (Basic): WO 9221703 A

A method for preparing a microcrystalline starch compsn. useful as a fat substitute in reduced calorie foods, comprises partially hydrolysing granular starch to form a microporous granular starch and disintegrating the prod. into crystalline starch particles. Also claimed is the microcrystalline starch compsn. produced.

Pref. the microporous granular starch is formed by action of an amylase enzyme on granular starch and the microporous granular starch is mechanically or chemically disintegrated to form the starch compsn.

USE/ADVANTAGE—The compsn. can be opt. treated with starch reactive cross-linking agents and/or other surface modifying agents to optimise its rheological properties and organoleptic qualities of processed foods contg. the compsn. The compsn. imparts the sensory perception of fattiness with less calorie content and without compromising other organoleptic qualities of the food prod.

Starch—Meat Product 9

Food fat substitute compsn. having good mouthfeel—comprising aq. soln. of alginate and complex carbohydrate having texture resembling that of fat when dissolved in water.

Patent Assignee: TIVALL USA INC (TIVA-N)
Inventor: SHEMER M; SHEMER S
Number of Countries: 032 Number of Patents: 002
Patent No Kind Date Applicat No Kind Date Main IPC Week
WO 9202147 A 19920220 199210 B
AU 9185030 A 19920302 AU 9185030 A 19910801 A23L-001/05 199224
WO 91US5444 A 19910801
Abstract (Basic): WO 9202147 A

A food fat substitute compsn. comprises an aq. soln. of alginate and complex carbohydrate having a texture resembling that of fat when dissolved in water. Also claimed is a food prod. contg. the fat substitute.

The complex carbohydrate is a plant derived water soluble fibre or starch prod. consisting essentially of partially hydrolysed starch. The starch prod. is selected from SHP, PASELLI SA2(RTM), MALTRIN MO40(RTM), and N-OIL(RTM). The compsn. is in powdered or granulated form. The compsn. comprises 1–20 wt. (esp. 5–15) wt.% alginate. Alternatively the compsn. is in aq. soln. form and comprises 4–25 (esp. 10–15) wt.% of the complex carbohydrate and 0.3–5 (esp. 1 to 1.5) wt.% of alginate.

USE/ADVANTAGE—The fat substitute is made entirely of natural prods. and has improved fat-like properties and gives improved mouthfeel to food prods. esp. meat substitutes contg. it. The food prod. contg. the substitute is selected from soup, gravy, sauce and dressing.

Starch—Meat Product 10

Low calorie meat prod.—comprises comminuted lean meat free from visible fat, specified vegetable fat replacement and opt. salt.

Patent Assignee: DANISH CROWN INC AS (DACR-N); SLAGTERISELSK WENBO (SLAG-N); STAGTERISELSK WENBO (WENB-N); SLAGTER SKABET WENB (SLAG-N); SLAGTERISELSKABET WEMBO AMBA (SLAG-N); DANISH CROWN INC (DACR-N); SLAGTERISELSKABET WENBO AMBA (SLAG-N)

Inventor: CHRISTENSEN B; MOGENSEN F; CHRISTENSE B

Number of Countries: 039 Number of Patents: 022

Patent No Kind Date Applicat No Kind Date Main IPC Week

WO 9108680 A 19910627 WO 90DK312 A 19901130 199128 B
FR 2655517 A 19910614 FR 9015481 A 19901211 199135
AU 9169165 A 19910718 199142
PT 96121 A 19910930 PT 96121 A 19901207 199142
ZA 9009702 A 19911030 ZA 909702 A 19901203 199148
CN 1052419 A 19910626 CN 90109842 A 19901211 199214
NO 9200174 A 19920310 WO 90DK312 A 19901130 A23L-001/31 199223
NO 92174 A 19920114
FI 9202693 A 19920610 WO 90DK312 A 19901130 A23L-000/00 199237
FI 922693 A 19920610
EP 505412 A1 19920930 WO 90DK312 A 19901130 A23L-001/314 199240
EP 91900743 A 19901130
BR 9007913 A 19921006 BR 907913 A 19901130 A23L-001/314 199245
WO 90DK312 A 19901130
NZ 236384 A 19930428 NZ 236384 A 19901207 A23L-001/317 199320
HU 62186 T 19930428 WO 90DK312 A 19901130 A23L-001/314 199322
HU 921269 A 19901130
ES 2035764 A1 19930416 ES 903154 A 19901210 A23L-001/317 199324
JP 5505098 W 19930805 WO 90DK312 A 19901130 A23L-001/31 199336
JP 91501197 A 19901130
AU 641202 B 19930916 AU 9169165 A 19901130 A23L-001/317 199344
ES 2035764 B1 19931216 ES 903154 A 19901210 A23L-001/317 199403
IT 1241028 B 19931227 IT 9067994 A 19901211 A23L-000/00 199422
EP 505412 B1 19940817 WO 90DK312 A 19901130 A23L-001/314 199432
EP 91900743 A 19901130
DE 69011691 E 19940922 DE 611691 A 19901130 A23L-001/314 199437
WO 90DK312 A 19901130
EP 91900743 A 19901130
IL 96520 A 19950831 IL 96520 A 19901130 A23L-001/317 199543
US 5468510 A 19951121 US 90517663 A 19900501 A23L-001/317 199601

US 90566223 A 19900813
US 90597719 A 19901016
US 90623747 A 19901219
US 94186028 A 19940125
IE 67971 B 19960515 IE 904443 A 19901210 A23L-001/314 199630
Abstract (Basic): WO 9108680 A

A low calorie meat prod. comprises: (a) a mixt. comprising (1) comminuted lean meat substantially free from visible fat in an amt. of 20–95 wt.% of the mixt.; (2) a vegetable fat replacement ingredient comprising dietary fibre and starch in a wt. ratio of 1:32 to 1:1. The dietary fibre is at least 5 wt.% of the fat replacement ingredient dry matter when determined as non-starch polysaccharide (NSP) and the proportion of starch is at least 50 wt.% of the fat replacement ingredient. The proportion of vegetable fat replacement ingredient is 5–80 wt.% of the mixt.; (b) opt. added salt in an amt. of 0.1–4 wt.% of the mixt.; (c) opt. added water in an amt. of 5–50 wt.% of the mixt.; and (d) opt. one or more further ingredient.

USE/ADVANTAGE—The low calorie meat prod. is a pet food or a ready to cook or ready to eat consumer meal etc. (hamburger, sausage, spreadable prods. etc.); when the prod. is a hamburger prod. the content of fat is at the most 15 wt.% and in other prods. the fat content is at most 10 wt.%; when the lean meat is fish meat the prod. does not comprise hardened fat and the dietary fibre is not Konjak mannan. The prods. have same taste, texture, appearance and water binding capacity as conventionally prepd. high fat meat prods.

Starch—Meat Product 11

Gel-forming starch hydrolysate prepn.—comprises two-stage addn. of amylolytic enzyme to starch milk concentrate and heating.
Patent Assignee: ODESS BAKERY IND (ODBA-R); ODESS FOOD IND TECHN (ODFO)
Inventor: DUDKIN M S; KAPRELYANT L V; SEREDNITSK P V
Number of Countries: 001 Number of Patents: 001
Patent No Kind Date Applicat No Kind Date Main IPC Week
SU 1616588 A 19901230 SU 4414589 A 19880421 199146 B
Abstract (Basic): SU 1616588 A

A gel-forming starch hydrolysate is obtd. more efficiently by concentrating starch milk, which is a side prod. of bread making, to solids content of 15–30% and adding an amylolytic enzyme. The enzyme is added in two stages. In the first stage 45–55% of the enzyme is added. The suspension is heated to 50–52°C at the rate of 0.5–1.0°C/min., and left to be heated for 5 min. at the max. temp. Subsequent heating to 71°C is followed by addn. of the remaining enzyme.

USE/ADVANTAGE—Used in food industry as a cheaper method of producing maltodextrins, which can replace fat in food preparations.

Starch—Snack 1

Fat free corn snacks—comprise corn, fat free filler e.g., starch, non-digestible fibre and fat free ingredients e.g., salt.

Patent Assignee: PROCTER & GAMBLE CO (PROC)
Inventor: BIEDERMANN D T; JENSEN J M; JOHNSTON R W; RECE R D
Number of Countries: 026 Number of Patents: 002
Patent No Kind Date Applicat No Kind Date Main IPC Week
WO 9639865 A1 19961219 WO 96US8541 A 19960604 A23L-001/164 199705 B
AU 9659747 A 19961230 AU 9659747 A 19960604 A23L-001/164 199716
Abstract (Basic): WO 9639865 A

Fat free corn snacks comprise: (a) 20–50% corn; (b) 20–62% fat free filler comprising starch, protein and/or non-digestible fibre; (c) 1–35% non-digestible fat substitute and (d) 0–10% fat free ingredients comprising salt, emulsifiers and/or fat free seasonings.

USE—The corn snacks are digestible fat free corn chips e.g., fried, baked and/or extruded salted snacks such as corn chips and sticks, tortilla chips, corn curls and puffs, pellet snacks, half products and crackers.

ADVANTAGE—The low moisture triglyceride or digestible fat free corn snacks have good taste and mouthfeel lubriciousness and acceptable greasiness impressions.

Starch—Spread & Salad Dressing 1

Shortening substitute for use in foodstuffs and its prepn.—useful in baked goods, candy and icing and esp. as a roll-in fat substitute.

Patent Assignee: AMERICAN MAIZE PROD CO (AMEM); CERESTAR USA INC (CERE-N)
Inventor: MAURO D; STANKUS C; TREECE T
Number of Countries: 020 Number of Patents: 002
Patent No Kind Date Applicat No Kind Date Main IPC Week
US 5576043 A 19961119 US 95478509 A 19950607 A23L-001/0522 199701 B
WO 9639863 A1 19961219 WO 96US9859 A 19960607 A23L-001/0522 199705
Abstract (Basic): US 5576043 A

A shortening substitute comprises a mixt. of (a) 1–10 wt.% pregelatinised, unmodified starch; (b) 5–15 wt.% pregelatinised, modified, high amylopectin starch selected from pregelatinised, crosslinked, hydroxypropylated starch and pregelatinised, crosslinked esterified starch; (c) 5–10 wt.% emulsifier comprising at least a monoglyceride; (d) 5–25 wt.% shortening; and (e) the remainder (greater than or equal to 60 wt.%) water.

Also claimed is (i) process for making the shortening substitute; and (ii) reduced fat foodstuffs in which shortening is replaced by the shortening substitute.

USE—The shortening substitute is used to replace at least a portion of the shortening in a foodstuff (e.g., in a wt. ratio of 1:1) to make a fat-reduced foodstuff (claimed), partic. in baked goods and esp. laminated pastry made with roll-in shortening where all the shortening is substd., danish, pie crust, cake and biscuits, candy and icing (all claimed).

ADVANTAGE—The shortening substitute has a caloric content = 2 calories/g while that of conventional shortening = 9 calories/g. It has the necessary texture to act as a roll-in fat substitute. It works well in frozen doughs. It has been found, in some instances, to produce baked goods with superior taste to those produced with conventional shortening. The substitute provides cost savings over conventional shortenings.

Starch—Spread & Salad Dressing 2

Reduced fat peanut butter prod.—comprises ground peanuts and native starch which reduces or replaces the fat and/or sugar content.

Patent Assignee: OPTA FOOD INGREDIENTS INC (OPTA-N)
Inventor: FINNOCHIARO E T
Number of Countries: 001 Number of Patents: 001
Patent No Kind Date Applicat No Kind Date Main IPC Week
US 5549923 A 19960827 US 94219983 A 19940330 A23L-001/38 199640 B
Abstract (Basic): US 5549923 A

A reduced fat peanut butter prod. (I) comprises: (a) ground peanuts in a continuous oil phase; and (b) 5–50 wt.% native starch derived from corn, pea, potato, garbanzo bean, wheat, rice, tapioca, sorghum, barley, waxy maize, milo, arrow root, waxy rice or waxy milo.

USE—(I) is useful as a peanut butter, peanut spread or imitation peanut butter, having a creamy, crunchy, old-fashioned or natural form.

ADVANTAGE—(I) has the flavour and consistency of conventional peanut butter, and does not exhibit phase or oil sepn.

Starch—Spread & Salad Dressing 3

Fat free spread with the spreadability, body, texture and taste of ordinary margarine—comprising gellan gum, water, non-gelling starch, gelling salt, and non-fat milk solids.

Patent Assignee: MONSANTO CO (MONS)
Inventor: CHALUPA W F; SANDERSON G R
Number of Countries: 018 Number of Patents: 003
Patent No Kind Date Applicat No Kind Date Main IPC Week
EP 685170 A2 19951206 EP 95870062 A 19950531 A23L-001/054 199602 B
EP 685170 A3 19960501 EP 95870062 A 19950531 A23L-001/054 199626
US 5534286 A 19960709 US 94252307 A 19940601 A23L-001/0522 199633
Abstract (Basic): EP 685170 A

Spreads comprise 81–95.9% water, 2–11% non-gelling starch, 1–3% gelling salt, 1–3% non-fat milk solids and 0.1–1.0% gellan gum.

Gellan gum and most of the starch are added to most of the water and hydrated by heating to 180–212 (pref. 200) deg. F while mixing. The salt and milk solids are mixed in and the mixt. cooled to 150–160°F. The rest of the starch and water are added and blended until uniform, and the mixt. poured into a container and allowed to cool and set. The initial starch and water are at least 70 and at least 88% of the total amounts.

USE—The spreads are useful as margarine substitutes that are fat free yet have the spreadability, body, texture and taste of ordinary margarine.

Starch—Spread & Salad Dressing 4

Non-fat food prods. e.g., fruit spreads and pie fillings—contg. pectin, starch, cellulose or protein based fat mimetic having improved texture and spreadability.

Patent Assignee: SMUCKER J M CO (SMUC-N)
Inventor: BRAIN C H; GAITHER K S; MUENZ D J
Number of Countries: 001 Number of Patents: 001
Patent No Kind Date Applicat No Kind Date Main IPC Week
US 5451420 A 19950919 US 92857254 A 19920325 A23L-001/0524 199543 B
US 93115825 A 19930903
Abstract (Basic): US 5451420 A

A non-fat food prod. comprises: (a) a mixt. of whole fruit, fruit purée, fruit juice, fruit juice concentrate, cocoa, tomatoes, tomato juice, tomato paste, tomato paste concentrate and/or tomato sauce; (b) one of water and a sweetener; and (c) one of a stabiliser and a gel promoting agent; (d) a fat mimetic as an additional ingredient providing the physical and organoleptic characteristics of fat, selected from pectin based, starch based, cellulose based and/or protein based fat mimetics.

The fat mimetic is a low methoxyl pectin forming 0.1 wt.% of the mixt. The prod. has a soluble solids content of 5–80% and consists of particle 5–100 μm.

USE—Used in non-fat food prods. e.g., fruit spreads, bakery fillings, flavoured syrups, pie glazes and fillings etc.

ADVANTAGE—The food prods. have improved texture and enhanced spread ability, flavour and mouthfeel. Bakery filling prods. also have improved water retention and bake stability.

Starch—Spread & Salad Dressing 5

Non-fat or low-fat spreadable or squeezable margarine—comprises fat mimetic, bulky agent, inulin and/or gum and water.

Patent Assignee: KRAFT GEN FOODS INC (KRFT); KRAFT FOODS INC (KRFT)

Inventor: BULIGA G S; LIS D G; MILLER M S; POWELL W F; KRISHNAMURTHY R G; TOMSKI S J; WITTE V C; TOMSKI S

Number of Countries: 019 Number of Patents: 005

Patent No Kind Date Applicat No Kind Date Main IPC Week
EP 648425 A2 19950419 EP 94307646 A 19941018 A23D-007/00 199520 B
CA 2132502 A 19950419 CA 2132502 A 19940920 A23D-007/02 199529
EP 648425 A3 19950705 EP 94307646 A 19941018 A23D-007/00 199612
CA 2150086 A 19951209 CA 2150086 A 19950524 A23D-007/015 199614
US 5501869 A 19960326 US 92997689 A 19921228 A23D-007/015 199618
US 93138734 A 19931018
US 94255454 A 19940608

Abstract (Basic): EP 648425 A

Margarine comprises: (a) a fat mimetic selected from waxy maize starch, mixts. of the starch with gelling type maltodextrins and/or modified by acid hydrolysis to remove amorphous regions from it; (b) opt. a bulking agent selected from non-gelling maltodextrins, polydextrose and corn syrup solids; (c) inulin and/or gum; and (d) water.

The bulking agent is present in an amt. of 0–5 (esp. 1–5)% and component (c) is inulin. The compsn. also comprises a sweetness masking agent selected from Ca-citrate and/or microreticulated microcrystalline cellulose present in an amt. of 0.75–3 wt.% on a dry solids basis or Na-salt of racemic 2-(4-methoxyphenoxy) propionic acid present at a level of 50–200 ppm. The fat mimetic is present at a level of 3.5–8% and the inulin at a level of 10–23%.

USE—The margarine contains no fat or low-fat, and it is spreadable or squeezable.

ADVANTAGE—The prod. has rheological properties similar to solid margarine or squeezable margarine. The prod. has no fat and substantially fewer calories compared to margarine.

Starch—Spread & Salad Dressing 6

Macro-colloidal starch particles as fat or cream substitutes—for use in ice cream, sauces, spreads, whipped toppings, salad dressing, cheese, cream cheese or icing.

Patent Assignee: NUTRASWEET CO (NUTR-N)
Inventor: SINGER N S
Number of Countries: 001 Number of Patents: 001
Patent No Kind Date Applicat No Kind Date Main IPC Week
US 5370894 A 19941206 US 88211494 A 19880624 A23L-001/307 199503 B
US 89367322 A 19890620 US 91678897 A 19910328
US 92956788 A 19921005
Abstract (Basic): US 5370894 A

A water-dispersible macrocolloid comprises particles of starch that are non-aggregated, spheroidal, of mean particle size distribution 0.1–4 μm with less than 2% (by number) over 5 μm and in a hydrated state. They form macrocolloids of smooth organoleptic character like an oil-in-water emulsion. They are selected from taro, Saponaria vaccaria, Amaranthus retroflexus, Maranta arundinacea, or buckwheat starches.

USE—The macrocolloid is used as an analogue for ice cream, salad dressing, mayonnaise, cheese, cream cheese, icing, spreads, whipped topping or sauce.

ADVANTAGE—The compsn. simulates the mouthfeel of fat and/or cream in the prod. when used to replace all or part of the fat and/or cream.

Starch—Spread & Salad Dressing 7

Compsn. prepn. for replacing fat and/or oil in foods—comprises gelatinising starch contg. amylopectin, de-branching amylopectin using ultrasonic, forming ppte. of de-branched prod. and fragmenting to form gel.

Patent Assignee: STALEY MFG CO A E (STAL)
Inventor: LITTLE J A; SCOBELL H D; HARRIS D W
Number of Countries: 018 Number of Patents: 003
Patent No Kind Date Applicat No Kind Date Main IPC Week
WO 9418850 A1 19940901 WO 94US698 A 19940118 A23L-001/05 199436 B
US 5372835 A 19941213 US 90483208 A 19900220 199504
US 90578994 A 19900906 US 91746381 A 19910816
US 91798291 A 19911126 US 92908728 A 19920706
US 92918862 A 19920730 US 9319130 A 19930216
US 5395640 A 19950307 US 90483208 A 19900220 A23L-001/0522 199515 N

US 90578994 A 19900906 US 91746381 A 19910816
US 91798291 A 19911126 US 92908728 A 19920706
US 92908728 A 19920706 US 92918862 A 19920730

Abstract (Basic): WO 9418850 A

Prodn. of a compsn. of matter useful in replacing fat and/or oil in food formulation comprises: (a) gelatinising a starch having amylopectin component; (b) debranching the amylopectin in the gelatinised starch in a debranching medium comprising ultrasonic waves at a frequency 20–100 kHz. The debranching is effective to convert more than 80 wt.% of the amylopectin to short chain amylase and form a debranched amylopectin starch in the medium; (c) ceasing the prodn. of ultrasonic waves in the medium and allowing the medium to form a ppte. of debranched amylopectin starch; and (d) fragmenting a minor amt. of the debranched or amylopectin starch ppte. in a major amt. of an aq. liquid. The fragmenting is effective to form a particle gel of the compsn.

USE/ADVANTAGE—The debranched starch ppte. allows for replacement of a substantial portion (10–100 wt.%) of fat and/or oil in food formulations such as frostings, icings, ice-cream, margarine, dressing, meat prods., cheese prods., puddings, sauces, toppings, etc. The ppte. will also have utility as a thickener, bodying agent, etc. Replacement of fat and/or oil enables redn. in calories of the food prods. of at least one third per customary serving without adversely affecting the organoleptic properties of the prod.

Starch—Spread & Salad Dressing 8

Reduced fat shortening substitute for bakery prods.—comprises emulsion with fat and emulsifier as oil phase in aq. phase contg. viscosifier and humectant.

Patent Assignee: UNILEVER PLC (UNIL); UNILEVER NV (UNIL); VAN DEN BERGH FOODS CO (VBER-N)

Inventor: BODOR J; DESAI G; DESAI G N

Number of Countries: 046 Number of Patents: 009

Patent Family:

Patent No Kind Date Applicat No Kind Date Main IPC Week
WO 9412039 A1 19940609 WO 93EP3155 A 19931110 A21D-002/16 199424 B
AU 9454648 A 19940622 AU 9454648 A 19931110 A21D-002/16 199436
US 5360627 A 19941101 US 92982929 A 19921130 A23D-009/00 199443
ZA 9308668 A 19950726 ZA 938668 A 19931119 A23D-000/00 199535
EP 673201 A1 19950927 WO 93EP3155 A 19931110 A21D-002/16 199543
EP 94900126 A 19931110
EP 673201 B1 19960724 WO 93EP3155 A 19931110 A21D-002/16 199634
EP 94900126 A 19931110

DE 69303829 E 19960829 DE 603829 A 19931110 A21D-002/16 199640
WO 93EP3155 A 19931110
EP 94900126 A 19931110
JP 8503372 W 19960416 WO 93EP3155 A 19931110 A21D-002/16 199645
JP 94512690 A 19931110
ES 2089903 T3 19961001 EP 94900126 A 19931110 A21D-002/16 199645
Abstract (Basic): WO 9412039 A

Shortening substitutes are emulsions of 10–40% fat phase (I) and 90–60% aq. phase (II). (I) contain a triglyceride and at least 3 wt.% (w.r.t. emulsion) of emulsifier (II), at least 4.5 wt.% of (III) being propylene glycol monoester of fats and fatty acids. (II) contains 5–30 wt.% starch, starch deriv. and/or gum as viscosifier (IV) and 10–50 wt.% polyol humectant (V).

Pref. emulsions are oil-in-water. (I) and (II) are 15–35 and 65–85 wt.% resp. (III) is 30–45% alpha monoglyceride and 45—70% propylene glycol monoester. It esp. also contains lecithin. Prods. contain not over 20% fat. The ratio triglyceride : emulsifier is 4–1 : 1. The triglyceride has solid fat index at 10°C 20–70, 21°C 10–60, 33°C 5–50 and 40°C 1–20. (IV) is low DE-maltodextrin, tapioca dextrin or pregelatinised tapioca dextrin. (V) is hydrolysed corn starch or high fructose corn syrup.

USE/ADVANTAGE—The prods. are used in bakery prods. and give reduced fat, reduced caloric baked goods without introducing problems such as reduced cake volume.

Starch—Spread & Salad Dressing 9

Fat-free margarine compsn. having reduced calorie content—comprises inulin and/or gum, water, modified starch or gelling-type maltodextrin fat mimetic and opt. bulking agent.

Patent Assignee: KRAFT GEN FOODS INC (KRFT); KRAFT FOODS INC (KRFT)
Inventor: BULIGA G S; LIS D G; MILLER M S; POWELL W F; DANIEL G L
Number of Countries: 020 Number of Patents: 005
Patent No Kind Date Applicat No Kind Date Main IPC Week
EP 605217 A2 19940706 EP 93310499 A 19931223 A23D-007/00 199426 B
NO 9304824 A 19940629 NO 934824 A 19931227 A23L-001/307 199429
FI 9305870 A 19940629 FI 935870 A 19931227 A23D-000/00 199433
CA 2110195 A 19940629 CA 2110195 A 19931129 A23D-007/00 199434
EP 605217 A3 19950503 EP 93310499 A 19931223 A23D-007/00 199545
Abstract (Basic): EP 605217 A

Non-fat margarines comprise (a) a fat mimetic, (b) opt. a bulking agent, (c) inulin and/or gum and (d) water. Fat mimetic (a) is a gelling type maltodextrin or is starch with the amorphous regions removed by hydrolysis.

The bulking agent is at 0–5 wt.%. Component (c) is inulin. The margarine is spreadable. The margarine esp. contains calcium citrate, esp. at 0.75–3.0%. It also contains a gum, esp. xanthan, guar or acacia gum, alginate, carrageenan, pectin or gelatin, esp. at 0.1–2.0%. The fat mimetic is at 3.5–8 or 5–10%. The bulking agent is at 1.0–5%. The inulin is at 10–23%, esp. 15–25%. If (b) is present, (c) is gum and the margarine is squeezable. (b) is at 5–10%. Compsns. also contain 1.0–2.5% salt. They also contain 0.5–15% fat or oil.

ADVANTAGE—Compsns. have the appearance and taste of margarine or squeezable margarine with no fat and reduced calorie content.

Starch—Spread & Salad Dressing 10

Carbohydrate replacers for fat or oil in foods e.g., icing, glazes, margarine etc.—is made of gelatinised, fragmented and retrograded amylose starch in particulate gel form.

Patent Assignee: STALEY MFG CO A E (STAL)
Inventor: HARRIS D W; LITTLE J A; STANLEY K D
Number of Countries: 047 Number of Patents: 007
Patent No Kind Date Applicat No Kind Date Main IPC Week
WO 9409645 A1 19940511 WO 93US10321 A 19931028 A23L-001/05 199420 B
AU 9455411 A 19940524 WO 93US10321 A 19931028 199434
AU 9455411 A 19931028
US 5387426 A 19950207 US 90483208 A 19900220 A23L-001/0522 199512
US 90578994 A 19900906 US 91746381 A 19910816
US 91746432 A 19910816 US 91798291 A 19911126
US 91798292 A 19911126 US 92908728 A 19920706
US 92918861 A 19920730 US 92918862 A 19920730
US 92918951 A 19920730 US 92918952 A 19920730
US 92968979 A 19921030 US 5436019 A 19950725
US 90483208 A 19900220 A23L-001/05 199535 N
US 90578994 A 19900906 US 91798292 A 19911126
US 92908728 A 19920706 US 92918951 A 19920730
EP 666715 A1 19950816 WO 93US10321 A 19931028 A23L-001/05 199537
EP 94900410 A 19931028
JP 8502888 W 19960402 WO 93US10321 A 19931028 A23L-001/05 199645
JP 94511295 A 19931028
EP 666715 A4 19970205 EP 94900410 A 19940000 A23L-001/05 199722
Abstract (Basic): WO 9409645 A

Heat-treated and fragmented amylose starch hydrolysates are prepd. by

(i) gelatinising and retrograding an amylose starch to a degree that permits physical degradation to form a particle gel; (iii) physically sepg. the treated amylose from the aq. medium at elevated temp. to remove a water-soluble hydrolysate fraction and the aq. medium, leaving hydrolysed, retrograded amylose and (iv) physically fragmenting some of this in an aq. medium to produce a particle gel.

The temp. in (iii) is over 90°C. The particle gel exhibits, at a shear strain of under 50 millistrain, a transition from constant to decreasing dynamic elastic modulus. The starch is derived from Zea mays. The starch is derived from a starch of at least 40 wt.% amylose. the starch after treatment has only a low content of 90°C water solubles.

Also claimed are foodstuffs contg. the prods. and aq. dispersions of the prods.

USE—The gels act as carbohydrate replacements for some of the fat and/or oil in food compsns., e.g., icings, glazes, creme fillings, frozen desserts, dressings, meat prods., cheese prods., margarine, fruit butters, other imitation dairy prods., puddings, sweets, sauces, toppings and syrups.

Starch—Spread & Salad Dressing 11

Viscous salad dressing with reduced fat—having proteinaceous water-dispersible macrocolloid of denatured non-dairy whey protein as fat substitute.

Patent Assignee: LABATT LTD JOHN (LABA)
Inventor: LATELLA J; SINGER N S; YAMAMOTO S
Number of Countries: 001 Number of Patents: 001
Patent No Kind Date Applicat No Kind Date Main IPC Week
US 5139811 A 19920818 US 84606959 A 19840504 A23L-001/24 199236 B
US 87127955 A 19871202 US 89367261 A 19890616
US 90568745 A 19900817
Abstract (Basic): US 5139811 A

Some or all of the fat and/or oil of a viscous salad dressing is replaced by a proteinaceous, water-dispersible macrocolloid comprising non-aggregated particles of denatured non-dairy whey protein.

In a dry state the particles have mean dia. ranging from 0.1–2.0 microns with less than 2% (in number) over 3.0 microns. They are generally spheroidal viewed under an 800x microscope. In a hydrated state they form a macrocolloid with smooth, emulsion-like, organoleptic character.

USE—Prods. have texture like mayonnaise or starch-based salad dressings and can be formulated to give sandwich spreads, tartar sauce or refigerated spoonable salad dressing.

Starch—Spread & Salad Dressing 12

Reduced calorie salad dressing—contains fat mimetic, microcrystalline cellulose, cold water swelling starch and gum giving fat-like properties.
Patent Assignee: LIPTON CO THOMAS J (LIPT-N)
Inventor: BAUER R; CUCCURULLO J A; DAZO P E; KOCHAKJI D J; RIKON S M; RUBOW R E
Number of Countries: 001 Number of Patents: 001
Patent No Kind Date Applicat No Kind Date Main IPC Week
US 5286510 A 19940215 US 92957492 A 19921007 A23L-001/0522 199407 B
Abstract (Basic): US 5286510 A

Fat mimetic compsns. are an intimate admixt. of 30–70 wt.% colloidal microcrystalline cellulose (I); 30–70% cold water swelling starch (II); 1–15 % xanthan, carrageenan, locust bean and/or guar gums (III); 0–5 % alginate or alginate deriv. and (IV); 0–5% opacifier (V). (V) is TiO_2 and/or milk solids. The mimetic imparts organoleptic props. similar to fat at 1–10% in a dressing contg. up to 30% fat.

Pref., (I) is at 50–60 (56%); (II) at 40–50 (32%); (III) at 3–5 (4%); (IV) at 1–3 (or 5%) and (V) at 0.5–4 (3)%. (IV) is propylene glycol alginate and (V) is TiO_2.

70–99 pts. water are put in a vessel and agitation started. A dry mixt. of 0.3–5.6 pts. microcrystalline cellulose, 0.3–6 pts. starch, 0.1–0.5 pts. xanthan gum, 0.1–0.5 pts. propylene glycol alginate and 0.04–0.52 pts. TiO_2 is prepd. and added under agitation. In a second vessel contg. 21–45 pts. water, 8–10 pts. vinegar, 12–27 pts. sweetener, 5–25 pts. flavour cocktail, and 0–30 pts. oil are added and agitated until homogeneous. 25–30 pts. of the fat mimetic is then dispersed in the compsn. in the second vessel.

USE/ADVANTAGE—Mimetics are used in low or no fat, reduced calorie salad dressings. Dressings have smooth, creamy mouthfeel and texture and lubricity like edible fat-contg. prods.

Starch—Spread & Salad Dressing 13

Reduced calorie food compsns. useful for salad dressings, etc.—comprise extended polyvinyl alcohol fatty acid ester(s) as fat mimetics.
Patent Assignee: NABISCO INC (NATY)
Inventor: DAMELIA R P; JACKLIN P T; JANES L E; SCIMONE A
Number of Countries: 001 Number of Patents: 001
Patent No Kind Date Applicat No Kind Date Main IPC Week
US 5240996 A 19930831 US 89312618 A 19890217 C08F-008/00 199336 B
US 89446220 A 19891205 US 92865565 A 19920409
Abstract (Basic): US 5240996 A

Food compsn. comprises (as fat mimetic) an extended polyvinyl alcohol ester polymer of formula $H(CH_2\text{-}CH((CH_2)mOH)\text{-})nH$ (I) (where m is 1–8; n is 5–100; X is H or RCO; and R is 1-20C aliphatic).

The compsn. is pref. a bakery or snack prod. (pref. also comprising flour or starch), a candy (pref. also comprising a sweetener), or an emulsion (a fat phase contg. (I), and an aq. phase). The compsns. may also comprise a proteinaceous or sucrose polyester fat replacement. Pref. in the food compsns., (I) is used to replace at least 10% esp. at least 25% of the conventional fat. A pref. (I) is prepd. by polymerising 4-penten-1-yl acetate with a catalytic amt. of $(PhCO)_2O_2$ under N_2; removing unreacted acetate ester by distn., interesterification with Me oleate in the presence of NaOMe; then purifying the resulting (I).

USE/ADVANTAGE—The fat replacement polymers (I) may be individually tailored to provide different polyvinyl alcohol esters having desirable functional props. in a range of food prods. Thus (I) are useful in emulsions (salad dressings and margarines), in high natural fat foods (dairy, meat, nut and egg prods.), in all types of leavened baked goods, in snack prods., and as frying oils.

Starch—Spread & Salad Dressing 14

Fat mimetic compsns. for reduced calorie salad dressings—comprise microcrystalline cellulose, cold water swelling starch, gum, alginate, opacifier and water.

Patent Assignee: UNILEVER PLC (UNIL); UNILEVER NV (UNIL); LIPTON CO THOMAS J (LIPT-N); UNILEVER LTD (UNIL)
Inventor: BAUER R; CUCCURULLO J A; DAZO P E; KOCHAKJI D J; RIKON S M; RUBOW R E
Number of Countries: 023 Number of Patents: 013
Patent No Kind Date Applicat No Kind Date Main IPC Week
US 5209942 A 19930511 US 91799583 A 19911127 A23C-001/24 199320 B
AU 9229619 A 19930603 AU 9229619 A 19921125 A23L-001/24 199329
CA 2083806 A 19930528 CA 2083806 A 19921125 A23L-001/24 199333
EP 558832 A2 19930908 EP 92203669 A 19921127 A23L-001/24 199336
JP 5236906 A 19930917 JP 92341215 A 19921127 A23L-001/24 199342
HU 63752 T 19931028 HU 923728 A 19921126 A23L-001/29 199348
CZ 9203496 A3 19940216 CS 923496 A 19921126 A23L-001/24 199413
ZA 9209221 A 19940727 ZA 929221 A 19921127 A23C-000/00 199431
SK 9203496 A3 19950208 CS 923496 A 19921126 A23L-001/24 199525
EP 558832 A3 19940831 EP 92203669 A 19921127 A23C-001/24 199531
JP 95095932 B2 19951018 JP 92341215 A 19921127 A23L-001/24 199546
AU 667203 B 19960314 AU 9229619 A 19921125 A23L-001/24 199618

CA 2083806 C 19960528 CA 2083806 A 19921125 A23L-001/24 199633
Abstract (Basic): US 5209942 A

Fat mimetic compsn. comprises: (a) 30–70% colloidal microcrystalline cellulose (I); (b) 30–70% cold H_2O swelling starch (II); (c) 1–15% gum (III) (xanthan, carrageenan, locust bean or guar gums or mixts.); (d) 0–5% alginate (IV) (or deriv.); and (e) 0–5% opacifier (V) (TiO_2 and/or milk solids). The compsn. imparts organoleptic properties similar to fat when formulated at 1–10% in a dressing contg. up to 7% fat.

Pref. compsn. comprises 50–60% esp. 56% (I), 40–50% (II), 3–5% esp. 4% (III) (esp. xanthan gum), 1–3% esp. 5% (IV) (esp. as propylene glycol alginate), and 0.5–4% esp. 3% (V) (esp. as TiO_2).

USE/ADVANTAGE—The fat mimetic compsns. allow the prodn. of low fat/no fat reduced calorie salad dressings with the taste and functionality of full fat dressings. In addn., the dressings may be prepd. using relatively low energy processes.

Starch—Spread & Salad Dressing 15

Milk fat substitute particles for food spread—contg. insol. hydrophilic inner matrix, bonded hydrophobic layer of fatty acid and outer lipidic or amphiphilic cpd. for low fat paste.

Patent Assignee: BIOVECTOR THERAPEUTICS SA (BIOV-N); A & S BIOVECTEURS (ASBI-N); BIOVECTOR THERAPEUTICS SA (ASBI-N)
Inventor: GIBILARO J; SAMAIN D
Number of Countries: 019 Number of Patents: 007
Patent No Kind Date Applicat No Kind Date Main IPC Week
WO 9221251 A1 19921210 WO 92FR497 A 19920604 A23L-001/308 199252 B
FR 2677225 A1 19921211 FR 916744 A 19910604 A23L-001/307 199306
EP 542965 A1 19930526 EP 92911690 A 19920604 A23L-001/308 199321
WO 92FR497 A 19920604
JP 6500697 W 19940127 JP 92510770 A 19920604 A23C-011/00 199409
WO 92FR497 A 19920604
EP 542965 B1 19960508 EP 92911690 A 19920604 A23L-001/308 199623
WO 92FR497 A 19920604
DE 69210549 E 19960613 DE 610549 A 19920604 A23L-001/308 199629
EP 92911690 A 19920604 WO 92FR497 A 19920604
US 5534501 A 19960709 US 93978685 A 19930402 A01N-043/04 199633
US 95479539 A 19950607
Abstract (Basic): WO 9221251 A

Particles comprise (a) an insol. hydrophilic matrix surrounded by (b) a 1st hydrophobic layer of fatty acids bonded to the matrix by covalent bonds, and (c) a 2nd layer of lipidic or amphiphilic cpds. Pref. the matrix is a polysaccharide, naturally insol. or chemically or physically insolubilised, esp. naturally insol. polysaccharides, cellulose, certain starches and dextrans, carragenenes, and sol. polysaccharide gels rendered insol. by chemical crosslinking. The fatty acids are bonded to the matrix by ester functions, esp. esterification on the OH gps. of the matrix, using natural fatty acids. (c) The amphiphilic cpds. are phospholipids or proteins, (milk components).

Starch—Spread & Salad Dressing 16

Cold swellable granulated starch for calorie reduced food—combined with mayonnaise, Hollandaise, salad cream, etc., without requiring synthetic prod.

Patent Assignee: CPC INT INC (CORP); MELWITZ A (MELW-I); MAIZENA GMBH (CORP)
Inventor: MELWITZ A; SEEWI G; SPITZFADEN K; STUTE R
Number of Countries: 022 Number of Patents: 013
Patent No Kind Date Applicat No Kind Date Main IPC Week
DE 4117327 C 9920903 DE 4117327 A 19910527 A23L-001/0522 199236 B
EP 516107 A1 19921202 EP 92108989 A 19920527 A23L-001/0522 199249
AU 9217170 A 19921203 AU 9217170 A 19920526 A23L-001/0522 199304
NO 9202095 A 19921130 NO 922095 A 19920526 A23L-001/29 199305
CA 2069463 A 19921128 CA 2069463 A 19920522 A23L-001/308 199307
FI 9202406 A 19921128 FI 922406 A 19920526 A23L-001/0522 199308
JP 5252906 A 19931005 JP 92135334 A 19920527 A23L-001/307 199344
AU 660978 B 19950713 AU 9217170 A 19920526 A23L-001/0522 199535
EP 516107 B1 19950920 EP 92108989 A 19920527 A23L-001/0522 199542
TW 254846 A 19950821 TW 92104083 A 19920525 A23L-001/19 199543
DE 69204904 E 19951026 DE 604904 A 19920527 A23L-001/0522 199548
EP 92108989 A 19920527
ES 2077293 T3 19951116 EP 92108989 A 19920527 A23L-001/0522 199551
IE 67896 B 19960501 IE 921629 A 19920701 A23L-001/0522 199629
Abstract (Basic): DE 4117327 C

Use is claimed of cold-swellable, granulated starch as a substitute for fat or oil in foodstuffs, pref. fat-reduced emulsions, esp. mayonnaise, hollandaise, salad cream and dips.

Pref. ratio of starch to fat or oil in the whole prod. is 2:1–1:15, and the amt. of starch in the whole prod. is 2–12 (3–7) wt.%. The prod. pref. contains 10–60 (15–50) wt.% fat or oil.

USE/ADVANTAGE—For calorie-reduced foods. The prod. has good taste, consistency and feeling, without requiring the use of a synthetic prod. The emulsion is formed without requiring large amts. of starch.

Starch—Spread & Salad Dressing 17

Edible plastic dispersion esp. for use in low fat prods.—has a non-fat continuous phase, and includes at least two condensed phases comprising gel-forming compsns. contg. different gelling agents.
Patent Assignee: UNILEVER NV (UNIL); UNILEVER PLC (UNIL)
Inventor: CAIN F W; CLARK A H; DUNPHY P J; JONES M G; NORTON I T; ROSS-MURPH S B; ROSS-MURPHY S B
Number of Countries: 016 Number of Patents: 008
Patent No Kind Date Applicat No Kind Date Main IPC Week
EP 298561 A 19890111 EP 88201405 A 19880705 198902 B
AU 8818750 A 19890112 198909
JP 1086831 A 19890331 JP 88169982 A 19880707 198919
ZA 8804936 A 19900328 ZA 884936 A 19880708 199017
US 4956193 A 19900911 US 88215009 A 19880705 199039
EP 298561 B1 19950517 EP 88201405 A 19880705 A23L-001/307 199524
DE 3853796 G 19950622 DE 3853796 A 19880705 A23L-001/307 199530
EP 88201405 A 19880705
JP 96029047 B2 19960327 JP 88169982 A 19880707 A23D-007/015 199617
Abstract (Basic): EP 298561 A

An edible plastic dispersion not having a continuous fat phase and including at least two condensed phases at least one of which is continuous comprises (i) a gel-forming compsn. (A) contg. 1–8 times the critical concn. of a gelling agent (I), and (ii) a gel-forming compsn. (B) contg. 1–8 times the critical concn. of a gelling agent (b).

At least one of (a) and (b) is an aggregate-forming gelling agent and at least one is not a starch. (a) and (b) are different and neither is a non-waxy intact starch.

Also claimed are use of the dispersion in the prepn. of a food prod., and a food prod. contg. the dispersion.

USE/ADVANTAGE—The dispersion can be used to replace margarine or halvarine, or as dessert topping or filling, or can be used in the prepn. of other food prods. to reduce their fat content, e.g., in mayonnaise-like food prods. or pate.

Starch—Spread & Salad Dressing 18

Converted gelling starch—of use as replacement for fat or oil in foodstuffs.
Patent Assignee: NAT STARCH & CHEM CORP (NATT)
Inventor: HOFFMAN S; LENCHIN J; TRUBIANO P C
Number of Countries: 017 Number of Patents: 011
Patent No Kind Date Applicat No Kind Date Main IPC Week

US 4510166 A 19850409 US 84572266 A 19840119 198517 B
EP 149258 A 19850724 EP 84116504 A 19841229 198530
AU 8436972 A 19850725 198537
ZA 8409843 A 19850613 ZA 849843 A 19841218 198539
JP 60164449 A 19850827 JP 856013 A 19850118 198540
DK 8500259 A 19850720 198603 CA 1226167 A 19870901 198739
EP 149258 B 19910508 199119 DE 3484562 G 19910613 199125
JP 93037007 B 19930601 JP 856013 A 19850118 A23L-001/0522 199324
JP 6105652 A 19940419 JP 92310583 A 19921119 A23D-009/00 199420

Abstract (Basic): US 4510166 A

Converted gelling starch (I) has a dextrin equivalent (DE) less than 5; aq. dispersions at 10–50 wt.% starch solids have a hot flow viscosity of at least 10 secs. at 55°C and are capable of forming gels having a strength of at least 25 g within 24 hrs. at 4°C.

Pref. (I) is a dextrin, or an acid-converted or enzyme-converted starch, e.g., tapioca, corn or potato; it is esp. a tapioca dextrin of DE 1.5 or less, hot flow viscosity 15–80 secs. and gel strength 65–150 g at 25% solids.

USE/ADVANTAGE—(I) forms with water a gel of neutral taste and creamy smooth consistency; it is readily prepd. by conventional means. (I) may be used to replace oil or fat partially or completely, e.g., in ice cream, salad dressing, margarine, whipped topping or sauce.

Starch—Method 1

New method of prodn. of high amylose starch-based texturising agent—useful in foods and in drug and cosmetic formulations.

Patent Assignee: OPTA FOOD INGREDIENTS INC (OPTA-N)
Inventor: FINOCCHIARO E T; MALLEE F M; STONE J A
Number of Countries: 001 Number of Patents: 001
Patent No Kind Date Applicat No Kind Date Main IPC Week
US 5547513 A 19960820 US 92900899 A 19920618 C13K-001/06 199639 B
US 93138541 A 19931015
WO 94US11654 A 19941014
US 95459401 A 19950602

Abstract (Basic): US 5547513 A

A new method of producing a high amylose starch-based texturising agent comprises: (a) heating a slurry of high amylose starch in an aq. acidic medium for a temp., pressure and time sufficient to substantially disrupt starch granules to produce a solubilised starch soln.; (b) filtering the resultant soln. to remove impurities; and (c) drying the solubilised starch soln. by a suitable means to preserve the amorphous structure and produce a starch-based texturising agent that is non-retrograded and non-crystalline.

USE—The texturising agent functions to provide several fat-like attributes such as structure, viscosity, smoothness and opacity to reduce and/or essentially replace the fat content in foods. Additionally the texturising agent can be used in full fat foods as a stabiliser. The texturising agent can also be incorporated into drug and cosmetic formulations.

Starch—Method 2

Prepn. and packaging of frozen, instant mashed potato prod.—by heating slurry contg. fat-contg. ingredient or substitute and water, mixing with dehydrated potato solids, dispensing into ovenable trays, sealing and freezing.
Patent Assignee: CONAGRA INC (CONA-N)
Inventor: JONSON S H; MOGILEVSKY S; SCHERPF D H
Number of Countries: 001 Number of Patents: 001
Patent No Kind Date Applicat No Kind Date Main IPC Week
US 5536525 A 19960716 US 95550890 A 19951031 A23L-001/216 199634 B
Abstract (Basic): US 5536525 A

A frozen instant mashed potato prod. is prepd. and packaged, by: (a) heating a slurry contg. a fat-contg. ingredient (or fat substitute) and water at above the gelatinisation temp. of potato starch but below the b.pt. of the slurry; (b) mixing the heated slurry with dehydrated potato solids in a high-speed mixer processor; and (c) dispensing the instant mashed potato prod. into an ovenable container, sealing it, and freezing the contents.

The slurry is obtd. by combining (wt.%) 0.5–10 butter, margarine, and/or fat substitute; 0–30 liq. milk; 0–3 dry milk cream; 0–8 seasonings and 50–85 water.

USE—The process is useful in the prodn. of a frozen meal which only needs heating before eating.

ADVANTAGE—The same flavour and texture is obtd. as mashed potatoes prepd. from fresh-cooked potatoes.

The batch cycle time is reduced, allowing a high speed packaging line of 250–300 meals/min.

Starch—Method 3

Prepn. of non-fat foodstuffs, esp. fruit and vegetable based products—involving adding fat mimetic based on starch, pectin or protein to improve texture and other properties.
Patent Assignee: SMUCKER J M CO (SMUC-N)
Inventor: BRAIN C H; GAITHER K S; MUENZ D J
Number of Countries: 001 Number of Patents: 001

Patent No Kind Date Applicat No Kind Date Main IPC Week
US 5503863 A 19960402 US 92857257 A 19920325 A23L-001/29 199619 B
US 93115825 A 19930903
US 95488686 A 19950607
Abstract (Basic): US 5503863 A

A non-fat food product (I) comprising a mixt. of (a) a food ingredient selected from whole fruit, fruit puree, fruit juice or concentrate, cocoa, tomatoes or tomato juice, sauce, paste or paste concentrate; (b) water and/or sweetener; (c) a stabiliser and/or gel promoting agent; and (d) a fat mimetic which is pectin, starch and/or protein based.

A range of compsns. contg. particular food ingredients is claimed, e.g., a prod. contg. up to 55 wt.% fruit puree or fruit juice, 10–75% sweetener, up to 80% water, food acid, gel promoter, stabiliser and 0.1–4.0% pectin based mimetic where the soluble solids are 20–80% and the particle size is 5–100 μm.

USE—The products (I) are not fat imitation products but are similar to the traditional products comprising (a)–(c).

ADVANTAGE—(d), added as additional ingredient rather than as fat substitute, improves the texture of (I), enhances the spreadability, flavour and mouthfeel of some fruit spreads and improves the water retention and bake stability of bakery filled products.

Starch—Flavor 1

Fat substitute for processed foods—prepd. by enzymatic hydrolysis of small granule starch to give partial solubilisation.

Patent Assignee: LAFAYETTE APPLIED CHEM INC (LAFA-N)
Inventor: WHISTLER R L
Number of Countries: 065 Number of Patents: 002
Patent No Kind Date Applicat No Kind Date Main IPC Week
WO 9610586 A1 19960411 WO 95US12466 A 19950929 C08B-030/00 199621 B
AU 9537600 A 19960426 AU 9537600 A 19950929 C08B-030/00 199631
Abstract (Basic): WO 9610586 A

Mfr. of granular starch-based fat substitutes for processed foods comprises (i) hydrolysing a small granule starch until at least 5 wt.% solubilised and (ii) recovering the prod. The starch used has average dia. <5 μm. Hydrolysis is with an amylase in an aq. medium at below the starch gelatinisation temp.

USE—The prods. have the rheological props. of fat and can be used in low calorie processed foods as fat mimetics.

Starch—Fruits & Vegetables 1

Prodn. of starch hydrolysis prod. contg. partly gelatinised starch granules—by heating aq. starch suspension, treating with alpha-amylase and deactivating enzyme, for use as oil or fat substitutes.

Patent Assignee: CPC INT INC (CORP)
Inventor: DEA I C M; ROLLER S
Number of Countries: 009 Number of Patents: 007
Patent No Kind Date Applicat No Kind Date Main IPC Week
EP 704169 A2 19960403 EP 95305834 A 19950822 A23L-001/0522 199618 B
CA 2159039 A 19960328 CA 2159039 A 19950925 C12P-019/14 199628
ZA 9507478 A 19960731 ZA 957478 A 19950906 C08L-000/00 199635
JP 8176202 A 19960709 JP 95246436 A 19950925 C08B-031/00 199637
EP 704169 A3 19960821 EP 95305834 A 19950822 A23L-001/0522 199641
BR 9504171 A 19961022 BR 954171 A 19950926 A23L-001/24 199648
SG 34269 A1 19961206 SG 951348 A 19950913 A23L-001/09 199706
Abstract (Basic): EP 704169 A

Starch hydrolysis prods. contg. partly gelatinised starch granules are produced by: (i) preparing. an aq. starch suspension contg. 10–30 wt.% starch (dry wt.); (ii) heating to 58–80°C which is not significantly over the starch gelatinisation temp.; (ii) treating with porcine pancreatic alpha-amylase at 58–63°C until the required dextrose equiv. (DE) or mol. wt. for the water-soluble fraction is reached; and (iv) deactivating the enzyme.

USE—The prods. are usable as oil or fat substitutes in food compsns., esp. salad dressing (claimed).

ADVANTAGE—Prods. are partly soluble in cold water, are not pourable at 90°C, contain partly gelatinised starch granules, exhibit birefringence under cross-polarised light and can form aq. gels of concn. 20% with gel strength at least 25 g/mm in 24 hrs. at 4°C (claimed).

Starch—Fruits & Vegetables 2

Fruit spread—contains fat mimetic of low methoxy pectin or modified corn starch improving texture and flavour and decreasing dissipation rate in the mouth.

Patent Assignee: SMUCKER J M CO (SMUC-N)
Inventor: BRAIN C H; GAITHER K S; MUENZ D J
Number of Countries: 003 Number of Patents: 004
Patent No Kind Date Applicat No Kind Date Main IPC Week
US 5260083 A 19931109 US 92857254 A 19920325 A23L-001/06 199346 B
AU 9335368 A 19930930 AU 9335368 A 19930319 A23L-001/064 199347
CA 2082751 A 19930926 CA 2082751 A 19921112 A23L-001/06 199351

AU 9517852 A 19950629 AU 9335368 A 19930319 A23L-001/064 199533
AU 9517852 A 19950503

Abstract (Basic): US 5260083 A

Fruit spreads with improved texture and flavour comprise a microparticulated blend of (a) up to 55 wt.% fruit ingredient; (b) sweetener, to a soluble solids content of 20–70 wt.%; (c) up to 80 wt.% water and (d) a fat mimetic. Ingredient (a) is whole fruit, fruit puree or fruit juice.

Pref. fat mimetic (d) is a low methoxyl pectin or a modified corn starch. It is esp. at least 0.5 (0.5–3.0) wt.% low methoxyl pectin, and the blend has particle size 5–100 microns; or is 5–20 wt.% modified corn starch, and the blend has particle size 2–15 microns, opt. aggregated to not over 100 microns. The spreads are produced by mixing the ingredients, cooking to a desired solids content and homogenising under high shear.

USE/ADVANTAGE—Spreads are jelly- or jam-like. They have improved texture and flavour characteristics and decreased dissipation rate in the mouth.

Starch—Bakery & Grain 1

Starch-prune premixes for flour-based food prods.—useful as fat replacements to give food prods. of good taste, improved shelf-life and healthy eating characteristics.

Patent Assignee: CADEN J A (CADE-I); WOLKE M (WOLK-I)
Inventor: CADEN J A; WOLKE M
Number of Countries: 001 Number of Patents: 001
Patent No Kind Date Applicat No Kind Date Main IPC Week
US 5484622 A 19960116 US 93105395 A 19930812 A21D-010/00 199609 B
US 95404506 A 19950315

Abstract (Basic): US 5484622 A

Starch-prune premixes are used for making flour-based food prods. They comprise amylopectin starch (I), amylose starch (II) and prunes (III). All three are mixed together to form the premix, to which flour and other components may be added to make the food prods.

ADVANTAGE—The prods. are low in fat, all natural, low cholesterol, low Na, mould resistant, economical, resistant to microwave-induced loss of texture and taste, have good taste and have good shelf life.

Starch—Bakery & Grain 2

Low fat, low calorie fat substitute emulsions—contg. only natural ingredients which require no other change in a recipe, e.g., baked goods.

Patent Assignee: MRS BATEMAN'S BAKERY LC (BATE-N)
Inventor: BATEMAN K

Number of Countries: 037 Number of Patents: 002
Patent No Kind Date Applicat No Kind Date Main IPC Week
WO 9526641 A1 19951012 WO 95US4153 A 19950404 A23L-001/052 199546 B
AU 9522063 A 19951023 AU 9522063 A 19950404 A23L-001/052 199605
Abstract (Basic): WO 9526641 A

Low fat, low calorie fat substitutes are emulsions of 40–90 wt.% polysaccharide (I) in 5–60 wt.% water.
The emulsions can be substituted 1-to-1 for fat in food prods. without any other changes in the recipe and without altering the texture of the prod.

Also claimed are substitutes made from 1–40 wt.% baking fat, 40–80% (I) and 5–40% water.

A second polysaccharide (II), pref. a water soluble starch, is present at 1–15%. A flavouring, esp. butter or an artificial flavouring, is present at up to 10%. The flavouring is oil or butter, olive, peanut, canola, corn or safflower oil flavouring, or is up to 1% dried butter. A food colouring, esp. beta-carotene or a yellow dye is pref. present. (I) is a maltodextrin of DE < 20, esp. corn, rice, potato or tapioca starch.

Shelf-life is improved by adding up to 1% preservative. Up to 4% whey protein and/or xanthan gum is added to enhance texture. The pH is also adjusted.

USE—The compsns. can replace, e.g., shortening, margarine, butter, oil, lard, and cream cheese.

ADVANTAGE—The compsns. are made only of natural prods. and need no emulsifiers.

Starch—Bakery & Grain 3

Fat reduced laminated doughs—using aq. gel of maltodextrin and beta-glucan and/or pentosan in water as fat replacer.
Patent Assignee: UNILEVER PLC (UNIL); CONOPCO INC (CONO-N); VAN DEN BERGH FOODS CO (VBER-N); UNILEVER NV (UNIL)
Inventor: BOODE-BOISSEVAIN K; VAN HOUDT-MOREE J D; VAN HOUDT-MOREE J
Number of Countries: 054 Number of Patents: 006
Patent No Kind Date Applicat No Kind Date Main IPC Week
WO 9421128 A1 19940929 WO 94EP698 A 19940308 A21D-013/08 199439 B
AU 9463753 A 19941011 AU 9463753 A 19940308 A21D-013/08 199504
ZA 9401855 A 19951129 ZA 941855 A 19940316 A21D-000/00 199601
US 5480662 A 19960102 US 94217521 A 19940324 A21D-002/00 199607
EP 700251 A1 19960313 EP 94911121 A 19940308 A21D-013/08 199615
WO 94EP698 A 19940308

JP 8507920 W 19960827 JP 94520594 A 19940308 A21D-002/18 199702
WO 94EP698 A 19940308
Abstract (Basic): WO 9421128 A

Laminated doughs comprise alternating layers of dough and of another ingredient. The layers of other ingredient at least partly comprise an aq. gel contg. 20–50 wt.% maltodextrin, esp. amylodextrin and 0–30 wt.% of beta-glucan and/or pentosans, with the balance water.

USE/ADVANTAGE—Doughs are used for puff pastry, laminated snacks, or for croissants. They may be frozen or baked. The aq. gel acts as a fat replacer giving reduced fat content in the final baked dough.

Starch—Bakery & Grain 4

Edible compsns. with reduced calorie value—in which fat is partially replaced by partially digestible N-acylated esterified amino acid derivs.
Patent Assignee: NABISCO INC (NATY)
Inventor: FINLEY J W; KLEMANN L P; YARGER R G
Number of Countries: 001 Number of Patents: 001
Patent No Kind Date Applicat No Kind Date Main IPC Week
US 5190782 A 19930302 US 89409254 A 19890919 A23L-001/29 199315 B
US 91690732 A 19910424
Abstract (Basic): US 5190782 A

Edible compsn. contg. fat has at least 5% of the fat comprising an acylated amino acid of formula R1OCOA(Xa)NHCOr (I) (where A is 1-6C hydrocarbyl; X is opt. acylated amino acid side chain with 1-25C; n is 0 or 1; each R is 1-29C aliphatic, 2029C R2OR3- or R3OCOR3- or R2CO2R3; R2 and R3 are aliphatic gps.; and each R1 is 1-30C aliphatic, or 2-30C R2OR3- or R3OCOR2- or R2CO2R3-.

Pref. compsn. is a bakery prod. also contg. flour starch; a candy also contg. a sweetener, and an emulsion comprising an aq. phase, and a fat phase including (I). Pref. compsns. may also comprise a sucrose polyester or proteinaceous fat replacement. Pref. compsns. have at least 20% esp. at least 25% of the fatty ingredient replaced by (I). Pref. (I) are fatty acid acylated, fatty alcohol esterified amino acids selected from arginine, histidine, tyrosine, cysteine, asparagine, glutamine, glycine, alanine, valine, (iso)leucine, methionine, proline, phenylalanine, and tryptophan, esp. aspartic or glutamic acid (or derivs.), lysine, ornithine, serine, and threonine, partic. an N-acrylated aspartic acid diester (3-23C acyl; 4-24C ester gps.). Pref. (I) deliver 0.5–3 kcal/g on being metabolised.

ADVANTAGE—Pref. acylated amino acid ester derivs. (I) contain 1 side chain, and are partially digestible, achieving reduced calorie value and reducing problems associated with non-metabolisable fat substitutes (gastrointestinal upsets, including diarrhoea and anal leakage etc.). (I) may also be tailored to include essential or desired fatty acids if desired.

Starch—Bakery & Grain 5

Fat replacer for mfg. low or zero fat content foods—contains phospholipid liposome(s) in water and reinforcing carbohydrate.
Patent Assignee: AMERICAN LECITHIN CO (AMLE-N)
Inventor: BUCCINO J; FIERRO J; JODLBAUER H; SILVA R F
Number of Countries: 001 Number of Patents: 001
Patent No Kind Date Applicat No Kind Date Main IPC Week
US 5120561 A 19920609 US 91691357 A 19910425 A23L-001/30 199226 B
Abstract (Basic): US 5120561 A

Low (or zero)-fat food contains as fat replacer liposomes contg. at least 5% phospholipid (I) and water, with water to (I) ratio 2–20:1. (I) is at least 35% phosphatidyl choline (Ia) with (Ia): phosphatidyl ethanolamine (Ib) ratio 2–10:1, and the liposomes also include an edible reinforcing material (II) which stabilises them. (II) is starch, cellulose and/or gum, and the (Ii): (I) ratio is 0.5–4:1.

The fat replacer is new.

(Ia) is pref. 40–90% and (Ia): (Ib) is 3–6:1. (II) is potato maltodextrin; pregelatinised wheat starch and/or xanthan gum.

USE/ADVANTAGE—Apart from replacing (some of) the fat in the food, the liposomes can also serve as carriers (for colours, vitamins, flavours, etc.), encapsulating or moisturising agents, or depanner. These replacements are partic. used in baking and can be used in smaller amts. than the fats which they replace.

Starch—Bakery & Grain 6

Low-fat dry mix based on sweetened cereal—comprising polydextrose, cellulosic material, non-fat milk solid, emulsifier, modified food starch and xanthan, guar or locust bean gum.
Patent Assignee: NELSON K J (NELS-I); PILLSBURY CO (PILL)
Inventor: NELSON K J; HAHN P W
Number of Countries: 033 Number of Patents: 006
Patent No Kind Date Applicat No Kind Date Main IPC Week
WO 9200012 A 19920109 A21D-002/18 199205 B
AU 9174470 A 19920227 199218
EP 536139 A1 19930414 EP 91905226 A 19910121 A21D-002/18 199315
WO 91US407 A 19910121

US 5262187 A 19931116 US 90546017 A 19900628 A23L-001/10 199347
US 91722710 A 19910628 US 92918945 A 19920722
EP 536139 B1 19940824 EP 91905226 A 19910121 A21D-002/18 199433
WO 91US407 A 19910121
DE 69103633 E 19940929 DE 603633 A 19910121 A21D-002/18 199438
EP 91905226 A 19910121 WO 91US407 A 19910121

Abstract (Basic): WO 9200012 A

Mix comprises: a sweetened cereal-grain ingredient base with a fat-mimetic system of (i) less than 0.1 to 5 wt.% of a polydextrose or its buffered form, (ii) less than 0.1 to 15 wt.% of a cellulosic material, (iii) less than 0.1 to 8 wt.% of a non-fat milk solid or substitute (IV), less than 0.1 to 4 wt.% of each of an emulsifier and a modified food starch (V) and less than 0.1 to 2 wt.% of a mixt. of xanthan gum and guar or locust bean gum. The wt.% are relative to the total wt. of the dry-mix.

Also claimed is a baked, low-fat food compsn. contg. the dry mix and a low-fat ready-to-use butter contg. the dry mix.

Pref. the ingredient base includes sugar and flour at a ratio of 2:1 to 1:1 pts. wt. (Pbw). The dry mix also includes flavourings colouring, salt, leavening agent, and/or preservatives.

USE/ADVANTAGE—The baked compsn. contg. the dry mix is moist, tender, crumbly with good mouth feel and pref. contains one-third fewer calories than a similar full fatted compsn. The dry mix produces substantially homogeneously distributed small air cells throughout the volume of the baked compsn.

Starch—Bakery & Grain 7

Food prod. with moisture contg. filling—enclosed in bread-like casing and intermediate layer sepg. filling from casing made of cake material of specific vol.

Patent Assignee: UNILEVER NV (UNIL); DIJKSHOORN J (DIJK-I); UNILEVER PLC (UNIL); VAN DEN BERGH FOODS CO (VBER-N)
Inventor: DIJKSHOORN J; HOLSCHER E J
Number of Countries: 016 Number of Patents: 008
Patent No Kind Date Applicat No Kind Date Main IPC Week
EP 421509 A 19910410 EP 90202466 A 19900918 199115 B
CA 2026614 A 19910403 199125
JP 3119945 A 19910522 JP 90263698 A 19901001 199127
US 5145699 A 19920908 US 90585859 A 19900919 A23D-001/08 199239
EP 421509 B1 19950201 EP 90202466 A 19900918 A21D-013/00 199509
DE 69016555 E 19950316 DE 616555 A 19900918 A21D-013/00 199516
EP 90202466 A 19900918

ES 2069671 T3 19950516 EP 90202466 A 19900918 A21D-013/00 199526
JP 2528734 B2 19960828 JP 90263698 A 19901001 A21D-002/26 199639
Abstract (Basic): EP 421509 A

A food prod. comprises a moisture contg. filling enclosed in a bread-like casing and an intermediate layer sepg. the filling from the casing made of a cake material-having a specific volume of 1.5–4.0 m^3/kg.

The cake material has a specific volume of 2–3 m^3/kg and has a fully developed cellular crumb structure. The bread-like casing is based on a whole meal flour. The material of the intermediate layer is formed from a batter of which the oil and fat phase in the form of an oil-in-water emulsion comprising water soluble proteins and a combination of emulsifier comprising 12-24C fatty acid acyl lactylate together with a) a polyglycerol ester of an unsatd. 12-24C fatty acid, or b) a monoglyceride of an unsatd. 12-24C fatty acid, or c) a mixt. of a monoglyceride of satd. and unsatd. 12-24C fatty acids. The water soluble proteins are selected from whole eggs, egg white, non-fat dry milk solids, skimmed milk powder and/or whey protein and is used in an amt. of 0.5–10 wt.% based on the wt. of the cake batter. At least part of the fat or oil is replaced by a low-calorie fat replacer, esp. an edible polyester or polyhydric alcohol having at least 4 free OH gps. of which at least 70% is esterified with a satd. or unsatd. alkyl chain 8-24C fatty acid. A liquid oil is incorporated into the batter absorbed in expanded at least partly gelatinised starch. The 12-24C fatty acid acyl lactate is selected from free acid, alkali metal salts and/or alkaline earth metal salts.

USE/ADVANTAGE—The intermediate cake layer has a fat content of at most 20 wt.% based on the total recipe of the cake batter and acts as a moisture migration controlling agent and as a softness imparting agent. The filling is a savoury filling, a meat based filling, a fermented sausage, or sweet filling, or a fruit based filling.

Starch—Beverage 1

Flavour carrier for forming emulsions of flavour oils—comprises beta-limit dextrin obtd. from duwx starch obtd. from starch bearing plant with dull waxy homozygous genotype.

Patent Assignee: AMERICAN MAIZE PROD CO (AMEM); AMERICAN MAIZE TECHNOLOGY INC (AMEM)
Inventor: AMMERAAL R; FRIEDMAN R; AMMERAAL R N; FRIEDMAN R B
Number of Countries: 005 Number of Patents: 005
Patent No Kind Date Applicat No Kind Date Main IPC Week
US 5482560 A 19960109 US 94281408 A 19940727 C08B-031/00 199608 B
GB 2291882 A 19960207 GB 9515174 A 19950724 C08B-030/18 199609

AU 9523342 A 19960208 AU 9523342 A 19950629 C08B-030/18 199613
FR 2723106 A1 19960202 FR 958093 A 19950705 C12P-019/04 199613
BE 1008583 A3 19960604 BE 95648 A 19950725 C08B-000/00 199632
Abstract (Basic): US 5482560 A

Flavour carrier comprises a beta-limit dextrin having a DE of < 1 and a polymerisation degree as determined by a wt. ave. of 15,000–20,000. The dextrin is obtd. from a duwx starch obtd. from a starch bearing plant with a dull waxy homozygous genotype.

USE—The beta-limit dextrin is used as a beverage clouding agent, thickener for gum candies, carrier for volatile ingredients for spray drying, and bulking agent and in low fat food prods. as a fat replacer and extruded prods. The beta-limit dextrin is also used as a slow release agent for delivery of non-caloric sweeteners and drugs and for accelerating wound healing.

ADVANTAGE—The beta-limit dextrin has good water holding activity at low viscosity, low dextrose equiv., limited enzyme susceptibility and cold water solubility and reaches equilibrium slowly on dissolution.

Starch—Beverage 2

Prepn. of maltose and a novel limit dextrin—by treatment of starch with a specific amylase below the gelatinisation temp. followed by prod. recovery by ultrafiltration.

Patent Assignee: NOVO-NORDISK AS (NOVO)
Inventor: CHRISTENSEN T R; CHRISTOPHERSEN C; PEDERSEN S
Number of Countries: 059 Number of Patents: 002
Patent No Kind Date Applicat No Kind Date Main IPC Week
WO 9510627 A1 19950420 WO 94DK383 A 19941013 C12P-019/22 199521 B
AU 9478532 A 19950504 AU 9478532 A 19941013 C12P-019/22 199536
Abstract (Basic): WO 9510627 A

Prodn. of maltose and limit dextrin comprises: (i) treating raw starch with amylase, which is a hydrolase with the enzyme classification EC 3.2.1.133; and (ii) recovering the maltose and limit dextrin by ultrafiltration, where the maltose is the permeate and the limit dextrin is produced as the solid phase by liq.-solid sepn. of the retentate. The method is carried out at a temp. lower than the lowest temp. at which the raw starch is gelatinised. Also claimed is the limit dextrin produced by this method.

ADVANTAGE—The method is simpler and cheaper than known methods for the prodn. of (I), and affords (I) or purity above 90%. The prepd. inexpensive (II) is useful as a fat replacer in foods (claimed), when it has the same good organoleptic properties as traditional fat replacers. (II) may also be used in confections with a gum structure, in soft drinks, in viscous dairy prods., and as a carrier for dried liqs.

Starch—Dairy 1

Food additive contg. synthetic sweetener and cream flavouring—comprising fatty acid or ester, methyl ketone, diketone, hydroxy-ketone, aldehyde or lactone, with low calorie value.

Patent Assignee: WILD GMBH & CO KG RUDOLF (WILD-N)
Inventor: WILD R
Number of Countries: 001 Number of Patents: 001
Patent No Kind Date Applicat No Kind Date Main IPC Week
DE 4305874 A1 19940915 DE 4305874 A 19930225 A23L-001/226 199436 B
Abstract (Basic): DE 4305874 A

A food additive contains a synthetic sweetener and a flavour with the taste of cream, comprising a 3-20 C opt. satd. fatty acid or ester with a 1-4C alcohol, a 4-14C methyl ketone, a diketone, a hydroxyketone, a 4-14C opt. satd. aldehyde, or a gamma- or delta-lactone.

Pref., the additive contains 1–10 pts. of sweetener, 0.5–20 pts. of cream flavouring, and opt. a fat substitute, comprising starch, pectin, insulin or protein cpds., esp. 10–1000 pts. of starch cpd., 10–2000 pts. of fruit pectin and/or 2–500 pts. of non-fruit pectin, or 1–1000 pts. of protein cpd. The sweetener is, e.g., aspartame, saccharin. The additive may contain a dearomatised and concd. fruit compsn. with 60–80 deg. Brix. The fatty acid has 8-12 C, with 1 or 2 unsatns., and the alcohol is glycerol. The starch cpd. is enzymatically modified potato or tapioca starch, opt. enzymatically modified potato starch, enzymatically modified tapioca starch and whey protein in ratio of 0.3 : 1 : 1–1 : 4 : 10. The pectin prod. is low or high esterified citrus pectin, and the protein is whey protein.

USE—The additive is used domestically or industrially in prepn. of dairy or ice prods. (claimed), esp. in skimmed milk prods., e.g., fruit yoghurt and fruit curd with reduced sugar and fat content.

ADVANTAGE—Although the additive has low nutritional value, it has a creamy taste.

Starch—Dairy 2

Low fat dairy prods. prepn.—by replacing part of the milk fat by hydrated or pregelatinised starch particles before aggregation of the casein.

Patent Assignee: UNILEVER NV (UNIL); UNILEVER PLC (UNIL)
Inventor: KLOOSTERMAN J; TORENVLIET L; VISSER J; KLOOSTERMA J
Number of Countries: 013 Number of Patents: 003
Patent No Kind Date Applicat No Kind Date Main IPC Week
EP 427310 A 19910515 EP 90202761 A 19901017 199120 B

EP 427310 B1 19930609 EP 90202761 A 19901017 A23C-019/05 199323
DE 69001883 E 19930715 DE 601883 A 19901017 A23C-019/05 199329
EP 90202761 A 19901017
Abstract (Basic): EP 427310 A

Prepn. of improved low fat dairy prods. aggregation of casein in milk is effected by replacing at least part of the milk fat by hydrated or pregelatinised starch particles, of particle size = 4–20 microns, before aggregation of the casein is carried out. The prods. obtd. by this process are claimed. A low fat cheese contains hydrated starch or pregelatinised starch particles of size = 4–20 microns.

USE/ADVANTAGE—To prepare yoghurt, hard, semi-hard, processed, fresh or soft cheeses. Addn. of the starch particles induces a mouthfeel similar, e.g., that of fat in cheese-like prods.

Starch—Dairy 3

Imitation cheese compsn.—comprises water, vegetable fat or oil, and caseinate replaced in part or whole with debranched starch.
Patent Assignee: ABLESTIK LAB (ABLE-N); NAT STARCH & CHEM INVESTMENT (NATT); NAT STARCH & CHEM CORP (NATT)
Inventor: CHIU C; ZALLIE J P; CHIU C W
Number of Countries: 011 Number of Patents: 007
Patent No Kind Date Applicat No Kind Date Main IPC Week
EP 363741 A 19900418 EP 89117943 A 19890928 199016 B
US 4937091 A 19900626 US 88258237 A 19881014 199028
AU 8942502 A 19900426 199033
JP 2211827 A 19900823 JP 89255355 A 19891002 199040
EP 363741 B1 19930331 EP 89117943 A 19890928 A23C-020/00 199313
DE 68905743 E 19930506 DE 605743 A 19890928 A23C-020/00 199319
EP 89117943 A 19890928
CA 1336245 C 19950711 CA 611940 A 19890919 A23C-020/00 199535
Abstract (Basic): EP 363741 A

Imitation cheese consists of H_2O, an edible vegetable fat or oil, cheese additives, and one or more edible caseinates (I) or starches suitable for replacing (I). The cheese is prepd. by replacing up to 80% of (I) with a gelatinised starch (II) which has been enzymatically treated to partially debranch it and yield a mixt. comprising partially debranched amylopectin and short-chain amylose.

USE/ADVANTAGE—The specific gelatinised starch (II) is an inexpensive substitute for caseinates in the imitation cheeses, and provides the reqd. texture, thermoreversibility and emulsificn. characteristics.

Starch—Dairy 4

Dairy food substitutes from vegetable oil and malto-dextrin—for use as substitutes for milk, cream or butter in wide variety of foods.
Patent Assignee: MELKRIDGE PTY LTD (MELK-N)
Inventor: STRONG M J
Number of Countries: 031 Number of Patents: 003
Patent No Kind Date Applicat No Kind Date Main IPC Week
WO 8908988 A 19891005 WO 89AU131 A 19890330 198942 B
AU 8934132 A 19891016 199008
ZA 8902330 A 19901128 ZA 892330 A 19890329 199101
Abstract (Basic): WO 8908988 A

New dairy substit. formulation comprises 6–10 pts. wt. oil in a carbohydrate or protein matrix, 4–8 pts. wt. maltodextrin, sufficient emulsifier to give a stable emulsion at 16g formulation per 250 ml water, and an effective amt. of antioxidant. The maltodextrose is prod. by partial hydrolysis of tuber or cereal starch. It is of formula $(C_6H_{10}O_5)_n$, where n = 300–1000, and has dextrose equiv. (DE) 2–5, and pH 5.5–7 in 25% aq. soln.

USE/ADVANTAGE—Formulations can replace milk or butter fat in, e.g., custards, cream, substits. ice creams, soft serve creams, coffe whiteners, yoghurt, cakes, pastries, biscuits or butter replacers. They have realistic mouthfeel, taste and appearance.

Starch—Emulsifier, Stabilizer, and Suspending Agent 1

Dry, water-dispersible fine cellulose compsn. used e.g., as stabiliser for food or medicines—comprises fine cellulose and water-soluble gums and/or hydrophilic substances.
Patent Assignee: ASAHI KASEI KOGYO KK (ASAH)
Number of Countries: 001 Number of Patents: 001
Patent No Kind Date Applicat No Kind Date Main IPC Week
JP 7173332 A 19950711 JP 93318322 A 19931217 C08L-001/02 199536 B
Abstract (Basic): JP 7173332 A

Dry, water-dispersible fine cellulose compsn. consists of at least 20 wt.% and less than 50 wt.% of (A) fine cellulose and more than 50 wt.% and up to 80 wt.% of (B) water-soluble gums and/or hydrophilic substances. When the compsn. is dispersed in water, it has average particle size of up to 8 microns, contains up to 40% of particles having size of at least 10 microns and has colloid fraction of at least 65%.

The water-soluble gums are, e.g., CMC-Na xanthan gum, carrageenan, pectin, karaya gum, gelatin and arabic gum. The hydrophilic substances are starch hydrolysates, dextrin, glucose, fructose, sucrose, maltose, lactose, polydextrose, mannitol and sorbitol.

USE/ADVANTAGE—The compsn. is used as stabilisers for food and medicine, dietary fibre and substitute for fats and oils. When the compsn. is dispersed in water, a colloidal dispersion is obtd. which has smooth feeling.

Starch—Emulsifier, Stabilizer, and Suspending Agent 2

New starch which can be used as a thickener—obtd. from grain homozygous recessive for the waxy and amylose extender genes and heterozygous for dull gene.

Patent Assignee: DU PONT DE NEMOURS & CO E I (DUPO)
Inventor: PEARLSTEIN R W; ULRICH J F; PEARLSTEIN R; ULRICH J
Number of Countries: 053 Number of Patents: 005
Patent No Kind Date Applicat No Kind Date Main IPC Week
WO 9422291 A1 19941013 WO 94US3398 A 19940329 A01H-005/10 199441 B
AU 9464181 A 19941024 AU 9464181 A 19940329 A01H-005/10 199505
EP 691807 A1 19960117 EP 94911740 A 19940329 A01H-005/10 199608
WO 94US3398 A 19940329
BR 9406183 A 19960206 BR 946183 A 19940329 A01H-005/10 199612
WO 94US3398 A 19940329
US 5502270 A 19960326 US 9340333 A 19930330 A01H-005/00 199618
Abstract (Basic): WO 9422291 A

(A) Grain produced by a starch bearing plant is claimed in which the genotype of the grain comprises a genome which is homozygous recessive for the waxy gene and the amylose extender gene and heterozygous for the dull gene.

(B) Also claimed is a pure starch extracted from a grain as in (A). To produce the grain, homozygous recessive ae du wx plants are cross pollinated with homozygous recessive ae wx plants or vice versa. The ae wx plants used to make the cross pollination are homozygous dominant for the du gene.

USE/ADVANTAGE—The starch can be used as a thickener without being chemically modified. The starch can be cooked with a foodstuff and water to produce a thickened foodstuff (claimed). The starch has a creamy texture when cooked, making it suitable as a fat substitute. The starch can also be used in, e.g., paper, plastics, adhesives or paint. The starch has a higher paste viscosity, greater shear resistance and greater acid resistance than normal maize starch.

Starch—Emulsifier, Stabilizer, and Suspending Agent 3

Ready-to-eat, low–no fat pudding—comprises water, calcium source, thickening and sweetening agents, emulsifier, and calcium-sensitive, irreversible gelling hydrocolloid.

Patent Assignee: KRAFT GEN FOODS INC (KRFT); KRAFT FOODS INC (KRFT)
Inventor: KING L D; LESHIK R R
Number of Countries: 004 Number of Patents: 006
Patent No Kind Date Applicat No Kind Date Main IPC Week
GB 2261805 A 19930602 GB 9224485 A 19921123 A23L-001/187 199322 B
DE 4239590 A1 19930603 DE 4239590 A 19921125 A23L-001/187 199323
CA 2082969 A 19930528 CA 2082969 A 19921116 A23L-001/187 199333
US 5238699 A 19930824 US 91800617 A 19911127 A23L-001/187 199335
GB 2261805 B 19950802 GB 9224485 A 19921123 A23L-001/187 199534
CA 2082969 C 19960507 CA 2082969 A 19921116 A23L-001/187 199628
Abstract (Basic): GB 2261805 A

Compsn. for the prepn. of a packaged ready-to-eat pudding comprises: less than 3% fat; H_2O; a source of soluble Ca (I); thickening agent (II); sweetener; emulsifier/stabiliser (III) and/or polyphosphate; and 0.01–1.5% by wt. of an ungelled, Ca-sensitive, irreversible, gelling hydrocolloid (IV) as fat replacement.

Pref. compsn. comprises 0–3%, esp. 0% fat. Pref. (I) is milk solids. Pref. sweetener is sugar-free. Pref. (IV) is algin (or salts), low methoxyl pectin, gellan gum or mixts., esp. Na alginate; and is pref. the only non-starch hydrocolloid present.

ADVANTAGE—The low/no fat, ready-to-eat pudding-like desserts may be UHT sterilised, when they are stable to storage for prolonged periods, or may be prepd. under controlled conditions and stored at refrigeration temps. The prods. have a smooth, creamy texture and mouthfeel, and the weak, soft gel structure of full-fat, ready-to-eat puddings.

Starch—Emulsifier, Stabilizer, and Suspending Agent 4

Ultrafine lupin flour used as substitute for starch, fat etc.—obtd. by cleaning white lupin seeds, shelling and pre-grinding to obtain particles of a specified size.

Patent Assignee: LA NOELLE SERVICES (NOEL-N); LA NOELLE SERVICES COOP INTERET COLLECTI (NOEL-N); LA NOELLE SERV COOP (NOEL-N); LA NOELLE SERVICES COOP INTERET (LNOE-N)
Inventor: AUGER I; CORRE V
Number of Countries: 012 Number of Patents: 008
Patent No Kind Date Applicat No Kind Date Main IPC Week
EP 449697 A 19911002 EP 91400714 A 19910315 199140 B
FR 2660163 A 19911004 FR 904205 A 19900328 199150
PT 97206 A 19911129 199201
AU 9180457 A 19930211 AU 9180457 A 19910717 A23L-001/20 199313 N

AU 642509 B 19931021 AU 9180457 A 19910717 A23L-001/20 199349 N
EP 449697 B1 19940601 EP 91400714 A 19910315 A23L-001/20 199421
DE 69102184 E 19940707 DE 602184 A 19910315 A23L-001/20 199427
EP 91400714 A 19910315
ES 2054456 T3 19940801 EP 91400714 A 19910315 A23L-001/20 199432
Abstract (Basic): EP 449697 A

Flour produced from shelled lupin seeds has a particle size distribution such that at least 90% of the particles are smaller than 100 microns and at least 60% are smaller than 30 microns.

At least 98% of the particles are smaller than 100 microns, at least 75% are smaller than 30 microns, and at least 50% are smaller than 10 microns.

White lupin (Lupinus albus) seeds are cleaned, opt. heat-treated by fluidisation in air at 85–170°C for 0.5–12 min., shelled, preground to 500–2000 microns in a hammer mill, and finally ground by passage through a series of three pairs of counter-rotating rolls under a pressure of 10 bar.

USE/ADVANTAGE—The flour is finer than known lupin flours and has better functional properties, e.g., emulsifying, gelling and thickening power. Used in foodstuffs, e.g., as partial caseinate substitute or a starch or fat substitute.

Starch—Emulsifier, Stabilizer, and Suspending Agent 5

Particulate free-flowing peanut butter material—contg. expanding gelatinised starch material for prodn. of sauces.
Patent Assignee: UNILEVER NV (UNIL); UNILEVER PLC (UNIL)
Inventor: VAN ROOIJEN A; VANROOIJEN A
Number of Countries: 013 Number of Patents: 004
Patent No Kind Date Applicat No Kind Date Main IPC Week
EP 414290 A 19910227 EP 90202045 A 19900726 199109 B
EP 414290 B1 19930922 EP 90202045 A 19900726 A23L-001/38 199338
DE 69003494 E 19931028 DE 603494 A 19900726 A23L-001/38 199344
EP 90202045 A 19900726
ES 2045765 T3 19940116 EP 90202045 A 19900726 A23L-001/38 199407
Abstract (Basic): EP 414290 A

New particulate food compsns. comprise peanut butter and 5–35 wt.% expanded (partially) gelatinised starch material.

The starch material is at 10–25 wt.%. Compsns. contain up to 10 wt.% of additive(s). These are herbs, spices, flavourants, colourants, emulsifiers, antioxidants, vegetable, fruits, dairy prods., meat from mammals, poultry or fish, animal, vegetable or fungal protein, animal, vegetable or synthetic oil or fat (fraction) and/or low-calorie fat replacer.

USE/ADVANTAGE—Prods. are free flowing and can be used for the mfr. of peanut butter based sauces (e.g., satay) for meat dishes and meals.

Starch—Emulsifier, Stabilizer, and Suspending Agent 6

Starch natural gum composite—processed so that polysaccharide components are completely solubilised, are useful in foods as thickening and suspending agents.

Patent Assignee: US SEC OF AGRIC (USDA)
Inventor: CHRISTIANSON D D; FANTA G F
Number of Countries: 003 Number of Patents: 006
Patent No Kind Date Applicat No Kind Date Main IPC Week
WO 9414887 A2 19940707 WO 93US11862 A 19931208 C08L-003/02 199428 B
AU 9465479 A 19940719 AU 9465479 A 19931208 C08L-003/02 199439
WO 9414887 A3 19940915 WO 93US11862 A 19931208 C08L-003/02 199518
US 5424088 A 19950613 US 92991811 A 19921217 A23L-001/05 199529
EP 674682 A1 19951004 WO 93US11862 A 19931208 C08L-003/02 199544
EP 94913248 A 19931208
JP 8505170 W 19960604 WO 93US11862 A 19931208 C08L-003/02 199648
JP 94515201 A 19931208

Abstract (Basic): WO 9414887 A

Compsn. comprises a water-solubilised blend of polysaccharide components of starch and of a natural gum, the starch polysaccharide components:natural gum polysaccharide components dry wt. ratio is in the range 99:1–90:10.

Pref. the highest mol. wt. polysaccharide components of the blend have significant molecular wt. redn.

USE/ADVANTAGE—Compsns. are useful in foods as thickening agents, suspending agents and fat substitutes. When placed in water, the compsns. hydrate rapidly and yield dispersions that are not only smooth and viscous but also possess considerable lubricity. Aq. dispersions of certain blends show little or none of the undesirable tendency of cooked starches to form rigid gels on standing or to exude water when frozen and thawed.

In an example, 400 g. wheat starch was dry blended with 20 g. guar gum. The blend was dispersed in 3 l. of water and the pH adjusted to 7. Steam jet cooking was then carried out at 140°C with a steam pressure of 40 psig. within the cooker. The cooked soln. was drum dried and ground. An emulsion formed by adding 30–35 wt.% corn oil to a 10 wt.% aq. dispersion the compsn. was smooth and spreadable and remained stable under refrigeration and/or room temp. conditions during extended storage.

Starch—Emulsifier, Stabilizer, and Suspending Agent 7

Emulsifying starch degradation prod. used in low calorie foods—comprises acidolysis of starch or acid roasting starch without degrading particle structure.

Patent Assignee: SANMATSU KOGYO CO (SANM-N)
Number of Countries: 001 Number of Patents: 001
Patent No Kind Date Applicat No Kind Date Main IPC Week
JP 5301903 A 19931116 JP 92134237 A 19920427 C08B-030/00 199350 B
Abstract (Basic): JP 5301903 A

Emulsifying starch degradation prod. (I) comprises acidolysis of starch (II) or acid roasting of (II) without degradation of the starch particle structure. (I) has a dextrose equiv. (DE) of 0.04–0.30, viscosity of 10–1,000 cps, and emulsification above 0.3.

Low calorie emulsion foods contg. (I) as substitute oils and/or fats are also claimed. Pref. the starch has ratio of amylopectin/amylose = 80/20–85/15, and is esp. sweet potato starch and/or tapioca starch.

(II) is added to acid soln. (e.g., 1% hydrochloric acids). The mixt. is stirred at 45°C for a few hr. to obtain (I), or a mixt. of (II) and acid (pref. 1% to (II)) is heated at 130°C in a rotary kiln to obtain (I).

USE/ADVANTAGE—(I) is a good emulsifying agent used to emulsify fats and oils, and is useful as a substitute for fats and oils. (I) is prepd. simply and easily.

Starch—Emulsifier, Stabilizer, and Suspending Agent 8

Water-dispersible starch materials—produced by microwave cooking and drying.

Patent Assignee: INRA INST NAT RECH AGRONOMIQUE (INRG)
Inventor: COLONNA P; DELLAVALLE G; TAYEB J
Number of Countries: 013 Number of Patents: 004
Patent No Kind Date Applicat No Kind Date Main IPC Week
WO 8909793 A 19891019 WO 89FR153 A 19890404 198944 B
FR 2629684 A 19891013 FR 884528 A 19880406 198948
AU 8934192 A 19891103 199003
EP 374208 A 19900627 EP 89904573 A 19890404 199026
Abstract (Basic): WO 8909793 A

New starch materials (I) have a particle size of 0.5–5mm, a water-solubility (S) of 15–65% and water-swellability (G) of 15–45 ml/g, where S and G are calcd. from following formulae using 0.5g samples stirred in 50 ml H_2O at 65°C for 30 min.: S = Wi–Wg/Wi × 100, G = Vw–Vs/Wg, where Wi is the initial wt. of the sample (dry basis); Wg is the wt. of gel formed; Vs is the initial vol. of water, Vs is the vol. of supernatant.

USE/ADVANTAGE—(I) are useful as fat substitutes in foodstuffs, e.g., cooked dishes, sausages and sauces. They are readily dispersed in water at any temp. and have a high thickening power.

Starch—Dessert 1

Food modifying compsns. for fat-free cake icing—comprise edible micro-milled soy fibre in aq. liq.

Patent Assignee: KRAFT GEN FOODS INC (KRFT); KRAFT FOODS INC (KRFT)

Inventor: ANDERSON W A; DULIN D A; LOH J P; DULIN D; LOH J

Number of Countries: 019 Number of Patents: 005

Patent Family:

Patent No Kind Date Applicat No Kind Date Main IPC Week

US 5230918 A 19930727 US 92865593 A 19920409 A23L-001/308 199331 B

EP 565260 A1 19931013 EP 93302133 A 19930322 A23L-001/29 199341

CA 2091973 A 19931010 CA 2091973 A 19930318 A23G-003/00 199402

EP 565260 B1 19951011 EP 93302133 A 19930322 A23L-001/29 199545

DE 69300611 E 19951116 DE 600611 A 19930322 A23L-001/29 199551

EP 93302133 A 19930322

Abstract (Basic): US 5230918 A

(A) Food modifying compsn. comprises (by wt.) 1–15% of an edible soy fibre (I) of particle size 0.1–20 micron dispersed in 85–99% of an aq. liq.

(B) Cake icing comprises 10–100% of the compsn. (A).

Pref. compsn. (A) comprises 7–12% (I) and 88–93% aq. liq.; and pref. also comprises 0.001–1.5% of a non-gelling, non-abrasive hydrocolloid as whitening enhancer (esp. 0.3–0.9% gum arabic; 0.01–0.05% CMC, locust bean gum, or carrageenan; or 0.001–0.01% guar gum), and 0.1–2%, esp. 0.5–1.5% TiO_2. Pref. (I) has particle size 2–7 microns. Pref. aq. liquids are H_2O, milk, or an aq. sugar soln. (esp. comprising 30–70% sugar and 40–75% H_2O; sugar pref. sucrose, fructose, dextrose, corn syrup solids, high fructose corn syrup solids, glycerol, sorbitol, or other liq. or solid sugars).

Pref. cake icing compsns. (B) comprise sugar, H_2O and compsn. (A) and opt. starch, pref. (concns. independent of sugar and H_2O content of (A)) 25–80% sugar, 25–50% H_2O, 2–10% starch and compsn. (A).

Cake icing compsns. (B) are prepd. by wet-milling a blend of sugar, H_2O and compsn. (A) ((I) of particle size above 20 microns) to the desired (I)-particle size.

USE/ADVANTAGE—The fat-free food modifying compsn. (A) contg. micromilled soy fibres is an effective fat substitute, and is esp. useful in cake icing compsns. to provide these with a creamy taste and a flavour profile that resembles fat-contg. icing.

Starch—Dessert 2

Prodn. of non-fat non-milk ice cream—from aq. mix. contg. sucrose and starch hydrolysate.

Patent Assignee: AKAD WISSENSCHAFTEN DDR (DEAK)
Inventor: ANTER E; AUGUSTAT S; GROSCHNER P; POESCHEL W; RICHTER M; SCHIERBAUM F; SCHULZ P; SELLMER I
Number of Countries: 001 Number of Patents: 001
Patent No Kind Date Applicat No Kind Date Main IPC Week
DD 161178 A 19850502 DD 215086 A 19790821 198535 B
Abstract (Basic): DD 161178 A

Prodn. of ice-cream substitutes free of fat and milk protein is effected by preparing a mix contg. 15.7 wt.% sucrose, 7–9 wt.% of a gel-forming starch hydrolysate with a D.E. of 5–8%, water, fruit prods. and stabilisers. The mix is then pasteurised, cooled and frozen while whipping to incorporate 50% air, opt. followed by hardening.

ADVANTAGE—The prods. have better whipping, melting and mouth-feel properties than conventional water-ice.

Starch—Dessert 3

Frozen desserts contg. rice and/or oat starch as fat substitute—giving good texture, smoothness and mouth-feel, reducing fat content to below 2%.

Patent Assignee: CONAGRA INC (CONA-N)
Inventor: BOST R; CHIGURUPATI S R; SCHERPF D
Number of Countries: 018 Number of Patents: 002
Patent No Kind Date Applicat No Kind Date Main IPC Week
WO 9213465 A1 19920820 WO 92US727 A 19920128 A23G-009/00 199236 B
AU 9214344 A 19920907 AU 9214344 A 19920128 A23G-009/00 199249
WO 92US727 A 19920128
Abstract (Basic): WO 9213465 A

Frozen desserts comprise 1–4 wt.% rice starch and/or oat starch. Rice starch has particle dia. less than 10 microns. The starch content is about 2% and fat less than 10 (not over 2). Desserts comprise 1–4% starch, 0–10% edible fat, 5–40% non fat solids, 0–40% flavouring, 25–80% water and an effective amount of a sweetener, esp. 1–4% flavouring, 25–80% water and an effective amount of a sweetener, esp. 1–4% starch, 0–10% butterfat, 8–14%

non-fat milk solids, 10–30% sweetener solids, 0–40% flavouring and 25–80% water. The butterfat is esp. not over 2%, milk solids 11–13%, sweetener 18–23% and starch 2%. Compsns. also contain 0.3% stabiliser solids. Desserts comprise 1–4% starch, 0–10% (0–2%) butterfat, 10–14% (11–13%) non-fat milk solids. 10–17% (12–15%) cane sugar solids, 5–10% (6–9%) corn sugar syrup solids, 0.1–0.5 (0.3) % stabiliser solids, 0–40% flavourings and 25–80 (60–65)% water.

USE/ADVANTAGE—The starch acts as a fat substitute, allowing fat to be reduced to under 2% in ice cream, frozen yogurt, ice milk, soft ice, soft frozen yogurt, novelties etc. Prods. have good texture, smoothness and mouth-feel.

DIETARY FIBER (DF)-BASED FAT SUBSTITUTES

DF—General 1

Prodn. of beta glucanase-treated, water-soluble dietary fibre compsn.—involves treating aq. dispersion of beta-glucan with enzyme to form compsn. with improved fat mimicking properties, i.e., similar taste.

Patent Assignee: QUAKER OATS CO (QUAK)
Inventor: SMITH J J
Number of Countries: 001 Number of Patents: 001
Patent No Kind Date Applicat No Kind Date Main IPC Week
US 5458893 A 19951017 US 92847258 A 19920306 A23L-001/10 199605 B
US 93156134 A 19931122
Abstract (Basic): US 5458893 A

Prodn. of beta glucanase-treated, water-soluble, dietary fibre compsn. where aq. dispersion of a gelatinised, milled, beta-glucan contg. grain is treated with alpha-amylase under conditions that will hydrolyse it and yield both soluble and insol. fraction. Soluble fraction is sepd. and from it is recovered the water-soluble dietary fibre mainly free of water-insol. fibre. The improvement comprises: (a) treating beta-glucans released from the grain with beta-glucanase. The wt. ratio of beta-glucanase to initial beta-glucan contg. grain is 4×10 power -6:1 to 2×10 power -2 to 1; (b) treatment of the beta-glucans with the beta-glucanase is carried out at 30–60°C for 5–120 minutes at a pH of 5–7.

USE—Used as food additive or as a fat substitute in food prods.

ADVANTAGE—Compsn. has improved fat-mimicking properties. Prods. made with them have same or similar taste, feel, texture, heat stability and cooking properties as those made from fats.

DF—General 2

Water-soluble dietary fibre compsn. prepn., useful as fat mimetic—comprises treating beta-glucan(s) released from substrate with beta-glucanase, providing food additives, e.g., meat, dairy goods etc.

Patent Assignee: QUAKER OATS CO (QUAK)
Inventor: SMITH J J
Number of Countries: 017 Number of Patents: 005
Patent No Kind Date Applicat No Kind Date Main IPC Week
EP 634106 A1 19950118 EP 93111393 A 19930715 A23L-001/105 199507 B
NO 9302621 A 19950123 NO 932621 A 19930720 A23L-001/308 199511 N
BR 9302977 A 19950301 BR 932977 A 19930723 A23L-001/307 199515 N
FI 9303331 A 19950124 FI 933331 A 19930723 A23L-001/308 199516 N
CA 2100848 A 19950120 CA 2100848 A 19930719 A23L-001/308 199516 N
Abstract (Basic): EP 634106 A

Water-soluble dietary fibre compsn. (I) is prepd. by treating an aq. dispersion of a gelatinised, milled, beta-glucan-contg. grain-based substrate with an alpha-amylase under hydrolysis conditions; sepg. the soluble and insol. fractions; and recovering (I), free from insol. fibre, from the soluble fraction. The obtd. beta-glucans released from the substrate, are then treated with beta-glucanase under hydrolysis conditions.

USE (claimed)—(I) Is used as a fat mimetic or a fibre additive in food, esp. processed meat, meat prods., dairy prods., baked goods; doughs or dry mixes for preparing baked goods, fillings for baked goods or griddle prods., doughnuts, condiments, confectioneries, desserts, egg substitutes, dry mixes, snack foods, soft drinks, malt beverages, sports beverages, dietary beverages, salad dressings, spreads, soups, sauces, gravies, juice drinks, frozen food or solidified foods.

DF—General 3

Water-dispersing compsn. for use in food, paint, medicine industry, e.g., thickening stabiliser—comprises fine cellulose and hydrophilic substance.

Patent Assignee: ASAHI KASEI KOGYO KK (ASAH)
Number of Countries: 001 Number of Patents: 001
Patent No Kind Date Applicat No Kind Date Main IPC Week
JP 7070365 A 19950314 JP 93218436 A 19930902 C08L-001/02 199519 B
Abstract (Basic): JP 7070365 A

Water dispersing compsn., which is a dry compsn., consists of 50–95 wt.% of fine cellulose and 5–50 wt.% of hydrophilic substance. Ratio of particles with particle size of at least 10 microns is less than 40% and colloid graduation is at least 50% when compsn. is dispersed again into water.

USE/ADVANTAGE—Used for food, medicine, cosmetics, paint, ceramics, resin, industrial products, etc. as suppression stabiliser, emulsion stabiliser, thickening stabiliser, cloudy agent, foam stabiliser, fluidity improver, shape retaining agent, water-leaving agent, ground modifier, powdering base, and further, food-fibre base, oil and fat substitute, etc. The water dispersing compsn. can be dispersed to original fine cellulose particles and shows low viscosity when dispersed into water, which provides good feel when passing through throat, and acts.

DF—General 4

Water dispersible, colloid generating cellulose complex—is used in food and drinks, is free from sandy taste, is low calorie and provides fibre.

Patent Assignee: ASAHI KASEI KOGYO KK (ASAH); MINAMI Y (MINA-I)
Inventor: MINAMI Y; MIYOMOTO H; MIYAMOTO H
Number of Countries: 005 Number of Patents: 006
Patent No Kind Date Applicat No Kind Date Main IPC Week
AU 9225398 A 19930401 AU 9225398 A 19920929 C08L-001/02 199320 B
CA 2079558 A 19930331 CA 2079558 A 19920930 C08B-037/00 199324
AU 647968 B 19940331 AU 9225398 A 19920929 C08L-001/02 199418
TW 239864 A 19950201 TW 92107480 A 19920922 C08B-037/00 199516
JP 7268129 A 19951017 JP 92259396 A 19920929 C08L-001/02 199550
CN 1078481 A 19931117 CN 92112829 A 19920930 C08L-001/02 199710
Abstract (Basic): AU 9225398 A

Water dispersible complex, comprising: (a) 50–98% by wt. of fine cellulose particles; and (b) 2–50% by wt. of water-soluble gum and/or hydrophilic material; and in which the compsn. is such that an aq. dispersion of it comprises; (i) not more than 5% by vol. of particles at least 10 microns in size; and (ii) a colloid fraction of at least 65%; is new.

USE/ADVANTAGE—The complex is useful as a suspension, emulsion, thickening or cloudiness stabiliser in foods, medicaments, cosmetics, coating materials, ceramics, resins, and other industrial prods. It generates a large amt. of colloidal particles on dispersion, is free from a sandy, rough taste, and does not increase viscosity, the last two being partic. important in food and drinks, in addition to improving taste. Examples of use in the food industry are in beverages, soups, ice and soft cream, coffee whitener, mayonnaise and other dressings, breads, cakes, noodles and pasta, and toppings and fillings. The prod. is low-calorie, provides fibre, and can substitute for fats and oils in diets.

DF—Beverage 1

High fibre low calorie beverage—prepd from rice bran, honey and whey protein concentrate opt. with sweeteners or flavourings.
Patent Assignee: UNIV RES & MARKETING INC (UYRE-N)
Inventor: HAMMOND N A
Number of Countries: 001 Number of Patents: 001
Patent No Kind Date Applicat No Kind Date Main IPC Week
US 5153019 A 19921006 US 91707468 A 19910530 A23L-002/02 199243 B
Abstract (Basic): US 5153019 A

Powdered beverage prods. comprise (i) rice bran which has been stabilised against the prodn. of fatty acids; (ii) honey which has not been degraded by heating and (iii) whey protein concentrate. Honey (ii) is free from coliform bacteria, spores and/or protein, all of which come from the intestinal tract of the honeybee.

Prods. contain powdered milk, esp. non-fat milk or soya based milk substitute. Powdered fruit juice is also present. Bran (i) is defatted and stabilised. Prods. also contain a sweetener and/or flavouring esp. aspartame. The wt. ratio (i):(ii) is 1.3–3:1, esp. 1:2–2:1. Prods. comprises 30–70 wt.% (i), 30–60% (ii) and 30–70% (iii).

Liq. beverages from the prod. are new and contain 3–7 wt.% (i), 3–6% (ii) and 3–7% (iii), esp. sweetened by aspartame, saccharin or liquorice root extract.Reduced calorie beverages are new and contain 3–6 wt.% (i), 3–5% (ii) and 3–4% (iii), totalling not over 25 wt.%, and water to 100%. The water can be replaced by non-fat milk, esp. defatted soya milk, or by fruit juice.

USE/ADVANTAGE—Prods. give reduced calorie beverages which are high in fibre and protein. The powders are resistant to bacterial spoilage.

DF—Bakery 1

Reduced fat deep-fried doughnuts—incorporating water-soluble dietary fibre made from gelatinised cereal by amylase hydrolysis to avoid fat take-up and act as fat replacement.
Patent Assignee: QUAKER OATS CO (QUAK)
Inventor: BABBITT L; BRODIE J; BURKE R; KACHER J
Number of Countries: 066 Number of Patents: 003
Patent No Kind Date Applicat No Kind Date Main IPC Week
WO 9618304 A2 19960620 WO 95US16941 A 19951214 A21D-002/36 199630 B
AU 9646097 A 19960703 AU 9646097 A 19951214 A21D-002/36 199642
WO 9618304 A3 19960822 WO 95US16941 A 19951214 A21D-002/36 199643
Abstract (Basic): WO 9618304 A

Reduced-fat deep fried doughnuts are prepd. by (a) preparing raw doughnut material, (b) forming it into a doughnut shape, (c) deep frying and (d) removing the cooked doughnut from the hot frying fat. The doughnut material contains sufficient soluble dietary fibre to prevent some or all fat absorption during frying. The fibre is prepd. by (i) treating an aq. dispersion of a gelatinised, milled cereal with an alpha-amylase under hydrolysis conditions and (ii) sepg. soluble and insol. fractions.

ADVANTAGE—The fibre component both prevents fat absorption and acts as a fat replacementas a stabiliser by the colloidal property of fine cellulose.

DF—Bakery 2

Reduced fat roll-in shortening spreads—giving baked goods with taste etc. at least as good as full-fat prods.
Patent Assignee: BUNGE FOODS CORP (BUNG-N)
Inventor: KINCS F R; MINOR M P
Number of Countries: 001 Number of Patents: 001
Patent No Kind Date Applicat No Kind Date Main IPC Week
US 5395638 A 19950307 US 9389711 A 19930709 A21D-013/08 199515 B
Abstract (Basic): US 5395638 A

Reduced fat roll-in shortening spreads have oil-soluble phase (I) and water-soluble phase (II) which are blended together. (I) is 48–65 wt.% shortening and 0.5–5% emulsifier, both w.r.t. spread. (II) is 30–47% water and 0.5–4% fat substitute. The fat substitute (III) is whey protein concentrate and/or oat fibre derivs. and contains not over 5% fat w.r.t. (III).

(III) is at 0.5–2 wt.% w.r.t. spread. The shortening has m.pt. 103–122°C and SFI 16–34 at 70°C. At least 2 (10–30)% of the shortening is beta′ tending fat, the rest being beta tending fat. The emulsifier is a water-in-oil combination of 0.5–2 pts. wt. lecithin per pt. wt. monoglycerides. Combinations of the spread and dough are new. Baked prods. from these combinations are new.

USE—Spreads are used to make reduced fat baked goods of equal or improved organoleptic props. and taste to their full fat equivalents.

DF—Meat Product 1

Low calorie food—contains dietary fibre of specified max. average particle dia. and min. moisture content.
Patent Assignee: AJINOMOTO KK (AJIN)
Number of Countries: 001 Number of Patents: 001
Patent No Kind Date Applicat No Kind Date Main IPC Week
JP 2057161 A 19900226 JP 88208562 A 19880823 199014 B

Abstract (Basic): JP 2057161 A

0.7–10 wt.% of dietary fibres of ave. particle dia. 80 microns or less and having a moisture content of 9 or more are contained as a protein, carbohydrate or fat substitute.

USE—Used in sausages, ham and other foods. Its calorie content is

DF—Meat Product 2

Reduce fat comminuted meat compsns.—contg. cereal hydrolysate, oat bran, corn syrup solids and opt. yeast and encapsulated salt as fat mimetic.

Patent Assignee: RHONE POULENC SPECIALTY CHEM CO (RHON)
Inventor: JENKINS R K; RHONE-POULENC SPECIALTY
Number of Countries: 023 Number of Patents: 007
Patent No Kind Date Applicat No Kind Date Main IPC Week
EP 619083 A1 19941012 EP 94302221 A 19940328 A23L-001/317 199439 B
AU 9459045 A 19941006 AU 9459045 A 19940324 A23L-001/307 199441
BR 9401367 A 19941018 BR 941367 A 19940330 A23L-001/317 199443
NO 9401190 A 19941006 NO 941190 A 19940330 A23L-001/10 199443
CA 2120382 A 19941006 CA 2120382 A 19940331 A23L-001/308 199501
JP 6303943 A 19941101 JP 9453533 A 19940324 A23L-001/314 199503
CN 1095557 A 19941130 CN 94103973 A 19940401 A23L-001/105 199547
Abstract (Basic): EP 619083 A

Cereal hydrolysate compsns. are for use as fat mimetics in foods. They comprise (a) cereal hydrolysate, (b) oat bran and (c) corn syrup solids in amounts that, when intimately mixed with food, give a fat reduced prod. with the texture and mouthfeel of the full fat prod. Hydrolysate (a) is prepd. by hydrolysing an aq. dispersion of a cereal with an amylase to give a water soluble fraction (I) and an insoluble fraction (II) that contains the cereal protein. It, (a), is (I) and/or (II) or water soluble dietary fibre solids from (I).

USE—Compsns. are used to give reduced fat comminuted meat.

DF—Fruit Paste 1

Low fat high fibre natural bread—with fat replaced by high fibre fruit paste esp. contg. citrus pulp.

Patent Assignee: FAHLEN A E (FAHL-I)
Inventor: FAHLEN A E
Number of Countries: 001 Number of Patents: 001
Patent No Kind Date Applicat No Kind Date Main IPC Week
US 4971823 A 19901120 US 89375536 A 19890630 199049 B
Abstract (Basic): US 4971823 A

High fibre baked prods. comprise yeast; flour and high-fibre fruit paste, but no added fat. Most of the flour is high fibre flour and 7–10 % of it is vital wheat gluten. The fruit paste is at 5–15 wt% wrt flour dry wt. and is intimately mixed with the flour.

USE/ADVANTAGE—By using the fruit paste instead of fat, high-fibre bread is obtd. with increased fibre content and reduced fat.

DF—Low Calorie Foods 1

Flour compsns. with high gluten and soluble dietary fibre—comprising milled oat groat prod. and having good staling resistance and low calorie content.

Patent Assignee: RUDEL H W (RUDE-I)
Inventor: RUDEL H W
Number of Countries: 022 Number of Patents: 013
Patent No Kind Date Applicat No Kind Date Main IPC Week
WO 9005453 A 19900531 199025 B
CA 2002223 A 19900522 199031
AU 9047441 A 19900612 199036
US 4961937 A 19901009 US 88276408 A 19881122 199043
ZA 9003737 A 19910327 ZA 903737 A 19900516 199117 N
EP 438536 A 19910731 EP 90901231 A 19891114 199131
JP 4023942 A 19920128 JP 9012893 A 19900518 199210 N
IL 91755 A 19920906 IL 91755 A 19890924 199242
AU 641628 B 19930930 AU 9047441 A 19891114 199347
EP 438536 B1 19941005 WO 89US5207 A 19891114 199438
EP 90901231 A 19891114
DE 68918702 E 19941110 DE 618702 A 19891114 199444
WO 89US5207 A 19891114
EP 90901231 A 19891114
EP 438536 A4 19920102 EP 90901231 A 19900000 199520
CA 2002223 C 19950704 CA 2002223 A 19891103 199534
Abstract (Basic): WO 9005453 A

Flour compsns. contain sufficient gluten flour to give a vital gluten content of at least 17% of the dry mix, and a milled oat groat prod. giving 0.2–56.0% soluble oat dietary fibre w.r.t. the vital gluten content.

The vital gluten content is at least 75% and the soluble oat dietary fibre content is 8.0–56.0 (0.2–10.6)%. The oat groat prod. includes milled oat bran and/or milled rolled oats. Baking flour is at 10–90% and vegetable germ at 0.5–3.5% w.r.t. dry mix. The baking flour includes wheat flour, rye flour, milled corn meal flour, whole wheat flour and/or milled miller's bran flour. The vegetable gum is guar gum.

USE/ADVANTAGE—Baked goods produced from the compsns. do not

stale and have extended keep qualities, have high protein and dietary fibre. content and have reduced calories.

APPLICATION OF HYDROCOLLOIDS/GUMS TO LOW-FAT AND LOW-CALORIE FOOD PRODUCT DEVELOPMENT

Hydrocolloid—General 1

Smooth, low fat or fat-free emulsion-simulating food prod.—has opaque appearance and has additive of tricalcium phosphate and gum esp. xanthan gum.

Patent Assignee: RHONE POULENC INC (RHON); COUTANT A F (COUT-I); RHONE POULENC SPECIALTY CHEM CO (RHON)
Inventor: COUTANT A F; WONG P
Number of Countries: 022 Number of Patents: 007
Patent No Kind Date Applicat No Kind Date Main IPC Week
EP 551170 A1 19930714 EP 93300008 A 19930104 A23L-001/0522 199328 B
AU 9331075 A 19930708 AU 9331075 A 19930106 A23L-001/05 199334
CA 2085381 A 19930708 CA 2085381 A 19921215 A23L-001/03 199339
US 5292544 A 19940308 US 92818690 A 19920107 A23L-001/05 199410
US 92984155 A 19921202
JP 6038705 A 19940215 JP 93545 A 19930106 A23L-001/24 199411
NZ 245627 A 19950224 NZ 245627 A 19930106 A23L-001/0522 199513
AU 661358 B 19950720 AU 9331075 A 19930106 A23L-001/05 199537
Abstract (Basic): EP 551170 A

Smooth low fat, very low fat or fat-free emulsion-simulating food prod. with an opaque appearance and non-gloppy texture having up to 15% fat mimetic additive comprises: (i) greater than 1 to 10 wt.% of tricalcium phosphate; and (ii) 0.1–5 wt.% gum. Also claimed is a method of preparing the food prod.

The prod. is fat-free and contains up to 10% fat mimetic additive. The amt. of tricalcium added is 1.2–5% and the prod. contains 50–95% water. The fat mimetic comprises xanthan gum esp. oatrim.

Preparing the prod. comprises adding to the food specified amts. of tricalcium phosphate and the gum.

USE/ADVANTAGE—The prod. is esp. an emulsion-simulated dairy prod. contg. sweetener and milk solids or a salad dressing. The prod. can be used in foods such as salad dressing, ice cream, ice milk prods., fat-free milk prods. etc. Tricalcium phosphate improves the opacity of the food giving it an improved smoother texture and prevents stringiness or gloppiness in many food prods. employing gums esp. xanthan gum.

Hydrocolloid—General 2

Low calorie, low fat spoonable ice prod.—contg. sugar alcohol, glycerine, gelling agent, bulking agent, synthetic sweetener, water and opt. minor ingredients.

Patent Assignee: MAMA TISH'S ITAL SPECIALTIES INC (MAMA-N)
Inventor: FISHER T L; KATZ S N
Number of Countries: 001 Number of Patents: 001
Patent No Kind Date Applicat No Kind Date Main IPC Week
US 5246725 A 19930921 US 92829422 A 19920203 A23G-009/00 199339 B
Abstract (Basic): US 5246725 A

Low fat frozen ice prods. are spoonable at temps. above 4°C. They comprise 5:5–9:5 wt.% sugar alcohol, 0.85–2.0 wt.% glycerine, 0.5–1.15 wt.% gelling agent, 3–10 wt.% bulking agent, 0.03–0.1 wt.% sweetener and water to 100%.

Pref. the sugar alcohol is sorbitol, mannitol and/or xylitol. The gelling agent is pectin, agar-agar, gelatin, carrageenan, alignate, gum arabic and/or gum tragacanth. The bulking agent is maltodextrin, hydrolysed cereal solids, corn syrup solids, polydextrose, xanthan gum, locust bean gum and/or CMC. It esp. has DE 10-18.The synthetic sweetener is aspartame, thaumatin, acesulphame K, glycyrrhizin, saccharin, chalcone, miracin, sucralose and/or stevioside.

USE/ADVANTAGE—The prods. have a low calorie content.

Hydrocolloid—General 3

Complexed cpd. of microorganism cellulose—comprises microorganism cellulose or their derivs. and high polymer material.

Patent Assignee: NAKANO SU-MISE KK (NAKA-N)
Number of Countries: 001 Number of Patents: 001
Patent No Kind Date Applicat No Kind Date Main IPC Week
JP 3157402 A 19910705 JP 89294808 A 19891115 199133 B
Abstract (Basic): JP 3157402 A

Complexed cpd. of micro-organism cellulose, comprises micro-organism cellulose or their derivs. and high polymer material as main component.

Pref. useful micro-organism to produce cellulose are aceto bacterium, gluco b., pseudomonus b., agro b. etc. One of desirable cultivate bed is well known Hestria-Schramm, and whose pH is 5–9, temp. 20–40°C. Optional high polymers to be used are chitin, carboxymethyl chitin, chitosan, carboxymethyl cellulose, hydroxyethyl cellulose etc. Similar said micro-fibril structure of cellulose produced by micro-organism and active high polymer can be produced mechanically by mixing pure both materials, and can be shaped into film or filaments.

USE/ADVANTAGE—Cellulose produced by micro-organism is useful as food-stuffs, low calories adducts and stabiliser, but they are not enough to provide their functions, and are desirable to be modified with chemicals or physical devices, which have still various troubles in practical uses. Present invention has succeeded to improve these disadvantages by adding high polymer material to the cultivate bed of micro-organism to produce complexed microfibril of cellulose and high polymer, under mutual activities. So the prod. has excellent functions and is useful as food-base, additive, and modifier, high polymer material and medical uses.

Hydrocolloid—General 4

Low calorie fat substitute—having low calorie or calorie-free core with outer coating of digestible fat.

Patent Assignee: PFIZER INC (PFIZ); CULTOR LTD (CULT-N)
Inventor: HENDRICK M E; REIMER R A
Number of Countries: 022 Number of Patents: 015
Patent No Kind Date Applicat No Kind Date Main IPC Week
EP 380225 A 19900801 EP 90300428 A 19900116 199031 B
AU 9048843 A 19900802 199038
CA 2008314 A 19900725 199041
JP 2242656 A 19900927 JP 9015936 A 19900125 199045
ZA 9000520 A 19910828 ZA 90520 A 19900124 199139
EP 380225 A3 19921014 EP 90300428 A 19900116 199340
KR 9207007 B1 19920824 KR 90829 A 19900124 199406
US 5356644 A 19941018 US 89301576 A 19890125 199441
US 90607216 A 19901029
US 92957648 A 19921006
JP 95028696 B2 19950405 JP 9015936 A 19900125 199518
EP 380225 B1 19960228 EP 90300428 A 19900116 199613
DE 69025480 E 19960404 DE 625480 A 19900116 199619
EP 90300428 A 19900116
ES 2083997 T3 19960501 EP 90300428 A 19900116 199625
PH 27047 A 19930201 PH 39934 A 19900125 199635
IE 71931 B 19970312 IE 90265 A 19900124 199727
CA 2008314 C 19970527 CA 2008314 A 19900123 199733
Abstract (Basic): EP 380225 A

Free-flowing microparticulate compsns. comprise an outer shell of a digestible (semi)solid fat compsn. surrounding a low calorie or calorie-free core material. If the core material is cellulose it is nm-fibrous.

The core material is a solid, liq., gel-forming compsn., foam and/or gas. The mean particulate dia. is less than 250 microns. The core material is polydextrose, non-fribrous cellulose deriv., erythritol, micronised bran or a wax, esp. polydexlose. The core material is an aq. gel-forming compsn., esp. formed by combining in an aq. medium, a gel-forming alginate, CMC, succinoglycan, xanthan, gelatin, pectin or scleroglucan with a cross-linking amount of Ca (II) or Mg(II) salt. A layer is present between the core and shell and is of cellulose methylcellulose, cellulose acetate, phthalate, albumin, casein, zinc, agar, gelatin, pectin, or gum arabic, but not the same as the core material.

Prodn. of the compsns. by encapsulating such cores in such shells is new. The coating is esp. by pan coating, spin disc coating, gas suspension coating, centrifugal coextrusion, rotational suspension, coaceration, inclusion complexation spray coating or spray drying.

USE/ADVANTAGE—Compsns. are used as low calorie fat substitutes which are insol. under food formulation conditions.

Hydrocolloid—General 5

A two-phase emulsion useful as a low calorie fat substitute—comprises specified amts. of aq. phase rendered non-flowable by addn. of suitable gel-forming compsn., oil phase compsn. and emulsifier.

Patent Assignee: PFIZER INC (PFIZ); PFIZER CORP (PFIZ)
Inventor: FUNG F; MILLER J W; WUESTHOFF M T; FUNG F N
Number of Countries: 023 Number of Patents: 018
Patent No Kind Date Applicat No Kind Date Main IPC Week
EP 441495 A 19910814 EP 91300482 A 19910122 199133 B
AU 9170239 A 19910808 199139
NO 9100421 A 19910806 199141
CA 2035529 A 19910806 199142
FI 9100534 A 19910806 199143
PT 96660 A 19911031 199148
US 5082684 A 19920121 US 90475576 A 19900205 199206
ZA 9100805 A 19920930 ZA 91805 A 19910204 A23L-000/00 199244
US 5158798 A 19921027 US 90475576 A 19900205 A23D-009/00 199246
US 91636549 A 19910111
EP 441495 A3 19920916 EP 91300482 A 19910122 199339
AU 640200 B 19930819 AU 9170239 A 19910204 A23D-007/02 199340
AU 9341519 A 19930902 AU 9170239 A 19910204 A23D-007/02 199342
AU 9341519 A 19930625
US 5308639 A 19940503 US 90475576 A 19900205 A23D-007/00 199417
US 92823800 A 19920117
IL 97093 A 19940412 IL 97093 A 19910129 A23D-007/02 199422
KR 9304456 B1 19930527 KR 911909 A 19910204 A23D-009/00 199423

JP 7067577 A 19950314 JP 9114539 A 19910205 A23L-001/307 199519
AU 660812 B 19950706 AU 9170239 A 19910204 A23D-007/02 199534
AU 9341519 A 19930625
CA 2035529 C 19951031 CA 2035529 A 19910201 A23L-001/30 199603
Abstract (Basic): EP 441495 A

A two-phase emulsion useful as a low calorie fat substitute comprises: (a) 1–95% of an aq. phase rendered non-flowable by the addition of a suitable amt. of a gel-forming compsn., and (b) from 5–99% of an oil phase comprising a fat or oil and an emulsifier. The interaction between the non-flowable aq. phase and the oil phase results in the two phase emulsion being pourable.

Also claimed is a foodstuff contg. the two-phase emulsion and a method of reducing fat content of a food contg. triglyceride using the emulsion, and a fat substitute contg. in addn. to (a) and (b) specified amts. of a fat extender.

USE/ADVANTAGE—The emulsions are useful as fat substitutes, replacing at least a portion of the normally present triglycerides. Pref. foods into which the emulsion can be incorporated are salad dressings, frozen desserts, soups, mayonnaise, fillings for cookies and cakes, whipped desserts, etc.

Abstract (Equivalent): US 5082684 A

2-Phase emulsion comprises (a) 1–95% of single aq. phase rendered non-flowable by addn. of gel-forming compsn.; and (b) 5–99% of oil phase comprising solid or semi-solid fat or oil, and an emulsifier. Interaction between (a) and (b) causes emulsion obtd. to be pourable. Gel-forming compsn. comprises agar, gelatin, pectin, or carrageenan, and opt. a crosslinking agent.

USE—A low calorie fat substitute.

Hydrocolloid—General 6

Dispersion-type food or drug compsn.—contg. parenchymal cell cellulose as stabiliser.

Patent Assignee: SBP INC (SBPS-N)
Inventor: MYERS C D; WEIVBEL M K
Number of Countries: 001 Number of Patents: 001
Patent No Kind Date Applicat No Kind Date Main IPC Week
US 4923981 A 19900508 US 89334596 A 19890406 199023 B
Abstract (Basic): US 4923981 A

A food or drug comestible consisting of at least one first material dispersed in at least one second material is stabilised using parenchymal cell cellulose (PCC), pref. in amt. at least 0.02 wt.%, esp. 0.02–20, partic. 0.02–10 wt.%.

USE/ADVANTAGE—PCC is used for stabilising food prods. in the form of emulsions (e.g., mayonnaise), foams (e.g., whipped cream), batters and doughs, and for stabilising liq. or solid pharmaceutical prods. The stabilised compsn. has reduced caloric content, reduced fat content, improved texture, improved flavour release and/or improved mouthful. PCC is a superior replacement for microcrystalline cellulose or xanthan gum normally used in such compsns.

Hydrocolloid—General 7

Fragmented anisotropic xanthan-protein complex dispersions mfr.—comprises passing complex of the complex fibres through high shear.

Patent Assignee: KRAFT INC (KRFT); KRAFT GENERAL FOODS (KRAF-N)

Inventor: BAER C C; BALMACEDA E A; BORWANKAR R P; CHEN C; CHEN W; GAUD S M; HASENHEUTTL G L; HELLGETH L C; HENRY G A; KAISER J M; KERWIN P J; KRATOCHVIL J F; LLOYD W L; MILLER M S; MORGAN R G; STRANDHOLM J J; BALMADECA E A; MORGAN R G A; WENSHERNG C

Number of Countries: 036 Number of Patents: 013

Patent No Kind Date Applicat No Kind Date Main IPC Week
EP 340035 A 19891102 EP 89304316 A 19890428 198944 B
WO 8910068 A 19891102 198946
PT 90413 A 19891110 198950
AU 8935742 A 19891124 199016
CN 1038571 A 19900110 199042
FI 9005303 A 19901026 199107
EP 414776 A 19910306 EP 89905909 A 19890428 199110
DK 9002597 A 19901227 199112
NO 9004619 A 19901227 199112
BR 8907406 A 19910423 199121
JP 3505814 W 19911219 JP 89505929 A 19890428 199206
US 5104674 A 19920414 US 90548950 A 19900428 199218
CA 1334354 C 19950214 CA 598326 A 19890501 A23J-003/00 199514

Abstract (Basic): EP 340035 A

Microfragmented anisotropic xanthan (I)/protein (II) complex dispersion is produced as follows: (a) an aq. suspension of molecularly intimately complexed (I)/(II) fibres is prepd. (contg. at least 10 wt.% (I) gum based on total solids); and (b) the aq. fibre suspension is passed through a high shear zone so that the fibres are fragmented to the title microfragments of max dimension less than 15 micron.

Step (a). The aq. suspension pref. comprises 1–10 by wt. (I)/(II)

complex fibres, and is pref. heated to stabilise the complex. Step (b). The dispersion is pref. concd. by centrifugation (at the isoelectric pH), or by evapn. of at least some of the aq. phase. In an extension of the above method, a syneresed molecularly entangled complexed ionic polysaccharide (III)/(II) complex ppt is treated as above, where (III) is an anisotropic carboxymethyl cellulose or carrageenan. Prefd. (II) include whey proteins and egg albumen. The microfragments are pref. coated at least in part with Ca alginate or Ca pectinate.

USE/ADVANTAGE—The microfragmented xanthan/protein dispersion have desirable rheological props., including a stable lubricity and creamy mouthfeel. The dispersions are useful as fat or oil substitutes in food prods. (frozen desserts, spreads, dressings, baked goods and sauces, etc.), esp. as replacements for edible triglycerides.

Hydrocolloid—General 8

Sugar beet pectin for use in food or drug comestibles—has low mol. wt., is highly acetylated, hydrophobic domains, specific ferulic acid content and low viscosity.

Patent Assignee: SBP INC (SBPS-N); SLR INC (SLRS-N); WESTERN SUGAR CO (WSUG-N); ST LAWRENCE REACTORS (SLAW-N); WEIBEL M K (WEIB-I)
Inventor: WEIBEL M K
Number of Countries: 018 Number of Patents: 008
Patent No Kind Date Applicat No Kind Date Main IPC Week
US 5008254 A 19910416 US 89430166 A 19891101 199118 B
EP 426434 A 19910508 EP 90311886 A 19901030 199119
AU 9065641 A 19910509 199126
CA 2029022 A 19910502 199128
JP 3197502 A 19910828 JP 90295185 A 19901031 199141
EP 426434 B1 19961211 EP 90311886 A 19901030 C08B-037/06 199703
DE 69029365 E 19970123 DE 629365 A 19901030 C08B-037/06 199709
EP 90311886 A 19901030ES 2098257 T3 19970501 EP 90311886 A 19901030 C08B-037/06 199724
Priority Applications (No Type Date): US 89430166 A 19891101; US 82414931 A 19820903; US 83512940 A 19830712; US 8762445 A 19870615; US 89334596 A 19890406
Abstract (Basic): US 5008254 A

Sugar beet pectin is claimed have at least one of the following properties: (a) low molecular weight; (b) highly acetylated; (c) many hydrophobic domains; (d) ferulic acid content up to 3 wt.%; and (e) relatively low viscosity at 10 wt.%.

The sugar beet pectin is prepd. by: suspending sugar beet plant material in an aq. medium to form a suspension; adjusting the pH to less than 4.5 or greater than 9.0; maintaining at a temp. greater than 125°C for 15–600 sec.; subjecting the suspension to mechanical shearing; and isolating the sugar beet pectin from the suspension.

Also claimed is a food or drug comestible, other than fruit spreads, having at least one of the following properties; (a) reduced caloric content; (b) reduced fat content; (c) improved texture; (d) improved flavour release; or (e) improved mouthfeel. The comestible being comprised of at least one first material, at least second material, and the sugar beet pectin as above in amt. sufficient to input at least one of the properties to be comestible.

USE/ADVANTAGE—The sugar beet pectin can be incorporated into food or drug prods. to give improved properties, including physicochemical, rheological and nutritional properties. Dietetic or other speciality comestibles may also be prepd. in view of the fact that sugar beet pectin has a negligible food value and is devoid of fat or cholesterol. The sugar beet pectin also impedes the development of the ageing process so that, e.g., ice cream creaminess is prolonged during storage and bread maintains a fresh elastic leaf texture for longer periods of time.

Hydrocolloid—General 9

A fat substitute—comprises microparticulate beads of hydrous hydrocolloid gel produced by emulsion gelation.

Patent Assignee: MARS GB LTD (MRSC); MARS INC (MRSC)

Inventor: IZZO M T; JEROME R A; NACE J A; SPEIRS C; WHITE K E; SPIERS C

Number of Countries: 034 Number of Patents: 006

Patent No Kind Date Applicat No Kind Date Main IPC Week

WO 9119424 A 19911226 199203 B

AU 9180011 A 19920107 199217

EP 533815 A1 19930331 EP 91912025 A 19910619 A23L-001/308 199313

WO 91GB983 A 19910619

EP 533815 B1 19960207 EP 91912025 A 19910619 A23L-001/308 199610

WO 91GB983 A 19910619

DE 69117059 E 19960321 DE 617059 A 19910619 A23L-001/308 199617

EP 91912025 A 19910619

WO 91GB983 A 19910619

ES 2084171 T3 19960501 EP 91912025 A 19910619 A23L-001/308 199625

Abstract (Basic): WO 9119424 A

A fat substitute comprises microparticulate beads of a hydrous hydrocolloid gel which is a prod. of emulsion gelation. Also claimed is a food prod. contg. the fat substitute and a heat resistant chocolate comprising the fat substitute. Pref. the beads comprise 0.1–10 wt.% gelling agent and contain the reaction prod. of a gellable ionic polysaccharide and a physiologically tolerable metal capable of gelation of the polysaccharide. The ionic polysaccharide comprises at least one of alginate, pectate and sodium carboxymethyl cellulose.

USE/ADVANTAGE—The microparticulate beads are usable as fat substitutes, as food additives with differing mouthfeel sensations in food prods. such as ice cream, pudding, cheesecake, chocolate, dips, salad dressings, etc. The beads can also be used for encapsulation of drugs, enzymes, etc.

Hydrocolloid—General 10

Hydrophilic colloid as foam stabiliser—polyglycerol fatty ester emulsifiers in low calorie food topping spreads and ice creams.

Patent Assignee: BRISTOL-MYERS CO (BRIM); DRACKETT CO (DRAK)
Number of Countries: 002 Number of Patents: 002
Patent No Kind Date Applicat No Kind Date Main IPC Week
US 3809764 A 19740507 197420 B
CA 969417 A 19750617 197527
Abstract (Basic): US 3809764 A

0.2–3.0 wt.% hydrophilic colloid (acacia or xanthan gum, carboxymethyl cellulose, gelatin, starch or a water-soluble protein) is used as a foam stabilizer for a low calorie food such as imitation butter, margarine, cheese spreads, dips, frozen desserts, ice creams, salad dressings and sauces obtained from 0–5 wt.% fat, 0.33–7.5 wt.% polyglycerol ester as foaming agent, and ≤45 wt.% flavouring, colouring, bodying and texturizing ingredients. The polyglycerol ester contains 3–10 glycerol units and 1 or 2 saturated fatty acyl ester gps (16-20C).

Triglycerol monostearate, hexaglycerol distearate and decaglycerol distearate as foaming agents

Hydrocolloid—General 11

Edible dispersion esp. used as fat substitute—with continuous and gelled disperse phases contg. different hydrocolloids, e.g., galactomannan and gelatin.

Patent Assignee: TESSENDERLO CHEMIE NV (TESS-N)
Inventor: MUYLDERMANS G
Number of Countries: 019 Number of Patents: 002
Patent No Kind Date Applicat No Kind Date Main IPC Week

WO 9317582 A1 19930916 WO 93BE12 A 19930308 A23L-001/05 199338 B
BE 1005742 A3 19940111 BE 92236 A 19920309 A23L-000/00 199407
Abstract (Basic): WO 9317582 A

Edible dispersion for providing a plastic texture contains at least two hydrocolloids (HC) or HC systems and comprises a first phase (P1) and a second gelled phase (P2). P1 forms a continuous phase in which P2 is dispersed at at leat one temp. in the range of 0–40 (pref. 5–20, esp. 10-15)°C. The concn. of the first HC or HC system is sufficient to form a continuous phase which is immiscible with P2, such that P2 is dispersed in P1. The concn. of the first HC or HC system is such that the continuous phase is non-gelled.

Also claimed is a mixt. for forming the dispersions, contg. at least two HCs or HC systems, where the first HC (system) has critical temp. below 5°C and the second HC (system) has critical temp. above 15°C. Wt. ratio of first HC (system) to second HC (system) is 0.1–1:1.

USE/ADVANTAGE—Use of the dispersions or mixts. in prodn. of food prods. and compsns., esp. as fat substitutes, is claimed. The dispersions are transparent or translucid (due to the almost constant size of the dispersed phase particles), and do not adversely affect the colour of food compsns., e.g., chocolate pastes. Typical applications are in salad sauces, butter creams, ice creams, chocolate pastes and pates. The dispersions provide texture, plasticity and cuttability, and act as thickeners. They give good mouthfeel and improved release of aroma, and have no unpleasant taste.

Hydrocolloid—General 12

Powdery edible material in aq. suspension—comprises cellulose material regenerated from edible polysaccharide in suspension, for use as edible fat substitute.

Patent Assignee: ASAHI CHEM IND CO LTD (ASAH)
Number of Countries: 001 Number of Patents: 001
Patent No Kind Date Applicat No Kind Date Main IPC Week
JP 5023119 A 19930202 JP 91198232 A 19910715 A23L-001/0534 199310 B
Abstract (Basic): JP 5023119 A

The material comprises cellulose regenerated from aq. alkali metal hydroxide and edible polysaccharide, homogeneous mixt. of both ingredients being at least 10% in the continuous form and its particle size of 50% of accumulated vol. being 50 microns or less. Water suspension contains the material in an amt. of 3 to 40 wt.%.

Pref. the edible polysaccharide comprises gum arabicum, alginic acid, carrageenan, pectin, pluran, mannan, starch, etc. The polysaccharide is 10% or more in the material. The cellulose is dissolved in alkaline soln. and then polysaccharide followed by mixing and kneading, to give dope. The dope is extruded in water to coagulate, and it is washed and dried.

USE/ADVANTAGE—Material has good touch and feeling and bitter taste is reduced, used as substitute for edible fat material, etc.

Hydrocolloid—General 13

Foodstuff compsn.—comprises mixt. of oligomers derived from degradation of a polysaccharide deriv.

Patent Assignee: ALKO LTD (ALKO-N); ALKO OY AB (ALKO-N)
Inventor: LAHTINEN T; RHA C; TIMONEN M; VAARA R; VAARA T
Number of Countries: 017 Number of Patents: 005

Patent No	Kind	Date	Applicat No	Kind	Date	Main IPC	Week
EP 470870	A	19920212	EP 91307416	A	19910812		199207 B
AU 9181742	A	19920213					199217
CA 2042559	A	19920211					199218
FI 9103094	A	19920211	FI 913094	A	19910625	A23L	199219
JP 4229157	A	19920818	JP 91224889	A	19910810	A23L-001/307	199240

Abstract (Basic): EP 470870 A

A foodstuff compsn. comprises a mixt. of oligomers derived from degradation of a polysaccharide deriv., a majority of the oligomers having mol. wt. such that the oligomer has a rod-like configuration. A method for preparing a reduced caloric food prod. comprising the mixt. of oligomers, and a mixt. of oligomers derived from the degradation of the polysaccharide deriv.

Pref. the compsn. comprises a mixt. of oligomers derived from degradation of a polysaccharide deriv., other than a cellulose deriv. The mixt. of oligomers have an average degree of polymerisation of 3–500. The polysaccharide deriv. includes one or more carboxymethyl, hydroxyethyl methyl, methyl, hydroxypropyl, methyl ethyl, hydroxyethyl, hydroxypropyl methyl, sulphate, carboxylic acid, carboxylic acid ester and/or pyruvate substituents. The polysaccharide contains 0.5 to 3 substituents per saccharide unit. The polysaccharide deriv. is a starch deriv., carragmeenan, pullulan, pustulan, alginate, laminarin, guar gum, gum arabic, inulin, pectin, whelan, rhamsan, gellan, xanthan, zooglan, methylan, chitin, cyclodextrin or chitsan (esp. the deriv. consists substantially of glucose units). The mixt. of oligomers has an average degree of polymerisation of 5–100 (esp. 5–50). The mixt. has a polydispersibility less than 2 and contains less than 25 wt.% of mono- and disaccharides. The mixt. has average mol. wt. less than 15,000 (esp. 10,000).

USE/ADVANTAGE—The fat substitute is fat free and has fat-like properties such that eating quality of the new prods. or high calorie ingredient-replaced footstuff is desirable or substantially maintained.

Hydrocolloid—General 14

Fructose polymer-contg. food with improved taste and flavour—where the polymer is added as substitute for gelling material, low calorie saccharide and/or fat.
Patent Assignee: AJINOMOTO KK (AJIN)
Number of Countries: 001 Number of Patents: 001
Patent No Kind Date Applicat No Kind Date Main IPC Week
JP 4356169 A 19921209 JP 91226638 A 19910529 A23L-001/307 199305 B
Abstract (Basic): JP 4356169 A

Gelling material, thickener, low calorie saccharide, high sweetness sweetener and/or fat is added to the food. A part or all of gelling material, low calorie saccharide and fat is substd. by fructose polymer. The fat is cream, cream cheese, butter and/or vegetable fat. Gelling material and/or thickener is gelatin, gum, pectin, starch, egg yolk, and/or egg white. The food is cream, jelly, jam, ice-cream, sauce, chocolate, pudding, sponge-cakes, bread, spread or ham and sausage.

USE—Gel property and creamy feel are improved. Flavour and taste of the food is increased.

Hydrocolloids—General 15

Non-aggregating hydrocolloid micro-particulates—are used as foodstuff fat replacers or as carriers, e.g., drugs, herbicides, detergent, surfactants, enzymes, fertilisers etc.
Patent Assignee: FMC CORP (FMCC)
Inventor: CROSBY G A; DUMONT L E; RENN D W; RILEY P J; SEWALL C J; THOMAS W R
Number of Countries: 052 Number of Patents: 003
Patent No Kind Date Applicat No Kind Date Main IPC Week
WO 9505939 A1 19950302 WO 94US8860 A 19940804 B32B-009/00 199514 B
AU 9475210 A 19950321 AU 9475210 A 19940804 B32B-009/00 199526
US 5624612 A 19970429 US 93111800 A 19930825 B01J-013/02 199723
US 95476989 A 19950607
Abstract (Basic): WO 9505939 A

Dry, rehydratable, water-dispersible, gel-forming, porous hydrocolloid microparticulates comprise (a) a gel-forming hydrocolloid as the matrix; and (b) at least one water-soluble, non-gelling, hydration-enhancing hydrocolloid. Matrix (a) contains (b) within its porous structure and may also have (b) as a full or partial coating around the microparticulates. Pref., when rehydrated, the microparticulates have average particle dia. of 0.1–150 (esp.10–30) microns. They are esp. spherical. The matrix (a) is, e.g., agar, agarose, algin, low methyl pectin, gellan, kappa-carrageenan, furcellaran, beta-carrageenan, curdlan, konjac, glucomannan (or its derivs.) etc. Colloid (b) is a galactomannan, glucomannan, starch, cellulose deriv., lambda-carrageen, algin, pectin, xanthan and/or a synthetic polymer. It is esp Na CMC, and (a) is esp heat-stable, cold-melt konjac.

USE—Prods are fat replacers in foodstuffs or carriers for drugs herbicides, detergents, enzymes, etc.

Hydrocolloid—Bakery & Grain 1

Low-fat dry mix based on sweetened cereal—comprising polydextrose, cellulosic material, non-fat milk solid, emulsifier, modified food starch and xanthan, guar or locust bean gum.

Patent Assignee: NELSON K J (NELS-I); PILLSBURY CO (PILL)
Inventor: NELSON K J; HAHN P W
Number of Countries: 033 Number of Patents: 006
Patent No Kind Date Applicat No Kind Date Main IPC Week
WO 9200012 A 19920109 A21D-002/18 199205 B
AU 9174470 A 19920227 199218
EP 536139 A1 19930414 EP 91905226 A 19910121 A21D-002/18 199315
WO 91US407 A 19910121
US 5262187 A 19931116 US 90546017 A 19900628 A23L-001/10 199347
US 91722710 A 19910628
US 92918945 A 19920722
EP 536139 B1 19940824 EP 91905226 A 19910121 A21D-002/18 199433
WO 91US407 A 19910121
DE 69103633 E 19940929 DE 603633 A 19910121 A21D-002/18 199438
EP 91905226 A 19910121
WO 91US407 A 19910121
Abstract (Basic): WO 9200012 A

Mix comprises: a sweetened cereal-grain ingredient base with a fat–mimetic system of (i) less than 0.1 to 5 wt.% of a polydextrose or its buffered form, (ii) less than 0.1 to 15 wt.% of a cellulosic material, (iii) less than 0.1 to 8 wt.% of a non-fat milk solid or substitute (IV), less than 0.1 to 4 wt.% of each of an emulsifier and a modified food starch (V) and less than 0.1 to 2 wt.% of a mixt. of xanthan gum and quar or locust bean gum. The wt.% are relative to the total wt. of the dry-mix.

Also claimed is a baked, low-fat food compsn. contg. the dry mix and a low-fat ready-to-use butter contg. the dry mix.

Pref. the ingredient base includes sugar and flour at a ratio of 2:1 to 1:1 pts. wt. (Pbw). The dry mix also includes flavourings colouring, salt, leavening agent, and/or preservatives.

USE/ADVANTAGE—The baked compsn. contg. the dry mix is moist, tender, crumbly with good mouthfeel and pref. contains one-third fewer calories than a similar full fatted compsn. The dry mix produces substantially homogeneously distributed small air cells throughout the volume of the baked compsn.

Hydrocolloid—Bakery & Grain 2

Low fat, low calorie fat substitute emulsions—contg. only natural ingredients which require no other change in a recipe, e.g., baked goods.
Patent Assignee: MRS BATEMAN'S BAKERY LC (BATE-N)
Inventor: BATEMAN K
Number of Countries: 037 Number of Patents: 002
Patent No Kind Date Applicat No Kind Date Main IPC Week
WO 9526641 A1 19951012 WO 95US4153 A 19950404 B 199546 B
AU 9522063 A 19951023 AU 9522063 A 19950404 B 199605
Abstract (Basic): WO 9526641 A

Low fat, low calorie fat substitutes are emulsions of 40–90 wt.% polysaccharide (I) in 5–60 wt.% water. The emulsions can be substituted 1-to-1 for fat in food prods. without any other changes in the recipe and without altering the texture of the prod.

Also claimed are substitutes made from 1–40 wt.% baking fat, 40–80% (I) and 5–40% water.

A second polysaccharide (II), pref. a water soluble starch, is present at 1–15%. A flavouring, esp. butter or an artificial flavouring, is present at up to 10%. The flavouring is oil or butter, olive, peanut, canola, corn or safflower oil flavouring, or is up to 1% dried butter.

A food colouring, esp. beta-carotene or a yellow dye is pref. present. (I) is a maltodextrin of DE < 20, esp. corn, rice, potato or tapioca starch.

Shelf-life is improved by adding up to 1% preservative. Up to 4% whey protein and/or xanthan gum is added to enhance texture. The pH is also adjusted.

USE—The compsns. can replace, e.g., shortening, margarine, butter, oil, lard, and cream cheese.

ADVANTAGE—The compsns. are made only of natural prods. and need no emulsifiers.

Hydrocolloid—Beverage 1

Low-calorie beverage contg. hydro-colloidal polysaccharide—saccharin salt and aspartame, with texture and sweetness similar to prods. sweetened with fructose syrup.
Patent Assignee: PEPSICO INC (PEPS)

Inventor: HAVEKOTTE M J; SHARKASI T; HAVEKOTTS M J
Number of Countries: 010 Number of Patents: 010
Patent No Kind Date Applicat No Kind Date Main IPC Week
US 5126158 A 19920630 US 90564012 A 19900807 A23L-002/38 199229 B
US 91758225 A 19910909
GB 2259438 A 19930317 GB 9119530 A 19910911 A23L-001/236 199311 N
DE 4131084 A1 19930325 DE 4131084 A 19910918 A23L-002/38 199313 N
AU 9183752 A 19930311 AU 9183752 A 19910909 A23L-001/236 199317 N
FR 2681220 A1 19930319 FR 9111318 A 19910913 A23L-002/00 199320 N
ES 2034895 A1 19930401 ES 912096 A 19910923 A23L-002/38 199323 N
AU 643557 B 19931118 AU 9183752 A 19910909 A23L-001/236 199402 N
ES 2034895 B1 19931216 ES 912096 A 19910923 A23L-002/38 199403 N
JP 6090721 A 19940405 JP 91274534 A 19910926 A23L-002/00 199418 N
GB 2259438 B 19950301 GB 9119530 A 19910911 A23L-001/236 199512 N
Abstract (Basic): US 5126158 A

Beverage contains at least one acceptable hydrocolloid polysaccharide (I) at 25–800 mg/L; a saccharin salt (II) and aspartame (III), with the (III):(II) ratio being 25–50:1.

More specifically, (I) is at least one of natural or modified gum (esp. xanthan or guar); an alkyl cellulose either (e.g, methylcellulose); pectin and propylene glycol alginate. (II) is the Na and/or Ca salt.

USE/ADVANTAGE—These dietetic beverages have improved mouthfeel and sweetness, i.e., in these respects they closely ressemble beverages sweetened with high-fructose corn syrup (HFC5)

Hydrocolloid—Dairy 1

Making low calorie butter made from dairy cream—by phase reversion on scraped surface heat exchanger using unsatd. distilled monoglyceride and hydrocolloids.

Patent Assignee: ANONYMOUS (ANON)
Number of Countries: 001 Number of Patents: 001
Patent No Kind Date Applicat No Kind Date Main IPC Week
RD 303053 A 19890710 198933 B
Abstract (Basic): RD 303053 A

Low calorie butter can be made form dairy cream by phase reversion on a scraped surface heat exchanger, using unsaturated distilled monoglyceride and hydrocolloids added to the cream.

In an example, 94.4% dairy cream 38% fat; 4.0% gelatin; 0.5% salt; 0.1% K-sorbate and 1.0% unsaturated distilled monoglyceride, high iodine value. In all samples were used 7 ppm flavour, 4 ppm beta-carotene and pH was adjusted to 6.0. The dairy cream was heated to 50°C and the additives were added during intensive agitation. Phase reversion was achieved in a laboratory perfector using 2 cooling cylinders approx. 40% of normal capacity and ammonia temperature −10°C. The speed of the rotor in the cooling cylinders was approx. 950 rpm and outlet temperature of the low calorie butter approx. 18°C. The low calorie butter sample has no loose water by spreading after storage at 5 and 18°C and has an agreeable butter-like taste.

Hydrocolloid—Dairy 2

Low calorie, palatable frozen food compsns.—contg. poly-dextrose, fructose, guar gum and emulsifier.

Patent Assignee: MINGHELLAS ISLE OF (MING-N)
Inventor: MINGHELLA E
Number of Countries: 001 Number of Patents: 002
Patent No Kind Date Applicat No Kind Date Main IPC Week
GB 2193873 A 19880224 GB 86619827 A 19860814 198808 B
GB 2193873 B 19900214 GB 8619827 A 19860814 199007
Abstract (Basic): GB 2193873 A

Frozen food compsn. (contg. at least 5% by wt. fat, and at least 7.5 % by wt. milk solids) comprises (per 500 wt. pts. of compsn). 50–70 wt. pts. polydextrose (I), 20–30 pts. fructose (II), 0.75–1.5 pts. guar gum (III), and 0.75–1.25 pts. of an emulsifier (IV).

ADVANTAGE—The particular combination of milk prods. and sweetening agents affords a low calorie, low carbohydrate prod. which is extremely palatable. By virtue of the fat and milk solids content, the prod. can be called "ice-cream."

Hydrocolloid—Dairy 3

Low calorie virtually fat-free processed cheese—produced from skimmed milk cheese, microcrystalline cellulose, corn syrup solids, anionic hydrophilic gum, emulsifier and opacifier.

Patent Assignee: KRAFT GEN FOODS INC (KRFT); KRAFT FOODS INC (KRFT)
Inventor: BAER C C; BULIGA G S; HASSENHEUTTL G L; HENRY G A; HETH A A; JACKSON L K; KENNEDY-TOLSTEDT J M; KERWIN P J; MILLER M S; PARKER E M; PAUL N K; PECHAK D G; SMITH G F; WITTE V C; DAVISON B C; HAMANN A C; PROSTKO L J; SCHWIMMER W H; DAVIDSON B C; SMITH W H; NEELA K P; SMITH G G F
Number of Countries: 023 Number of Patents: 022
Patent No Kind Date Applicat No Kind Date Main IPC Week
WO 9102461 A 19910307 199112 B

PT 95027 A 19910418 199118
PT 95028 A 19910418 199118
US 5011701 A 19910430 US 89395800 A 19890818 199119
AU 9063525 A 19910403 199125
AU 9064282 A 19910403 199125
FI 9200673 A 19920217 WO 90US4619 A 19900816 A23C 199221
FI 92673 A 19920217
FI 9200674 A 19920217 WO 90US4621 A 19900816 A23L 199221
FI 92674 A 19920217
EP 487649 A1 19920603 EP 90914330 A 19900816 A23C-019/00 199223
WO 90US4619 A 19900816
NO 9200581 A 19920326 WO 90US4619 A 19900816 A23C-019/00 199226
NO 92581 A 19920214
NO 9200582 A 19920409 WO 90US4621 A 19900816 A23L 199228
NO 92582 A 19920214
JP 4507349 W 19921224 JP 90513382 A 19900816 A23C-019/082 199306
WO 90US4619 A 19900816
US 5215778 A 19930601 US 89395800 A 19890818 A23C-019/00 199323
US 90462606 A 19900109
US 93758462 A 19930601
NZ 234705 A 19930727 NZ 234705 A 19900730 A23L-001/24 199333
NZ 234706 A 19930727 NZ 234706 A 19900730 A23C-019/09 199333
AU 638751 B 19930708 AU 9063525 A 19900816 A23L-001/308 199334
AU 643706 B 19931125 AU 9064282 A 19900816 A23C-019/082 199403
EP 487649 B1 19960515 EP 90914330 A 19900816 A23C-019/00 199624
WO 90US4619 A 19900816
DE 69027034 E 19960620 DE 627034 A 19900816 A23C-019/00 199630
EP 90914330 A 19900816
WO 90US4619 A 19900816
PH 26991 A 19921228 PH 41041 A 19900816 A23L-001/0534 199635
ES 2088433 T3 19960816 EP 90914330 A 19900816 A23C-019/00 199639
CA 2059544 C 19961001 CA 2059544 A 19900816 A23L-001/052 199650
Abstract (Basic): WO 9102461 A

Fat-free processed cheese prods. are prepd. by (a) blending comminuted natural skimmed milk cheese (I) with an aq. slurry of porous particulate microreticulated microcrystalline cellulose (contg. 5–12 wt.% solids), 15–28 DE corn syrup solids, anionic hydrophilic gum, emulsifying salt and TiO_2 opacifier to form a fat-free processed cheese blend, (b) injecting 6–17 wt.% steam with mixing into the blend to form a homogeneous fluidised cheese melt at 165–270°F, (c) keeping it at 220°F for 85 sec. or an equiv. time-temp. relationship, (d) flash cooling into a vacuum zone (30 in. Hg or less) to a temp. of 140–170 deg and (e) packaging.

(I) contains 50–60 wt.% water, under 1.67 wt.% fat and 40–50 wt.% non-fat dairy solids. The prod. contains under 1.67 wt.% fat.

ADVANTAGE—Prods. are low calorie and fat-free. They have texture and mouthfeel like conventional processed cheese slices.

Hydrocolloid—Dairy 4

Non gelatin-contg. powder compsns. for ice cream and milk drinks—contains acid, starch milk powder, sweetener, colour, flavour, dried cultured milk powder and gums.

Patent Assignee: BEN-GURION UNIV OF NEGEV (UYNE)
Inventor: DEVSHONY S
Number of Countries: 015 Number of Patents: 003
Patent No Kind Date Applicat No Kind Date Main IPC Week
EP 242056 A 19871021 EP 87302238 A 19870316 198742 B
JP 62275653 A 19871130 JP 8758714 A 19870313 198802
IL 78146 A 19890928 199002
Abstract (Basic): EP 242056 A

A powdered compsn for use in making tart during drinks and soft ice cream comprises (a) 1–15% edible acid, (b) 0–6% pretreated starch, (c) 0–10% dried, cultured milk powder, (d) 0.3–90% sweeteners (e) 0–7% colours and flavours (f) 0–50% milk powder, and (g) at least two of guar, carot and xanthan gum, each of the two or more being present in an amt. of 0.3–4%, and in a total quantity of 2.3–8%.

USE/ADVANTAGE—The compsn. may be mixed with water or milk to produce a stable, low calarie tart dairy drink or mixed with milk in a soft ice cream machine to produce a stable, soft, low calorie ice cream. Sepn. does not occur, nor does syneresis after 5–6 days in the refrigerator. The compsns. are kosher, being free of gelatin, so Jews can enjoy them.

Hydrocolloid—Dairy 5

Low fat, low cholesterol process cheese prepn.—by adding cheese culture to liq. milk having low fat content, processing soln., processing obtd. curd, sepg. whey and ripening curd.

Patent Assignee: FIRST WORLD CHEESE (FIRS-N); ALPINE LACE BRANDS INC (ALPI-N); GAMAY A (GAMA-I)
Inventor: GAMAY A
Number of Countries: 035 Number of Patents: 007
Patent No Kind Date Applicat No Kind Date Main IPC Week
WO 9117664 A 19911128 199150 B
AU 9178897 A 19911210 199212
US 5225220 A 19930706 US 90522203 A 19900511 A23C-019/032 199328

US 92877953 A 19920430
NZ 238107 A 19941222 NZ 238107 A 19910510 A23C-019/00 199505
US 5395630 A 19950307 US 90522203 A 19900511 A23C-019/032 199515
US 92877953 A 19920430 US 9367455 A 19930523 US 94250336 A 19940527
US 5549916 A 19960827 US 90522203 A 19900511 A23C-019/32 199640
US 92877953 A 19920430 US 9367455 A 19930525 US 94250336 A
19940527 US 95378515 A 19950126 US 95475143 A 19950607
US 5612073 A 19970318 US 90522203 A 19900511 A23C-019/032 199717
US 92877953 A 19920430 US 9367455 A 19930527 US 94250336 A
19940527 US 95378515 A 19950126
Abstract (Basic): WO 9117664 A

Mfg. a low fat cheese starting material for process cheese mfg. comprises: a) preparing a starting liq. milk having a fat content of 0–0.3%; b) adding a selected cheese culture to the liq. milk and forming a starting cheese formulation soln.; c) processing the cheese formulation soln. for reacting and coagulating the soln. and forming the curd; d) cutting and processing the curd at elevated temp until achieving a preselected pH range for the curd; e) sepg. whey from the curd and controlling pH of the curd during further curd development. The whey includes calcium dissolved during achievement of the preselected pH range; and f) processing and ripening the curd to form the cheese starting material.

Also claimed is a method of mfg. a real process cheese prod. and a low fat prod.

USE/ADVANTAGE—The cheese produced is fat free, cholesterol free and low in calorie content. Flavours can be used to mask bitter and unpalatable tastes and for imparting acceptable cheese flavours.

Hydrocolloid—Dairy 6

Low fat, low cholesterol cheese mfr.—by mixing and dissolving carrageenan to low fat milk, adding selected cheese culture, processing, separating whey and ripening the curd.

Patent Assignee: FIRST WORLD CHEESE (FIRS-N); ALPINE LACE BRANDS INC (ALPI-N); ALPINE LACE BRANDS (ALPI-N)
Inventor: GAMAY A
Number of Countries: 035 Number of Patents: 004
Patent No Kind Date Applicat No Kind Date Main IPC Week
WO 9117663 A 19911128 199150 B
US 5080913 A 19920114 US 90522527 A 19900511 199206
AU 9178795 A 19911210 199212
NZ 238108 A 19941222 NZ 238108 A 19910510 A23C-019/00 199505
Abstract (Basic): WO 9117663 A

Mfr. of low fat cheese comprises: a) preparing a starting liq. milk having a fat content of 0.01–0.3%; b) mixing and dissolving a carrageenan with the starting milk; c) adding a selected cheese culture to the liq. milk and dissolved carrageenan and forming a cheese formulation soln.; d) processing the formulation soln. for reacting and coagulating the soln and forming a curd; e) cutting and processing the cord at elevated temp until achieving a preselected pH range for the curd; f) sepg. whey from the curd and controlling the water content in association with the curd for controlling pH during curd development; and g) processing and ripening the curd to form the low fat cheese.

USE/ADVANTAGE—The method affords cheese with texture, mouthfeel and flavour similar to higher fat natural cheese. The prod is of low fat, low cholesterol and low calorie. The cheese produced is selected from Cheddar cheese, Colby cheese, mozzarella cheese, Jack cheese, Muenster cheese, Gouda cheese, Swiss cheese, blue cheese, Romano cheese, Parmesan cheese and Camembert cheese.

Hydrocolloid—Dairy 7

Non-dairy frozen dessert compsns.—give ice cream substitutes with usual appearance, texture and melt but low lactose, cholesterol, satd. fat and calorie content.

Patent Assignee: KOHLMANN H G (KOHL-I)
Inventor: MINGIONE A
Number of Countries: 001 Number of Patents: 001
Patent No Kind Date Applicat No Kind Date Main IPC Week
US 5478587 A 19951226 US 93109707 A 19930820 A23G-009/02 199606 B
Abstract (Basic): US 5478587 A

Non-dairy compsns. for frozen dessert prepn. comprise 14.00–78.26% (as dry wt.) non-dairy creamer (I), 3.48–52.17% sweetener (II), 2.5–42.98% filler (III), 0.14–6.96% stabiliser (IV) and 0.01–0.29% smoother (V).

Pref. (ii) is sucrose with corn syrup solids (VI), aspartame (VII), polydextrose (VIII), or (VI) and (VII) or (VII) and (VIII), or is (VIII) with (VI) and/or (VII). (III) is maltodextrin. (V) is a vegetable gum, esp. xanthan, guar, xanthan and guar, or carrageenan gum. Compsns. also contain a source of dietary Ca. They also contain a partially hydrogenated vegetable oil, esp. olive or canola oil, having mono-unsatd.: satd. fat ratio > 2:1 and mono-: poly-unsatd. fat ratio > 1:19. Compsns. also contain 50–70 wt.% water. They also contain 50–70 vol.% fruit juice.

USE—Prods. give lactose-free, low satd. fat, low cholesterol, low calories desserts with the appearance, texture and melting characteristics of ice cream.

Hydrocolloid—Dairy 8

Non-fat natural cheese prepn.—by combining skim milk, fat substitute additive, starter culture and milk coagulating enzyme, coagulating obtd. substrate, etc.

Patent Assignee: KRAFT GEN FOODS INC (KRFT)
Inventor: BORWANKAR R P; CARRELL N A; HAMANN A C; HYNES J T; JACOBSON K A; KERRIGAN G L; NATH K R; REDDY D S; ALM W L
Number of Countries: 017 Number of Patents: 002
Patent No Kind Date Applicat No Kind Date Main IPC Week
WO 9206598 A1 19920430 WO 91US7100 A 19910927 A23C-019/05 199220 B
AU 9187405 A 19920520 AU 9187405 A 19910927 A23C-019/05 199233
WO 91US7100 A 19910927
Abstract (Basic): WO 9206598 A

Mfr. comprises combining skim milk, a fat substitute additive, a starter culture and a milk coagulating enzyme to provide a non-fat milk substrate, coagulating the substrate, cutting the coagulation to provide curd particles and whey, draining the whey, pressing the curd and curing the curd to form a non-fat natural cheese.

Also claimed is the natural cheese prod. formed.

The fat substitute additive is pref. a microgel, a hydrocolloid or a microfragment anisotropic polysaccharide/protein complex. The additive has an average particle size of 0.5 to 30 microns and is present at a level of 0.5–50 wt.% on dry solids basis (the fat substitute additive is esp. a fragmented calcium alginate gel, a hydrocolloid selected from guar, agar, xanthan and carrageenan or a microfragmented anisotropic xanthan (protein complex more esp. xanthan/whey or xanthan/egg albumin complex).

USE/ADVANTAGE—The method enables preparation of non-fat natural cheese. The additives added serve to provide the same function as the fat particles usually associated with the protein matrix of cheese. The additives provide particles which do not integrate with the casein network of the cheese, but remain detached and provide mouthfeel resembling fat-contg. cheeses.

Hydrocolloid—Dairy 9

Paste used as fat substitute, contg. carrageenan and potassium ions—for food such as low calorie ice cream and mayonnaise, suitable for diet foods.

Patent Assignee: AJINOMOTO CO INC (AJIN); AJINOMOTO KK (AJIN)
Inventor: FUSEYA Y; KONISHI M; KONOIKE T; MARUYAMA K;

MORITA Y; TAKAGAKI Y; TSUJIMURA H; YAMAGATA M
Number of Countries: 001 Number of Patents: 004
Patent No Kind Date Applicat No Kind Date Main IPC Week
WO 9504480 A1 19950216 WO 94JP1288 A 19940804 A23L-001/307 199512 B
JP 7046965 A 19950221 JP 93194687 A 19930805 A23L-001/05 199517
EP 664084 A1 19950726 EP 94923071 A 19940804 A23L-001/307 199534
WO 94JP1288 A 19940804
EP 664084 A4 19960703 EP 94923071 A 19940000 A23L-001/307 199644
Abstract (Basic): WO 9504480 A

A paste for use in a food product contains 1.5–10 wt.% of carrageenans mainly comprising kappa-carrageenan and 2–30 wt.% (based on the carrageenan) of potassium ions. The paste has a viscosity of 300–25000 cP at 25°C. An aqueous solution contg. 1 wt.% of the carrageenans can pass completely through a sieve having a JIS opening of 20 micron.

USE—The paste is used in salad dressing, mayonnaise and food products contg. mayonnaise, and in ice cream and whipped cream (claimed) as a partial or complete substitute for the fat component of a fat-contg. emulsion food. It is useful in diet foods.

ADVANTAGE—The paste does not have an unpleasant effect on the taste or appetising quality of food contg. it. Mayonnaise contg. the paste has excellent viscosity characteristics, preservability, physical properties for mixing with vegetables, etc.

Hydrocolloid—Dairy 10

Low fat or fat-free powdered coffee whitener—using reformed casein micelles as fat substitute.

Patent Assignee: NESTEC SA (NEST)
Inventor: MELACHOURIS N; MOFFITT K R; RASILEWICZ C E; TONNER G F
Number of Countries: 001 Number of Patents: 001
Patent No Kind Date Applicat No Kind Date Main IPC Week
US 5318793 A 19940607 US 91760663 A 19910916 A23C-011/08 199422 B
US 92937574 A 19920831
Abstract (Basic): US 5318793 A

Powdered coffee whitener comprises a spray-dried dispersion of reformed casein micelles formed in situ by the sequential addn. of a soluble source of Ca ions and a soluble source of phosphate ions to an aq. medium contg. processed casein but no casein micelles.

The process casein material is acid casein and/or alkali metal caseinate; the Ca source and phosphate source are each soluble salts. The spray-dried dispersion of reformed casein micelles is blended with a carbohydrate, 0.05–1 wt.% hydrophilic colloid and sufficient buffer to give a pH of 6.3–6.8.

USE—The coffee whiteners use the casein as a replacement for the fat component. They have the same functional and organoleptic properties as conventional whiteners.

In an example, 96.9g of 8.87% $CaCl_2$ soln. was mixed into 1 l. of 55°C water contg. 126g Na caseinate. Then 60.0g of soln. contg. 17.1% di K phosphate and 1.8% NaOH was mixed in. After ultrafiltering, 1 × dilution and ultrafiltering, the micelle suspension (96g) was mixed with a dry blend of 3.0g sucrose and 0.5g locust bean gum, homogenised, pasteurised and opt. mixed with maltodextrin and spray dried.

Hydrocolloid—Dairy 11

Low fat natural cheese mfr. for body and texture of full-fat cheese—by adding gel-forming fat mimetic of methylcellulose gum to skimmed milk, setting. cutting, cooking and draining substrate, and curing.

Patent Assignee: KRAFT GEN FOODS INC (KRFT); KRAFT FOODS INC (KRFT)
Inventor: CRAWFORD S I; MEHNERT D; MEIBACH R L; MILLER M S; SURBER K J; WREZEL P
Number of Countries: 022 Number of Patents: 005
Patent No Kind Date Applicat No Kind Date Main IPC Week
WO 9521534 A1 19950817 WO 95US518 A 19950113 A23C-019/00 199538 B
AU 9516801 A 19950829 AU 9516801 A 19950113 A23C-019/00 199548
EP 693881 A1 19960131 EP 95908508 A 19950113 A23C-019/00 199609
WO 95US518 A 19950113
US 5532018 A 19960702 US 94195270 A 19940214 A23C-019/00 199632
EP 693881 A4 19960612 EP 95908508 A 19950000 A23C-019/00 199644
Abstract (Basic): WO 9521534 A

The mfr. comprises:

(a) adding a gel-forming fat mimetic to skimmed milk;
(b) setting, cutting, cooking and draining the substrate formed;
(c) curing the cheese curd formed;
(d) comminuting the skimmed milk cheese obtd. and heating to 140–180°F;
(e) holding for 0.5–8 min. to give a homogeneous cheese mass; and
(f) packaging.

Also claimed is a method for mfr. of a low-fat natural cheese comprising providing a mixt. comprising a skimmed milk cheese, a gel-forming fat mimetic, emulsifying salt and water.

USE—Used for mfr. of a low-fat natural cheese.

ADVANTAGE—The prod. emulates the body and texture of fat-contg. natural cheeses.

Hydrocolloid—Dessert 1

Dry blend shortening substitute for bakery prods.—comprising xanthan gum, guar gums and emulsifiers, for complete fat replacement in, e.g., cakes.
Patent Assignee: MERCK & CO INC (MERI)
Inventor: LAWSON M A; LIN S W
Number of Countries: 014 Number of Patents: 004
Patent Family:
Patent No Kind Date Applicat No Kind Date Main IPC Week
EP 468552 A 19920129 EP 91201304 A 19910530 199205 B
CA 2043764 A 19911207 199209
JP 4252134 A 19920908 JP 91134695 A 19910606 A21D-008/00 199243
EP 468552 A3 19931222 EP 91201304 A 19910530 199515
Abstract (Basic): EP 468552 A

Substitute comprises xanthan gum(s) and ingredient(s) of (a) other gum(s) of gum arabic, propylene glycol alignate, guar-, locust bean or gellan-gum, alginates, carrageenan, maltodextrin and carboxymethyl cellulose, and (b) emulsifier(s) of monodiglycerides, sodium stearoyl lactylate, lecithin, sorbitan monostearate, poly(oxy-1,2-ethanediyl) derivs. of lactylate, lecithin, sorbitan monooctadecanoate and diacetyl tartaric acid ester of monoglycerides. A fat-reduced baking compsn. comprises 0.01–0.8 wt.% of the fat substitute.

USE/ADVANTAGE—Used to replace up to 100% of the fat in bakery prods. such as layer cakes, muffins, devils food cake, cookies and doughnuts. Prods. esp. cakes, contg. the fat substitutes have similar baking vols. and cake densities, fine and uniform cell structures and comparable organoleptic properties to full-fat cakes.

Hydrocolloid—Dessert 2

Reduced calorie, low acid dessert toppings—comprises carrageenan gum blend, powdered cellulose bulking agent, non-heat thinning cellulose gum bulking agent, corn syrups etc.
Patent Assignee: SMUCKER J M CO (SMUC-N)
Inventor: ROCKLAND L B
Number of Countries: 001 Number of Patents: 001
Patent No Kind Date Applicat No Kind Date Main IPC Week
US 5132128 A 19920721 US 91686810 A 19910417 A23G-003/00 199232 B
Abstract (Basic): US 5132128 A

Reduced calorie, fat-contg., low acid dessert topping compsn. comprises:

a carrageenan gum (I) blend, a powdered cellulose bulking agent (II), a non-heat thinning cellulose gum bulking agent (III), high fructose corn syrups (IV), an edible humectant (V), and non-fat milk (VI). Compsn. has pH above 4.6, and has H_2O activity of less than 0.84 and contains at least 1/3rd less calories than standard toppings.

Comprise (by wt.) 0.75–1.75% (I), 3–4.5% (II), 50–60% (IV), 1–1.5% (V), 6.5–8.5% (VI), and 30–40% H_2O; and pref. also comprise 4–15% cocoa powder as a flavour constituent (prim. agent a mixt. of Dutch and natural cocoa powders). Pref. (I) blend includes a gelling gum and a viscosity control gum in ca eq. amts., esp. carrageenan with added gelling agents and carrageenan with guar gum. Pref. (III) is a microcrystalline cellulose. Pref. (V) is propylene glycol.

ADVANTAGE—Low acid topping compsns. have the physical characteristics of conventional standard toppings, but have ca 1/3rd of the calories of a normal prod. Compsns. are esp. hot fudge toppings. In addn. the compsns. have smooth uniform texture at ambient temps. and on cold surfaces.

Hydrocolloid—Dessert 3

Aerated ice confections—with gas cells of high stability and capable of acting as fat replacers.

Patent Assignee: UNILEVER PLC (UNIL); UNILEVER NV (UNIL); GOOD HUMOR CORP (GOOD-N)

Inventor: BEE R D; NEEDHAM D; SMALLWOOD K

Number of Countries: 049 Number of Patents: 017

Patent No Kind Date Applicat No Kind Date Main IPC Week

WO 9412050 A1 19940609 WO 93EP3319 A 19931125 A23G-009/02 199424 B

AU 9456947 A 19940622 AU 9456947 A 19931125 A23G-009/02 199436

FI 9502694 A 19950602 WO 93EP3319 A 19931125 A23G-000/00 199536
FI 952694 A 19950602

NO 9502179 A 19950728 WO 93EP3319 A 19931125 A23G-000/00 199540
NO 952179 A 19950601

ZA 9309041 A 19950830 ZA 939041 A 19931202 A23G-000/00 199540

EP 675685 A1 19951011 WO 93EP3319 A 19931125 A23G-009/02 199545
EP 94902657 A 19931125

CN 1095555 A 19941130 CN 93121654 A 19931202 A23G-009/02 199547

US 5472726 A 19951205 US 93160536 A 19931201 A23G-009/00 199603

SK 9500733 A3 19951108 WO 93EP3319 A 19931125 A23G-009/02 199605
SK 95733 A 19931125

CZ 9501431 A3 19951213 CZ 951431 A 19931125 A23G-009/02 199606

NZ 258873 A 19960625 NZ 258873 A 19931125 A23G-009/02 199631
WO 93EP3319 A 19931125
JP 8503608 W 19960423 WO 93EP3319 A 19931125 A23G-009/02 199645
JP 94512765 A 19931125
AU 671703 B 19960905 AU 9456947 A 19931125 A23G-009/02 199647
EP 675685 B1 19970507 WO 93EP3319 A 19931125 A23G-009/02 199723
EP 94902657 A 19931125
DE 69310545 E 19970612 DE 610545 A 19931125 A23G-009/02 199729
WO 93EP3319 A 19931125 EP 94902657 A 19931125
ES 2102189 T3 19970716 EP 94902657 A 19931125 A23G-009/02 199735
HU 71934 T 19960228 WO 93EP3319 A 19931125 A23G-009/02 199740
HU 951589 A 19931125

Abstract (Basic): WO 9412050 A

Ice confections comprise gas cells having a stability in excess of 2 weeks and having a D3,2 (sic) particle size of less than 20 microns.

The D3,2 size of the gas cells is 0.1–10, esp. 0.5–3, microns. The gas cells have a surface of edible surface active material. The gas cells are prepd. separately in bulk and added to the ice confection during or after its prepn.

ADVANTAGE—Compsns. have good creaminess, whiteness and flavour. The gas cells replace some of the fat in the compsns.

In an example, low fat ice cream was prepd. from 57.33 wt.% water, 3.00% butter oil, 0.11% locust bean gum, 10.00% skimmed milk powder, 8.00% maltodextrin of D.E. 17–19, 0.50% glycerol monostearate, 0.06% guar gum, 6.00% maltodextrin of D.E. 40 and 15.00% gas cell mixt.

Hydrocolloid—Dessert 4

Sweetening compsn., useful for sugar-coated prods., e.g., chewing gum, confectionery etc.—contains erythritol, non-erythritol saccharide(s) and thickening stabiliser, e.g., agar.

Patent Assignee: NIKKEN CHEM CO LTD (NIKM); NIKKEN KASEI KK (NIKK-N)

Number of Countries: 001 Number of Patents: 001

Patent No Kind Date Applicat No Kind Date Main IPC Week

JP 8322504 A 19961210 JP 95154101 A 19950530 A23L-001/22 199708 B

Abstract (Basic): JP 8322504 A

Compsn. contains 35–65 w/w% of erythritol and 0.03–0.7 w/w% of thickening stabilising agent comprised of polysaccharides selected from one or more of carrageenan, agar, farcelan, pectin, curdlan, gellan gum, xanthan gum, alginic acid sodium salt, tamarind gum. Saccharides other than erythritol are in the amt. 43 pts. wt. of less (w.r.t. 100 pts. wt. of erythritol). Obtd. compsn. is coated on surface of core material and dried.

USE/ADVANTAGE—Used for chocolate, tablet, chewing gum, candy and medicinal products. Low calorie and non-cariogenic sweetening is preserved for long term. Confectionery and medicinal products have improved taste.

Hydrocolloid—Emulsifier, Stabilizer, & Suspending Agent 1

Roughage rich diet supplement made from natural materials—comprises soy bran and guar bean meal stored dry and finely ground and may be added to, e.g., liquid foods including fruit juices.

Patent Assignee: DESAGA H (DESA-I)
Number of Countries: 001 Number of Patents: 001
Patent No Kind Date Applicat No Kind Date Main IPC Week
DE 29611879 U1 19970807 DE 96U2011879 U 19960709 199737 B
Abstract (Basic): DE 29611879 U

Roughage rich composition for human nourishment, or at least as a food supplement, comprises soy bran and guar bean meal. Preferably, the soy husk residues (2) have the maximum possible surface area; they may be half husks. The bran is roasted. Components of this material are stored dry, and may be finely ground. The guar meal acts as a thickener or swelling agent.

USE—The roughage rich foodstuff is useful as a low-calorie food supplement.

ADVANTAGE—The roughage-rich material controls digestion in a calorie-reduced diet. It may be mixed, e.g., with fluid foods such as, e.g., fruit juice, soups, gravy, yoghurt or porridge, where the guar meal acts as a thickener.

Hydrocolloid—Emulsifier, Stabilizer, & Suspending Agent 2

Ready-to-eat, low–no fat pudding—comprises water, calcium source, thickening and sweetening agents, emulsifier, and calcium-sensitive, irreversible gelling hydrocolloid.

Patent Assignee: KRAFT GEN FOODS INC (KRFT); KRAFT FOODS INC (KRFT)
Inventor: KING L D; LESHIK R R
Number of Countries: 004 Number of Patents: 006
Patent No Kind Date Applicat No Kind Date Main IPC Week
GB 2261805 A 19930602 GB 9224485 A 19921123 A23L-001/187 199322 B
DE 4239590 A1 19930603 DE 4239590 A 19921125 A23L-001/187 199323
CA 2082969 A 19930528 CA 2082969 A 19921116 A23L-001/187 199333

US 5238699 A 19930824 US 91800617 A 19911127 A23L-001/187 199335
GB 2261805 B 19950802 GB 9224485 A 19921123 A23L-001/187 199534
CA 2082969 C 19960507 CA 2082969 A 19921116 A23L-001/187 199628
Abstract (Basic): GB 2261805 A

Compsn. for the prepn. of a packaged ready-to-eat pudding comprises: less than 3% fat; H_2O; a source of soluble Ca (I); thickening agent (II); sweetener; emulsifier/stabiliser (III) and/or polyphosphate; and 0.01–1.5% by wt. of an ungelled, Ca-sensitive, irreversible, gelling hydrocolloid (IV) as fat replacement.

Pref. compsn. comprises 0–3%, esp. 0% fat. Pref. (I) is milk solids. Pref. sweetener is sugar-free. Pref. (IV) is algin (or salts), low methoxyl pectin, gellan gum or mixts., esp. Na alginate; and is pref. the only non-starch hydrocolloid present.

ADVANTAGE—The low/no fat, ready-to-eat pudding-like desserts may be UHT sterilised, when they are stable to storage for prolonged periods, or may be prepd. under controlled conditions and stored at refrigeration temps. The prods. have a smooth, creamy texture and mouthfeel, and the weak, soft gel structure of full-fat, ready-to-eat puddings.

Hydrocolloid—Emulsifier, Stabilizer, & Suspending Agent 3

Starch natural gum composite—processed so that polysaccharide components are completely solubilised, are useful in foods as thickening and suspending agents.

Patent Assignee: US SEC OF AGRIC (USDA)
Inventor: CHRISTIANSON D D; FANTA G F
Number of Countries: 021 Number of Patents: 007
Patent No Kind Date Applicat No Kind Date Main IPC Week
WO 9414887 A2 19940707 WO 93US11862 A 19931208 B 199428 B
AU 9465479 A 19940719 AU 9465479 A 19931208 B 199439
WO 9414887 A3 19940915 WO 93US11862 A 19931208 B 199518
US 5424088 A 19950613 US 92991811 A 19921217 B 199529
EP 674682 A1 19951004 WO 93US11862 A 19931208 B 199544
EP 94913248 A 19931208
JP 8505170 W 19960604 WO 93US11862 A 19931208 B 199648
JP 94515201 A 19931208
AU 679740 B 19970710 AU 9465479 A 19931208 B 199736
Abstract (Basic): WO 9414887 A

Compsn. comprises a water-solubilised blend of polysaccharide components of starch and of a natural gum, the starch polysaccharide components: natural gum polysaccharide components dry wt. ratio is in the range 99:1–90:10.

Pref. the highest mol. wt. polysaccharide components of the blend have significant molecular wt. redn.

USE/ADVANTAGE—Compsns. are useful in foods as thickening agents, suspending agents and fat substitutes. When placed in water, the compsns. hydrate rapidly and yield dispersions that are not only smooth and viscous but also possess considerable lubricity. Aq. dispersions of certain blends show little or none of the undesirable tendency of cooked starches to form rigid gels on standing or to exude water when frozen and thawed.

In an example, 400 g. wheat starch was dry blended with 20 g. guar gum. The blend was dispersed in 3 l. of water and the pH adjusted to 7. Steam jet cooking was then carried out at 140°C with a steam pressure of 40 psig. within the cooker. The cooked soln. was drum dried and ground. An emulsion formed by adding 30–35 wt.% corn oil to a 10 wt.% aq. dispersion the compsn. was smooth and spreadable and remained stable under refrigeration and/or room temp. conditions during extended storage.

Hydrocolloid—Fruits & Vegetables 1

Fruit spread—contains fat mimetic of low methoxy pectin or modified corn starch improving texture and flavour and decreasing dissipation rate in the mouth.

Patent Assignee: SMUCKER J M CO (SMUC-N)
Inventor: BRAIN C H; GAITHER K S; MUENZ D J
Number of Countries: 003 Number of Patents: 001

Patent No	Kind	Date	Applicat No	Kind	Date	Main IPC	Week
US 5260083	A	19931109	US 92857254	A	19920325		199346 B
AU 9335368	A	19930930	AU 9335368	A	19930319		199347
CA 2082751	A	19930926	CA 2082751	A	19921112		199351
AU 9517852	A	19950629	AU 9335368	A	19930319		199533
			AU 9517852	A	19950503		
AU 678698	B	19970605	AU 9335368	A	19930319		199731
			AU 9517852	A	19950503		

Abstract (Basic): US 5260083 A

Fruit spreads with improved texture and flavour comprise a microparticulated blend of (a) up to 55 wt.% fruit ingredient; (b) sweetener, to a soluble solids content of 20–70 wt.%; (c) up to 80 wt.% water and (d) a fat mimetic. Ingredient (a) is whole fruit, fruit purée or fruit juice.

Pref. fat mimetic (d) is a low methoxyl pectin or a modified corn starch. It is esp. at least 0.5 (0.5–3.0) wt.% low methoxyl pectin, and the blend has particle size 5–100 microns; or is 5–20 wt.% modified corn starch, and the blend has particle size 2–15 microns, opt. aggregated to not over 100 microns. The spreads are produced by mixing the ingredients, cooking to a desired solids content and homogenising under high shear.

USE/ADVANTAGE—Spreads are jelly- or jam-like. They have improved texture and flavour characteristics and decreased dissipation rate in the mouth.

Hydrocolloid—Fruits & Vegetables 2

Prepn. of non-fat foodstuffs, esp. fruit and vegetable based products—involving adding fat mimetic based on starch, pectin or protein to improve texture and other properties.

Patent Assignee: SMUCKER J M CO (SMUC-N)
Inventor: BRAIN C H; GAITHER K S; MUENZ D J
Number of Countries: 001 Number of Patents: 001
Patent No Kind Date Applicat No Kind Date Main IPC Week
US 5503863 A 19960402 US 92857257 A 19920325 A23L-001/29 199619 B
US 93115825 A 19930903
US 95488686 A 19950607
Abstract (Basic): US 5503863 A

A non-fat food product (I) comprising a mixt. of (a) a food ingredient selected from whole fruit, fruit puree, fruit juice or concentrate, cocoa, tomatoes or tomato juice, sauce, paste or paste concentrate; (b) water and/or sweetener; (c) a stabiliser and/or gel promoting agent; and (d) a fat mimetic which is pectin, starch and/or protein based.

A range of compsns contg. particular food ingredients is claimed, e.g., a prod. contg. up to 55 wt% fruit puree or fruit juice, 10–75% sweetener, up to 80% water, food acid, gel promoter, stabiliser and 0.1–4.0% pectin based mimetic where the soluble solids are 20–80% and the particle size is 5–100 μ.

USE—The products (I) are not fat imitation products but are similar to the traditional products comprising (a)–(c).

ADVANTAGE—(d), added as additional ingredient rather than as fat substitute, improves the texture of (I), enhances the spreadability, flavour and mouthfeel of some fruit spreads and improves the water retention and bake stability of bakery filled products.

Hydrocolloid—Fruits & Vegetables 3

Starch-prune premixes for flour-based food prods.—useful as fat replacements to give food prods. of good taste, improved shelf-life and healthy eating characteristics.

Patent Assignee: CADEN J A (CADE-I); WOLKE M (WOLK-I)
Inventor: CADEN J A; WOLKE M
Number of Countries: 001 Number of Patents: 001
Patent No Kind Date Applicat No Kind Date Main IPC Week
US 5484622 A 19960116 US 93105395 A 19930812 A21D-010/00 199609 B
US 95404506 A 19950315
Abstract (Basic): US 5484622 A

Starch-prune premixes are used for making flour-based food prods. They comprise amylopectin starch (I), amylose starch (II) and prunes (III). All three are mixed together to form the premix, to which flour and other components may be added to make the food prods.

ADVANTAGE—The prods. are low in fat, all natural, low cholesterol, low Na, mould resistant, economical, resistant to microwave-induced loss of texture and taste, have good taste and have good shelf life.

Hydrocolloid—Fruits & Vegetables 4

Non fat food prods., e.g., fruit spreads and pie fillings—contg. pectin, starch, cellulose or protein based fat mimetic having improved texture and spreadability.

Patent Assignee: SMUCKER J M CO (SMUC-N)
Inventor: BRAIN C H; GAITHER K S; MUENZ D J
Number of Countries: 001 Number of Patents: 001
Patent No Kind Date Applicat No Kind Date Main IPC Week
US 5451420 A 19950919 US 92857254 A 19920325 A23L-001/0524 199543 B
US 93115825 A 19930903
Abstract (Basic): US 5451420 A

A non-fat food prod. comprises: (a) a mixt. of whole fruit, fruit purée, fruit juice, fruit juice concentrate, cocoa, tomatoes, tomato juice, tomato paste, tomato paste concentrate and/or tomato sauce; (b) one of water and a sweetener; and (c) one of a stabiliser and a gel promoting agents; (d) a fat mimetic as an additional ingredient providing the physical and organoleptic characteristics of fat, selected from pectin based, starch based, cellulose based and/or protein based fat mimetics.

The fat mimetic is a low methoxyl pectin forming 0.1 wt.% of the mixt. The prod. has a soluble solids content of 5–80% and consists of particle 5–100 μm.

USE—Used in non-fat food prods., e.g., fruit spreads, bakery fillings, flavoured syrups, pie glazes and fillings etc.

ADVANTAGE—The food prods. have improved texture and enhanced spread ability, flavour and mouthfeel. Bakery filling prods. also have improved water retention and bake stability.

Hydrocolloid—Snack 1

Xanthan gum and dextrin for puffed snacks—with less calories and more stable structure than gun puffed fat and starch complexes.
Patent Assignee: GENERAL FOODS CORP (GENO)
Number of Countries: 002 Number of Patents: 002
Patent No Kind Date Applicat No Kind Date Main IPC Week
US 3821428 A 19740628 197428 B
CA 978015 A 19751118 197549
Abstract (Basic): US 3821428 A

1-2 wt. pts. xanthan gum and 2-1 wt. pts. dextrin, are mixed and formed into a paste with H_2O until the dough is shiny and stringy. After stranding for >18 hrs. pref. 24 hrs the dough is rolled into 0.125 inch sheets, seasoned and baked, pref. for 15 mins at 400°F. The process is used to make low calorie, puffed sticks, pretzels or fillings with a cheese, onion, bacon, garlic or peanut. butter flavour.

Hydrocolloid—Spread & Salad Dressing 1

Water-in-oil emulsion low fat spread—contg. combination of linear and spherical gel structure hydrocolloids in aq. phase.
Patent Assignee: UNILEVER NV (UNIL)
Inventor: MILO B T; REISSMANN H A W
Number of Countries: 014 Number of Patents: 006
Patent No Kind Date Applicat No Kind Date Main IPC Week
EP 52899 A 19820602 EP 81201222 A 19811030 198223 B
US 4389426 A 19830621 198327
ZA 8108060 A 19830520 198329
CA 1168923 A 19840612 198428
EP 52899 B 19850102 198502
DE 3168085 G 19850214 198508
Abstract (Basic): EP 52899 A

A water-in-oil emulsion spread has a fat content of 25–65 wt.% and comprises a dispersed aq. phase contg. a gelling system contg. one or more hydrocolloids selected from maltodextrins of DE at least 20, pectin, lambola carrageen and alginates, and at least one hydrocolloid selected from guar gum, locust bean gum and iota carrageenan.

The gelling system pref. comprises a mixt. of guar gum and highly esterified pectin in wt. ratio at least 4, pref. 6 or more. The compsn. pref. contains 0.1–1.0, esp. 0.2–0.5 wt.% guar gum and 0.01–0.3, esp. 0.03–0.075 wt.% pectin, and 0.01–8, esp. 1–5 wt. protein, e.g., milk, vegetable or microbial protein. The fat is pref. a plastic fat blend having the following solids contents at the given temps.:—N10 20–30; N20 10–18; N30 1–8.

Use of a combination of linear gel structure and spherical gel structure hydrocolloids yields a low calorie spread which is stable in storage but breaks down pleasantly in the mouth.

Hydrocolloid—Spread & Salad Dressing 2

Low calorie spread contg. high-methoxylated pectin—to replace gelatin as emulsion stabiliser.

Patent Assignee: GRINDSTED PROD AS (GRIN)
Number of Countries: 001 Number of Patents: 001
Patent No Kind Date Applicat No Kind Date Main IPC Week
RD 217009 A 19820510 198222 B
Abstract (Basic): RD 217009 A

In a 40% fat calorie spread, milk protein destabilises the emulsion which gives a spread with coarse water dispersion and poor microbiological shelf life. Gelatin is known to stabilise the emulsion in the prod. at a dosage of, e.g., 2.5% gelatin 120 bloom calculated on the low calorie spread.

In trying to replace gelatine with pectin, the following trials were made with high-methoxylated pectin. Water phase contained 1.0% whey powder, 1.0% salt and 53.9–55.4% water at pH 6.5. (1) 2.5% Gelatin 120 bloom; (2) 1.0% Mexpectin SS 200 (slow set); (3) 2.0% Mexpectin SS 200 (slow set); (4) 1.0% Mexpectin MS 300 (medium set); (5) 2.0% Mexpectin MS 300 (medium set); (6) 1.0% Mexpectin RS 400 (rapid set); (7) 2.0% Mexpectin RS 400 (rapid set); fat phase contained 0.5% DIMODAN OT (unsatd. distilled monoglyceride); 0.1% sorbic acid; 0.3% colour; 39.2% fat blend; 24 pts. hardened soya, 41°C, 76 pts. liq. soya-bean oil. The spreads were produced on a 2-tube laboratory Perfector with low capacity and moderate cooling.

Evaluation after storage at 5°C showed that the spreads with Mexpectin had a satisfactory water dispersion and shelf life.

Hydrocolloid—Spread & Salad Dressing 3

Fat-free margarine compsn. having reduced calorie content—comprises inulin and/or gum, water, modified starch or gelling-type maltodextrin fat mimetic and opt. bulking agent.

Patent Assignee: KRAFT GEN FOODS INC (KRFT); KRAFT FOODS INC (KRFT)
Inventor: BULIGA G S; LIS D G; MILLER M S; POWELL W F; DANIEL G L
Number of Countries: 020 Number of Patents: 005
Patent No Kind Date Applicat No Kind Date Main IPC Week

EP 605217 A2 19940706 EP 93310499 A 19931223 A23D-007/00 199426 B
NO 9304824 A 19940629 NO 934824 A 19931227 A23L-001/307 199429
FI 9305870 A 19940629 FI 935870 A 19931227 A23D-000/00 199433
CA 2110195 A 19940629 CA 2110195 A 19931129 A23D-007/00 199434
EP 605217 A3 19950503 EP 93310499 A 19931223 A23D-007/00 199545
Abstract (Basic): EP 605217 A

Non-fat margarines comprise (a) a fat mimetic, (b) opt. a bulking agent, (c) inulin and/or gum, and (d) water. Fat mimetic (a) is a gelling type maltodextrin or is starch with the amorphous regions removed by hydrolysis.

The bulking agent is at 0–5 wt.%. Component (c) is inulin. The margarine is spreadable. The margarine esp. contains calcium citrate, esp. at 0.75–3.0%. It also contains a gum, esp. xanthan, guar or acacia gum, alginate, carrageenan, pectin or gelatin, esp. at 0.1–2.0%. The fat mimetic is at 3.5–8 or 5–10%. The bulking agent is at 1.0–5%. The inulin is at 10–23%, esp. 15–25%. If (b) is present, (c) is gum and the margarine is squeezable. (b) is at 5–10%. Compsns. also contain 1.0–2.5% salt. They also contain 0.5–15% fat or oil.

ADVANTAGE—Compsns. have the appearance and taste of margarine or squeezable margarine with no fat and reduced calorie content.

Hydrocolloid—Spread & Salad Dressing 4

Prodn. of low-fat salad dressing—contg. oil or fat and fresh cheese.
Patent Assignee: VER COOP MELKIND (VEME-N)
Number of Countries: 001 Number of Patents: 001
Patent No Kind Date Applicat No Kind Date Main IPC Week
NL 8203425 A 19840402 NL 823425 A 19820901 198417 B
Abstract (Basic): NL 8203425 A

Mayonnaise-like dressings with a lower fat content than normal mayonnaise are prepd. by blending an edible oil or fat with ingredients conventionally used in mayonnaise, salad creams and other dressings. The novel feature comprises incorporating fresh cheese in the mixt.

The mixt. pref. contains 5–40 wt.% oil or fat and 10–60% cheese, esp. cottage cheese, opt. enriched with whey protein. The mixt. is pref. pasteurised. A specifically claimed dressing comprises 48.2% cottage cheese (with 20% whey protein concentrate), 20.0% vegetable oil, 18.0% water, 6.5% sugar, 2.25% starch, 1.65% salt, 1.2% powdered egg, 1.2% lactic acid, 0.5% flavour and colour, 0.25% K sorbate and 0.2% guar.

The dressings have a low calorific value (e.g., 700–1030 KJ/100 g) and good storage stability, texture and flavour.

Hydrocolloid—Spread & Salad Dressing 5

Fat spread-type fermented milk used on bread and cracker—comprises fermented milk, gelling type water-soluble polymer, iota carrageenan, starch and thickening water-soluble polymer.
Patent Assignee: OYAMA NYUGYO NOGYO KYODO KUMIAI (OYAM-N)
Number of Countries: 001 Number of Patents: 001
Patent No Kind Date Applicat No Kind Date Main IPC Week
JP 9172961 A 19970708 JP 95335030 A 19951222 199737 B
Abstract (Basic): JP 9172961 A

A milk containing composition of raw materials comprises fermented milk, two or more of gelling-type water-soluble polymer for food containing at least iota carrageenan and starch and one or more thickening water-soluble polymer for food.

USE—The product is used by spreading to bread and cracker.

ADVANTAGE—The product is smoothly spread to bread. Decoration is easily made. Whey does not separate. Low fat and low calorie product is obtained.

Hydrocolloid—Spread & Salad Dressing 6

Low fat spread prodn. with continuous aq. phase—which is gelled with gelatin, a gelling hydrolysed starch and a gelling polysaccharide.
Patent Assignee: UNILEVER PLC (UNIL); UNILEVER NV (UNIL)
Inventor: NORTON I T; UNDERDOWN J
Number of Countries: 010 Number of Patents: 005
Patent No Kind Date Applicat No Kind Date Main IPC Week
WO 9535036 A2 19951228 WO 95EP2354 A 19950619 A23D-007/015 199606 B
AU 9528850 A 19960115 AU 9528850 A 19950619 A23D-007/015 199620
WO 9535036 A3 19960201 WO 95EP2354 A 19950619 A23D-007/015 199622
EP 753996 A1 19970122 EP 95924270 A 19950619 A23D-007/015 199709
WO 95EP2354 A 19950619
ZA 9505181 A 19970226 ZA 955181 A 19950622 A23D-000/00 199714
Abstract (Basic): WO 9535036 A

Low-fat spread contains 0–40% fatty phase in a continuous aq. phase. The aq. phase is water contg. (wt.%): (a) 0.1–7 gelatin; (b) 2–30 gelling hydrolysed starch, and (c) 0.3–5 (pref. 0.5–5) gelling polysaccharide (I). (I) is agar, kappa- or iota-carrageenan, gellan, furcelleran, alginate and/or pectin and the levels of (a), (b) and (c) are all w.r.t. the wt. of water. The spread is produced by preparing a premix of (a), (b) and (c) in water, gelling (c) and opt. (b) in the presence of shear at >50°C, and then cooling to <30°C.

USE—The spreads are low fat for low-calorie or other dietetic considerations.

Hydrocolloid—Spread & Salad Dressing 7

Low fat water-in-oil emulsion spreads with margarine-like properties—using co-processed microcrystalline cellulose and galactomannan as fat substitute.

Patent Assignee: FMC CORP (FMCC)
Inventor: HUMPHREYS W M
Number of Countries: 045 Number of Patents: 008
Patent No Kind Date Applicat No Kind Date Main IPC Week
WO 9412043 A1 19940609 WO 93US11195 A 19931118 A23D-007/00 199424 B
US 5338562 A 19940816 US 92981649 A 19921125 A23D-009/04 199432
AU 9456124 A 19940622 AU 9456124 A 19931118 A23D-007/00 199436
EP 670678 A1 19950913 WO 93US11195 A 19931118 A23D-007/00 199541
EP 94901582 A 19931118
EP 670678 A4 19951011 EP 94901582 A 19940000 A23D-007/00 199620
AU 668632 B 19960509 AU 9456124 A 19931118 A23D-007/00 199626
JP 8501702 W 19960227 WO 93US11195 A 19931118 A23D-007/00 199643
JP 94513246 A 19931118
JP 2652085 B2 19970910 WO 93US11195 A 19931118 A23D-007/015 199741
JP 94513246 A 19931118
Abstract (Basic): WO 9412043 A

Low fat water-in-oil emulsions (I) contain at least 56 wt.% water; a fat substitute (II); a stabiliser (III); a gum; a continuous phase of not more than 28% oil and an emulsifier (IV). (II) is co-processed microcrystalline cellulose (MCC) and galactomannan and has mean particle size 8–35 microns.

Pref. the emulsion contains 15–25% oil, 67% or more water, 0.5–4% stabiliser and 0.1% or more gum. The stabiliser is MCC of mean particle size 0.05–0.5 microns, or 0.1–0.6 microns. the gum is xanthan and (IV) is a fatty acid ester of an 8–18C fatty acid with glycerol, diglycerol or polyglycerol. (IV) is esp. a mixt. of esters, esp. including a monoglyceride or polyglycerol ester of an 8–18C (12–18) (14–18) fatty acid. (II) is a co-processed MCC/guar or it has mean particle size 16–24 (18–22) microns and is at 0.5–1.5 wt.% and is co-processed MCC/galactomannan. (IV) has HLB 3–7 (4–6).

USE—Emulsions mimic the taste, thickness, smoothness, waxiness, cohesiveness, physiological effect and mouth coating ability of full fat margarine.

Hydrocolloid—Spread & Salad Dressing 8

Fat substitute for addn. to foods as a salad dressing—comprises particles contg. microcrystalline cellulose and galactomannan gum.

Patent Assignee: FMC CORP (FMCC)
Inventor: MCGINLEY E J; TUASON D C
Number of Family:
Patent No Kind Date Applicat No Kind Date Main IPC Week
US 5192569 A 19930309 US 89359065 A 19890526 A23L-001/0526 199321 B
US 90519693 A 19900507
US 91809857 A 19911218
Abstract (Basic): US 5192569 A

Compsn. comprises dry, water-dispersible, water-stable, spheroidal-shaped particles having an average particle size in the range of about 0.1–100 microns, each particle consisting of an aggregate of about 60–99 wt.% of microcrystalline cellulose and about 40–1 wt.% galactomannan gum, the aggregate remains impact if dispersed in an aq. medium. The particle size is pref. about 5–15 microns. The microcrystalline cellulose is of colloidal size and the galactomannan gum is pref. guar gum or locust bean gum.

USE/ADVANTAGE—The compsn., in colloidal form, when added to foods as salad dressings or dairy prods. as a fat substitute, imparts a fat-like mouth-feel and consistency without the calorific value of fat.

Hydrocolloid—Spread & Salad Dressing 9

Fat mimetic compsns. for reduced calorie salad dressings—comprise microcrystalline cellulose, cold water swelling starch, gum, alginate, opacifier and water.

Patent Assignee: UNILEVER PLC (UNIL); UNILEVER NV (UNIL); LIPTON CO THOMAS J (LIPT-N); UNILEVER LTD (UNIL)
Inventor: BAUER R; CUCCURULLO J A; DAZO P E; KOCHAKJI D J; RIKON S M; RUBOW R E
Number of Countries: 023 Number of Patents: 015
Patent No Kind Date Applicat No Kind Date Main IPC Week
US 5209942 A 19930511 US 91799583 A 19911127 A23C-001/24 199320 B
AU 9229619 A 19930603 AU 9229619 A 19921125 A23L-001/24 199329
CA 2083806 A 19930528 CA 2083806 A 19921125 A23L-001/24 199333
EP 558832 A2 19930908 EP 92203669 A 19921127 A23L-001/24 199336
JP 5236906 A 19930917 JP 92341215 A 19921127 A23L-001/24 199342
HU 63752 T 19931028 HU 923728 A 19921126 A23L-001/29 199348
CZ 9203496 A3 19940216 CS 923496 A 19921126 A23L-001/24 199413
ZA 9209221 A 19940727 ZA 929221 A 19921127 A23C-000/00 199431

SK 9203496 A3 19950208 CS 923496 A 19921126 A23L-001/24 199525
EP 558832 A3 19940831 EP 92203669 A 19921127 A23C-001/24 199531
JP 95095932 B2 19951018 JP 92341215 A 19921127 A23L-001/24 199546
AU 667203 B 19960314 AU 9229619 A 19921125 A23L-001/24 199618
CA 2083806 C 19960528 CA 2083806 A 19921125 A23L-001/24 199633
CZ 282656 B6 19970813 CS 923496 A 19921126 A23L-001/24 199739
SK 278504 B6 19970806 CS 923496 A 19921126 A23L-001/24 199740
Abstract (Basic): US 5209942 A

Fat mimetic compsn. comprises: (a) 30–70% colloidal microcrystalline cellulose (I); (b) 30–70% cold H2O swelling starch (II); (c) 1–15% gum (III) (xanthan, carrageenan, locust bean or guar gums or mixts.); (d) 0–5% alginate (IV) (or deriv.); and (e) 0–5% opacifier (V) (TiO_2 and/or milk solids). The compsn. imparts organoleptic properties similar to fat when formulated at 1–10% in a dressing contg. up to 7% fat.

Pref. compsn. comprises 50–60% esp. 56% (I), 40–50% (II), 3–5% esp. 4% (III) (esp. xanthan gum), 1–3% esp. 5% (IV) (esp. as propylene glycol alginate), and 0.5–4% esp. 3% (V) (esp. as TiO_2).

USE/ADVANTAGE—The fat mimetic compsns. allow the prodn. of low fat/no fat reduced calorie salad dressings with the taste and functionality of full fat dressings. In addn., the dressings may be prepd. using relatively low energy processes.

Hydrocolloid—Spread & Salad Dressing 10

Improving flavour release in low calorie spread—by addn. of hydrocolloid, e.g., sodium alginate, without protein.
Patent Assignee: GRINDSTED PROD AS (GRIN)
Number of Countries: 001 Number of Patents: 001
Patent No Kind Date Applicat No Kind Date Main IPC Week
RD 281062 A 19870910 198741 B
Abstract (Basic): RD 281062 A

Flavour release in a low calorie spread is improved by incorporation of a hydrocolloid (I), e.g., Na alginate or gelatin.

ADVANTAGE—(I), normally added as stabilisers, improve flavour release without the need to incorporate proteins (usually milk proteins) as in known compsns.

Hydrocolloid—Spread & Salad Dressing 11

Edible plastic dispersion esp. for use in low fat prods.—has a non-fat continuous phase, and includes at least two condensed phases comprising gel-forming compsns. contg. different gelling agents.
Patent Assignee: UNILEVER NV (UNIL); UNILEVER PLC (UNIL)

Inventor: CAIN F W; CLARK A H; DUNPHY P J; JONES M G; NORTON I T; ROSS-MURPH S B; ROSS-MURPHY S B
Number of Countries: 016 Number of Patents: 008
Patent No Kind Date Applicat No Kind Date Main IPC Week
EP 298561 A 19890111 EP 88201405 A 19880705 198902 B
AU 8818750 A 19890112 198909
JP 1086831 A 19890331 JP 88169982 A 19880707 198919
ZA 8804936 A 19900328 ZA 884936 A 19880708 199017
US 4956193 A 19900911 US 88215009 A 19880705 199039
EP 298561 B1 19950517 EP 88201405 A 19880705 A23L-001/307 199524
DE 3853796 G 19950622 DE 3853796 A 19880705 A23L-001/307 199530
EP 88201405 A 19880705
JP 96029047 B2 19960327 JP 88169982 A 19880707 A23D-007/015 199617
Abstract (Equivalent): US 4956193 A

New edible plastic dispersion without continuous fat phase, but with 2+ different condensed phases at least one being continuous, comprises 0.1–99 %wt. gel-forming compsn. (A) contg. 1-8 (1-5) X critical conc. of gelling agent (A) (gelatin, kappa- or iota-carrageenan, alginate, agar, gellan, pectin, or mixts.) and 0.1–99.9 %wt. gel-forming compsn. (B) contg. 1-8 (1-5) X critical conc. of gelling agent (b) (whey protein, starch, denatured bovine serum protein or soy protein, microcrystalline cellulose, or mixt.). Disposal is at below 70 (20)°C. Continuous phase melts at 20–45°C. Fat phase and thickening agents (xanthan gum) may be present. Aggregates are of mean size 0.01–10 microns. Mean diam. of fat globules if below 10 microns.

USE—Dietetic non- or low-fat replacement dispersions resembling butter, margarine etc. without brittleness or too much elasticity.

Hydrocolloid—Spread & Salad Dressing 12

Edible plastified dispersion used as spread—comprises continuous fat phase and aq. phase contg. protein and/or hydrocolloid.

Patent Assignee: UNILEVER NV (UNIL); VAN DEN BERGH FOODS CO (VBER-N)
Inventor: CAIN F W; DAY J I; JONES M G; NORTON I T; SALGADO E Y
Number of Countries: 015 Number of Patents: 007
Patent No Kind Date Applicat No Kind Date Main IPC Week
EP 279499 A 19880824 EP 88200283 A 19880216 198834 B
AU 8811786 A 19880825 198843 FI 8800713 A 19880819 198848
EP 279499 B 19911204 199149 DE 3866555 G 19920116 199204
FI 93601 B 19950131 FI 88713 A 19880216 A23D-007/00 199510
US 5451422 A 19950919 US 88157209 A 19880217 A23D-007/04 199543
US 89324962 A 19890316 US 91663755 A 19910301

Abstract (Basic): EP 279499 A

An edible plastified dispersion of fat content less than 30 wt.% comprises a continuous fat phase, and an aq. phase containing protein and/or hydrocolloid. The aq. phase has viscosity less than 400 cps at 35°C, shear rate 1000 sec power 1. The content of amino acid residues is less than 200 ppm, based on the wt. of the aq. phase.

Pref. fat content is 15–25 wt.%. 0.1–0.5% emulsifier, e.g., monoglyceride compsn. derived from partially hydrogenated sunflower oil, is present. The aq. phase contains 95–99.9% water and 0.4–1% hydrocolloid, e.g., kappa or iota carrageenan; it may be gelled. Droplet dia. is 5–25 microns.

USE/ADVANTAGE—The product is a spread, i.e., butter or margarine replacement. It has a thick mouthfeel and not the watery feel of prior spreads of low fat content. It is stable, and prepd. by conventional methods. These results are achieved by having an aq. phase of relatively low viscosity, and a very low content of amino acids.

Hydrocolloid—Spread & Salad Dressing 13

Low fat low calorie water-continuous spread——contains oligofructose, another biopolymer and small amt. of oil phase.
Patent Assignee: UNILEVER NV (UNIL); UNILEVER PLC (UNIL)
Inventor: ALDERLIESTEN L; CASTENMILLER W A M; SCHOTEL R A; VERSCHUREN J J; DE FOUW N J; VAN AMELSVOORT J M M; AMELSVOORT J M M; DE FOUW MW N J; CASTENMILLER W A; MATEUS J; NANNEKE JOKE DE FOUW M W; VAN AMELSVOORT M
Number of Countries: 045 Number of Patents: 008
Patent No Kind Date Applicat No Kind Date Main IPC Week
EP 596546 A1 19940511 EP 93201727 A 19930616 A23L-001/236 199419 B
WO 9409647 A1 19940511 WO 93EP2837 A 19931012 199420
AU 9453338 A 19940524 WO 93EP2837 A 19931012 A23L-001/236 199434
AU 9453338 A 19931012
AU 9453723 A 19940524 WO 93EP3010 A 19931028 A23L-001/236 199434
AU 9453723 A 19931028
ZA 9307870 A 19950628 ZA 937870 A 19931022 A23L-000/00 199531
ZA 9308104 A 19950726 ZA 938104 A 19931029 A23D-000/00 199535
SK 9500556 A3 19950914 WO 93EP2837 A 19931012 A23L-001/236 199544
SK 95556 A 19931012
CZ 9501122 A3 19951213 CZ 951122 A 19931028 A23L-001/05 199606
Abstract (Basic): EP 596546 A

Water-continuous spreads comprise 10–50 wt.% oligofructose, 0.05–30 wt.% other bipolymer and less than 20% of an oil phase.

Pref., the second biopolymer is a gum, starch microcrystalline cellulose and/or protein. The gum is agar, algin, arabic, carrageenan, furcellaran, gellan, ghatti, guar, karaya, larch, locust bean, pectin, trigacanth or xanthan gum and is at 0.05–5 wt.%. The starch is a gelling, esp. hydrolysed starch at 5–20 wt.%. The protein is a gelling protein, esp. gelatin, at 0.05–10 wt.%. The stress strain relation has a maximum stress of 0.01–100 kPa, esp. 0.3–60 kPa, and a ratio of plastic stress to maximum stress of 0.1–1, esp. 0.2–0.95, at 5°C. The spread has Stevens value of over 50 g at 5°C. It has hardness over 12 N, gumminess over 0.7 and/or chewiness over 0.7, as measured by TPA. It is non-thixotropic. The ratio of initial hardness at 260 seconds as measured by CUC (40 second cycle time) is less than 1.5.

USE—Spreads are low fat, low calorie spreads.

Hydrocolloid—Spread & Salad Dressing 14

Reduced calorie salad dressing—contains fat mimetic, microcrystalline cellulose, cold water swelling starch and gum giving fat-like properties.

Patent Assignee: LIPTON CO THOMAS J (LIPT-N)

Inventor: BAUER R; CUCCURULLO J A; DAZO P E; KOCHAKJI D J; RIKON S M; RUBOW R E

Number of Countries: 001 Number of Patents: 001

Patent No Kind Date Applicat No Kind Date Main IPC Week

US 5286510 A 19940215 US 92957492 A 19921007 A23L-001/0522 199407 B

Abstract (Basic): US 5286510 A

Fat mimetic compsns. are an intimate admixt. of 30–70 wt.% colloidal microcrystalline cellulose (I); 30–70% cold water swelling starch (II); 1–15 % xanthan, carrageenan, locust bean and/or guar gums (III); 0–5 % alginate or alginate deriv. (IV) and 0–5% opacifier (V). (V) is TiO_2 and/or milk solids. The mimetic imparts organoleptic props. similar to fat at 1–10% in a dressing contg. up to 30% fat.

Pref., (I) is at 50–60 (56%); (II) at 40–50 (32%); (III) at 3–5 (4%); (IV) at 1–3 (or 5%) and (V) at 0.5–4 (3)%. (IV) is propylene glycol alginate and (V) is TiO_2.

70–99 pts. water are put in a vessel and agitation started. A dry mixt. of 0.3–5.6 pts. microcrystalline cellulose, 0.3–6 pts. starch, 0.1–0.5 pts. xanthan gum, 0.1–0.5 pts. propylene glycol alginate and 0.04–0.52 pts. TiO_2 is prepd. and added under agitation. In a second vessel contg. 21–45 pts. water, 8–10 pts. vinegar, 12–27 pts. sweetener, 5–25 pts. flavour cocktail and 0–30 pts. oil are added and agitated until homogeneous. 25–30 pts. of the fat mimetic is then dispersed in the compsn. in the second vessel.

USE/ADVANTAGE—Mimetic are used in low or no fat, reduced

calorie salad dressings. Dressings have smooth, creamy mouth feel and texture and lubricity like edible fat-contg. prods.

In an example, fat mimetic comprise 5.6 pts. Avicel CL-611 (RTM), 0.4 pts. Keltrol T (RTM), 3.2 pts. Mira-Thik 468 (RTM), 0.5 pts. Kelcoloid LVF (RTM), 0.3 pts. (13 white dispersion S. (RTM) and 85% water.

Hydrocolloid—Spread & Salad Dressing 15

Low calorie water-in-oil spread compsn.—comprises continuous oil-and-fat phases including emulsifier and decentralised water phases including water-soluble hemicellulose.

Patent Assignee: TAIYO OIL & FAT MFG (TAIY); TERUMO CORP (TERU)
Number of Countries: 001 Number of Patents: 001
Patent No Kind Date Applicat No Kind Date Main IPC Week
JP 5168402 A 19930702 JP 91296324 A 19911015 A23D-007/00 199331 B
Abstract (Basic): JP 5168402 A

A water-in-oil spread compsn. is composed of continuous oil-and-fat phases and decentralised water phases. The oil-and-fat phases are 20–33 wt.% based on the total amt. of the compsn. and includes emulsifier. The water phases contain 10–20 wt.% water-soluble hemicellulose derived from cereals based on the total amt. of the compsn. The water-soluble hemicellulose is an extract from hull of cereals, and more than 60 wt.% of the extract has mol.wt. 10,000 or less and viscosity of its 10 wt.% soln. is below 30cp.

USE—Compsn. gives good applying property, flavour, texture smoothness and stability, etc., and prevents increase of cholesterol.

Hydrocolloid—Spread & Salad Dressing 16

Low calorie, non-fat viscous dressing prepn.—by addn. of starch base to premix contg. gum- and spice-blends and micro reticulated microcrystalline cellulose

Patent Assignee: KRAFT GEN FOODS INC (KRFT)
Inventor: BARBERA B D; COMBES R C; SCHWIMMER W H
Number of Countries: 001 Number of Patents: 001
Patent No Kind Date Applicat No Kind Date Main IPC Week
US 5087471 A 19920211 US 90626733 A 19901213 199209 B
Abstract (Basic): US 5087471 A

Mixt. is prepd. of (i) a blend of gum (I) and a diluent, (ii) a blend of H_2O, salt, sweetener (II), and spice, and (iii) an aq. dispersion of a microreticulated microcrystalline cellulose (III); and (b) obtd. premix is blended with a starch base (IV) to give dressing comprising 0.25–4% (II), 0.2–2% (I), 60–80% H_2O, 2–20% carbohydrates, 0–10% protein and less than 4% triglycerides. Gum blend pref. contains 25–500% diluent by wt. of

(I). (I) is pref. xanthan, locust bean or guar gum, carboxymethyl cellulose, carrageenan, or alginates or mixts., esp. xanthan gum; and amt. is pref. 40–60% by wt. w.r.t. (III). The diluent is pref. a dry H_2O-soluble component of the dressing, or a liq. triglyceride oil, fluid at room temps. (II) is pref. sucrose, dextrose, fructose, maltose, triose, high DE corn syrup solids, or a synth. sweetener; esp. 3–25% corn syrup solids. Pref. the process is continuous.

USE/ADVANTAGE—Smooth and creamy oral texture and lubricity closely simulating the texture and taste of edible fat contg. prods. Also used for operation on a continuous basis.

Hydrocolloid—Spread & Salad Dressing 17

Reduced fat emulsion-type foods—with curdlan gel particles as fat replacement.

Patent Assignee: TAKEDA CHEM IND LTD (TAKE)
Inventor: NAKAO Y; OKURA Y; TAWADA T
Number of Countries: 018 Number of Patents: 004
Patent No Kind Date Applicat No Kind Date Main IPC Week
EP 520747 A1 19921230 EP 92305764 A 19920623 A23L-001/314 199301 B
CA 2072060 A 19921225 CA 2072060 A 19920623 A23L-001/054 199316
JP 6189700 A 19940712 JP 91151791 A 19910624 A23L-001/054 199432
US 5360624 A 19941101 US 92902239 A 19920623 A23L-001/054 199443
Abstract (Basic): EP 520747 A

Emulsion-type foods have part or all of the fat components substituted by a curdlan gel (I). They are prod. by mixing finely divided (I) with the other raw materials.

(I) is pulverised to not larger than 100 microns. It contains 0.6–10 wt.% curdlan. At least 20 wt.% of the fat component is replaced by (I). The curdlan content of the food is 0.5–3 wt.%. (I) is thermo(ir)reversible.

USE/ADVANTAGE—Low calorie mayonnaise, spreads, dressings, desserts, whipped cream, cheeses, dairy prods., confectioneries, white sauces, etc., can be obtd. They have good appearance.

Hydrocolloid—Spread & Salad Dressing 18

Reduced-calorie butter-like spread—is produced from wet concn. and dry butter-fat and an aq. phase worked to give water-in-oil emulsion.

Patent Assignee: UNILEVER PLC (UNIL); UNILEVER NV (UNIL)
Inventor: CAIN F W; ERNSTING P B; HOLEMANS P M J; NIEMEYER T R J
Number of Countries: 018 Number of Patents: 008
Patent No Kind Date Applicat No Kind Date Main IPC Week
EP 385541 A 19900905 EP 90200425 A 19900223 199036 B
AU 9050505 A 19900906 199043

CA 2011412 A 19900903 199047
ZA 9001612 A 19911127 ZA 901612 A 19900302 199201
AU 640124 B 19930819 AU 9050505 A 19900227 A23C-015/04 199340
EP 385541 B1 19940427 EP 90200425 A 19900223 A23C-015/16 199417
DE 69008393 E 19940601 DE 608393 A 19900223 A23C-015/16 199423
EP 90200425 A 19900223
IE 63415 B 19950419 IE 90707 A 19900227 A23C-015/16 199523
Abstract (Basic): EP 385541 A

Edible oil-and-water emulsion comprises 30–70 wt.% of an aq. phase (sic.) comprising wet-concentrated and dry butterfat. The wet-conc. butterfat is either butter or conc. cream, having over 40 wt.% fat. Pref. the wet concd. butterfat component comprises at least 40 wt.% whole butterfat triglycerides. It is dairy butter or cream of fat content over 40 wt.%. The dry butterfat is a butterfat fraction, esp. an olefin fraction, esp. of m. pt. less than 20°C. The emulsion contains a gelling or thickening agent, esp. milk protein, gelatin, locust bean gum, guar gum, xanthan gum, alginate, carrageenan and/or pectin. The emulsion contains a non-milk fat. It contains 30–50 wt.% fat phase and 70–50 wt.% aq. phase. The emulsion is prepd. by (a) admixing the butterfat at 1:10–10:1 and opt. including a thickener and (4) working under high shear conditions that a stable edible water-in-oil emulsion is formed. Step (a) is esp. admixing dairy cream, butter olefin and a non-dairy aq. phase.

USE/ADVANTAGE—Butter-like spreads have reduced calorie and fat content, good spreadability and buttery taste.

Hydrocolloid—Spread & Salad Dressing 19

Emulsified fat compsn. used for, e.g., food dressing—contains edible fat, water, xanthan gum, phospholipid mixt. or diglyceride.

Patent Assignee: KAO CORP (KAOS)
Number of Countries: 001 Number of Patents: 001
Patent No Kind Date Applicat No Kind Date Main IPC Week
JP 5146270 A 19930615 JP 91337704 A 19911126 A23L-001/24 199328 B
Abstract (Basic): JP 5146270 A

Compsn. contains edible fat and water component. 0.055 wt.% or less of xanthan gum and phospholipid mixt. of wt. ratio of phospholipid not contg. nitrogen atom to phospholipid contg. nitrogen atom to phospholipid contg. nitrogen atom 1.0 or more of diglyceride are further compounded.

USE—The compsn. is suitably used for dressing. It has smooth taste without oiliness. It contains low calorie. Gelling after preservation does not occur.

Hydrocolloid—Spread & Salad Dressing 20

Low-calorie mayonnaise prodn.—from aq. mixt. of dairy protein and pectin, sugar, salt, mustard paste, vegetable oil and acetic acid.

Patent Assignee: DAIRY RAW METLS USE RES (DAIR-R); FOOD IND CORRSP INS (FOOD-R)
Inventor: BABAK V G; MOLOCHNIKO V V; VOSKANYAN O S
Number of Countries: 001 Number of Patents: 001
Patent No Kind Date Applicat No Kind Date Main IPC Week
SU 1648321 A 19910515 SU 4712042 A 19890510 199206 B
Abstract (Basic): SU 1648321 A

The method comprises prepn. of an aq. mixt. of a complex of dairy proteins with pectin or edible carboxy-methyl cellulose, in amt. 0.7–0.8% at ratio (1:5)–(1:6), respectively pH 7.5–8.0 and temp. 35–40°C with mixing for 5–10 min., adding 1.5–2.5% sugar, 1.0–1.5% salt and 0.05% soda pasteurising at 60–65°C for 15–20 min., cooling to 30–35°C, mixing with separately prepd. mustard paste (I) and adding with continuous mixing, 30–40% of vegetable oil, at 20–25°C and 12–14% of 6% vinegar, followed by homogenising.

Mustard paste (I) is prepd. from 1.0–1.5% mustard powder and water, by mixing at 35–40°C and ratio 1:(3.5–4.0), pasteurising obtd. paste at 90–95°C for 15–20 min. and cooling to 35–40°C.

Tests show that obtd. prod. has viscosity 2.2–2.5 Pa. sec. at relative shear rate 27/sec. and improved stability to centrifuging (1.5% of water separates during centrifuging at 3000 rpm for 5 min.).

USE/ADVANTAGE—In oil and fat industry, as the method of prodn. of mayonnaise of reduced calorific value. Produced low calorie low-calorie mayonnaise has improved nourishing properties and increased stability on storage.

Hydrocolloid—Spread & Salad Dressing 21

Reduced calorie fruit spread—contg. sucralose high intensity sweetener, low methoxy pectin or carrageenan, CMC, guar gum and locust bean gum.

Patent Assignee: MCNEIL-PPC INC (MCNI)
Inventor: ANTENUCCI R N; SHARP S E
Number of Countries: 019 Number of Patents: 007
Patent No Kind Date Applicat No Kind Date Main IPC Week
US 5270071 A 19931214 US 92900643 A 19920618 A23L-001/06 199350 B
EP 575179 A2 19931222 EP 93304745 A 19930617 A23L-001/06 199351

CA 2098673 A 19931219 CA 2098673 A 19930617 A23L-001/064 199410
NZ 247788 A 19941125 NZ 247788 A 19930603 A23L-001/0532 199501
EP 575179 A3 19940608 EP 93304745 A 19930617 A23L-001/06 199526
EP 575179 B1 19970514 EP 93304745 A 19930617 A23L-001/06 199724
DE 69310613 E 19970619 DE 610613 A 19930617 A23L-001/06 199730
EP 93304745 A 19930617

Abstract (Basic): US 5270071 A

Fruit spread, contg. not more than 9 calories per teaspoon, comprises the gelled prod. of (a) water, (b) fruit, (c) sucralose high intensity sweetener, (d) low methoxy pectin or carrageenan gelling agent, (e) carboxymethylcellulose, (f) guar gum, and (g) locust bean gum.

USE/ADVANTAGE—The spread is comparable in organoleptic quality to full-calorie, high-solids prods. It has good sweetness intensity and quality, and good texture.

Abstract (Equivalent): EP 575179 B

A fruit spread having not more than 7.5 kJ/ml (9 calories per teaspoon), said fruit spread comprising the gelled product of: (a) water; (b) fruit or fruit flavouring; (c) sucralose high intensity sweetener; (d) low methoxy pectin having a degree of methylation below 50% or carrageenan gelling agent; (e) carboxymethylcellulose.

Hydrocolloid—Spread & Salad Dressing 22

Prepn. of low fat food prods.—by heating-shearing aq. microcrystalline cellulose, then mixing with xanthan gum then food components.

Patent Assignee: KRAFT GEN FOODS INC (KRFT)

Inventor: BAER C C; BULIGA G S; HASSENHEUTTL G L; HENRY G A; HETH A A; JACKSON L K; KENNEDY-TOLSTEDT J M; KERWIN P J; MILLER M S; PARKER E M; PAUL N K; PECHAK D G; SMITH G F; WITTE V C; BAER C; BULIGA G; HASSENHEU G L; HENRY G; HETH A; JACKSON L; KENNEDYTOL J; KERWIN P

Number of Countries: 019 Number of Patents: 003

Patent No Kind Date Applicat No Kind Date Main IPC Week
WO 9102463 A 19910307 199112 B
EP 487639 A1 19920603 EP 90913618 A 19900816 A23L-001/0534 199223
WO 90US4621 A 19900816
JP 4507348 W 19921224 JP 90512721 A 19900816 A23L-001/24 199306
WO 90US4621 A 19900816

Abstract (Basic): WO 9102463 A

Low fat or fat-free prods. are prepd. as follows: (a) an aq. dispersion comprising (by wt.) 3–10% microcrystalline cellulose (I) and 90–97% H_2O is heated and repeatedly sheared in a high shear zone having a pressure drop at least 12,000 psi to fragment (I) to submicron sized fragments; (b) the (I) fragments are re-agglomerated under high shear conditions to afford an aq. dispersion of porous microreticulated microcrystalline cellulose (II) particles having void vol. at least 25 vol.%, mean particle size 5–20 micron, and particle size distribution such that at least ca 75 wt.% of the particles have max. dimension less than 25 micron; (c) the dispersion is combined with 2–33% of a xanthan gum (III) (based on (II) dry wt.); and (d) the xanthan-stabilised (II) dispersion is blended with additional food components to provide the title food comprising 0.25–4% (II), 50–99 H_2O, 1–35% carbohydrates, 0–10% protein, and less than 7% triglycerides.

ADVANTAGE—The process affords a range of nutritious, low calorie, fat-free foods (frozen desserts, and food dressings, etc.) which have exceptional, smooth, creamy, oil-like textures and well rounded fat mimetic mouthfeel characteristics.

Hydrocolloid—Spread & Salad Dressing 24

Low-calorie spread contg. fibre from de-hulled peas—has oil and/or water phase(s) contg., e.g., mono-(di-)glyceride, gelatin, and up to 20 percent fibre.

Patent Assignee: ANONYMOUS (ANON)
Number of Countries: 001 Number of Patents: 001
Patent No Kind Date Applicat No Kind Date Main IPC Week
RD 313011 A 19900510 199023 B
Abstract (Basic): RD 313011 A

A low-calorie spread with dietary fibre has been developed, a typical recipe could be: Water Phase: 68.8% water; 10.0% pea fibre; 1.0% gelatin; 0.1% salt; 0.1% K-sorbate; Fat Phase: 1.0% distilled monoglyceride, iodine value 105; 19.0% fat blend; 25 pts. hardened soya, m. pt. 41°C; 75 pts. soya oil; 4 ppm beta-carotene; plus flavouring. The pea fibre used was a fine-powdered highly functional fibre prod. made from dehulled peas. A typical analysis is: Dietary fibre 35%; Starch 45%; Protein 11%; Fat 0.0%; Ash 2.0%; Moisture 7%; pH (10% suspension) 6.8. The low-calorie spread can be produced under standard conditions on a tube-chiller system. Trials made on pilot plant tube-chiller have shown that the recipe can be varied considerably and still a spreadable and stable prod. can be obtd., e.g., water content 0–88%, fat content from 0–90%, distilled monoglyceride or mono-diglyceride with iodine value from 1–134 and dosage from 0–5%; and hydrocolloids from 0–4%. The content of the pea fibre prod. can be up to 20%.

Hydrocolloid—Spread & Salad Dressing 25

Water-in-oil emulsion low fat spread—contg. combination of linear and spherical gel structure hydrocolloids in aq. phase.
Patent Assignee: UNILEVER NV (UNIL)
Inventor: MILO B T; REISSMANN H A W
Number of Countries: 014 Number of Patents: 006
Patent No Kind Date Applicat No Kind Date Main IPC Week
EP 52899 A 19820602 EP 81201222 A 19811030 198223 B
US 4389426 A 19830621 198327
ZA 8108060 A 19830520 198329
CA 1168923 A 19840612 198428
EP 52899 B 19850102 198502
DE 3168085 G 19850214 198508
Abstract (Basic): EP 52899 A

A water-in-oil emulsion spread has a fat content of 25–65 wt.% and comprises a dispersed aq. phase contg. a gelling system contg. one or more hydrocolloids selected from maltodextrins of DE at least 20, pectin, lambda carrageenan and alginates, and at least one hydrocolloid selected from guar gum, locust bean gum and iota carrageenan.

The gelling system pref. comprises a mixt. of guar gum and highly esterified pectin in wt. ratio at least 4, pref. 6 or more. The compsn. pref. contains 0.1–1.0, esp. 0.2–0.5 wt.% guar gum and 0.01–0.3, esp. 0.03–0.075 wt.% pectin, and 0.01–8, esp. 1–5 wt. protein, e.g., milk, vegetable or microbial protein. The fat is pref. a plastic fat blend having the following solids contents at the given temps.:—N10 20-30; N20 10-18; N30 1-8.

Use of a combination of linear gel structure and spherical gel structure hydrocolloids yields a low calorie spread which is stable in storage but breaks down pleasantly in the mouth.

Hydrocolloid—Spread & Salad Dressing 26

Low calorie spread contg. high-methoxylated pectin—to replace gelatin as emulsion stabiliser.
Patent Assignee: GRINDSTED PROD AS (GRIN)
Number of Countries: 001 Number of Patents: 001
Patent No Kind Date Applicat No Kind Date Main IPC Week
RD 217009 A 19820510 198222 B
Abstract (Basic): RD 217009 A

In a 40% fat calorie spread, milk protein destabilises the emulsion which gives a spread with coarse water dispersion and poor microbiological shelf life. Gelatin is known to stabilise the emulsion in the prod. at a dosage of, e.g., 2.5% gelatin 120 bloom calculated on the low calorie spread.

In trying to replace gelatin with pectin, the following trials were made with high-methoxylated pectin. Water phase contained 1.0% whey powder, 1.0% salt and 53.9–55.4% water at pH 6.5. (1) 2.5% Gelatin 120 bloom; (2) 1.0% Mexpectin SS 200 (slow set); (3) 2.0% Mexpectin SS 200 (slow set); (4) 1.0% Mexpectin MS 300 (medium set); (5) 2.0% Mexpectin MS 300 (medium set); (6) 1.0% Mexpectin RS 400 (rapid set); (7) 2.0% Mexpectin RS 400 (rapid set); fat phase contained 0.5% DIMODAN OT (unsatd. distilled monoglyceride); 0.1% sorbic acid; 0.3% colour; 39.2% fat blend; 24 pts. hardened soya, 41°C, 76 pts. liq. soya-bean oil. The spreads were produced on a 2-tube laboratory Perfector with low capacity and moderate cooling.

Evaluation after storage at 5°C showed that the spreads with Mexpectin had a satisfactory water dispersion and shelf life.

Hydrocolloid—Spread & Salad Dressing 27

Fat-like agent compsn—comprises dry, water-dispersible particles of an agglomerate of micro-reticulated or micro-fibrillated microcrystalline cellulose and a readily water dispersible hydrocolloid.

Patent Assignee: FMC CORP (FMCC)
Inventor: HEESE S; RUSZKAY T A; TUASON D C
Number of Countries: 046 Number of Patents: 004
Patent No Kind Date Applicat No Kind Date Main IPC Week
WO 9502966 A1 19950202 WO 94US6830 A 19940616 A23L-001/05 199510 B
AU 9473552 A 19950220 AU 9473552 A 19940616 A23L-001/05 199521
EP 716571 A1 19960619 EP 94922440 A 19940616 A23L-001/05 199629
WO 94US6830 A 19940616
EP 716571 A4 19970305 EP 94922440 A 19940000 A23L-001/05 199729
Abstract (Basic): WO 9502966 A

A compsn. comprises dry, water-dispersible particle comprising an agglomerate of components comprising microreticulated or micro-fibrillated microcrystalline cellulose in a predominant amt. by wt., and a hydrocolloid selected from carboxymethylcellulose and xanthan gum to provide effective coverage of the cellulose. The agglomerate readily disperses in water into its component pts. under aq. food processing conditions.

Also claimed are (i) prepn. of the compsn.; (ii) a food compsn. contg the compsn and (iii) a process for imparting fat-like properties to a low-calorie aq. based foodstuff.

USE—The compsn provides fat-like properties to low-calorie aq. based foodstuffs, such as salad dressings, dairy prods. such as frozen desserts etc.

Other food stuffs such as candies, frostings, gravies, margarines, puddings, soups, spreads etc. may also be improved using the compsn.

ADVANTAGE—The agglomerate readily disperses in water into its component parts.

Hydrocolloid—Low Calorie Foods: Satiety/Weight Control 1

Low calorie liq. food for patients having obesity or diabetes mellitus—contains pectin with specific degree of esterification, gels at pH less than 3, has good taste and long retention time in stomach.

Patent Assignee: TERUMO CORP (TERU)
Number of Countries: 001 Number of Patents: 001
Patent No Kind Date Applicat No Kind Date Main IPC Week
JP 6030729 A 19940208 JP 92192491 A 19920720 A23L-001/307 199410 B
Abstract (Basic): JP 6030729 A

Liq. food contains a pectin with a degree of esterification of less than 40% and has ability to gel at a pH of less than 3.

USE—As a low calorie food, for preventing obese patients from overeating and protecting patients of diabetes mellitus from abrupt increase in blood glucose values. It has a good taste and a long retention time in the human stomach.

Hydrocolloid—Low Calorie Foods: Satiety/Weight Control 2

Low calorie jelly contg. glucomannan—which swells in stomach giving feeling of fullness.

Patent Assignee: ENNAGRAM SARL (ENNA-N)
Inventor: LERMONTOFF A
Number of Countries: 001 Number of Patents: 001
Patent No Kind Date Applicat No Kind Date Main IPC Week
FR 2684848 A1 19930618 FR 913589 A 19910325 A23L-001/307 199337 B
Abstract (Basic): FR 2684848 A

Glucomannan is used in the prepn. of an eatable jelly giving a feeling of fullness.

The glucomannan is pref. derived from Amorphophallus Konjak, 15–30 g. being used per 1000 g. of jelly. The remainder of the jelly is water, but it may further contain stabilisers, esp. 0.5–2 g. of pectin and citric acid, preservatives, esp. 0.5–1.5 g. methyl p-hydroxy benzoate and flavourings. Other additives which may be included are sweeteners, such as Aspartame, fructose, sucrose, or saccharin and colours. They are packed in 25 g. sachets for use.

USE—A low calorie aid to dieting.

Hydrocolloid—Low Calorie Foods: Satiety/Weight Control 3

An improved diet food for controlling calorie intake—suitable for patients suffering from obesity or diabetes.

Patent Assignee: TERUMO CORP (TERU); OHTA A (OHTA-I)
Inventor: OHTA A; WATANABE H
Number of Countries: 012 Number of Patents: 009
Patent No Kind Date Applicat No Kind Date Main IPC Week
WO 8802992 A 19880505 WO 87JP821 A 19871026 198819 B
AU 8781045 A 19880520198833
JP 62506676 X 19881006 JP 87506676 A 19870000 198846
EP 333858 A 19890927 EP 87906943 A 19871026 198939
JP 92020585 B 19920403 JP 87506676 A 19871026 199218
US 5122379 A 19920616 WO 87JP821 A 19871026 A23L-001/182 199227
US 89350701 A 19890426
EP 333858 B1 19930203 EP 87906943 A 19871026 A23L-001/307 199305
WO 87JP821 A 19871026
DE 3784076 G 19930318 DE 3784076 A 19871026 A23L-001/307 199312
EP 87906943 A 19871026
WO 87JP821 A 19871026
EP 333858 A4 19901227 EP 87906943 A 19870000 199514
Abstract (Basic): WO 8802992 A

Improved diet food for controlling calorie intake, has a reduced content of carbohydrate and contains low-calorie cereals, water-soluble edible fibres, and proteins in predetermined amts. corres. to an intended intake. The proteins are specified to have an isoelectric point in acid region. The amts. of the water-soluble edible fibres and the proteins are adjusted so that when an aq. soln. of this food comes into contact with a gastric juice the soln. become a gel. The weight ratio of the water-soluble edible fibres to the proteins is specified to be 1:0.5–1:8 (pref. 1:0.5–1:2). The weight ratio of the total amt. of the water-soluble edible fibres and the proteins to the amt. of the low-calorie cereals is specified to be 1:1–100. The low-calorie cereals are sugar-free cereals produced by removing sugar materials from boiled rice through extraction. Pref. water-soluble edible fibres are carrageenan and guar gum. An example of this diet food is rice gruel. The diet food can contain condiments such as soy sauce, bean paste, sodium glutamate.

USE/ADVANTAGE—The diet food contains 50% or less calories than usual foods and can stay for a prolonged time in the stomach. Useful as food for patients suffering from obesity or diabetes.

Hydrocolloid—Low Calorie Foods: Satiety/Weight Control 4

Low calorie protein based compsns.—that expand in the stomach to firm gelatinous masses which reduce appetite by mechanical action.
Patent Assignee: BATTISTA O A (BATT-I)
Inventor: BATTISTA O A
Number of Countries: 021 Number of Patents: 006
Patent No Kind Date Applicat No Kind Date Main IPC Week
WO 9001879 A 19900308 WO 89US3538 A 19890818 199013 B
AU 8941804 A 19900323 199033
EP 403597 A 19901227 EP 89909670 A 19890818 199101
HU 54880 T 19910428 199123
JP 3502047 W 19910516 JP 89509055 A 19890818 199126
EP 403597 A4 19920205 EP 89909670 A 19890000 199520
Abstract (Basic): WO 9001879 A

Very low calorie edible produce that expands to at least five times its original vol. when in contact with stomach juices is produced by (i) dry blending 10–50% animal or vegetable protein, at least 5% alpha cellulose, 10–50% microcrystalline cellulose and 10–25% edible gum and (ii) compressing into a shaped form. The gum is in dry powder form and the other components in dry, solid particulate form.

The total non-foamed non-crosslinked protein is pref. 10–50 (30)% of the blend. The blend is shaped by compressing at 2–20% or more kg. The components are at at least 20, at least 5, 20–40 and 10–20% resp. The shaped forms are circular elliplical, oblong or round-edged rectangular prods. formed at 4–16 or more kg. The protein is gelatin the gum is carrageenan or guar gum. The protein and alpha cellulose are blended together before blending with the other ingredients. The prod. comprises 10% carrageenan, 10% guar gum, 20% alpha cellulose, and non-foamed non-crosslinked protein, microcrystalline celluloses RC581 and PH101 (or their commercial equivs. or analogues) to 100%. The protein is animal protein, gelatin or soybean protein.

USE/ADVANTAGE—The prods. provide feeling a satiety without using drugs yet have good taste, easy intestinal tract absorption and are pleasant to consume.

Hydrocolloid—Low Calorie Foods: Satiety/Weight Control 5

Prepn. of high fibre, zero-calorie expandable compsns.—by compressing dry mix of microcrystalline cellulose(s), alpha-cellulose, and edible gums.

Patent Assignee: BATTISTA O A (BATT-I)
Inventor: BATTISTA O A
Number of Countries: 015 Number of Patents: 004
Patent No Kind Date Applicat No Kind Date Main IPC Week
EP 317079 A 19890524 EP 88309767 A 19881019 198921 B
AU 8824524 A 19890525 198929
JP 1296954 A 19891130 JP 88291115 A 19881119 199003
US 5032415 A 19910716 US 90545708 A 19900629 199131
Abstract (Basic): EP 317079 A

Zero-calorie edible prods. are prepd. by: (a) dry blending a mixt. of dry, solid (non-foamed) particulate ingredients comprising 40–80% microcrystalline celluloses (I), at least 5% alpha-cellulose (II), and 8–20% fine, powdered, edible gums (III); and (b) the dry compsn. is compressed into a shaped form. The prod. can expand to at least 5 times its original vol. when contacted with gastric juices.

USE/ADVANTAGE—The compsns. do not swell significantly until they reach the stomach, when they form a heavy, liq., swollen mass of ca zero calorie content.

Hydrocolloid—Low Calorie Foods: Satiety/Weight Control 6

Low calorie, boiled, granular cereal—with reduced carbohydrate levels, useful for obesity and diabetes.

Patent Assignee: TERUMO CORP (TERU); THERMO KK (THER-N)
Inventor: OHTA A
Number of Countries: 009 Number of Patents: 007
Patent No Kind Date Applicat No Kind Date Main IPC Week
EP 251925 A 19880107 EP 87401510 A 19870630 198801 B
JP 63112959 A 19880518 JP 87161095 A 19870630 198826
US 4892747 A 19900109 US 88219055 A 19880712 199010
JP 92041580 B 19920708 JP 87161095 A 19870630 A23L-001/10 199231
EP 251925 B1 19920812 EP 87401510 A 19870630 A23L-001/10 199233
DE 3781051 G 19920917 DE 3781051 A 19870630 A23L-001/10 199239
EP 87401510 A 19870630

JP 4228043 A 19920818 JP 87161095 A 19870630 A23L-001/10 199239
JP 91133258 A 19870630

Abstract (Basic): EP 251925 A

Boiled, granular low-calorie cereal has a reduced carbohydrate content. Prod. is gruel-like, and pref. also contains a thickener/filler (pref. a dietary fibre, esp. highly soluble, e.g., carrageenan, pectin, xanthan gum), and seasonings (pref. salt, soybean sauce, miso, and Na glutamate). The prefd. cereal is rice.

By boiling a cereal, adding H_2O or dil. aq. acid heated to at least 60°C, warming the mixt. at not less than 60°C for 1–30 mins. while the viscosity of the H_2O or dil. aq. acid is kept at not more than 200 cP, then removing the soln.

USE/ADVANTAGE—The low-calorie, boiled cereal has a reduced carbohydrate (esp. saccharide) content, and is useful for the therapy and prevention of obesity, and the therapy of diabetes. The prod. has the taste, flavour and appearance of, e.g., plain rice gruel.

Hydrocolloid—Low Calorie Foods: Satiety/Weight Control 7

Formulation for use in treatment of obesity—complete hunger abating low-calorie diet comprising both liquid and solid components.

Patent Assignee: ABNEYCREST LTD (ABNE-N)

Inventor: CRAWFORD M

Number of Countries: 001 Number of Patents: 002

Patent No Kind Date Applicat No Kind Date Main IPC Week

GB 2169485 A 19860716 GB 8520330 A 19850814 198629 B

GB 2169485 B 19880713 GB 8520336 A 19850814 198828

Abstract (Basic): GB 2169485 B

A formulation of a daily diet for use in the treatment of obesity comprises 45–75 (pref. 45–60) g protein, 50–180 (pref. 50–150)g carbohydrate, 3–27 (pref. 3–15) g fat, at least 5g fibre and at least the min. recommended daily allowances of minerals and vitamins and contains 800–1200 KCals per daily dose. The formulation is administered partly in the form of a liquid dose and partly in the form of a solid dose. The formulation may further comprise at least 1g of tryptophan at least 10% of the fat may be medium-chain triglycerides (MCTs), the protein is vegetable protein and the fibre is slow-release guar gum coated with protein.

ADVANTAGE—The formulation is a complete, hunger-abating low calorie diet (LCD). MCTs reduce body adipose tissue, while tryptophan is converted in vivo to neurotransmitter serotonin which induces a feeling of insatiety thus leading to decreased food intake. The vegetable protein reduces blood cholesterol levels thus minimising the risk of heart disease. The guar gum coating of protein resists saliva which prevents the gum from swelling until it is in the stomach, where it can absorb cholesterol and triglyceride. The slow-release guar gum also prevents ''insulin rebound.'' Partial administration as a solid allows mastication, which reduces the feeling of hunger.

Hydrocolloid—Low Calorie Foods: Satiety/Weight Control 8

Diet compsn. for reducing body wt. and serum lipid level—contg. gelatin, bran and pectin, pref. protein and opt. additives.
Patent Assignee: BIOTEST SERUM INST GMBH (BIOT)
Inventor: BITTERMANN K H; BONHARD K; LISSNER R
Number of Countries: 012 Number of Patents: 005
Patent No Kind Date Applicat No Kind Date Main IPC Week
EP 28374 A 19810513 198121 B
DE 2944535 A 19810521 198122
DK 8004673 A 19810817 198137
EP 28374 B 19830316 198312
DE 3062369 G 19830421 198317
Abstract (Basic): EP 28374 A

Diet compsns. for reducing body wt. and lowering the serum lipid level contain gelatin in addn. to pectin and bran. Wt. ratio gelatin:pectin:bran is 100:5:80 to 100:43:28.

The diet compsn. is prepd. by dissolving gelatin and pectin in a little water, distributing the bran and opt. further additives in the viscous soln. and working the pasty compsn. to shaped articles.

The diet compsn. can replace 2 main meals for patients who are overweight or suffer from vascular disorders leading to myocardial infarct and arteriosclerosis.

Gelatin supplies amino acids required by the human body and prevents health hazards and catabolic effects setting in after 10 days on a bran/pectin mixt. diet. Central nervous system metabolic centres are stimulated to support the low calorie diet effects. The gelatin has a specific swelling activity, increases intestinal wall tone and overcomes the sensation of hunger.

Hydrocolloid—Low Calorie Foods: Laxative 1

Low calorie, high fibre laxative compsn.—comprising psyllium husk, apple fibre, fructose, gum arabic and flavourants.
Patent Assignee: MEER CORP (MEER-N)
Inventor: MEER F H; MOUNTAIN F; SCHULTZ H V

Number of Countries: 001 Number of Patents: 001
Patent No Kind Date Applicat No Kind Date Main IPC Week
US 5073370 A 19911217 US 91660406 A 19910222 199202 B
Abstract (Basic): US 5073370 A

Natural fibre laxatives contain psyllium husk, sweetener, gum arabic and flavourants. The prods. contain apple fibre, such that the apple fibre and psyllium husk together are at least 75 wt.% and are at 23–40 and 40–58 wt.% resp.

The psyllium husk is at about 48 wt.%. The apple fibre is at about 32 wt.%.

USE/ADVANTAGE—Prods. are mixable with water for use as a laxative and when used with a medically supervised dietary programme impart a feeling of satiety. The prods. are low in calories.

Hydrocolloid—Low Calorie Foods: Laxative 2

Low calorie high fibre laxative—comprising psyllium husk, apple fibre, fructose, gum arabic and flavourant.

Patent Assignee: MEER CORP (MEER-N)
Inventor: MEER E H; MOUNTAIN F; SCHULTZ H V
Number of Countries: 001 Number of Patents: 001
Patent No Kind Date Applicat No Kind Date Main IPC Week
US 4996051 A 19910226 US 88275714 A 19881123 199111 B
Abstract (Basic): US 4996051 A

Natural fibre laxatives consist of 40–58 wt.% psyllium husk, 23–40 wt.% apple fibre and the balance (up to 25 wt.%) fructose, gum arabic and flavourants.

The psyllium husk is at 48 wt.%. The apple fibre is at 32 wt.%. The fructose is at (12–24) 17 wt.%. The flavourant is natural apple flavour, esp. at 1–4.5 (2) wt.%. The gum arabic is at (0.3–2) 0.5 wt.%. All granular components are below a no. 40 mesh size esp. below a no. 50 mesh size.

ADVANTAGE—Compsns. are low calorie, high fibre laxatives which can be mixed with water or used with a medically supervised dietary programme to give a feeling of satiety.

Hydrocolloid—Misc. Low Calorie Foods 1

Gluten free biscuits contg. guar flour—are free from animal protein and fat, useful as appetite satisfiers for overweight people.

Patent Assignee: BIMBOSAN AG (BIMB-N)
Inventor: HOSANG A
Number of Countries: 001 Number of Patents: 001
Patent No Kind Date Applicat No Kind Date Main IPC Week

CH 684921 A5 19950215 CH 93125 A 19930114 A21D-013/08 199511 B
Abstract (Basic): CH 684921 A

Gluten-free biscuits contg. no animal protein and no animal fat are made using only gluten-free flours and with the addn. of guar flour.

USE—The biscuits can be taken by persons allergic to gluten, and are esp. useful as appetite satisfiers for overweight people.

ADVANTAGE—The guar acts as binder in the absence of gluten to maintain coherent biscuits. Guar has a very low calorie content and limits the uptake of cholesterol in the digestive system, and is thus a useful health-promoting ingredient.

Hydrocolloid—Misc. Low Calorie Foods 2

Prepn. of jelly food, e.g., low calorie pudding—contains mixt. of carrageenan and konjak powder.

Patent Assignee: SHIMIZU KAGAKU KK (SHIM-N)
Number of Countries: 001 Number of Patents: 001
Patent No Kind Date Applicat No Kind Date Main IPC Week
JP 8196218 A 19960806 JP 9531428 A 19950126 A23L-001/06 199641 B
Abstract (Basic): JP 8196218 A

Prodn. contains mixt. of carrageenan and konjak powder permeating 150 mesh at the ratio of 10:1–10:10 is 0.1–10 wt.%.

USE/ADVANTAGE—To prepare jelly food such as pudding of low calorie. Konjak powder and carrageenan can be used together in spite of their difference of swelling and gelling rate. Jelly food contg. low calorie is prepd. at low cost.

Hydrocolloid—Misc. Low Calorie Foods 3

Prepn. of low calorie bean-jam-like foods—comprises coagulating aq. soln. contg. gelling agent, gum or carrageenan and food additives and crushing.

Patent Assignee: SANEIGEN FFI KK (SANE-N)
Number of Countries: 001 Number of Patents: 001
Patent No Kind Date Applicat No Kind Date Main IPC Week
JP 8173087 A 19960709 JP 94328059 A 19941228 A23L-001/236 199637 B
Abstract (Basic): JP 8173087 A

Prepn. of low-calorie, bean-jam-like foods comprising preparing an aq. soln. contg. 0.4–5 wt.% gelling agent of gellan gum, agar and carrageenan and food additives, allowing the soln. to coagulate to gel and crushing finely to prepare bean-jam-like paste. Pref. the soln. contains a gelling agent comprising 0.4–2 wt.% gellan gum, 0.7–5 wt.% agar or 1–3 wt.% carrageenan.

ADVANTAGE—The foods are low-calorie and have a flavour like Japanese bean jam.

Hydrocolloid—Misc. Low Calorie Foods 4

New low-calorie soft drink having guava-like aroma—contains sugar substitute, pectin, colour reagent, protein hydrolysate from gelatin or casein, aromatising agent, fruit juice and carbonated water.

Patent Assignee: DIKOMA PROD CO (DIKO-R)
Inventor: ARTYUKOV A A; GOLOMPVZAYA E A; PARFENOVA T V
Number of Countries: 001 Number of Patents: 001
Patent No Kind Date Applicat No Kind Date Main IPC Week
RU 2044498 C1 19950927 RU 9345763 A 19930917 A23L-002/00 199623 B
Abstract (Basic): RU 2044498 C

Soft drink based on pectin juice, colourant, aromatising agent and water, additionally contains: (i) sugar substitute; (ii) protein hydrolysate from gelatin or casein; (iii) blueberry or blackcurrant juice; and (iv) carbonated water. The drink comprises (in kg per 100 dl of prod.): sugar substitute 0.2–0.5, pectin 0.5–2.0, and colour reagent 0.00001–0.00002, and (in litres) protein hydrolysate 1–3, aromatising agent 0.2–0.5, blueberry or blackcurrant juice 5–10 and balance carbonated water.

Soft drink is prepd. by mixing previously dissolved pectin with protein hydrolysate, sugar substitute, juice, colouring agent and aromatising agent, and carbonating the obtd. mixt. Drink has raspberry-red colour, a sweet-sour taste, aroma resembling guava fruit, dry substances content 2–3% and acidity 2.5–3.0 g/l.

ADVANTAGE—Provides new, low-calorie soft drink called ‘‘Farma’’ (RTM), having health improving-prophylactic properties, good appearance and original aroma with guava notes.

Hydrocolloid—Misc. Low Calorie Foods 5

Low calorie fruit spreads of good taste and texture—prepared by gelling water, fruit and sweeteners with gelling agent, carboxymethyl cellulose, guar gum and locust bean gum.

Patent Assignee: MCNEIL-PPC INC (MCNI); JOHNSON & JOHNSON (JOHJ)
Inventor: ANTENUCCI R N; DAVIS T R; MANIERE F Y; SHARP S E
Number of Countries: 023 Number of Patents: 009
Patent No Kind Date Applicat No Kind Date Main IPC Week
US 5397588 A 19950314 US 92900643 A 19920618 199516 B
US 93141166 A 19931021

EP 649601 A2 19950426 EP 94307704 A 19941020 199521
AU 9475840 A 19950511 AU 9475840 A 19941014 199527
CA 2130842 A 19950422 CA 2130842 A 19940825 199529
BR 9404173 A 19950627 BR 944173 A 19941020 199534
JP 7184570 A 19950725 JP 94273143 A 19941013 199538
EP 649601 A3 19960508 EP 94307704 A 19941020 199628
NZ 264668 A 19970324 NZ 264668 A 19941012 199719
AU 679110 B 19970619 AU 9475840 A 19941014 199733
Abstract (Basic): US 5397588 A

Low calorie fruit spreads comprise the gelled prod. of water, fruit or fruit flavouring, high intensity sweetener(s), low methoxy pectin or carrageenan gelling agent, CMC, guar gum and locust bean gum.

ADVANTAGE—The spreads have good sweetness intensity and quality and good texture.

Hydrocolloid—Misc. Low Calorie Foods 6

New isomalto-oligosaccharide cpd.—used as functional food material, prepd. by contacting new alpha-amylase with pullulan or panose.

Patent Assignee: OJI CORN STARCH CO LTD (OJIP); SAKANO Y (SAKA-I)
Number of Countries: 001 Number of Patents: 001
Patent No Kind Date Applicat No Kind Date Main IPC Week
JP 7025891 A 19950127 JP 93193881 A 19930712 C07H-003/06 199516 B
Abstract (Basic): JP 7025891 A

Isomalto-oligosaccharides of formula (I) are new. Also claimed is a novel alpha-amylase enzyme (AA), producing the isomalto-oligosaccharides of formulae (I) and (II). Properties of AA are as follows: (1) Action: (a) mainly produces maltose from starch; (b) produces panose from pullulan; (c) hydrolyses pullulan in the presence of glucose to produce (I) and (II). (2) Substrate specificity: hydrolyses the alpha-1,4-glucoside bonds of starch and pullulan to produce (respectively) maltose and panose, which panose is converted to (I) and (II) in the presence of glucose, and decomposes (II). (3) Optimal pH and stability: optimal at pH 6–7 for the pullulan substrate and stable at pH 6–9. (4) Optimal temp. and thermal stability: optimal at 45-55°C for the pullulan substrate and stable at at most 50°C. (5) Mol. wt.: about 60,000, measured by SDS polyacrylamide gel slab electrophoresis. Also claimed is prepn. of (I) by the action of AA on pullulan or panose.

USE—(I) are useful as functional food materials.

ADVANTAGE—The method and enzyme give the new isomalto-oligosaccharides (I) which have low sweetness, low calorie content, high tooth decay resistance and bifidus growth factor action, and are non-fermenting.

Hydrocolloid—Misc. Low Calorie Foods 7

Gum system for use in very low calorie table syrup, e.g., maple syrup—comprises carboxymethylcellulose, xanthan and propylene glycol alginate gums and imparts desirable viscosity, stability and taste profile.

Patent Assignee: QUAKER OATS CO (QUAK)
Inventor: JONES L J; RACICOT W F
Number of Countries: 057 Number of Patents: 003
Patent No Kind Date Applicat No Kind Date Main IPC Week
WO 9510197 A1 19950420 WO 94US11051 A 19941007 A23L-001/0534 199521 B
AU 9479228 A 19950504 AU 9479228 A 19941007 A23L-001/0534 199536
US 5478589 A 19951226 US 93134249 A 19931008 A23L-001/09 199606
Abstract (Basic): WO 9510197 A

A gum system for use in a stable, artificial sweetener-contg. very low calorie table syrup having an aftertaste comprises (a) carboxymethylcellulose gum, (b) xanthan gum, and (c) propylene glycol alginate gum. The combined amt. of carboxymethylcellulose gum and xanthan gum is sufficient to impart to the syrup a desired stable viscosity suitable for a table syrup. The amt. of propylene glycol alginate gum is sufficient to substantially mask the aftertaste of the syrup.

Also claimed are stable, artificially sweetened, very low calorie table syrups comprising the gum system.

Pref. the gum system comprises by wt. of the total syrup compsn. 1.00–1.40 wt.% carboxymethylcellulose, 0.14–0.22 wt.% xanthan gum, and 0.03–0.07 wt.% propylene glycol alginate gum. The wt. ratio of carboxymethylcellulose gum to xanthan gum is 5:1–8:1, and the wt. ratio of propylene glycol alginate gum to xanthan gum is 0.2:1–0.3:1.

ADVANTAGE—The gum system allows prepn. of synthetic table syrups, e.g., maple syrup, having desirable viscosity, mouthfeel, pourability, stability and taste profile.

Hydrocolloid—Misc. Low Calorie Foods 9

Reduced calorie sandwich biscuit fillings—has some fat/oil replaced by high solids sugar syrup contg. non- or low-calorie bulking agent.

Patent Assignee: FMC CORP (FMCC)
Inventor: LAAMAN T R; SEWALL C J
Number of Countries: 063 Number of Patents: 003
Patent No Kind Date Applicat No Kind Date Main IPC Week
WO 9601571 A1 19960125 WO 95US8371 A 19950630 A23L-001/0526 199610 B

AU 9529157 A 19960209 AU 9529157 A 19950630 A23L-001/0526 199619
US 5629041 A 19970513 US 94272891 A 19940708 A23L-001/0534 199725
Abstract (Basic): WO 9601571 A

Sandwich biscuit fillings are 35 wt.% fat/oil and 65% sugar with up to 5% additional flavouring and/or colouring. The calorie content is reduced by replacing fat/oil, such that its content is less than 25%, with a sugar syrup of at most 70% solids and a non-calorie or low calorie bulking agent of water absorptivity up to 200%. The water activity (Aw) of the filler is 0.2–0.7.

Water activity is 0.3–0.6 (pref. 0.51–0.59). The bulking agent has water absorptivity up to 150 (up to 100)% and is a cellulose, hemicellulose, inulin and/or polydextrose. The bulking agent is a sugar syrup of solids content at least 70% at 15–35% of the total filler. A polyhydric alcohol is present at up to 40 wt.%. A food grade emulsifier is present at up to 3.0 wt.%.

ADVANTAGE—Sugar in the filler is adequately bound, avoiding crumbling and loss of filler.

Hydrocolloid—Misc. Low Calorie Foods 10

Fine cellulose-contg. food compsn. for high vegetable fibre or low calorie food—comprises dried complex consisting of fine cellulose and water-soluble gum and/or hydrophilic material.

Patent Assignee: ASAHI KASEI KOGYO KK (ASAH)
Number of Countries: 001 Number of Patents: 001
Patent No Kind Date Applicat No Kind Date Main IPC Week
JP 6335365 A 19941206 JP 93318323 A 19931217 A23L-001/308 199508 B
Abstract (Basic): JP 6335365 A

Food compsn. comprises a dried complex consisting of 20–98 wt.%-fine cellulose, 2–80 wt.%-water soluble gums and/or a hydrophilic material. A fine cellulose-contg. food compsn. contains the water dispersible complex having average grain dia. of up to 8 microns when the complex is dispersed in water, and having grains of at least 10 microns, up to 40%, and a colloid fraction of at least 65%.

Pref., the water soluble gums comprise: low cost bean gum, gum arabic, agar, carrageenan, etc. the hydrophilic material comprises: starch hydrolysed material, dextrin, cane sugar, glucose, fructose, etc.

USE/ADVANTAGE—The compsn. is used for producing a high-vegetable fibre-contg. food or low-calorie food and drink, milk prod. or fat and oil-processed food. The use of the food compsn. for the drink, milk prod., or fat and oil-processed food enhances stability, texture, and appearance.

Hydrocolloid—Misc. Low Calorie Foods 11

Boiled rice grain type low calorie food—comprises water-soluble dispersion gel contg. glucomannan, starch, dietary fibre and alginic acid and/or carrageenan.

Patent Assignee: HOSODA SHOTEN KK (HOSO-N); SUGIYO CO LTD (SUGI-N)
Inventor: HOSODA S; HOSODA Y; KATO E
Number of Countries: 002 Number of Patents: 002
Patent No Kind Date Applicat No Kind Date Main IPC Week
JP 6315356 A 19941115 JP 93289529 A 19931118 A23L-001/0528 199505 B
US 5498435 A 19960312 US 93165855 A 19931214 A23L-001/05 199616
Abstract (Basic): JP 6315356 A

Water-soluble dispersion gel consisting of glucomannan, starch and dietary fibre forms a low calorie food. In addition, alginic acid and/or carrageenan is used.

USE—The appearance and mouthfeel are very close to boiled rice grains, and good resistance to freezing is obtd.

Hydrocolloid—Misc. Low Calorie Foods 12

Poly-dextrose prods. mfr. in commercially viable forms—by flash shearing polymerised prod. through spinning heads, used, e.g., addn. to low calorie foodstuffs.

Patent Assignee: FUISZ TECHNOLOGIES LTD (FUIS-N)
Inventor: FUISZ R C
Number of Countries: 002 Number of Patents: 003
Patent No Kind Date Applicat No Kind Date Main IPC Week
GB 2276173 A 19940921 GB 943075 A 19940217 C08B-037/00 199435 B
CA 2115808 A 19940819 CA 2115808 A 19940216 C07H-003/06 199439
GB 2276173 B 19970402 GB 943075 A 19940217 C08B-037/00 199717
Abstract (Basic): GB 2276173 A

Poly-dextrose is made by subjecting flowable poly-dextrose feedstock to flash shearing means in a spinning appts. This instantaneously disrupts the flowable stream into separate masses of poly-dextrose polymerisate.

Glucose and maltose polymers(poly-dextrose) are melt polymerised using edible acids as catalysts at temperatures of 140–180°C in a time/temp relationship.

The reaction takes place in a chamber (11) and the feedstock flows to a rotating (3500rpm) heated spinning head (32). A stream of air is also fed to the head to flash shear the product emerging from orifices in the spinning head. The material is collected in a fixed bin (34) for removal by other means.

USE/ADVANTAGE—To make poly-dextrose polymerise in a suitable form for adding to low calorie foodstuffs. Bioaffecting agents may be included with the poly-dextrose, e.g., (a) antitussives, such as dextromethorphan, and chlorphedianol hydrochloride; (b) antihistamines, such as chlorpheniramine maleate and terfenadine; decongestants, such as phenylephrine, phenylpropanolamine, pseudoephedrin and ephedrine; (d) various alkaloids, such as codeine and morphine; (e) mineral supplements such as potassium chloride; (f) laxative, vitamins and antacids; (g) ion-exchange resins such as cholestyramine; (h) anti-cholesterolemic and anti-lipid agents; (i) antiarrhythmics such as N-acetyl-procainamide; (j) antipyretics and analgesics such as acetaminophen, aspirin and ibuprofen; (k) appetite suppressants such as phenylpropanolamine hydrochloride or caffeine; (l) expectorants such as guaifenesin; (m) anti-anxiety agents such as diazepam; and (n) anti-ulcer agents such as sucralfate. It may also be used with cosmetic adjuvants, e.g., dimethyl siloxanes, mucopolysaccharides, methyl and propyl parabens, biotin, lanolin, aloe, glycerin, mineral oil, nicotinamide compounds, sunscreens, such as para-aminobenzoic acid, hair conditions, moisturisers, moisturising creams, astringents and powders such as talcs. The commercial material is formed ready to use without energy intensive milling operations.

Hydrocolloid—Misc. Low Calorie Foods 13

Prodn. of low calorie jelly sweets with high solid content—by replacing sugar with polydextrose and sorbitol, and using gellan gum as gelling agent.

Patent Assignee: GIBSON W (GIBS-I); KELCO INT LTD (KELC); ROLLEY N A (ROLL-I); SOFUYI O Y A (SOFU-I); WINWOOD R J (WINW-I)

Number of Countries: 001 Number of Patents: 001

Patent No Kind Date Applicat No Kind Date Main IPC Week

RD 361057 A 19940510 RD 94361057 A 19940420 A23G-000/00 199432 B

Abstract (Basic): RD 361057 A

Low calorie jelly sweets can be made by replacing most of the sugar with polydextrose and sorbitol; and gellan gum is used as gelling agent.

USE/ADVANTAGE—The firm jelly sweets (jubes) low total 80% solids or more and low calorie content (less than 70 KJ/15g). The addn. of up to 15% sorbitol lowers viscosity of the hot polydextrose-contg. confectionary mix sufficiently to allow deposition into moulds, and the gellan gum does not add to the viscosity of the depositing mix.

Hydrocolloid—Misc. Low Calorie Foods 14

Fat-free vitamin-C fortified yogurt and juice blend—mfd. by homogenising fat-free cultured un-flavoured yogurt and blending with pasteurised liq. contg. water, pectin-based fat substitute, citric and ascorbic acids and conc. juice flavouring.

Patent Assignee: NOHNER R (NOHN-I)
Inventor: NOHNER R; PARK P H
Number of Countries: 001 Number of Patents: 001
Patent No Kind Date Applicat No Kind Date Main IPC Week
CA 2077389 A 19930920 CA 2077389 A 19920902 A23C-009/133 199350 B
Abstract (Basic): CA 2077389 A

Mfg. a fat-free, vitamin C fortified yogurt and juice blended beverage having a smooth, full-bodied mouthfeel comprises: (a) culturing pasteurised skimmed milk to form fat-free unflavoured yogurt; (b) homogenising the unflavoured yogurt to eliminate lumps and curds; (c) preparing a liq. mixt. of water, a pectin-based fat substitute, citric acid and ascorbic acid to provide 100% of the U.S.R.A. (recommended daily allowances) of vitamin C in an 8 ounce serving of the resultant beverage; (d) pasteurising the liq. mixt. contg. the vitamin C before mixing it with the yogurt; and (e) blending together 40–50 pts.wt. of the liq. mixt., 10–25 pts.wt. of conc. juice flavouring, and 30–60 pts.wt. of the yogurt to form the fat-free vitamin C fortified beverage.

Also claimed is the beverage formed.

USE/ADVANTAGE—Addn. of the vitamin C to the liq. mixt. allows a substantial portion of it to survive pasteurisation. No pasteurisation of the yogurt occurs after culturing is initiated and the resulting beverage has active yogurt cultures which are believed to be beneficial to the digestive system. The vitamin C enrichment gives 100% of the US RDA for vitamin C, making the beverage a healthy portion of an overall balanced diet.

Hydrocolloid—Misc. Low Calorie Foods 15

Incorporating coagulable milk protein into flour based food prods.—gives improved nutritive value and reduced calorie content.

Patent Assignee: DUBOIS J (DUBO-I)
Inventor: DUBOIS J; DUBOIS J C
Number of Countries: 001 Number of Patents: 001
Patent No Kind Date Applicat No Kind Date Main IPC Week
FR 2661072 A 19911025 FR 905491 A 19900418 199202 B
Abstract (Basic): FR 2661072 A

Process allowing development of improved food prods. based on amylaceous substances comprises incorporating a coagulable milk protein into the formulation.

The coagulable milk protein is esp. casein or alkali(ne earth) salts of casein. Pref. the casein is in the form of a fine powder with a particle size of less than 500 micron. The casein may be incorporated as a technical additive in an amt. of 0.1–5% or as a substitute for part of the amylaceous material in an amt. of not less than 10%. Other materials which can be incorporated into the formulation as a replacement for part of the flour are inert non-calorific materials such as cereal residual prods., clays, coloidal kaolin, talc, vegetable or synthetic cellulose, hydrocolloids and mucilages; and protein hydrolysates, esp. where the overall level of substitution of the amylaceous material is 10–50%.

USE/ADVANTAGE—Incorporation of the milk protein into flour-based food prods. such as bread, cakes, biscuits, pancakes, pastry, etc., improves the nutritive value and flavour of the prod. and reduces the flour content and calorific value without affecting the normal character of the food prod.

Hydrocolloid—Misc. Low Calorie Foods 16

Polydextrose compsn. free of colour and bitter taste—prepd. by dissolving polydextrose in solvent, adjusting pH to 3.0 or higher, passing through ion-exchange column.

Patent Assignee: WARNER LAMBERT CO (WARN); WARNER-LAMBERT CO (WARN)
Inventor: BUNICK F J; LUO S J
Number of Countries: 010 Number of Patents: 012
Patent No Kind Date Applicat No Kind Date Main IPC Week
EP 458748 A 19911127 EP 91810374 A 19910516 199148 B
AU 9176301 A 19911128 199204
NO 9101954 A 19911125 199205
CA 2042920 A 19911123 199207
US 5091015 A 19920225 US 90527224 A 19900522 199211
PT 97731 A 19920228 199213
FI 9102443 A 19911123 199214
ZA 9103841 A 19920325 ZA 913841 A 19910521 199218
CN 1056697 A 19911204 CN 91103405 A 19910521 C08L-005/02 199235
JP 4227901 A 19920818 JP 91144033 A 19910521 C08B-037/00 199240
EP 458748 A3 19920311 EP 91810374 A 19910516 199326
PH 27202 A 19930504 PH 42497 A 19910522 C08B-037/00 199635
Abstract (Basic): EP 458748 A

A polydextrose compsn., substantially free of colour and bitter-tasting residual cpds. is made by a process comprising: (a) dissolving polydextrose in a solvent; (b) adjusting the pH of the soln. to 3.0 or higher; (c) passing the soln. through an ion exchange column; and (d) collecting and concentrating the eluate until a commercially useful polydextrose compsn. is recovered.

Pref. the solvent is water. The concn. of polydextrose in soln. is 5–90% esp. 30–40 wt.% of the soln. The ion exchange column is comprised by a resin selected from anionic exchange resins and/or cationic exchange resins (esp. derivs. of cellulose, chitin, silicate, dextrans, polyacrylamide gel and/or vinyl cross-linked resins). The polydextrose soln. is passed through the ion exchange column at room temp.; or at elevated temp. and pressure. The soln. is passed through the column more than once.

USE/ADVANTAGE—The compsn. is useful as a bulking agent for incorporation into low calorie food. The bulking agent may be combined with high intensity sweeteners as a replacement for sugar in foods to lower their calories without detracting from their texture and mouthfeel.

Hydrocolloid—Misc. Low Calorie Foods 17

Gum system for very low calorie table syrups—comprises carboxymethyl cellulose and xanthan gum.

Patent Assignee: QUAKER OATS CO (QUAK)
Inventor: GORDON W A; JONES L J
Number of Countries: 001 Number of Patents: 001
Patent No Kind Date Applicat No Kind Date Main IPC Week
US 5292545 A 19940308 US 90559121 A 19900726 A23L-002/00 199410 B
US 91784359 A 19911029
Abstract (Basic): US 5292545 A

Gum system comprises (by wt. of total syrup): (a) 1–1.75% carboxymethylcellulose (I); and (b) 0.1–0.27% xanthan gum (II); with wt. ratio (I):(II) = 5–21:1.

Very low calorie table syrups contg. the above gum system are also claimed.

Pref. gum systems and very low calorie table syrups comprise (by wt. of total syrup) 1–1.6% esp. 1–1.4% (I), 0.14–0.27% esp. 0.14–0.22% (II), and at least 75% deionised H_2O; and pref. also 0.01–0.1% of a chelating agent (esp. Na hexametaphosphate), and 0.01–0.1% of a preservative. The pref. syrups have pH 4–5, contain (I) and (II) in wt. ratio 5–8:1, and have viscosity 250–1000 esp. 400–700 cps. (''Broofield LVT'' (RTM) viscometer at ca. 25°C). Alternative pref. gum systems, and very low calorie table syrups comprise 1.2–2.6% (I) and 0.12–0.16% (II), in wt. ratio 9–12:1; at least 90% deionised H_2O, 0.01–0.1% chelating agent, and 0.01–0.1% preservative.

ADVANTAGE—The gum systems have a desirable mouthfeel, stability, viscosity and pourability, and may be used as a stable vehicle to provide palatable very low calorie synthetic table syrups which contain little or no sugar solids.

Hydrocolloid—Misc. Low Calorie Foods 18

Low calorie beverages—comprises aspartame, multi-vitamin(s), xanthan gum, citric or maleic acid and flavouring.

Patent Assignee: JANG D C (JANG-I)
Inventor: JANG D C
Number of Countries: 001 Number of Patents: 001
Patent No Kind Date Applicat No Kind Date Main IPC Week
CA 2098005 A 19931210 CA 2098005 A 19930608 A23L-002/00 199409 B
Abstract (Basic): CA 2098005 A

An aq. beverage compsn. contg. 1–40 calories per 11.5 oz. serving comprises: 200–600g aspartame; up to 200% of the recommended daily allowance (RDA) of multiple vitamins per serving; 30–250g of xanthan gum, 100–7000g of citric/maleic acid; and flavouring to produce a palatable beverage for a 250 gallon batch.

Also claimed is a process for making the compsn.

USE/ADVANTAGE—The beverages are useful as palatable, low calorie nutritious beverage. The beverage is pleasing to the eye as well as the palate and has a long shaft life, i.e., will not form precipitates for many months.

Hydrocolloid—Misc. Low Calorie Foods 19

Food modifying compsns. for fat-free cake icing—comprise edible micro-milled soy fibre in aq. liq.

Patent Assignee: KRAFT GEN FOODS INC (KRFT); KRAFT FOODS INC (KRFT)
Inventor: ANDERSON W A; DULIN D A; LOH J P; DULIN D; LOH J
Number of Countries: 019 Number of Patents: 005
Patent No Kind Date Applicat No Kind Date Main IPC Week
US 5230918 A 19930727 US 92865593 A 19920409 A23L-001/308 199331 B
EP 565260 A1 19931013 EP 93302133 A 19930322 A23L-001/29 199341
CA 2091973 A 19931010 CA 2091973 A 19930318 A23G-003/00 199402
EP 565260 B1 19951011 EP 93302133 A 19930322 A23L-001/29 199545
DE 69300611 E 19951116 DE 600611 A 19930322 A23L-001/29 199551
EP 93302133 A 19930322
Abstract (Basic): US 5230918 A

(A) Food modifying compsn. comprises (by wt.) 1–15% of an edible soy fibre (I) of particle size 0.1–20 micron dispersed in 85–99% of an aq. liq.

(B) Cake icing comprises 10–100% of the compsn. (A).

Pref. compsn. (A) comprises 7–12% (I) and 88–93% aq. liq.; and pref. also comprises 0.001–1.5% of a non-gelling, non-abrasive hydrocolloid as whitening enhancer (esp. 0.3—0.9% gum arabic; 0.01—0.05% CMC, locust bean gum, or carrageenan; or 0.001—0.01% guar gum), and 0.1—2%, esp. 0.5—1.5% TiO_2. Pref. (I) has particle size 2–7 microns. Pref. aq. liquids are H_2O, milk, or an aq. sugar soln. (esp. comprising 30–70% sugar and 40–75% H_2O; sugar pref. sucrose, fructose, dextrose, corn syrup solids, high fructose corn syrup solids, glycerol, sorbitol, or other liq. or solid sugars).

Pref. cake icing compsns. (B) comprise sugar, H_2O and compsn. (A) and opt. starch, pref. (concns. independent of sugar and H_2O content of (A)) 25–80% sugar, 25–50% H_2O, 2–10% starch and compsn. (A).

Cake icing compsns. (B) are prepd. by wet-milling a blend of sugar, H_2O and compsn. (A) ((I) of particle size above 20 microns) to the desired (I)-particle size.

USE/ADVANTAGE—The fat-free food modifying compsn. (A) contg. micromilled soy fibres is an effective fat substitute, and is esp. useful in cake icing compsns. to provide these with a creamy taste and a flavour profile that resembles fat-contg. icing.

Hydrocolloid—Misc. Low Calorie Foods 20

Low-calorie food used as fat substitute—contains polysaccharide and branched dextrin.

Patent Assignee: DAINIPPON PHARM CO LTD (DAIN)
Number of Countries: 001 Number of Patents: 001
Patent No Kind Date Applicat No Kind Date Main IPC Week
JP 5276898 A 19931026 JP 92112136 A 19920403 A23L-001/307 199347 B
Abstract (Basic): JP 5276898 A

Food contains polysaccharide(s), opt. xanthan, carageenan, alginates or cellulose and branched dextrin, e.g., enzymatically decomposed or acidified starch comprising amylopectin.

USE—Low-calorie food having reduced fat content is used as a substitute of fats.

Hydrocolloid—Misc. Low Calorie Foods 21

Stabilised low calorie table syrup—comprising water, artificial sweetener, and gum system comprising carboxymethyl cellulose gum and xanthan gum.

Patent Assignee: KRAFT GEN FOODS INC (KRFT); KRAFT FOODS INC (KRFT)
Inventor: ACKERMANN K R; SWALLOW N A

Number of Countries: 018 Number of Patents: 003
Patent No Kind Date Applicat No Kind Date Main IPC Week
US 5106646 A 19920421 US 91638581 A 19910108 199219 B
EP 494743 A1 19920715 EP 92300076 A 19920106 A23L-001/09 199229
CA 2058723 A 19920709 CA 2058723 A 19920103 A23L-001/09 199239
Abstract (Basic): US 5106646 A

Low calorie, aq. table syrup comprises (by wt.) at least 70% H_2O, less than 20 sugar solids (I), an artificial sweetener (II) and a gum system consisting of carboxymethyl cellulose gum (III) and a cellulose-free xanthan gum (IV). Amt. of (III) is to impart desired viscosity. Amt. of (IV) is 15–75 wt.% of (III). When the syrup is stored at 70°C its viscosity does not increase more than 40% after 7 months.

Pref. (III) has mol. wt. sufficient to give viscosity 500–6000, esp. 800–3100 cps. in a 2% aq. soln. at 25°C. Amt. of (III) is pref. to give syrup viscosity 200–2000, esp. 500–1600 cps. at 70°C pref. 0.3–3%, Amt. of (IV) is pref. 20–60 % by wt. of (III). (IV) pref. has a molecular wt. to give viscosity 1000–2000 cps. at 1 wt.% in a 1% soln. of KC1 in H_2O at 25°C.

ADVANTAGE—The reduced sugar content and reduced calorie table syrup is comparable in quality and stability to conventional table syrups.

Hydrocolloid—Misc. Low Calorie Foods 22

Dietetic ballast materials and pectin prodn. from dried plant residues—by treating with ammonia gas to foramido-pectin(s), extracting the amidated pectin and washing and drying the residue.

Patent Assignee: AMINO GMBH (AMIN-N)
Inventor: STEINMETZE W
Number of Countries: 001 Number of Patents: 001
Patent No Kind Date Applicat No Kind Date Main IPC Week
DE 4042405 A 19920326 DE 4042405 A 19900428 199214 B
Abstract (Basic): DE 4042405 A

Dietetic ballast or filler materials are prepd. from dried plant residues by first treating the dried plant residues with gaseous ammonia at room temp., after which the amidated pectin is extracted from the plant residues with water or dil. NaOH and the plant residues from which the pectin has been extracted are washed and neutralised and further processed into dietetic ballast or filler materials in the known way.

Pref. the dried plant residues, esp. sugar beet chips, are placed in a reaction tower and an atmos. of ammonia is introduced. The contact time between the dried residues and the ammonia gas is pref. 30 mins. to 10 hours, esp. 30–90 mins.

USE/ADVANTAGE—The process allows extraction of high grade

pectin from plant residues such as sugar beet chips, and also removes other water soluble impurities from the plant residues so that very pure cellulose- and hemicellulose-contg. residues are obtd. which can be processed into ballast and filler materials for incorporation into foodstuffs and dietary prods. such as reduced calorie foodstuffs.

Hydrocolloid—Misc. Low Calorie Foods 23

Prepn. of reduced calorie frozen dessert(s)—by enzyme treatment of aq. milk ingredients to hydrolyse polysaccharide(s) to mono-saccharide(s), heating, and adding sweetener.

Patent Assignee: SHAZER W H (SHAZ-I)
Inventor: ELLE ; KELLER S E; SHAZER W H
Number of Countries: 001 Number of Patents: 001
Patent No Kind Date Applicat No Kind Date Main IPC Week
US 5093137 A 19920303 US 90599219 A 19901017 199212 B
Abstract (Basic): US 5093137 A

Reduced calorie frozen dairy dessert prepn. comprises (a) a mixt. of milk ingredients (I) and H_2O is heated to effect pasturisation; (b) the mixt. is cooled and treated with an enzyme (II) for long enough to reduce milk polysaccharides to the monosaccharide components; (c) the mixt. is heated for 5–60 min. at 70–95°C; (d) a high potency sweetener (III) and flavours are added; and (e) the mixt. is frozen. The prod. contains no added sugars or bulking agents.

In step (1), (I) is pref. whole, skim, or condensed skim milk, or non-fat dry milk. Pasteurisation is pref. at 60–90°C. The (I)-H_2O mixt. pref. includes at least 10% by wt. lactose. In step (b), (II) may be added directly, or after immobilisation. A pref. (II) is beta-galactosidase. Step (d). (II) is pref. aspartame, cyclamate, acesulphame-K, sucralose, or salts or mixts. The frozen dessert pref. also comprises a stabiliser (esp. carrageenan, locust bean gum, xanthan gum, or microcryst cellulose). Opt. a cultured yogurt may be added to the dessert before it is frozen.

ADVANTAGE—The process affords sugar-free, reduced calorie frozen desserts that contain no additional bulking agents, but have superior consistency, palatability, and mouthfeel.

Hydrocolloid—Misc. Low Calorie Foods 24

Low calorie confectioneries—made from polydextrose by agglomerating into granules before tablet forming.

Patent Assignee: SOC EURO PROD REFRACTAIRES (SGPR); PFIZER INC (PFIZ); WARNER-LAMBERT CO (WARN); WARNER LAMBERT CO (WARN)

Inventor: BUNICK F J; SHAW J J
Number of Countries: 018 Number of Patents: 011
Patent No Kind Date Applicat No Kind Date Main IPC Week
EP 452262 A 19911016 EP 91810239 A 19910403 199142 B
AU 9174158 A 19911010 199148
NO 9101353 A 19911010 199150
CA 2039947 A 19911010 199201
FI 9101683 A 19911010 199203
ZA 9102593 A 19920129 ZA 912593 A 19910408 199210
JP 4228030 A 19920818 JP 91101775 A 19910408 A23G-003/00 199240
EP 452262 A3 19920408 EP 91810239 A 19910403 199328
EP 452262 B1 19960103 EP 91810239 A 19910403 A23L-001/308 199606
DE 69115974 E 19960215 DE 615974 A 19910403 A23L-001/308 199612
EP 91810239 A 19910403
ES 2082174 T3 19960316 EP 91810239 A 19910403 A23L-001/308 199618
Abstract (Basic): EP 452262 A

Reduced calorie confections are prepd. by (a) intimately contacting polydextrose with a binding soln. for long enough that the powder congeals into granules and (b) forming compressed tablets from the granules. The binding soln. is a sorbitol and/or alginate soln. It contains 50–80 (70)% sorbitol by wt. The alginate is Na or K alginate esp. 0.5–2.5 (2)% Na alginate soln. The granules have particle size 16–100 (20–70) (30–60) mesh. The polydextrose is homogeneously mixed with a bulking agent before contacting with the binding soln. The bulking agent is dextrose, sucrose, sugar alcohol, sugar alcohol oligomer, palatinite, dextrose and/or dextrose oligomers. The reduced calorie confections are new. Agglomerates were prepd. from 337.5g Pfizer improved polydextrose, 384.0g sucrose, 28.5g 42DE corn syrup, 15.5g breath freshener and 5.6g TiO_2, using 3.2g 2% algin soln. as binder. 300.00g of these were mixed with 2.25g Mg stearate, 1.25g aspartame and 2.25g spray dried flavour. The tablets were far better than controls with no binder: soln.

ADVANTAGE—Tablet forming is easy and tablets formed are uniform in wt. and appearance and are resistant to capping, chipping or crumbling in the mouth.

Hydrocolloid—Misc. Low Calorie Foods 25

Prepn. of low calorie dextrin—by heating starch with at least one of lactose, sugar or guar gum in presence of (in)organic acid.

Patent Assignee: NICHIDEN KAGAKU KK (NICH-N)
Number of Countries: 001 Number of Patents: 001
Patent No Kind Date Applicat No Kind Date Main IPC Week

JP 3084001 A 19910409 JP 89219703 A 19890825 199120 B
Abstract (Basic): JP 3084001 A

Prepn. comprises heating starch or partially hydrolysed starch with at least one sugar selected from lactose, sugar, guar gum and partially hydrolysed guar gum in the presence of (in)organic acid.

USE/ADVANTAGE—Low calorie food material which is hardly digestible is obtd.

In an example starch or partially hydrolysed starch is mixed with 10–30 wt.% of sugar. Inorganic acid or organic acid is added to the mixt. so that the pH of a sample of the soln. diluting to aq. 5% soln. shows 2.5–3.5. The acidic soln. is heated at 140–180°C for 1–3 hrs. to obtain dextrine soln. The dextrin soln. is purified with active carbon and spray-dried to obtain colourless and odorless dextrin. The acids are HCl, H_2SO_4, HNO_3, H_3PO_4, acetic acid or citric acid.

Hydrocolloid—Misc. Low Calorie Foods 26

Glucomannan prod.—comprises glucomannan with acidic material encapsulated with hydrophobic material.
Patent Assignee: NIPPON OILS & FATS CO LTD (NIOF); UNI COLLOID KK (UNIC-N)
Inventor: KENICHI H; KOICHI I; MASATSUGU I; SEIKI H
Number of Countries: 007 Number of Patents: 005
Patent No Kind Date Applicat No Kind Date Main IPC Week
EP 387899 A 19900919 EP 90105010 A 19900316 199038 B
JP 2245148 A 19900928 JP 8963538 A 19890317 199045
CN 1045982 A 19901010 199125
US 5049401 A 19910917 US 90496204 A 19900319 199140
JP 3247244 A 19911105 JP 9042420 A 19900226 199150
Abstract (Basic): EP 387899 A

Glucomannan prod. contains glucomannan (I) as the principal components and comprises an acidic material (II) encapsulated with a hydrophobic substance (III).

Pref. (II) are acetic, citric, fumaric, adipic, tartaric, malic, ascorbic, gluconic, succinic, or lactic acids. Opt. the glucomannan prod. may also contain an alkaline substance (esp. $Ca(OH)_2$, CaO, NaOH, KOH, K_2CO_3, Na_2CO_3, $NaPO_4$ or Na_2HPO_4) encapsulated with a hydrophobic material (IV) ((IV) of m. pt. less than the m. pt. of (III); esp. of m. pt. 5°C less than the (III) m. pt.), and/or cellulose, and/or a natural polysaccharide (esp. carrageenan, locust bean gum, guar gum, alginic acid, Na alginate, xanthan gum, cyclodextrin, tamarind seed polysaccharide, agar, pullulan, or pectin).

USE/ADVANTAGE—The prod. may be coagulated rapidly, when the tissues are not destroyed and a homogeneous material possessing better elasticity and H_2O-lowering props. is obtd. The coagulated material is used as a Konjak food, or it may be blended with other foods to produce low calorie comestibles or to improve their consistency.

Hydrocolloid—Misc. Low Calorie Foods 27

Low calorie ice pop formulation—contg. powdered cellulose and glycerine to prevent hardness and graininess.
Patent Assignee: JAMES RIVER CORP (JAME)
Inventor: ANG J F; MILLER W B
Number of Countries: 001 Number of Patents: 001
Patent No Kind Date Applicat No Kind Date Main IPC Week
US 4857352 A 19890815 US 8762517 A 19870616 198941 B
Abstract (Basic): US 4857352 A

New ice pop formulation comprises (a) at least 1 wt.% powdered cellulose of average particle size below 20 microns, (b) a polyhydric alcohol to lower the freezing point of the pop, (c) a gum to keep (a) suspended and (d) water.

The alcohol is propylene glycol or, esp., glycerine. The glycerine is at 1–5 (2–3) wt.%. Compsns. also contain 0.05–0.2 wt.% aspartame. The cellulose is at 1–5 wt.% and esp. has average particle size below 17.5 microns. The gum is xanthan, guar or locust bean gum, esp. at 0.2–0.6%. The formulation also contains flavouring agents, colouring and up to 0.5 wt.% souring agent. The souring agent is citric acid.

ADVANTAGE—The prod. is low calorie but not hard or lacking smoothness, which were problems with prior art low calorie pops.

Hydrocolloid—Misc. Low Calorie Foods 28

Low-calorie ice cream-type product—comprises milky protein, polyol, e.g., propylene glycol and stabiliser, e.g., gelatin.
Patent Assignee: GENERAL FOODS CORP (GENO)
Number of Countries: 001 Number of Patents: 001
Patent No Kind Date Applicat No Kind Date Main IPC Week
JP 1218553 A 19890831 JP 8843274 A 19880225 198941 B
Abstract (Basic): JP 1218553 A

The low-calorie ice cream-type prod. contg. less fat and no cane sugar comprises the following: (a) water, 70–75 wt.%: (b) Milky protein, 15–25 wt.%; (c) A polyol material, 3–7 wt.% of propylene glycol, glycerol, mannitol, sorbitol, glucose syrup hydride or starch hydrolysate hydride; and (d) a stabiliser, 1.0–2.0 wt.% of a component of gelatin, carrageenan, agar or pectin and a component of carboxy methyl cellulose, guar, locust bean gum, xanthan, gelatin, carragenane or acidolysis cellulose.

USE—The low-calorie ice cream-type prod. has ice cream-like taste and contains less fat and no cane sugar.

Hydrocolloid—Misc. Low Calorie Foods 29

Frozen fruit juice shake—comprising frozen mixt. of fruit juice, stabiliser(s), protein, flavour, acid, and water to give specified brix value.

Patent Assignee: OLYMPUS INDS INC (OLYM-N)
Inventor: WADE B; WADE T L
Number of Countries: 018 Number of Patents: 007
Patent No Kind Date Applicat No Kind Date Main IPC Week
EP 303374 A 19890215 EP 88306993 A 19880729 198907 B
AU 8820420 A 19890216 198915
US 4828866 A 19890509 US 88220283 A 19880720 198922
US 4830868 A 19890516 US 8785454 A 19870814 198923
JP 1231852 A 19890918 JP 88198763 A 19880808 198943
CN 1031468 A 19890308 199009
ZA 8805644 A 19900425 ZA 885644 A 19880801 199021
Abstract (Equivalent): EP 249446 B

A frozen, hard pack, fruit juice product comprising: at least one type of fruit juice; a fruit juice flavour enhancer selected from the group consisting of flavouring, spices, flavour enhancers and edible organic acids and mixtures thereof; from 0.5 percent to 1.5 percent by weight of at least one stabiliser based upon the total weight of said product with the provision that the product contains at least 0.02 percent xanthan gum; from 0.05 percent to 0.50 percent by weight of whipping agent protein based upon the total weight of said product; an amount of water to adjust the overall brix value of said product to the range of 10 to 35, and said product being essentially free of added sugar and corn sweetener additives and having overrun of at least 20 percent wherein said frozen fruit juice product has a smooth creamy appearance and good low temperature storage properties.

Hydrocolloid—Misc. Low Calorie Foods 30

Highly nutritional, vegetarian dry food supplement—comprising vegetable protein and lipid(s), psyllium husks as fibre and carbohydrate source.

Patent Assignee: KALOGRIS T P (KALO-I)
Inventor: KALOGRIS T P
Number of Countries: 001 Number of Patents: 001

Patent No Kind Date Applicat No Kind Date Main IPC Week
US 4737364 A 19880412 US 8711407 A 19870204 198817 B
Abstract (Basic): US 4737364 A

Known highly nutritional vegetarian dry food supplements (providing not more than 120 calories/15g) consisting of vegetable protein (I) (soy protein isolate and/or brewer's yeast; to give total protein content 35–65% by wt.), 10–20% by wt. total complex carbohydrate (II), at least 4% by wt. fibre (III), vegetable lipids (IV) (polyunsatd. vegetable oil or vegetable derived lecithin; to give total lipid content 10–20% by wt.), and 5–20% by wt. total vitamins and minerals are improved by using psyllium husks as the sole source of (II) and (III).

Hydrocolloid—Misc. Low Calorie Foods 31

Low calorie food and drink—contains gymnemaic acid and pullulan as suppressing agents for glucose absorption from the intestines.

Patent Assignee: HIJI Y (HIJI-I)
Inventor: HIJI Y
Number of Countries: 002 Number of Patents: 003
Patent No Kind Date Applicat No Kind Date Main IPC Week
JP 62236469 A 19871016 JP 8677725 A 19860404 198747 B
JP 91008188 B 19910205 JP 8677725 A 19860404 199109
US 5116820 A 19920526 US 8734957 A 19870406 A61K-031/70 199224
US 89418715 A 19891003
US 90563734 A 19900806
Abstract (Basic): JP 62236469 A

Food and drink contains gymnemaic acid and pullulan as the suppressing agent for the absorption of glucose from intestines.

USE/ADVANTAGE—Gymnemaic acid, the major ingredient of Gymnema sylvestre plant suppresses the absorption of glucose from the intestines. By using it together with pullulan, the amt. of gymnemaic acid can be saved.

Hydrocolloid—Misc. Low Calorie Foods 32

Carbonated beverage contg. low-calorie sweetener—with a cold water-soluble natural gum added to reduce carbon dioxide loss and improve palatability.

Patent Assignee: AJINOMOTO KK (AJIN)
Inventor: TAKIZAWA K; UEDA S
Number of Countries: 007 Number of Patents: 006
Patent No Kind Date Applicat No Kind Date Main IPC Week
EP 239938 A 19871007 EP 87104522 A 19870326 198740 B

JP 62232362 A 19871012 JP 8674834 A 19860401 198746
US 4956191 A 19900911 US 88275603 A 19881123 199039
EP 239938 B 19911204 199149
DE 3774912 G 19920116 199204
JP 93041222 B 19930622 JP 8674834 A 19860401 A23L-002/00 199327
Abstract (Basic): EP 239938 A

A carbonated beverage contains a low-calorie sweetener (I) as part or the whole of its sweetener content and a cold water-soluble natural gum (II). Pref. (I) is aspartame, Acesulphame, Stevia extract, or their derivs. and (II) is gum arabic.

Pref. the concn. of the natural gum in the carbonated beverage is 5–50 mg/dl. Pref. the amt. of (I) in the entire amt. of sweeteners is 30–90%, esp. 50–80%.

USE/ADVANTAGE—Carbonated beverages such as cola, cider-like soft drink and ginger ale and turbid carbonated beverages contg. fruit juices can be prepd. By including a natural gum into the carbonated beverage contg. the low-calorie sweetener in such a low concn. as to scarcely cause a thickening effect, there is obtd. a carbonate beverage having a high palatability comparable with a beverage contg. sugar and a reduced tendency toward the decrease of dissolved CO_2 gas after opening the bottle.

Hydrocolloid—Misc. Low Calorie Foods 33

Prepn. of low calorie instant noodle—by mixing soln. of arginic acid and carrageenan with starch and protein, and coagulating by contact with calcium salt or metal salts.

Patent Assignee: MISHOKUKEN KK (MISH-N)
Number of Countries: 001 Number of Patents: 002
Patent No Kind Date Applicat No Kind Date Main IPC Week
JP 62158466 A 19870714 JP 86865 A 19860107 198733 B
JP 89026665 B 19890524 198924
Abstract (Basic): JP 62158466 A

Soln. of arginic acid and carrageenan is mixed with starch and protein to make starch alpha state. The resultant is contacted with Ca salt or two or more valent metal strips to coagulate it, and the coagulated prod. is cut into lines and dried.

Hydrocolloid—Misc. Low Calorie Foods 34

Low-calorie powder for beverages—comprises powdered milk, beer yeast, saccharide and, e.g., pectin.

Patent Assignee: NIKKEN FOOD HONSHA (NIKK-N)

Number of Countries: 001 Number of Patents: 001
Patent No Kind Date Applicat No Kind Date Main IPC Week
JP 61242541 A 19861028 JP 8585686 A 19850422 198649 B
Abstract (Basic): JP 61242541 A

The powder comprises (1) 40%–70% (wt.) powdered milk, (1) 5%–20% (wt.) edible beer yeast, (3) 5%–20% fructooligosaccharide or isomerised lactose, and (4) 5%–30% (wt.) of pectin, alginic acid, guar gum, carrageenan, and/or an agar.

USE—The powder is used together with water or milk.

Hydrocolloid—Misc. Low Calorie Foods 35

Palatable reduced calorie chewing gum—contg. gum base, and low levels of polysaccharide and a sweetener.
Patent Assignee: WARNER-LAMBERT CO (WARN); WARNER LAMBERT CO (WARN)
Inventor: HRISCISEC F; SUBRAMAN R C; YOU C W; CHERUKURI S R; HRISCISCE F; WEI Y C
Number of Countries: 015 Number of Patents: 011
Patent No Kind Date Applicat No Kind Date Main IPC Week
AU 8771879 A 19871105 AU 8771879 A 19870423 198751 B
ZA 8702856 A 19871013 ZA 872856 A 19870422 198801
EP 252874 A 19880113 EP 87810267 A 19870428 198802
JP 62289149 A 19871216 JP 87106469 A 19870501 198805
PT 84797 A 19880527 198826
US 4765991 A 19880823 US 86859108 A 19860502 198836
EP 252874 B 19911016 199142
DE 3773772 G 19911121 199148
JP 92033427 B 19920603 JP 87106469 A 19870501 A23G-003/30 199226
ES 2026566 T3 19920501 EP 87810267 A 19870428 A23G-003/30 199228
CA 1321097 C 19930810 CA 535942 A 19870429 A23G-003/30 199338
Abstract (Basic): AU 8771879 A

Highly palatable, reduced calorie chewing gum comprises high levels (35–94%) of a non-styrene-butadiene copolymer/polyvinyl acetate chewing gum base, and low levels (5–10%) of a polysaccharide (I) and a sweetening agent (II). (I) is opt. modified polydextrose, or polymaltose, or mixts.

Pref. chewing gums contain (by wt.) 0.005–35% (II), 35–70% gum base, and pref. also 0.01–2% thickening agent (Me cellulose, alginate, carrageenan, xanthan gum, karaya, agar, gelatin, carob, tragacanth, locust bean gum, guar, gum arabic, pectin, (Na) carboxymethyl cellulose, hydroxypropyl cellulose, or mixts.), up to 7% cellulose, and up to 10% filler. The thickening agent is pref. added as a premix contg. (by wt.) 40–60% wetting agent, 12–18% H_2O, 22–48% (II), and 0.1–5% thickening agent. The prefd. (I) is polydextrose.

USE/ADVANTAGE—The low calorie chewing gum contains low levels of fillers, is highly palatable, has the necessary sweetness, and has a softer, more pleasant chew and mouthfeel.

Hydrocolloid—Misc. Low Calorie Foods 36

Prepn. of low-calorie, gelatin-free frozen confections—by dynamic freezing, with reduced hydrocolloid levels.

Patent Assignee: GENERAL FOODS CORP (GENO)
Inventor: GONSALVES A A; GRIFFIN J J; SMITH R A
Number of Countries: 002 Number of Patents: 002
Patent No Kind Date Applicat No Kind Date Main IPC Week
US 4582712 A 19860415 US 84667185 A 19841101 198618 B
CA 1249164 A 19890124 198911
Abstract (Basic): US 4582712 A

Low-calorie, gelatin-free frozen confection which is ready to eat at freezer temps. is prepd. as follows: (a) an aq. mixt. is formed comprising (by wt.) 2–5% f. pt. depressant (I), 0.1–1.8% hydrophilic colloid (II), stabiliser (III) (amt. (II)+(III) totals not more than 2%), 0.02–0.1% food acid, and 0.03–0.15% non-nutritive sweetener (IV); (b) the mixt. is dynamically cooled so that partial freezing is accomplished at 10–32°C; (c) the partially frozen mixt. is shaped; then (d) the shaped mixt. is frozen to less than 10°F. (II) is low methoxyl pectin, carrageenan, alginate, or mixts., and amt. used is to maintain the ice crystal structure produced during the partial freezing step (b).

ADVANTAGE—Elimination of gelatin from the compsns. affords a storage stable, high quality confection which is ready to eat at freezer temps. In addn., total hydrocolloid levels may be reduced. The prod. (which retains its shape on a stick, etc.) delivers a refreshing, texturally pleasing eating experience.

Hydrocolloid—Misc. Low Calorie Foods 37

Dietary fibre compsn. prepn.—by coating insoluble fibre with soluble fibre.

Patent Assignee: WARNER-LAMBERT CO (WARN)
Inventor: MORLEY R C; SHARMA S C
Number of Countries: 016 Number of Patents: 013
Patent No Kind Date Applicat No Kind Date Main IPC Week
ZA 8408391 A 19850429 ZA 848391 A 19841026 198539 B
EP 166825 A 19860108 EP 84304156 A 19840620 198602

PT 80576 A 19851206 198604
AU 8429735 A 19851212 198606
US 4565702 A 19860121 US 84616990 A 19840604 198606
JP 60262573 A 19851225 JP 84135352 A 19840702 198607
NO 8502230 A 19851230 198608
FI 8502188 A 19851205 198611
DK 8403025 A 19851205 198616
CA 1210630 A 19860902 198640
ES 8703728 A 19870516 ES 543821 A 19850603 198725
EP 166825 B 19880921 198838
DE 3474098 G 19881027 198844
Abstract (Basic): ZA 8408391 A

Dietary fibre prods. comprise (a) 40–60% sweetener, (b) a flavour source, and (c) 10–40% of a dietary fibre compsn. comprising insoluble fibre coated with soluble fibre, the insoluble fibre being purified and free of digestible components.

The insoluble fibre is purified wheat, maize, barley, rye and/or oat bran. The soluble fibre is a natural gum (e.g., arabic, tragacanth, karaya or ghatti), a seaweed extract (e.g., agar, alginate, carrageenan or furcellan) or a mucilage (e.g., psyllium).

ADVANTAGE—The prods. (e.g., tablets or snack bars) have a high ratio of fibre to digestable material without having a high calorie content. The unpleasant mouthfeel of the insoluble fibre is mashed by the soluble fibre rather than with fats or carbohydrates.

Hydrocolloid—Misc. Low Calorie Foods 38

High fibre food prod.—with coating contg. fat, sweetener, milk solids, yogurt and flavouring agents.

Patent Assignee: WARNER-LAMBERT CO (WARN)
Inventor: BAGAN J E; BECKER A J; MEDRI M W
Number of Countries: 014 Number of Patents: 010
Patent No Kind Date Applicat No Kind Date Main IPC Week
EP 128666 A 19841219 EP 84303155 A 19840510 198451 B
AU 8426420 A 19841115 198502
ZA 8402031 A 19840911 ZA 842031 A 19840319 198502
JP 59213361 A 19841203 JP 8491975 A 19840310 198503
US 4568557 A 19860204 US 83493451 A 19830511 198608
ES 8506986 A 19851201 198610
CA 1210632 A 19860902 198640
EP 128666 B 19870401 198713
DE 3462845 G 19870507 198719

US 4673578 A 19870616 US 85793369 A 19851031 198726
Abstract (Basic): EP 128666 A

High-fibre food prod. consists of (by wt. of prod.) 5–30% dietary fibre (I), coated with above 40% pref. not more than 70% of a coating compsn. The coating compsn. contains (by wt. of compsn.) 25–55% fat, 30–60% sweetener (II), up to 30% milk solids (III), up to 30% yogurt (IV), and up to 10% flavouring agent(s). (I) is suitably (hemi)cellulose, pectin or lignin from vegetables, fruit, grains, nuts or seeds (esp. bran or germ form pref. corn, wheat, oats, barley, soy, rye or rice; or oats). An esp. prefd. (I) is a mixt. of corn bran and corn germ used at 5–30% esp. 6–10 wt.% of total prod. (or 6–10% corn bran and up to 10% corn germ). The prod. contains pref. 40–65% esp. 45–50% partic. 45–47% of coating compsn. Fat is suitably a fractionated fat, an (opt. partially) hydrogenated fat, or an unsatd. fat, esp. coconut, palm, cottonseed, safflower, sunflower, soy or corn oils, partic. palm kernal oil. Amt. of fat is pref. 25–40% esp. 29–32% by wt. of compsn. (esp. 29–32% palm kernel oil with 0.5–0.6% palm oil). (II) is pref. saccharin or aspartame, esp. a mono- or di-saccharide, partic. granulated sugar, and amt. is 40–50% esp. 48% by wt. of compsn. (III) is pref. a solid of whole milk, non-fat milk, cream, whey, soy protein, casein, artificial creamer, pref. non-fat milk solids, and amt. is pref. 12–16% esp. 14% by wt. of compsn. Suitable flavouring agents include flavour oils, and flavouring foods (e.g., nuts, germs, fruits, etc.), esp. peanut butter at 7–16% by wt. of food prod. The coating compsn. has
H_2O-content pref. of 0.5–0.75%.

USE/ADVANTAGE—The ready-to-eat, nutritious, relatively low calorie snack prods. contain relatively large amts. of dietary fibre (I), but do not possess the dry taste and fibrous mouthfeel of conventional prods. In addn., the prod. tastes crunchy and crispy, but is not cooked or toasted, etc.

Hydrocolloid—Misc. Low Calorie Foods 39

High water content low calorie cake—contg. cellulose flour and opt. gum and emulsifier (SE 27.12.83).
Patent Assignee: GENERAL FOODS CORP (GENO)
Inventor: FROST J R; GLICKSMAN M; HEGEDUS E; SILVERMAN J E
Number of Countries: 002 Number of Patents: 002
Patent No Kind Date Applicat No Kind Date Main IPC Week
US 4451490 A 19840529 US 82355403 A 19820308 198424 B
CA 1182335 A 19850212 198511
Abstract (Basic): US 4451490 A

A cake comprises 40–65% water, 5–30% cake flour, 0–25% sugar, 1–6% shortening, 0–10% egg white solids, 0.5–6% leavening agent, 0–2%

emulsifier, 2–20% cellulose flour and 0–5% gum. The gum is, e.g., carrageenan, guar gum, locust bean gum, karaya gum, methyl cellulose, pectin, alginate or agar or their mixts. The emulsifier is pref. polyoxyethylene (20) sorbitan monooleate, Na stearoyl-2-lactylate mono- and diglycerides or mixts. of these. The leavening agent is pref. $NaHCO_3$ and NaAl phosphate. The compsn. pref. contains 45–60% water, 9–25% cake flour, 5–20% sugar, 1–5% shortening, 1–6% egg white solids, 1–5% leavening agent, 0.1–2% emulsifier, 5–15% cellulose flour and 0.1–3% gum.

The cake has high quality and excellent texture. It has a higher water content than conventional cakes, and a lower caloric value, typically below 2 cals/g.

Hydrocolloid—Misc. Low Calorie Foods 40

Low calorie cake prodn.—from mixt. contg. cellulose powder, citrus albedo, pineapple seed or sugar beet pulp.

Patent Assignee: GENERAL FOODS CORP (GENO)
Inventor: FROST J R; GLICKSMAN M; HEGEDUS E; SILVERMAN J E
Number of Countries: 003 Number of Patents: 003
Patent No Kind Date Applicat No Kind Date Main IPC Week
SE 8301234 A 19831227 SE 831234 A 19830307 198413 B
CA 1182334 A 19850212 198511
US 4503083 A 19850305 US 82355405 A 19820308 198512
Abstract (Equivalent): US 4503083 A

Cake comprises 40–65% water, 5–30% cake flour, 0–25% sugar, 1–6% shortening, 0–10% egg white solids, 0.5–6% leavening agent, 0–2% emulsifier, 1–10% of citrus albedo, sugar pulp, and/or pineapple core as bulking agent, and 0–10% gum, and contains less than 20 cals./g.

Pref. leavening agent is $NaHCO_3$, and/or sodium aluminium phosphate; and emulsifier is polyoxyethylene(20) sorbitan monooleate, sodium stearyl-2-lactylate and/or mono- and/or diglycerides. Gum is carrageenan, guar, gum arabic, locust bean gum, tragacanth, karaya, hydroxypropyl-cellulose, methylcellulose, carboxymethyl cellulose, xanthan, pectin, alginate and/or agar.

USE—Has high quality and excellent texture and is 40% or more calorie-reduced w.r.t. conventional cakes.

Hydrocolloid—Misc. Low Calorie Foods 41

Prepn. of low calorie, high fruit content marmalades, jams etc.—by mixing fruit, sucrose, pectin, thickener.

Patent Assignee: NYIREGYHAZI KONZERV (NYIR-N)
Inventor: BUGLYO T; GYORINE M; KOVACS P; NADASDI J

Number of Countries: 001 Number of Patents: 001
Patent No Kind Date Applicat No Kind Date Main IPC Week
HU 38041 T 19860428 HU 834247 A 19831213 198621 B
Abstract (Basic): HU 38041 T

Fruit or fruit juices, sugar (min. 30% sucrose), food acids, low degree ester pectin, one or more metallic salts and a fruit thickener are mixed together to produce low calorie, high fruit content marmalades, jams and jellies.

Hydrocolloid—Misc. Low Calorie Foods 42

Low calorie high moisture content cake prodn.—from batter contg. gum or bulking agent as water binding additive.
Patent Assignee: GENERAL FOODS CORP (GENO)
Inventor: FROST J R; GLICKSMAN M; HEGEDUS E
Number of Countries: 002 Number of Patents: 002
Patent No Kind Date Applicat No Kind Date Main IPC Week
US 4431681 A 19840214 US 82355404 A 19820308 198409 B
CA 1182683 A 19850219 198512
Abstract (Basic): US 4431681 A

Prepn. comprises forming a batter contg. 40–65 wt.% water, 5–30 wt.% cake flour, 0–25 wt.% sugar, 1–6 wt.% shortening, 0–10 wt.% egg white solids, 0.5–6 wt.% of a leavening agent, 0.2 wt.% emulsifier and 1–20 wt.% water binder; adjusting the viscosity of the batter to 15,000–50,000 cps. (Brookfield) and baking the batter at 300–450°F. for 10–60 mins. to produce a baking loss of 5–20%. The water binder is a gum, e.g., carrageenan, guar gum, locust bean gum, tragacanth, hydroxypropyl cellulose, CMC, xanthan, pectin, alginates or agar, or a bulking agent, e.g., citrus albedo, cellulose flour, sugar beet pulp, pineapple core, bran, sugar cane pulp or polydextrose. The emulsifier is, e.g., Tween 80 (RTM), Na stearoyl-2-lactylate or mono- or diglycerides. The batter may include minor amts. of other ingredients, e.g., salt, vanillin, non-fat milk solids, flavour or colouring. The viscosity of the batter is adjusted by addition of water.

The caloric value is at least 40% lower than that of conventional cakes. It contains 40% or more of water, but is not preceived to be excessively moist, and does not have a gritty or gummy texture.

Hydrocolloid—Misc. Low Calorie Foods 43

Vegetable and/or fruit juice preparations—are low-calorie, dietetic or diabetic prods. contg. pectin and magnesium.
Patent Assignee: KOZPONTI ELELMISZER (ELEL-N)

Inventor: BUGLYO T; HEGYI L; IVANICS L; NADASDI S; RICSO J; SCHLICK I; ZETELAKINE B
Number of Countries: 001 Number of Patents: 001
Patent No Kind Date Applicat No Kind Date Main IPC Week
HU 27810 T 19831128 HU 813945 A 19811223 198403 B
Abstract (Basic): HU 27810 T

Low-calorie, diet or diabetic vegetable/fruit juices; creams or cocktails are prepd. by (a) grinding the vegetable and/or fruit tissues; (b) treating with endopolygalacturonase, opt. in the presence of water; and (c) adding to the suspension, consisting of cell agglomerates of below 0.2 mm., a Mg source and opt. a stabiliser.

Hydrocolloid—Misc. Low Calorie Foods 44

Low-calorie, aerated, non-alcoholic medicinal drink—made by boiling and mincing dried apricots, adding sugar and pectin to part, and recombining the parts with steaming and cooling.
Patent Assignee: SAMARKAND COOP INST (SAMA-R)
Inventor: ABRAMOVA Z H I; RAIMOVA E G
Number of Countries: 001 Number of Patents: 001
Patent No Kind Date Applicat No Kind Date Main IPC Week
SU 891059 B 19811223 198242 B
Abstract (Basic): SU 891059 B

Method for manufacturing non-alcoholic aerated drinks for medicinal purposes, pref. by mixing dried apricots with water, heating the mixt. to boiling, mincing, and adding sugar. To extend the range of medicinal aerated low-calorie drinks, after mincing, part of the mixt. is separated, sugar and apple pectin are added in an amt. 0.25–0.5% of the total weight of the mixt. The prepd. mixt. is kept to allow the pectin to swell, it is boiled, cooled, mixed with the rest of the original mixture, casein hydrolysate is added (5% of the total weight), and then the mixture is whipped up.

Hydrocolloid—Misc. Low Calorie Foods 45

Non-nutritive flour substitutes for low calorie foods—contg. cellulose or starch deriv., xanthan gum and lecithin.
Patent Assignee: PFIZER INC (PFIZ)
Inventor: TORRES A
Number of Countries: 002 Number of Patents: 002
Patent No Kind Date Applicat No Kind Date Main IPC Week
US 4219580 A 19800826 198037 B
CA 1142387 A 19830308 198314
Abstract (Basic): US 4219580 A

Flour substitute comprises (a) cellulose and/or a non-digestible acid-treated starch deriv.; (b) 1–3.5 wt.% (based on (a)) xanthan gum and 2–7 wt.% (based on (a)) of lecithin, the amt. of lecithin being in addn. to lecithin that may be supplied by egg yolk present in food prods. contg. the substitute.

Substitute is non-nutritive and can replace ≦70% of the flour in low calorie baked goods.

Hydrocolloid—Misc. Low Calorie Foods 46

Low calorie spread contg. high-methoxylated pectin—to replace gelatin as emulsion stabiliser.

Patent Assignee: GRINDSTED PROD AS (GRIN)
Number of Countries: 001 Number of Patents: 001
Patent No Kind Date Applicat No Kind Date Main IPC Week
RD 217009 A 19820510 198222 B
Abstract (Basic): RD 217009 A

In a 40% fat calorie spread, milk protein destabilises the emulsion which gives a spread with coarse water dispersion and poor microbiological shelf life. Gelatin is known to stabilise the emulsion in the prod. at a dosage of, e.g., 2.5% gelatin 120 bloom calculated on the low calorie spread.

In trying to replace gelatin with pectin, the following trials were made with high-methoxylated pectin. Water phase contained 1.0% whey powder, 1.0% salt and 53.9–55.4% water at pH 6.5. (1) 2.5% Gelatin 120 bloom; (2) 1.0% Mexpectin SS 200 (slow set); (3) 2.0% Mexpectin SS 200 (slow set); (4) 1.0% Mexpectin MS 300 (medium set); (5) 2.0% Mexpectin MS 300 (medium set); (6) 1.0% Mexpectin RS 400 (rapid set); (7) 2.0% Mexpectin RS 400 (rapid set); fat phase contained 0.5% DIMODAN OT (unsatd. distilled monoglyceride); 0.1% sorbic acid; 0.3% colour; 39.2% fat blend; 24 pts. hardened soya, 41°C, 76 pts. liq. soya-bean oil. The spreads were produced on a 2-tube laboratory Perfector with low capacity and moderate cooling.

Evaluation after storage at 5°C showed that the spreads with Mexpectin had a satisfactory water dispersion and shelf life.

Hydrocolloid—Misc. Low Calorie Foods 47

Low calorie spread contg. high-methoxylated pectin—to replace gelatin as emulsion stabiliser.

Patent Assignee: GRINDSTED PROD AS (GRIN)
Number of Countries: 001 Number of Patents: 001
Patent No Kind Date Applicat No Kind Date Main IPC Week
RD 217009 A 19820510 198222 B
Abstract (Basic): RD 217009 A

In a 40% fat calorie spread, milk protein destabilises the emulsion which gives a spread with coarse water dispersion and poor microbiological shelf life. Gelatin is known to stabilise the emulsion in the prod. at a dosage of, e.g., 2.5% gelatin 120 bloom calculated on the low calorie spread.

In trying to replace gelatin with pectin, the following trials were made with high-methoxylated pectin. Water phase contained 1.0% whey powder, 1.0% salt and 53.9–55.4% water at pH 6.5. (1) 2.5% Gelatin 120 bloom; (2) 1.0% Mexpectin SS 200 (slow set); (3) 2.0% Mexpectin SS 200 (slow set); (4) 1.0% Mexpectin MS 300 (medium set); (5) 2.0% Mexpectin MS 300 (medium set); (6) 1.0% Mexpectin RS 400 (rapid set); (7) 2.0% Mexpectin RS 400 (rapid set); fat phase contained 0.5% DIMODAN OT (unsatd. distilled monoglyceride); 0.1% sorbic acid; 0.3% colour; 39.2% fat blend; 24 pts. hardened soya, 41°C, 76 pts. liq. soya-bean oil. The spreads were produced on a 2-tube laboratory Perfector with low capacity and moderate cooling.

Evaluation after storage at 5°C showed that the spreads with Mexpectin had a satisfactory water dispersion and shelf life.

Hydrocolloid—Misc. Low Calorie Foods 48

Low calorie diet bread—contg. added gluten, protein, alpha-cellulose flour and edible gum.

Patent Assignee: THOMPSON J B (THOM-I)
Inventor: THOMPSON J B
Number of Countries: 002 Number of Patents: 002
Patent Family:

Patent No	Kind	Date	Applicat No	Kind	Date	Main IPC	Week
GB 1538360	A	19790117					197909 B
US 4109018	A	19780822					197911

Abstract (Basic): GB 1538360 A

Dough composns. for bread making contain per 100 pts. wheat flour 3-9 pts. added vital wheat gluten, 5–12 pts. edible protein, 10–20 pts. alpha-cellulose flour and 0.5–6 pts. edible gum. The protein is esp. low fat soy flour,or soy flour with non-fat dried milk. The cellulose pref. has particle size 25–50 μm. The gum is a synthetic cellulose ether, esp. NaCMC, or guar gum or tragacanth.

The prod. has fewer calories, higher protein content and fibre content than conventional breads or diet breads.

Hydrocolloid—Misc. Low Calorie Foods 49

Flour substitute compsn. for reducing food calorie content—contains cellulose and/or non-digestible starch derivs., xanthan gum and emulsifier.

Patent Assignee: PFIZER INC (PFIZ)

Inventor: TORRES A
Number of Countries: 003 Number of Patents: 005
Patent No Kind Date Applicat No Kind Date Main IPC Week
DE 2804634 A 19780810 197833 B
JP 53099347 A 19780830 197840
GB 1580015 A 19801126 198048
DE 2804634 B 19810219 198109
JP 82005141 B 19820129 198208
Abstract (Basic): DE 2804634 A

Edible compsn. for use as flour substitute contains (a) ≥1 cellulose and/ or a non-digestible acid-treated starch deriv., and (w.r.t. wt. of (a)) (b) 1–3.5 (1–2)% xanthan gum and (c) 2–7 (3–5)% emulsifier(s).

The compsns. can be used as flour extenders in dietary reduced calorie foods, esp. for weight watchers, partic. for baking to bread, cakes, pastries, etc. Calorie content can be reduced by 30–35% on replacing 70% flour by the compsn.

Hydrocolloid—Misc. Low Calorie Foods 50

Edible fibrous cellulose coated with edible gum—as low calorie filler for foods and pharmaceuticals.
Patent Assignee: DOUGLAS D (DOUG-I); MAXFIBE INC (MAXF-N)
Number of Countries: 005 Number of Patents: 005
Patent No Kind Date Applicat No Kind Date Main IPC Week
DE 2729370 A 19780105 197803 B
JP 53003544 A 19780113 197808
US 4143163 A 19790306 197911
GB 1581841 A 19801230 198101
CA 1102698 A 19810609 198127
Abstract (Basic): DE 2729370 A

Low calorie, edible cellulose fibre product for human consumption contains corpuscular fibrous cellulose of average particle length <75 μm, the fibres being covered with an adherent soluble, smooth and palatable texture. The amt. of the exible gum comprises 2–15% of the fibrous cellulose.

Used as low calorie filler in foods, pharmaceuticals, etc. Low calorie and fat-free sour cream substitute, low calorie mayonnaise and margarine substitutes, etc. may be prepared with this prod. The prod. forms a stable, uniform gel-like suspension in water. The edible gum comprises sodium carboxymethyl cellulose, guar gum, xanthan gum or carob beam gum, etc.

Hydrocolloid—Misc. Low Calorie Foods 51

Stable jellied prods. from semi-manufactured fruit prods.—using xanthan, galactomannan, and pectin or water-sol., cellulose deriv.
Patent Assignee: BOCK W (BOCK-I)
Number of Countries: 001 Number of Patents: 001
Patent No Kind Date Applicat No Kind Date Main IPC Week
DD 121707 A 19760820 197641 B
Abstract (Basic): DD 121707 A

Jellied foods, esp. jams, preserves or jellies, are prepd. by heating liquid semi-manufactured fruit prods. with a pH esp. 2.5–3.5, with a jellying compsn. consisting of xanthan, galactomannan and pectin, or xanthan, galactomannan and a water-sol. cellulose hydrocolloid, in presence of saccharose and/or sugar substitute, followed by cooling to give a stable jellied prod. Prods. of high gel stability and high water-bonding capacity, with good clarity and brilliance are obtd. Low-calorie and dietetic foods can be prepd.

Hydrocolloid—Misc. Low Calorie Foods 52

Low calorie pasta prodn.—by adding polygalactomannan gum to vegetable protein and cereal material.
Patent Assignee: GEN MILLS INC (GENM)
Number of Countries: 002 Number of Patents: 002
Patent No Kind Date Applicat No Kind Date Main IPC Week
US 3843818 A 19741022 197444 B
CA 1016394 A 19770830 197737
Abstract (Basic): US 3843818 A

Title process comprises (a) mixing 15–50 pts. polygalacto-mannan gum, e.g., guar gum or locust bean gum, and 85–50 pts. of a mixt. of vegetable protein, e.g., vital gluten or soybean material and cereal material, e.g., durum flour, (b) adjusting the moisture content to 28–38 wt.% (c) working the hydrated mixt. in an extruder and raising the temp. to 55–98°C and (d) extruding to form a pasta. The moisture content of the product may be 80 wt.% and the calorie content reduced by ≥50% while the product has excellent taste and textural characteristics.

30

The Application of Complex Carbohydrates to Functional Food Development

SUSAN SUNGSOO CHO
The Kellogg Company, Battle Creek, Michigan

M. JENAB
University of Toronto, Toronto, Ontario, Canada

INTRODUCTION

"Let food be your medicine and medicine be your food"

Hippocrates, 400 BC (1)

Functional foods are defined as everyday foods and drinks that may provide identified health enhancing benefits due to their components (2,3). Japan is the birthplace of this concept and is so far the market leader in development and regulation of this emerging industry. The concept of functional foods has been adopted from the nutraceutical concept originated in the United States in the early 1980s after the Kellogg Company and the National Cancer Institute (NCI) made a joint campaign on the cancer preventive effects of certain types of fiber, in particular wheat bran fibers. NCI Stated on packages of All Bran, a wheat bran breakfast cereal, that certain types of dietary fiber help reduce the risk of certain types of cancer.

This campaign stimulated research into foods as an alternative medicine in prevention and the treatment of chronic diseases and the new concept on nutraceuticals was initiated to promote the development of foods of specified health benefits and to stimulate research activities in support of new product development. However, strict regulation by the U.S. Food and Drug Administration as well as the unavailability of an official process to implement such efforts have hindered the progress of marketing nutraceuticals in the U.S. However, Japan has modified the concept of nutraceuticals and has created the new concept ''functional foods'' or ''foods for specified use'' to improve the public health. It was possible since they created the third party association which can play a role between the industry and the government. The first functional food, now known as ''Yokult'' yoghurt, was developed in Japan in the 1930s and is currently consumed by over 23 million people worldwide (4). More such product successes will undoubtedly develop as the industry emerges from its infancy towards an estimated $100 billion worldwide market which translates to almost 5% of total food expenditure (2). Current markets for functional foods are estimated to be approximately 9, 28 and 30 billion dollars in the United States, Japan and European Union respectively.

The development of functional foods is driven by consumer lifestyle and attitude changes towards healthier eating. This is supported by both governments concerned about increasing health care costs of a growing and graying population and by constantly increasing knowledge and innovation on the link between nutrition and disease. After the establishment of the links between diet and disease, the development of functional foods aimed at reducing these risks and enhancing the diet seems only logical and natural in order to satisfy the growing consumer demands and interests that will develop. In fact, functional foods are the third generation of healthy foods to be placed on the market, following the introduction of products such as fruit juices and whole wheat bread in the mid-1970s and products with removed and lowered fat and sugar in the mid-1980s (4) all of which were also spurned due to increased consumer demand and technological and research advancements within the international food industry. Functional foods provide an ideal way in order to enact necessary dietary changes by providing a large variety of health conscious products that once carefully regulated, proven and trusted by consumers, will be used readily and effectively.

In general, functional foods fall into three categories: those that claim to reduce the risk of diseases such as coronary heart disease, cancer or diabetes; those that try to control or modulate immune function; and those that aim to improve or enhance mood and performance. Thus, the development of appropriate functional foods can have benefits to (a) the consumer, by enhancing their health and allowing longer, better and more productive lives, (b) governments, by reducing both health care costs and the burden on the system and (c) the industry, who research, develop and subsequently profit from products which are in high demand.

The development of functional foods relies heavily on the use of nutraceuticals, which are, according to the American Dietetic Association: ". . . substances that may be considered a food or part of a food and provide medical or health benefits, including the prevention and treatment of disease." (5) One such nutraceutical is dietary fiber, increased consumption of which may prevent a number of cancers (6), particularly colon cancer (7), as well as lowering cholesterol (8), important for coronary heart disease, and controlling blood sugar and insulin levels, of importance in diabetes (9). The need to increase the level of consumption of dietary fibers and the concomitant development of consumer friendly or palatable fibers and fiber mixtures along with consumer trends and increased pressures are pushing the development of more beneficial products containing high levels of dietary fibers or complex carbohydrates. Some examples of successful products containing these active ingredients are, in the UK: Ribena Fruit and Fiber, Fruit and Fiber Yoghurt, GAIO bioyoghurt and Shape Milk Drink; in Denmark: high oligosaccharide wine gums; and in France, high oligosaccharide smart drinks. Oligosaccharides, in particular resistant oligosaccharides, can be considered to be similar to fibers due to their indigestibility, increased fermentability and health benefits. They too can affect gut microflora, controlling the growth of undesirable bacterial strains while promoting the colonization by beneficial strains. In addition to soluble fibers, however, the oligosaccharides can also be employed as sweetening agents thus replacing sugars (10). These complex carbohydrates were the first functional ingredients. The ever-growing popularity of functional foods using these ingredients in Japan, Europe, and more recently in the United States, ensures that they will remain extremely important functional ingredients in the future.

FOOD PRODUCTION DEVELOPMENT PERSPECTIVES

The main reasons for the emergence of functional foods have come from three different avenues; first, from the consumer, who demands better and healthier products because of increased awareness and knowledge about nutrition and health in general; second, from governments, who are concerned about increased health care costs of populations that are increasingly living longer and getting older; and third, from the food industry who are anxious to apply new knowledge about nutrition and medicine to their products and to pursue opportunities in this sector. But different cultures and regions of the world may have varying perspectives and attitudes towards functional foods (2).

Functional food development essentially began in Japan, where functional foods have been welcomed and well accepted by eager consumers. For example, in Japan, functional beverage sales through vending machines rival those of soft drinks and beer. But these products may not be as popular in Western cultures (11). The Japanese approach to functional food development involves a thorough investigation of the safety and efficacy of the product as well as validity of the claims made. A close liaison between the government, industry, scientists, nutritionists and consumers takes place within a well developed legislative and regulatory framework (2).

Because of these varying perspectives of functional foods, the issues regarding business and product development in this sector differ between East and West. In Japan, the public acceptance and government/industry cooperation have allowed the quick development of a regulatory framework and thus of a multitude and large variety of functional food products, whereas in Europe and the United States, there is much debate on the need for or setup of any legislative and regulatory frameworks (2). Yet, despite this confused and complex situation in the West, many companies are trying to develop products with a single or overall health benefit in mind (2).

A central issue in functional food development is health claims. The opportunity to make health claims on foods can be a valuable marketing tool for the food industry in stimulating market growth and attracting consumer interest as well as allowing companies to gain a sustained competitive advantage. Since strong health claims carry important promises, a regulatory framework needs to clearly define if, when and how health claims can be made with a particular product and whether such claims need to be supported by extensive research to prove the efficacy as well as safety of the product (12). In general, the more health claims for foods move towards medical and physiological grounds, the greater the level of evidence that is required to support them.

In addition, if tougher health claim regulations become implemented, the product development and research costs will undoubtedly increase. At some point and with some products, the industry may find itself questioning whether the expense of developing functional food products is worthwhile. For example, if functional food health claims were to be supported in a system similar to the requirements for pharmaceuticals, it is estimated that a budget of a least $2 million would be required. Thus, ingredients which have already been extensively researched and tested for their beneficial effects may find great use in functional product development. For example, dietary fibers and complex carbohydrates have been the focus of decades of research throughout the world and are associated with a multitude of beneficial and healthful effects. Thus, existing or new fibers and fiber blends can and are being easily used in a wide variety of functional products such as bioyoghurts (oligosaccharides), high fiber breakfast cereals (wheat bran) and fiber enriched milk or soft drinks (polydextrose). In fact, in Japan, fiber rich drinks were the first commercially successful functional foods and dietary fibers and oligosaccharides are the two major ingredients currently used in functional foods (13).

Oligosaccharides can be used as functional ingredients for prebiotic or sweetening purposes. Some oligosaccharides used as functional ingredients, such as palatinose and coupling sugar, are digested completely and are absorbed from the small intestine. Other oligosaccharides, such as neosugar, however, are not hydrolyzed or poorly hydrolyzed in the small intestine and so reach the large intestine relatively intact. Once in the colon, they become active substrates for bacterial fermentation. It is this property that is associated with most of their health benefits (14,15).

There are also those oligosaccharides that improve the colonic bacterial milieu as well as providing energy for the host in the form of short chain fatty acids (SCFA). These SCFA also lower the pH in the lumen of the colon which promotes the growth of beneficial bacteria such as, Bifidobacterium and Lactobacillus, which are more resistant to an acidic environment, and decreases the numbers of less desirable and harmful bacteria such as Clostridium and Eubacterium strains (16,17). The beneficial strains of bacteria suppress the production of nitrogen derivatives (ammonia, indole), phenol and skatol and also decrease the production of potential carcinogens and mutagens due to their altered enzyme activities (18). Functionally, these oligosaccharides are perhaps the most important and have achieved wide use in functional food products in Japan and more increasingly in Europe and the United States (19). In fact, in Japan in 1996, of the 69 specific health use food items permitted by the Ministry of Health and Welfare, 40 use oligosaccharides such as neosugar, xylo-oligosaccharides, galacto-oligosaccharides, fructo-oligosaccharides, lacto-fructo-oligosaccharides, soybean oligosaccharides or isomalto-oligosaccharides (16). Currently, oligosaccharides are used widely in a variety of products in Japan, ranging from prebiotic soft drinks (Meiji Seika Co., Calpis Food Industry, Nichirei Co., Joban Yakuhin Kogyo Co., Asahi Breweries, Ostuka Pharmaceutical, Taisho Shokuhin Kogyo Co., Morinaga Milk Industry), table-top sweeteners (Meiji Seika Co., Hakubun Co., Calpis Food Industry, Taisho Pharmaceutical, Dainippon Seito Co., Showa Sangyo Co., Enuiko Sugar Co., Nissin Sugar Co., Nippon Oligo Co.), sugar confectionaries (Meiji Seika Co., Ezaki Glico Co.), chocolate confectionaries (Lotte Co., Ezaki Glico Co.), chewing gums (Lotte Co., Ezaki Glico Co.), biscuits (Ezaki Glico Co., Nippon Kayaku Co., Nippon Menado Katohin Co.), yoghurts (Suntory Co., Ezaki Glico Co., Takanashi Nyugyo Co., Morinaga Food Industry, Meiji Milk Products), vinegars (Morushige Ueda Co.), coffee drinks (Meiji Seika Co.), desserts (Meiji Milk Products), infant milk formulas and baby foods (Yakult Honsha Co.) (13).

Unlike Japan, the European consumer awareness of the benefits of oligosaccharides is much lower with between 3% (UK) to 16% (France) of survey respondents claiming to have heard of them (20) versus 70% in Japan (21). Only a few European products feature oligosaccharide ingredients. For example, a fermented milk drink called Fyos, launched in Belgium in 1994, and Fruit and Fiber Yoghurt sold by the Sainsbury chain in the UK both contain inulin, a functional oligosaccharide made from chicory (19). Much scientific evidence exists from a large number of international specialized university and corporate research centers to support the validity of these functions and also to document maximum allowable doses and the like (16). There are other benefits of oligosaccharides which as of yet do not merit functional claims due to the infancy of the experimentation levels. These effects, observed mostly for chicory oligosaccharides such as inulin, include improvement in the bioavailability of calcium, magnesium and iron as well as causing hypolipidemia (22). Thus oligosaccharides hold much promise as functional ingredients for current and future development of functional foods.

However perhaps the first functional ingredient was conventional dietary fiber ingredients which have historically been associated with various health benefits; wheat bran and psyllium in the prevention of constipation to prevention of colon cancer (6,7), improvement of glucose absorption (lowering of the glucose level and insulin response) (9), modulation of GI transit times, fecal bulking (23) and psyllium and oat bran in the prevention of cardiovascular disease and control of cholesterol bioavailability (8). Initially marketed with high success in bakery and cereal products, fiber sources such as polydextrose, added to milk and soft drinks are common practice in Japan (e.g. Fibe Mini from Otsuka Pharmaceutical, one of the most popular fiber functional drinks) and becoming popular in Europe where products such as Ribena Juice and Fiber (UK) have been extensively and successfully advertised and marketed with cholesterol lowering health claims (19). In Japan, the All Bran product, containing wheat bran (Nihon Kellogg Co.), was the first conventional dietary fiber product allowed to make a health claim. Dietary fibers have also been used in meat products such as sausages (Itoham Foods Co.), in pasta (Tokyo Tanebe Co.) and in soft drinks (Otsuka Pharmaceuticals, Pokka Corp., Fipro Seiyaku Co.). Dietary fibers commonly used in Japan are Wheat Bran, in the popular Kelloggs products, polydextrose, partially depolymerised guaran, indigestible dextrin, psyllium seed coat, pineapple fiber, konjak and tofu lees (13).

In the United States, awareness of the beneficial effects of fibers is increasing. The FDA now allows general health claims regarding the intake of foods containing certain amounts of dietary fiber and the risk of cancer and heart disease. Thus, functional products containing wheat bran and oat bran, classically associated with a decreased risk of colon cancer and heart disease respectively, will become more popular as awareness of the American public and acceptance of these products grows.

It is obvious that dietary fiber and oligosaccharides have become very popular functional ingredients. Thus, the functional food industry is dependent on a supply of these functional ingredients to be incorporated into functional foods. Such ingredients are produced from raw ingredients through either simple or very complex and often costly processing techniques. As the Japanese experience has clearly shown, their inclusion in the diet adds great value to a food by way of extra health benefits which attract consumer interest. This consumer interest has been a major driving factor in the functional food product development industry (24). The trends in the 1990's have been towards healthier natural and organic products such as low salt or low fat while the future trends in the next millennium are predicted to be towards health-enhancing, anti-cancer and preventative functional food products (24). Complex carbohydrates and dietary fibers are currently positioned as the major functional food ingredients and so the growth of this market will see an increase in the development and use of products containing them coupled to an increase in research about their benefits, necessary for the all important and sales driving health claims.

REGULATIONS, OPPORTUNITIES AND CONSTRAINTS

Japan

Regulation

In Japan, functional foods are regulated under the Foods for Specified Health Use (FOSHU). The legislation, brought about in 1991 due to a rise in the popularity of functional foods and due to concerns over the illegal marketing of some products, is an amendment to the Nutrition Improvement Law which was created shortly after World War II. In order to be licensed under FOSHU, a food must meet several criteria which will be discussed in detail later in the chapter. The FOSHU legislation licenses products with special dietary uses to bear a label claiming health promotion benefits (25). Often these claims are somewhat vague with statements such as ". . . need no anxiety on your decayed teeth? . . . ," ". . . useful for improving the dietary life of a person whose blood pressure is somewhat higher . . ." or ". . . it refreshes your intestines . . . ." However, foods making specific claims that they can prevent or treat disease are subject to regulation as medicines, which require much more supporting scientific data on the efficacy and safety of the product–a reasonable requirement. For example, the Kellogg's All Bran product is allowed under FOSHU to make the following claim: "Wheat bran is rich in dietary fiber, keeps your insides in good condition. A delicious food to refresh your body." The claim does not discuss the colon cancer protective effects of wheat bran which have been shown almost conclusively in a large number of international studies (7).

Constraints

FOSHU can be applied only to foods that have scientifically identified health benefits and not to isolated nutrients or supplements. FOSHU certification is not easy to obtain. Manufacturers must pass a stringent 3 stage approval process. This is easier for domestic manufacturers since they can use a self-regulated agency called the Japan Health Food Association (JHFA) to review the claimed health benefits of a product and to accelerate its approval. This is a major stumbling block for foreign manufacturers and food companies trying to access the volatile Japanese functional food market.

A second, perhaps more important constraint is that FOSHU accreditation will only be given to food products that can be consumed as part of the regular Japanese diet or in ''ordinary dietary patterns'' and have comparable nutrient compositions to similar foods. In other words, FOSHU controls foods traditionally found to be safe for consumption and to have ascertainable health benefits (26).

Despite this legislation, many problems, which are common throughout the world remain to be solved. These include: what distinguishes food from medicines, how to scientifically prove and judge the efficacy and safety of a product, how to monitor the appropriate marketing of a product or what type of a health claim to approve. It is clear that many of these constraints apply at the international level and so can best be considered and dealt with accordingly at that level.

Opportunities

Japan has a reasonable process for the approval of health claims and to provide a license to market the food product. This allows manufacturers some exclusivity and to gain a sustained competitive advantage by displaying an approved label to gain consumer confidence and trust. Despite the somewhat increased difficulty for foreign manufacturers to get FOSHU approval, this can be circumvented by forging partnerships and alliances with Japanese firms. Foreign firms may then seek membership in the JHFA which could then accelerate the approval of their product (26).

European Union

Legislation

Unlike Japan, the European Union has no regulation placing functional foods in a distinct food category. There is no legal definition for a functional food, let alone any regulations to deal with specific health claims. There has been some progress in government acceptance of the idea and concept of functional foods and the need for certain regulations and legislation particularly in the UK where the Ministry of Agriculture, Fisheries and Food has developed a working, but not legal, definition of a functional food (27). Similar to Japan, however, the European Union makes a clear distinction between food and medicine in that if specific health claims are made by a product suggesting that it can prevent, treat or cure disease, it must be dealt with as a medicine, thus requiring much more stringent regulation. There is debate over a distinction between a nutritional health claim and a medicinal health claim. The current legislation believes that the main function of a food is not to cure or prevent disease.

Constraints

The lack of a legal definition of functional foods and the delayed acceptance of functional foods as a separate category rather than an extension or better versions of current products are major constraints for the development of the functional foods industry in Europe. In addition, the lack of acceptance of health claims is also a major constraint for manufacturers. Although there is a European Union directive against health claims, it is up to member nations to adopt the directive or to legislate their own regulations. This causes a lack of harmonization where a product may be marketable in one area but not in another (26). The lack of appropriate and uniform legislation to cover functional foods may undermine consumer confidence and hurt the development of the functional foods market as manufacturers will be unwilling to invest in an unstable market.

Opportunities

Some health claims are being made in Europe mostly by high fiber breakfast cereals, probiotic dairy products, diabetic products and sports drinks (3). Opportunities exist for manufacturers willing to take the risk of marketing products only in certain regions and with selective labeling and careful advertising campaigns (26). As in Japan, opportunities exist with products historically or culturally associated with health benefits. This may allow the manufacturer to either make a subtle claim or to not make a claim at all.

The USA

Legislation

In the United States, as in Europe, there is no standard legislation governing nor even a direct definition of functional foods. The FDA only defines foods as articles used primarily for taste, aroma or nutritive value (28). However, the Nutrition Labeling Education Act (NLEA) may allow certain health claims as authorized by the FDA but only in the context of the whole diet, not just specific products, and only in cases where there is both strong available evidence and agreement among experts for a particular health benefit (27). The NLEA works to provide dietary recommendations to consumers by requiring that key sources of specific nutrients and their contribution to the recommended daily intake levels in every food product be identified on every pack (24). In addition, the NLEA defines terms such as light, low and reduced, commonly used by manufacturers to imply a healthier product. The act also regulates health claims that can be made by food products in relation to these terms and to their components. Currently in the United States, the FDA has authorized ten general health claims among which are those for intake of fiber containing grain products, fruits and vegetables and lowered cancer risk as well as intake of fiber containing grain products (especially soluble fiber, particularly from oat bran or oatmeal), fruits and vegetables and decreased coronary heart disease risk (29). However, the wording of these claims is very general.

Constraints

The biggest constraint to the growth of the U.S. functional food market is the lack of a definition and direct regulation of functional foods. In addition, the existing NLEA legislation requires strict and demanding scientific evidence for health claims of specific food or ingredients. In contrast, the DSHEA is a permissive piece of legislation than the NLEA. This disparity between the two may make the development and introduction of certain functional foods more challenging for the manufacturers.

Opportunities

In general the U.S. regulators seem to be accepting of functional foods and roles they can play in the health and well being of the American population. The FDA has mandated a Food Advisory Committee to debate the safety, efficacy and regulation of new food products, allowing expert input from industry, government, research institutions and organizations. This committee has often resulted in a consensus or strong majority of opinion and thus allowed the FDA to proceed more rapidly with approval of claims.

CONCLUSIONS

As research into the link between diet and disease intensifies, as newer links are found and old hypotheses proven, the educated public will demand high quality functional products and the food industry will meet their demands with new, popular, great tasting, safe, effective and health enhancing functional products. These large varieties of functional products will contain many functional ingredients and, as the Japanese experience shows, the bulk of these will be dietary fibers, oligosaccharides and other complex carbohydrates. Technological advancements in food science will allow the development of new fibers, fiber blends and oligosaccharides as well as more uses for existing ones. Thus, these ingredients will continue to play a vital role in functional product development throughout the world. The growing global functional food market will require international standardization and firm regulation of health claims, not only to protect the consumer from fraudulent claims but also to allow manufacturers to effectively develop, prove and market their products. The development of such legislation is critical for the global functional foods market which is still in its infancy.

Whoever gives these things [foods] no consideration and is ignorant of them, how can he understand the diseases of man?

Hippocrates, 400 BC (1)

REFERENCES

1. Jones, WHS. (1932) Hippocrates, p. 351.
2. Potter, D. (1996) Personal communication.
3. Young, J. (1997) Future opportunities for functional foods. Food Manufacture 70, 63.
4. Young, J. (1996) A perspective on functional foods. Food Science and Technol. 10, 18–21.
5. Anonymous. (1995) Position of the American Dietetic Association: phytochemicals and functional foods. J Am Diet Assoc. 95, 493–496.
6. Kritchevsky, D. (1996) Diet in heart disease and cancer. Adv Expt Med Bio 369, 201–209.
7. Wynder, EL., Reddy, BS., and Weisburger JH. (1992) Environmental dietary factors in colon cancer: some unresolved issues. Cancer 70, 1222–1228.
8. Anderson, JW. (1995) Dietary fiber, complex carbohydrate and coronary heart disease. Can J Cardiology 11Suppl.,55G–62G.
9. Nuttall, FQ. (1993) Dietary fiber in the management of diabetes. Diabetes 42, 503–508.
10. Blenford, D. (1995) Trends in functional foods and ingredients. Food Tech Europe, Dec 1995, 24–28.
11. Hollingsworth, P. (1995) Functional foods: fad or fact? Food Technology, 49, 32–35.
12. Brown, KS. (1996) Functional foods: a fruitful research field, but various regulatory obstacles persist. Scientist 10, 1–8.
13. Anonymous. (1997) Functional foods and drinks in Japan. JapanScan Food Industry Bulletin, Stratford-on-Avon, England.
14. Oku, T. (1994) Special physiological functions of newly developed mono- and oligosaccharides. In: Goldberg, I. (ed), Functional foods. New York, Chapman & Hall, 202–218.
15. Oku, T. (1992) Dietary fiber and new sugars. In: Baba, S., Akerele, O., Kawaguchi, Y. (eds). Natural resources and human health. Amsterdam, Elsevier, 159–170.
16. Oku, T. (1996) Oligosaccharides with beneficial health effects: a Japanese perspective. Nutrition Reviews 54Suppl., S59–S66.
17. Kumemura, M., Hashimoto, F., and Fiji, C. (1992) Effects of administration of 4G-B-D-galactosylsucrose on fecal microflora, putrefactive products, short-chain fatty acis, weight, moisture and pH, and subjective sensation of defecation in the elderly with constipation. J Clin Biochem Nutr 13, 199–210.
18. Gorbach, SL., and Goldin, BR. (1992) Nutrition and the gastrointestinal microflora. Nutrition Reviews 50, 378–381.
19. Hilliam, M. (1996) Functional foods: the Western consumer viewpoint. Nutrition Reviews 54Suppl., S189–S194.

20. Cathro, JS., and Hilliam, M. (1993) Future opportunities for functional and healthy foods in Europe: an in-depth consumer and market analysis. Leatherhead Food Research Association Multiclient Study.
21. Anonymous. (1993) Consumer survey on new foods. Japanscan 8, 16.
22. Roberfroid, MB. (1996) Functional effects of food components and the gastrointestinal system: chicory fructo-oligosaccharides. Nutrition Reviews 54Suppl., S38–S42.
23. Eastwood, MA. (1992) The physiological effect of dietary fiber: an update. Annu Rev Nutr 12:19–35.
24. Datamonitor (1996) Innovation on food ingredients. NY, NY.
25. Kojima, K. (1996) The Eastern consumer viewpoint: the experience in Japan. Nutrition Reviews 54Suppl., S186–S188.
26. Smith, BL., Marcotte, M., and Harrison, G. (1996) A comparative analysis of the regulatory framework affecting functional food development and commercialization in Canada, Japan, the European Union and the United States of America. Personal communication.
27. Richardson, DP. (1996) Functional foods–shades of gray: an industry perspective. Nutrition Reviews 54Suppl., S174–S185.
28. Federal Food, Drug and Cosmetic Act. (1938) 52 Stat 111.
29. Anonymous. (1993) The FDA's final regulations on health claims for foods. Nutrition Reviews 51, 90–93.
30. Federal Food, Drug and Cosmetic Act. (1938) 52 Stat 1040.
31. Hasler, CM. (1996) Functional foods: the Western perspective. Nutrition Reviews 54 Suppl., S6–S10.

Appendix I

Perspectives on Dietary Fiber Definition*

Consumer interest and public policy on dietary fiber has recently changed. The definition and method for determination of dietary fiber have evolved in Western countries over the past two decades. In the United States, the Food and Drug Amdinistration (FDA) and U.S. Department of Agriculture (USDA) issued final food labeling regulations in January 1993 (1,2). The regulations have mandated the labeling of dietary fiber with optional breakdown of soluble and insoluble dietary fiber on food packages. For nutritional labeling, AACC Methods 32-05 (corresponding to AOAC Method 985.29) and 32-07 (AOAC Method 991.43) (3–5) have been recommended for dietary fiber analysis by both agencies (1,2). Europe, the protocols for dietary fiber labeling are still being developed for the European common market.

It is important that regulatory agencies, researchers in nutritin and analytical areas, industry representatives, consumers, and health professionals have a common understanding of the definition of dietary fiber. The analytical methodologies should be developed and imporved to meet that definition.

Thus, we conducted two international surveys to determine wether a consenusus could be reached on the definition of dietary fiber and associated methodologies and to consider appropriate classification of oligosaccharides that are not

* Reprinted with permission from Cereal Foods World and American Association of Cereal Chemists, Inc. 1994.

hydrolyzed by human alimentary enzymes. Results of the survey should help international harmonization of acceptable definitions of dietary fiber and its components. The survey results will also provide insight for chemissts seeking to modify analytical methods and develop reference materials to meet the accepted definition.

In our first survey, initiated in December 1992, 144 professionals participated, representing 30 countries (3). Seventy percent of participants responded that the dietary fiber definition should reflect both chemical and physiological perspectives. The survey results indicated that 65% of respondents supported the current dietary fiber definition as polysaccharides and lignin that are not hydrolyzed by human alimentary exzymes. However, 59% supported the future expansion of the dietary fiber definition to include oligosaccharides that are resistant to hydrolysis by human alimentary exzymes.

Because inclusion of these unavailable oligosaccharides in the definition may influence future nutrition labeling and food technology research, a follow-up survey was sent in December 1993 along with the results form the first survey to find out if the first survey results could be confirmed. We specifically addressed the issure of the new definition that may include oligosaccharides that are not hydrolyzed by human alimentary enzymes. In the second survey (122 persons, representing 30 countries), 65% of the participants supported the inclusion of these oligosaccharides. Eighty percent supported the inclusion of resistant starches and lignin in addition to non-starch polysaccharides in the dietary fiber definition. It is noteworthy that 6% believed dietary fiber includes only non-starch polysaccharides or plant cell wall components (3). It appears that there is general agreement that the chemical entity of dietary fiber is not limited to nonstarch polysaccharides and plant cell wall components.

It is noteworthy that 78% of respondents believe the term *dietary fiber* should be preserved (3). Eighteen percent supported abolishing the term dietary fiber. It appears that scientists generally believe that the term dietary fiber should continue to be used in the scientific literature, although the exact definition of dietary fiber can evolve and be modified as long as scientific findings support such modifications.

Based on these scientific findings, we have propoed (5,6) the expansion of the definiton of dietray fiber to include resistant oligosaccharides, in addition to currently included nonstarch polysaccharides, resistant starch, and lignin. We have also proposed a new term, *resistant oligosaccharides*, which is defined as oligosaccharides that are resistant to hydrolysis by human alimentary enzymes (6). Tentatively, we propose that a minimum degree of polymerization (DP) unit for resistant oligosaccharides should be 3 or above. We want to point out that an exact cut-off DP unit can be developed in the future as a more common understanding on resistant oligosaccharides evolves. The term resistant oligosaccharides can be used synonymously with the term *unavailable oligosaccharides*.

Our proposals on the new dietary fiber difinition and the new term, resistant oligosaccharides, have been well received at the Sixth International Symposium on Biological and Environmental Reference Materials (7) and at the European dietary fiber symposium (8).

The addition of resistant oligosaccharides to the dietary fiber definition may open new avenues in the nutitional, analytical, and food technology research areas. Along this line, a common understanding on resistant oligosaccharides should be developed. We expect that certain types of oligosaccharides can be claimed for dietary fiber in the future, if the unavailability in the healthy human upper gastrointestinal tract and the resulting pyhsiological actions similar to other dietary fiber components are fully proven. We want to point out that oligosaccharides that are hydrolyzed in the upper GI tract of normal, healthy human subjects, such as lactose, maltotriose, and maltotetrose, cannot be classified as resistant oligosaccharides. It is noteworthy that most of the foods in today's market do not contain resistant oligosaccharides, with the exception of a few formulations, but new product development efforts as well as nutrition research could evolve. Along this line, analytical methodology should be fine tuned to fully recover resistant oligosaccharides as well as resistant starch in the dietary fiber analysis. In a previous article (9), we addressed the issue of incomplete recovery of resistant starch with the current dietary fiber methods. Until a reliable methodology is developed to meet the new definition of dietary fiber, currrent dietary fiber methods should continue to be used for dietary fiber labeling (9). We want to emphasize that this new definition would not affect the dietary fiber values of most food products.

REFERENCES

1. Food and Drug Administration. Food labeling, general provisions. Nutrition labeling. Label format. Nutrient content claims. Ingredient labeling state and local requirements. Exemptions, final rules. Fe. Reg. 58:2302, 1993.
2. Department of Agriculture. Food labeling, general provisions. Nutrition labeling. Label format. Nutrient content claims. Ingredient labeling, state and local requirements. Exemptions, final rules. Fed. Reg. 58:631, 1993
3. AACC Mehod 32-05, Total dietary fiber, app. October 1991; Mehtod 32-07, Determination of soluble, insoluble, and total dietary fiber in foods and food products, app. October 1991. *Approved Methods of the American Association of Cereal Chemists,* 8th ed. The Association, St. Paul, MN, 1983.
4. Prosky, L., Asp, N.-G., Schweizer, T. F., DeVries, J. W., and Furda, I. Determination of insoluble, soluble, and total dietary fiber in foods and food products: Interlaboratory study. J. Assoc. Off. Anal. Chem. 71:1017, 1988.
5. Lee, S. C., Prosky, L., and DeVries, J. W. Determination of insoluble, soluble, and total dietary fiber in foods: Collaborative study. J. AOAC Int. 75:395, 1992.

6. Lee, S. C., and Prosky, L. International survey on dietary fiber definition, analysis, and reference materials. J. AOAC Int. 79:in press.
7. Lee, S. C., and Prosky, L. International survey on dietary fiber reference materials. (Abstr.) Sixth Int. Symp. Biol. Environ. Ref. Materials, 1994.
8. Lee, S. C., and Prosky, L. International survey on dietary fiber definition. (Abstr.) Symp. Mech. Dietary Fiber Action, 1994.
9. Lee, S. C., and Prosky, L. Dietary fiber analysis for nutrition labeling. Cereal Foods World 37:765, 1992.

Appendix II

Total Carbohydrates and Total Dietary Fiber Content in Grain-Based Foods*

BAKERY

	Water	Carb.	% TDF	% FAT
Bagels, cinnamon-raisin	32	55.2	2.3	1.7
Bagels, cinnamon-raisin, toasted	26.9	59.3	2.5	1.8
Bagels, egg	32.7	53	2.3	2.1
Bagels, egg, toasted	27.7	57	2.5	2.2
Bagels, oat bran	32.9	53.3	3.6	1.2
Bagels, oat bran, toasted	27.9	57.3	3.8	1.3
Bagels, plain, enriched, with calcium propionate (includes onion, poppy, sesame)	32.6	53.4	2.3	1.6
Bagels, plain, enriched, without calcium propionate (includes onion, poppy, sesame)	32.6	53.4	2.1	1.6
Bagels, plain, toasted, enriched, with calcium propionate (includes onion, poppy, sesame)	27.6	57.5	2.5	1.7
Bagels, plain, toasted, enriched, without calcium propionate (includes onion, poppy, sesame)	27.6	57.5	2.5	1.7
Bagels, plain, toasted, unenriched, with calcium propionate (includes onion, poppy, sesame)	27.6	57.5		1.7
Bagels, plain, toasted, unenriched, without calcium propionate (includes onion, poppy, sesame)	27.6	57.5		1.7
Bagels, plain, unenriched, with calcium propionate (includes onion, poppy, sesame)	32.6	53.4	2.1	1.6
Bagels, plain, unenriched, without calcium propionate(includes onion, poppy, sesame)	32.6	53.4	2.1	1.6
Biscuits, mixed grain, refrigerated dough	37.8	47.4		5.6
Biscuits, mixed grain, refrigerated dough, baked	27.7	55.1	2.6	6.5

* Adopted from USDA Handbook No. 8 Electronic Release 11, 1997.

Biscuits, plain or buttermilk, commercially baked	26.7	48.5	1.3	16.5
Biscuits, plain or buttermilk, dry mix	9.2	63.3	2.1	15.4
Biscuits, plain or buttermilk, dry mix, prepared	28.9	48.4	1.8	12.1
Biscuits, plain or buttermilk, prepared from recipe	28.9	44.6	1.5	16.3
Biscuits, plain or buttermilk, refrigerated dough, higher fat	33.6	43.7	1.5	13.5
Biscuits, plain or buttermilk, refrigerated dough, higher fat, baked	27.8	47.5	1.6	14.7
Biscuits, plain or buttermilk, refrigerated dough, lower fat	37.9	47.6	1.6	4.5
Biscuits, plain or buttermilk, refrigerated dough, lower fat, baked	27.7	55.4	1.9	5.2
Bread crumbs, dry, grated, plain	6.2	72.5	2.4	5.4
Bread crumbs, dry, grated, seasoned	5.6	70.4	4.2	2.6
Bread sticks, plain	6.1	68.4	3	9.5
Bread stuffing, bread, dry mix	4.2	76.2	3.2	3.4
Bread stuffing, bread, dry mix, prepared	64.8	21.7	2.9	8.6
Bread stuffing, cornbread, dry mix	4.6	76.7	14.3	4.2
Bread stuffing, cornbread, dry mix, prepared	64.9	21.9	2.9	8.8
Bread stuffing, plain, prepared from recipe	65.2	22.2		7.2
Bread, banana, prepared from recipe, made with margarine	29.2	54.6	1.1	10.5
Bread, banana, prepared from recipe, made with vegetable shortening	27.8	55.1		11.8
Bread, Boston brown, canned	47.2	43.3	4.7	1.5
Bread, cornbread, dry mix, enriched (includes corn muffin mix)	7.8	69.5	6.5	12.2
Bread, cornbread, dry mix, prepared	31.9	48.1	2.4	10
Bread, cornbread, dry mix, unenriched (includes corn muffin mix)	7.8	69.5	6.4	12.2
Bread, cornbread, prepared from recipe, made with low fat (2%) milk	39.1	43.5		7.1
Bread, cornbread, prepared from recipe, made with whole milk	38.6	43.5	3.5	7.7
Bread, cracked-wheat	35.8	49.5	5.5	3.9
Bread, cracked-wheat, toasted	30.2	53.8	6	4.2
Bread, egg	34.7	47.8	2.3	6
Bread, egg, toasted	28.3	52.6	2.5	6.6
Bread, French or Vienna (includes sourdough)	34.3	51.9	3	3
Bread, French or Vienna, toasted (includes sourdough)	28.6	56.4	3.3	3.3
Bread, Indian (navajo) fry	26.5	53.3	1.8	9.5
Bread, Irish soda, prepared from recipe	30.1	56	2.6	5
Bread, Italian	35.7	50	2.7	3.5
Bread, Italian, toasted	29.4	55	2.9	3.9
Bread, mixed-grain (includes whole-grain, 7-grain)	37.7	46.4	6.4	3.8
Bread, mixed-grain, toasted (includes whole-grain, 7-grain)	32.3	50.4	6.6	4.1
Bread, oat bran	44	39.8	4.5	4.4
Bread, oat bran, toasted	38.5	43.7	4.9	4.8

Bread, oatmeal	36.7	48.5	4	4.4
Bread, oatmeal, toasted	31.2	52.7	4.3	4.8
Bread, pita, white, enriched	32.1	55.7	2.2	1.2
Bread, pita, white, unenriched	32.1	55.7	1.6	1.2
Bread, pita, whole-wheat	30.6	55	7.4	2.6
Bread, protein (includes gluten)	40	43.8	3	2.2
Bread, protein, toasted (includes gluten)	34	48.1	3.3	2.4
Bread, pumpernickel	37.9	47.5	6.5	3.1
Bread, pumpernickel, toasted	31.8	52.2	7.1	3.4
Bread, pumpkin, prepared from recipe	30.8	51.2		12.8
Bread, raisin, enriched	33.6	52.3	4.3	4.4
Bread, raisin, toasted, enriched	27.8	56.9	4.7	4.8
Bread, raisin, toasted, unenriched	27.8	56.9		4.8
Bread, raisin, unenriched	33.6	52.3		4.4
Bread, reduced-calorie, oat bran	46	41.3	12	3.2
Bread, reduced-calorie, oat bran, toasted	35.7	49.2	14.3	3.8
Bread, reduced-calorie, oatmeal	44	43.3		3.5
Bread, reduced-calorie, oatmeal, toasted	33.3	51.5		4.2
Bread, reduced-calorie, rye	46	40.5	12	2.9
Bread, reduced-calorie, rye, toasted	35.7	48.2		3.4
Bread, reduced-calorie, wheat	43.2	43.6	12	2.3
Bread, reduced-calorie, wheat, toasted	32.4	51.9		2.7
Bread, reduced-calorie, white	42.9	44.3	9.7	2.5
Bread, reduced-calorie, white, toasted	32	52.7		3
Bread, rice bran	41	43.5	4.9	4.6
Bread, rice bran, toasted	35.9	47.3	5.3	5
Bread, rye	37.3	48.3	5.8	3.3
Bread, rye, toasted	31	53.1	6.4	3.6
Bread, wheat (includes wheat berry)	37.1	47.2	4.3	4.1
Bread, wheat bran	37.8	47.8	4	3.4
Bread, wheat bran, toasted	31.6	52.5	4.4	3.7
Bread, wheat germ	37.1	48.3	2.078	2.9
Bread, wheat germ, toasted	29.3	54.3	2.336	3.3
Bread, wheat, toasted (includes wheat berry)	31.6	51.3	5.3	4.4
Bread, white, commercially prepared (includes soft bread crumbs)	36.7	49.5	2.3	3.6
Bread, white, commercially prepared, low sodium no salt	36.7	49.5	2.4	3.6
Bread, white, commercially prepared, toasted	30.4	54.4	2.5	4
Bread, white, commercially prepared, toasted, low sodium no salt	30.4	54.4		4
Bread, white, prepared from recipe, made with low fat (2%) milk	35.3	49.6	2	5.7
Bread, white, prepared from recipe, made with low fat (2%) milk, toasted	28.9	54.5	2.2	6.3
Bread, white, prepared from recipe, madc with nonfat dry milk	34.8	53.6	2	2.6
Bread, white, prepared from recipe, made with nonfat dry milk, toasted	28.3	58.9		2.9

Bread, white, prepared from recipe, made with whole milk	34.8	49.6		6.2
Bread, white, prepared from recipe, made with whole milk, toasted	28.4	54.5		6.9
Bread, whole-wheat, commercially prepared	37.7	46.1	6.9	4.2
Bread, whole-wheat, commercially prepared, toasted	30	51.7	7.4	4.8
Bread, whole-wheat, prepared from recipe	32.7	51.4	6	5.4
Bread, whole-wheat, prepared from recipe, toasted	26	56.4	6.7	5.9
Cake, angelfood, commercially prepared	33.2	57.8	1.5	0.8
Cake, angelfood, dry mix	2.8	85.1	0.31	0.4
Cake, angelfood, dry mix, prepared	32.9	58.7	0.216	0.3
Cake, angelfood, prepared from recipe	31.8	59.5		0.1
Cake, Boston cream pie, commercially prepared	45.4	42.9	1.4	8.5
Cake, Boston cream pie, prepared from recipe	34.5	46.2		13.2
Cake, carrot, dry mix, pudding-type	3.6	79.2		9.8
Cake, carrot, dry mix, pudding-type, prepared without frosting	30.9	46.7	2.038	15.7
Cake, carrot, prepared from recipe with cream cheese frosting	20.6	47.2	1.2	26.4
Cake, cherry fudge with chocolate frosting	46.1	38	1.23	12.5
Cake, chocolate, commercially prepared with chocolate frosting	22.9	54.6	2.8	16.4
Cake, chocolate, dry mix, pudding-type	3.9	78.7	3.48	9.2
Cake, chocolate, dry mix, pudding-type, prepared without frosting	30.2	44.4	1.951	18.6
Cake, chocolate, dry mix, regular	3.1	73	2.4	15.6
Cake, chocolate, dry mix, regular, prepared without frosting	32	49	2.2	11.7
Cake, chocolate, dry mix, special dietary	4.8	77.6		9.8
Cake, chocolate, dry mix, special dietary, prepared without frosting	24.4	60.6		7.7
Cake, chocolate, prepared from recipe without frosting	24.4	53.4	1.6	15.1
Cake, fruitcake, commercially prepared	25.3	61.6	3.7	9.1
Cake, fruitcake, prepared from recipe	18.6	64.8		11.5
Cake, German chocolate, dry mix, pudding-type	3.6	80.1	3.5	9.5
Cake, German chocolate, dry mix, pudding-type, prepared with coconut-nut frosting	26.9	49.7	1.367	18.6
Cake, gingerbread, dry mix	4.4	74.6	1.7	13.8
Cake, gingerbread, dry mix, prepared	33.1	50.7	1.16	10.2
Cake, gingerbread, prepared from recipe	28	49.2		16.4
Cake, marble, dry mix, pudding-type	3.1	79.3	2.9	11.7
Cake, marble, dry mix, pudding-type, prepared without frosting	29.8	47.3	1.725	17
Cake, pineapple upside-down, prepared from recipe	32.3	50.5	0.8	12.1
Cake, pound, commercially prepared, butter	24.6	48.8	0.496	19.9
Cake, pound, commercially prepared, fat-free	31	61	1.1	1.2
Cake, pound, commercially prepared, other than all butter, enriched	23.1	52.5	1	17.9
Cake, pound, commercially prepared, other than all butter, unenriched	23.1	52.5	1	17.9

Cake, pound, prepared from recipe, modified, made with butter	23.3	52.6		16.7
Cake, pound, prepared from recipe, modified, made with margarine	23.3	52.8		16.6
Cake, pound, prepared from recipe, old-fashioned, made with butter	20.4	47.6		24.7
Cake, pound, prepared from recipe, old-fashioned, made with margarine	20.3	47.8		24.5
Cake, shortcake, biscuit-type, prepared from recipe	28.4	48.5		14.2
Cake, snack cakes, creme-filled, chocolate with frosting	19.8	60.3	0.8	14.5
Cake, snack cakes, creme-filled, sponge	20.2	63.9	0.416	11.4
Cake, snack cakes, cupcakes, chocolate, with frosting, low-fat	22.8	67.2	4.3	3.7
Cake, sponge, commercially prepared	29.7	61.1	0.549	2.7
Cake, sponge, prepared from recipe	29.4	57.7		4.3
Cake, white, dry mix, pudding-type, enriched	3.5	81	0.7	9.5
Cake, white, dry mix, pudding-type, prepared without frosting	28.4	51.7	0.449	14.8
Cake, white, dry mix, pudding-type, unenriched	3.5	81		9.5
Cake, white, dry mix, regular	4	78	0.93	10.9
Cake, white, dry mix, regular, prepared without frosting	30.8	55.4	0.662	7.7
Cake, white, dry mix, special dietary (includes lemon-flavored)	6	79.6		8.4
Cake, white, dry mix, special dietary, prepared without frosting	26.4	61.3	0.61	6.5
Cake, white, prepared from recipe with coconut frosting	20.7	63.2	1	10.3
Cake, white, prepared from recipe without frosting	23.3	57.2	0.8	12.4
Cake, yellow, commercially prepared, with chocolate frosting	21.9	55.4	1.8	17.4
Cake, yellow, commercially prepared, with vanilla frosting	22.1	58.8	0.321	14.5
Cake, yellow, dry mix, light	3.1	84.1	1.3	5.5
Cake, yellow, dry mix, light, prepared no frosting, 3% fat	37.1	53.4	0.8	3.5
Cake, yellow, dry mix, light, prepared no frosting, 6% fat	34.4	53.2	0.8	5.3
Cake, yellow, dry mix, pudding-type	4	79.9	0.72	9.8
Cake, yellow, dry mix, pudding-type, prepared without frosting	30	48.1	0.428	15.9
Cake, yellow, dry mix, regular, enriched	3.7	78.1	1.1	11.6
Cake, yellow, dry mix, regular, prepared without frosting	29.8	54.4	0.8	9.4
Cake, yellow, dry mix, regular, unenriched	3.7	78.1		11.6
Cake, yellow, prepared from recipe without frosting	25.1	53	0.7	14.6
Cheesecake commercially prepared	45.6	25.5	0.42	22.5
Cheesecake prepared from mix, no-bake type	44.2	35.5	1.9	12.7
Cheesecake prepared from recipe	40.9	25.2		26

Cheesecake, plain, prepared from recipe, with cherry topping	49.2	26.5		18.5
Coffeecake, cheese	32.2	44.3	1	15.2
Coffeecake, cinnamon with crumb topping, commercially prepared, enriched	21.9	46.7	2	23.3
Coffeecake, cinnamon with crumb topping, commercially prepared, unenriched	21.9	46.7	3.3	23.3
Coffeecake, cinnamon with crumb topping, dry mix	3.3	77.7	1.82	12
Coffeecake, cinnamon with crumb topping, dry mix, prepared	30.5	52.8	1.199	9.6
Coffeecake, cinnamon with crumb topping, prepared from recipe	21	50.3		20.2
Coffeecake, creme-filled with chocolate frosting	29.1	53.8	2	10.8
Coffeecake, fruit	31.7	51.5	2.5	10.2
Cookies, animal crackers (includes arrowroot, tea biscuits,)	3.9	74.1	1.1	13.8
Cookies, brownies, commercially prepared	13.6	63.9	2.1	16.3
Cookies, brownies, dry mix, regular	2.8	76.6		14.9
Cookies, brownies, dry mix, regular, prepared	13	61.7	2.824	19.9
Cookies, brownies, dry mix, special dietary	3.5	80.4	4.2	12.5
Cookies, brownies, dry mix, special dietary, prepared	13	71.3	3.7	11.1
Cookies, brownies, prepared from recipe	12.6	50.2		29.1
Cookies, butter, commercially prepared, enriched	4.6	68.9	0.75	18.8
Cookies, butter, commercially prepared, unenriched	4.6	68.9	2.4	18.8
Cookies, chocolate chip, commercially prepared, reg, higher fat, enriched	4.1	66.8	2.5	22.6
Cookies, chocolate chip, commercially prepared, reg, higher fat, unenriched	4.1	66.8	2.5	22.6
Cookies, chocolate chip, commercially prepared, regular, lower fat	4.1	73.3	3.6	15.4
Cookies, chocolate chip, commercially prepared, soft-type	11.6	59.1	3.2	24.3
Cookies, chocolate chip, commercially prepared, special dietary	5.1	73.4	1.59	16.8
Cookies, chocolate chip, dry mix	3	66.1		25.2
Cookies, chocolate chip, dry mix, prepared	3.6	64.1	1.382	25.4
Cookies, chocolate chip, prepared from recipe, made with butter	5.7	58.2		28.4
Cookies, chocolate chip, prepared from recipe, made with margarine	5.7	58.4	2.8	28.3
Cookies, chocolate chip, refrigerated dough	12.7	61.4	1.49	20.4
Cookies, chocolate chip, refrigerated dough, baked	3	68.2	1.652	22.6
Cookies, chocolate sandwich, with creme filling, regular	2.3	70.3	3.2	20.6
Cookies, chocolate sandwich, with creme filling, regular, chocolate-coated	2	66.1	5.15	26.4
Cookies, chocolate sandwich, with creme filling, special dietary	4.2	67.7	4.14	22.1
Cookies, chocolate sandwich, with extra creme filling	1.6	68.1	2	25.2
Cookies, chocolate wafers	4.5	72.4	3.4	14.2

Cookies, coconut macaroons, prepared from recipe	10.6	72.2	1.8	12.7
Cookies, fig bars	16.5	70.9	4.6	7.3
Cookies, fortune	8	84	1.6	2.7
Cookies, fudge, cake-type (includes trolley cakes)	11.8	78.3	2.752	3.7
Cookies, gingersnaps	5.3	76.9	2.2	9.8
Cookies, graham crackers, chocolate-coated	2.6	66.5	3.1	23.2
Cookies, graham crackers, plain or honey (includes cinnamon)	4.4	76.8	2.8	10.1
Cookies, ladyfingers, with lemon juice and rind	19.5	59.7	1	9.1
Cookies, ladyfingers, without lemon juice and rind	19.5	59.7		9.1
Cookies, marshmallow, chocolate-coated (includes marshmallow pies)	10.1	67.7	2	16.9
Cookies, molasses	5.8	73.8	0.95	12.8
Cookies, oatmeal, commercially prepared, fat-free	12.5	78.6	7.3	1.5
Cookies, oatmeal, commercially prepared, regular	5.7	68.7	2.8	18.1
Cookies, oatmeal, commercially prepared, soft-type	11	65.7	2.7	14.7
Cookies, oatmeal, commercially prepared, special dietary	6.5	69.9	2.87	18
Cookies, oatmeal, dry mix	5.3	67.3		19.2
Cookies, oatmeal, dry mix, prepared	5.9	65.3	3.885	19.5
Cookies, oatmeal, prepared from recipe, with raisins	6.4	68.4		16.2
Cookies, oatmeal, prepared from recipe, without raisins	6.2	66.4		17.9
Cookies, oatmeal, refrigerated dough	15.3	59.1	2.51	18.9
Cookies, oatmeal, refrigerated dough, baked	5.8	65.7	2.787	21
Cookies, peanut butter sandwich, regular	2.8	65.6	1.9	21.1
Cookies, peanut butter sandwich, special dietary	3.7	50.8		34
Cookies, peanut butter, commercially prepared, regular	6.1	58.9	1.8	23.6
Cookies, peanut butter, commercially prepared, soft-type	11.5	57.7	1.7	24.4
Cookies, peanut butter, prepared from recipe	5.9	58.9		23.8
Cookies, peanut butter, refrigerated dough	12.6	52.1	1.14	25
Cookies, peanut butter, refrigerated dough, baked	4	57.3	1.248	27.5
Cookies, raisin, soft-type	13.1	68	1.2	13.6
Cookies, shortbread, commercially prepared, pecan	3.3	58.3	1.8	32.5
Cookies, shortbread, commercially prepared, plain	3.7	64.5	1.8	24.1
Cookies, shortbread, prepared from recipe, made with butter	3.1	56		33.4
Cookies, shortbread, prepared from recipe, made with margarine	3	56.4		33.2
Cookies, sugar wafers with creme filling, regular	1	70.1	0.6	24.3
Cookies, sugar wafers with creme filling, special dietary	4.4	66		25.7
Cookies, sugar, commercially prepared, regular (includes vanilla)	4.8	67.9	0.762	21.1
Cookies, sugar, commercially prepared, special dietary	5.7	76.8	0.89	13
Cookies, sugar, prepared from recipe, made with butter	8.9	59.8		23.6
Cookies, sugar, prepared from recipe, made with margarine	8.9	60	1.2	23.4
Cookies, sugar, refrigerated dough	14.5	59	0.68	20.7
Cookies, sugar, refrigerated dough, baked	5	65.6	0.8	23.1

Cookies, vanilla sandwich with creme filling	2.2	72.1	1.5	20
Cookies, vanilla wafers, higher fat	4.2	71.1	2	19.4
Cookies, vanilla wafers, lower fat	5.1	73.6	1.9	15.2
Cracker meal	7.6	80.9	2.56	1.7
Crackers, cheese, low sodium	3.1	58.2	2.4	25.3
Crackers, cheese, regular	3.1	58.2	2.4	25.3
Crackers, cheese, sandwich-type with peanut butter filling	3.8	57	2.82	23.2
Crackers, crispbread, rye	6.1	82.2	16.5	1.3
Crackers, matzo, egg	6.4	78.6	2.798	2.1
Crackers, matzo, egg and onion	7.2	77.1	5	3.9
Crackers, matzo, plain	4.3	83.7	3	1.4
Crackers, matzo, whole-wheat	4.8	78.9	11.8	1.5
Crackers, melba toast, plain	5.1	76.6	6.3	3.2
Crackers, melba toast, plain, without salt	5.1	76.6	6.3	3.2
Crackers, melba toast, rye (includes pumpernickel)	4.9	77.3	8	3.4
Crackers, melba toast, wheat	5.5	76.4	7.4	2.3
Crackers, milk	4.7	69.7	1.92	15.8
Crackers, rusk toast	5.5	72.3		7.2
Crackers, rye, sandwich-type with cheese filling	3.8	60.8	3.585	22.3
Crackers, rye, wafers, plain	5	80.4	22.89	0.9
Crackers, rye, wafers, seasoned	4	73.8	20.897	9.2
Crackers, saltines (includes oyster, soda, soup)	4.1	71.5	3	11.8
Crackers, saltines, fat-free, low-sodium	3.4	82.3	2.7	1.6
Crackers, saltines, low salt (includes oyster, soda, soup)	4.1	71.5	3	11.8
Crackers, saltines, unsalted tops (includes oyster, soda, soup)	4.1	71.5	2.7	11.8
Crackers, standard snack-type, regular	3.5	61	1.6	25.3
Crackers, standard snack-type, regular, low salt	3.5	61	1.6	25.3
Crackers, standard snack-type, sandwich, with cheese filling	3.9	61.7	1.851	21.1
Crackers, standard snack-type, sandwich, with peanut butter filling	3.1	58.7	2.756	23.9
Crackers, wheat, low salt	3.1	64.9	4.5	20.6
Crackers, wheat, regular	3.1	64.9	4.5	20.6
Crackers, wheat, sandwich, with cheese filling	3.2	58.2	3.076	25
Crackers, wheat, sandwich, with peanut butter filling	3.4	53.8	4.378	26.7
Crackers, whole-wheat	2.7	68.6	10.5	17.2
Crackers, whole-wheat, low salt	2.7	68.6	10.5	17.2
Cream puffs, prepared from recipe, shell (includes eclair)	40.5	22.8	0.8	25.9
Cream puffs, prepared from recipe, shell, with custard filling	53.5	22.9	0.4	15.5
Croissants, apple	45.6	37.1	2.5	8.7
Croissants, butter	23.2	45.8	2.6	21
Croissants, cheese	21	47	2.6	20.9
Croutons, plain	5.5	73.5	5.1	6.6
Croutons, seasoned	3.6	63.5	5	18.3
Danish pastry, cheese	31.4	37.2	0.97	21.9
Danish pastry, cinnamon, enriched	24.3	44.6	1.3	22.4

Danish pastry, cinnamon, unenriched	24.3	44.6	1.2	22.4
Danish pastry, fruit, enriched (includes apple, cinnamon, raisin, lemon, raspberry, strawberry)	27.1	47.8	1.9	18.5
Danish pastry, fruit, unenriched (includes apple, cinnamon, raisin, lemon, raspberry, strawberry)	27.1	47.8	1.9	18.5
Danish pastry, lemon, unenriched	27.1	47.8	1.9	18.5
Danish pastry, nut (includes almond, raisin nut, cinnamon nut)	20.4	45.7	2	25.2
Danish pastry, raspberry, unenriched	27.1	47.8	1.9	18.5
Doughnuts, cake-type, chocolate, sugared or glazed	16.3	57.4	2.2	19.9
Doughnuts, cake-type, plain (includes unsugared, old-fashioned)	20.8	49.7	1.5	22.9
Doughnuts, cake-type, plain, chocolate-coated or frosted	14.4	48	2	31
Doughnuts, cake-type, plain, sugared or glazed	19.6	50.8	1.5	22.9
Doughnuts, cake-type, wheat, sugared or glazed	29.8	42.6	2.22	19.3
Doughnuts, French crullers, glazed	17.9	59.5	1.2	18.3
Doughnuts, yeast-leavened, glazed, enriched (includes honey buns)	25.4	44.3	1.2	22.8
Doughnuts, yeast-leavened, glazed, unenriched (includes honey buns)	25.4	44.3	2.1	22.8
Doughnuts, yeast-leavened, with creme filling	38.2	30	0.77	24.5
Doughnuts, yeast-leavened, with jelly filling	35.6	39	0.85	18.7
Eclairs, custard-filled with chocolate glaze, prepared from recipe	52.4	24.2	0.6	15.7
English muffins, mixed-grain (includes granola)	40.2	46.3	2.79	1.8
English muffins, mixed-grain, toasted (includes granola)	35	50.3	3.04	1.9
English muffins, plain, enriched, with calcium propionate (includes sourdough)	42.1	46	2.7	1.8
English muffins, plain, enriched, without calcium propionate (includes sourdough)	42.1	46	2.7	1.8
English muffins, plain, toasted, enriched, with calcium propionate (includes sourdough)	37.1	50	2.9	2
English muffins, plain, toasted, enriched, without calcium propionate (includes sourdough)	37.1	50	2.9	2
English muffins, plain, toasted, unenriched, with calcium propionate (includes sourdough)	37.1	50		2
English muffins, plain, toasted, unenriched, without calcium propionate (includes sourdough)	37.1	50		2
English muffins, plain, unenriched, with calcium propionate (includes sourdough)	42.1	46		1.8
English muffins, plain, unenriched, without calcium propionate (includes sourdough)	42.1	46		1.8
English muffins, raisin-cinnamon (includes apple-cinnamon)	38.6	48.7	2.9	2.7
English muffins, raisin-cinnamon, toasted (includes apple-cinnamon)	33.3	53	3.1	2.9
English muffins, wheat	42.3	44.8	4.62	2
English muffins, wheat, toasted	37.2	48.7	5.03	2.1

English muffins, whole-wheat	45.7	40.4	6.7	2.1
English muffins, whole-wheat, toasted	41	44.1	7.3	2.3
French toast, frozen, ready-to-heat	52.6	32.1	1.11	6.1
French toast, prepared from recipe, made with low fat (2%) milk	54.7	25		10.8
French toast, prepared from recipe, made with whole milk	54.4	24.9		11.3
Hush puppies, prepared from recipe	29	46	2.8	13.5
Ice cream cones, cake or wafer-type	5.3	79	3	6.9
Ice cream cones, sugar, rolled-type	3	84.1	1.66	3.8
Leavening agents, baking powder, double-acting, sodium aluminum sulfate	5	27.7	0.2	0
Leavening agents, baking powder, double-acting, straight phosphate	4	24.1	0.2	0
Leavening agents, baking powder, low-sodium	6.2	46.9	2.2	0.4
Leavening agents, baking soda	0.2	0	0	0
Leavening agents, cream of tartar	1.7	61.5	0.2	0
Leavening agents, yeast, baker's, active dry	7.6	38.2	21	4.6
Leavening agents, yeast, baker's, compressed	69	18.1	8.1	1.9
Muffins, blueberry, commercially prepared	38.3	48	2.6	6.5
Muffins, blueberry, dry mix	20	63.2		10
Muffins, blueberry, dry mix, prepared	35.6	48.8	1.1	8.8
Muffins, blueberry, prepared from recipe, made with low fat (2%) milk	39.5	40.7		10.8
Muffins, blueberry, prepared from recipe, made with whole milk	39	40.6		11.3
Muffins, blueberry, toaster-type	30.8	53.3	1.8	9.5
Muffins, blueberry, toaster-type, toasted	26.4	56.7	1.9	10.1
Muffins, corn, commercially prepared	32.6	50.9	3.38	8.4
Muffins, corn, dry mix, prepared	30.5	49.1	2.37	10.2
Muffins, corn, prepared from recipe, made with low fat (2%) milk	33	44.2	12.3	
Muffins, corn, prepared from recipe, made with whole milk	32.5	44.2		12.9
Muffins, corn, toaster-type	23.6	57.9	1.6	11.3
Muffins, corn, toaster-type, toasted	18.7	61.6	1.7	12
Muffins, oat bran	35	48.3	4.6	7.4
Muffins, plain, prepared from recipe, made with low fat (2%) milk	37.7	41.4	2.7	11.4
Muffins, plain, prepared from recipe, made with whole milk	37.2	41.4	2.7	12
Muffins, wheat bran, dry mix	4.8	73		12
Muffins, wheat bran, dry mix, prepared	35.4	46.6	4.2	9.2
Muffins, wheat bran, prepared from recipe, made with low fat (2%) milk	35.4	41.9		12.2
Muffins, wheat bran, prepared from recipe, made with whole milk	34.9	41.8		12.8
Muffins, wheat bran, toaster-type with raisins	31.4	52.2	7.7	8.8
Muffins, wheat bran, toaster-type with raisins, toasted	27	55.5	8.2	9.4

Pancakes plain, frozen, ready-to-heat (includes buttermilk)	45.2	43.6	1.79	3.3
Pancakes, blueberry, prepared from recipe	53.2	29		9.2
Pancakes, buckwheat, dry mix, incomplete	9.1	71.3	8.47	2.7
Pancakes, buckwheat, dry mix, incomplete, prepared	53.7	28.2	2.3	7.6
Pancakes, buttermilk, prepared from recipe	52.5	28.7		9.3
Pancakes, plain, dry mix, complete (includes buttermilk)	8.8	71.3	2.7	4.9
Pancakes, plain, dry mix, complete, prepared	53	36.7	1.3	2.5
Pancakes, plain, dry mix, incomplete (includes buttermilk)	9.1	73.6	5.44	1.7
Pancakes, plain, dry mix, incomplete, prepared	52.9	28.9	1.86	7.7
Pancakes, plain, prepared from recipe	52.9	28.3		9.7
Pancakes, special dietary, dry mix	10.8	73.9		1.4
Pancakes, special dietary, dry mix, prepared	49	42.2		0.8
Pancakes, whole-wheat, dry mix, incomplete	8.8	71		1.5
Pancakes, whole-wheat, dry mix, incomplete, prepared	52.8	29.4	2.83	6.5
Phyllo dough	32.6	52.6	1.9	6
Pie crust, cookie-type, prepared from recipe, chocolate wafer, baked	5.5	55.5		31.7
Pie crust, cookie-type, prepared from recipe, chocolate wafer, chilled	7.3	54.4	1.5	31.1
Pie crust, cookie-type, prepared from recipe, graham cracker, baked	4.2	65.2	1.5	24.9
Pie crust, cookie-type, prepared from recipe, graham cracker, chilled	6.1	63.9	1.5	24.4
Pie crust, cookie-type, prepared from recipe, vanilla wafer, baked	6.7	51.2		37
Pie crust, cookie-type, prepared from recipe, vanilla wafer, chilled	8.5	50.2	0.1	36.2
Pie crust, standard-type, dry mix	7.6	52.1		31.4
Pie crust, standard-type, dry mix, prepared, baked	10.6	50.4	1.77	30.4
Pie crust, standard-type, frozen, ready-to-bake, baked	11.2	49.6	1	32.8
Pie crust, standard-type, frozen, ready-to-bake, enriched	21	44.1	0.89	29.2
Pie crust, standard-type, frozen, ready-to-bake, unenriched	21	44.1	0.89	29.2
Pie crust, standard-type, prepared from recipe, baked	9.8	47.5	1.68	34.6
Pie crust, standard-type, prepared from recipe, unbaked	19.7	42.3	3.4	30.8
Pie, apple, commercially prepared, enriched flour	52.2	34	1.6	11
Pie, apple, commercially prepared, unenriched flour	52.2	34	1.7	11
Pie, apple, prepared from recipe	47.3	37.1		12.5
Pie, banana cream, prepared from mix, no-bake type	50.9	31.6	0.62	12.9
Pie, banana cream, prepared from recipe	47.9	32.9	0.7	13.6
Pie, blueberry, commercially prepared	52.5	34.9	1.03	10
Pie, blueberry, prepared from recipe	51.2	33.5		11.9
Pie, butterscotch, pudding-type, prepared from recipe	46.3	33.3		14.3
Pie, cherry, commercially prepared	46.2	39.8	0.8	11
Pie, cherry, prepared from recipe	45.8	38.5		12.2
Pie, chocolate cream, prepared from recipe	46.6	31.2		16.1
Pie, chocolate creme, commercially prepared	43.5	33.6	2	19.4

Pie, chocolate mousse, prepared from mix, no-bake type	49.7	29.6		15.4
Pie, coconut cream, prepared from mix, no-bake type	49.7	28.5	0.5	17.6
Pie, coconut cream, prepared from recipe	43.7	34.2		16
Pie, coconut creme, commercially prepared	43.2	37.2	1.29	16.6
Pie, coconut custard, commercially prepared	49.2	30.2	1.8	13.2
Pie, egg custard, commercially prepared	60.9	20.8	1.6	11.6
Pie, egg custard, prepared from recipe	58.2	26.8		8.9
Pie, fried pies, cherry	37.6	42.6	2.6	16.1
Pie, fried pies, fruit	37.6	42.6	2.6	16.1
Pie, fried pies, lemon	37.6	42.6	2.6	16.1
Pie, lemon meringue, commercially prepared	41.7	47.2	1.2	8.7
Pie, lemon meringue, prepared from recipe	43.3	39.1		12.9
Pie, mince, prepared from recipe	37.4	48	2.6	10.8
Pie, peach	54.4	32.9	0.82	10
Pie, pecan, commercially prepared	19.3	57.2	3.5	18.5
Pie, pecan, prepared from recipe	19.5	52.2		22.2
Pie, pumpkin, commercially prepared	58.1	27.3	2.7	9.5
Pie, pumpkin, prepared from recipe	58.5	26.4		9.3
Pie, vanilla cream, prepared from recipe	47	32.6	0.6	14.4
Popovers, dry mix, enriched	11.7	71		4.3
Popovers, dry mix, prepared	54.6	31.6		4.5
Popovers, dry mix, unenriched	11.7	71		4.3
Popovers, prepared from recipe, made with low fat (2%) milk	54.5	28	0.9	7.6
Popovers, prepared from recipe, made with whole milk	53.8	27.9		8.5
Puff pastry, frozen, ready-to-bake	8.5	45.1	1.475	38.1
Puff pastry, frozen, ready-to-bake, baked	7.4	45.7	1.49	38.5
Rolls, dinner, egg	30.4	52	3.7	6.4
Rolls, dinner, oat bran	44	40.2	4.1	4.6
Rolls, dinner, plain, commercially prepared (includes brown-and-serve)	31.9	50.4	3	7.3
Rolls, dinner, plain, prepared from recipe, made with low fat (2%) milk	29.1	53.4	1.9	7.3
Rolls, dinner, plain, prepared from recipe, made with whole milk	28.6	53.4		7.8
Rolls, dinner, rye	30.1	53.1	4.87	3.4
Rolls, dinner, wheat	37	46	3.78	6.3
Rolls, dinner, whole-wheat	33.1	51.1	7.54	4.7
Rolls, French	34.8	50.2	3.2	4.3
Rolls, hamburger or hotdog, mixed-grain	38	44.6	3.81	6
Rolls, hamburger or hotdog, plain	34	50.3	2.7	5.1
Rolls, hamburger or hotdog, reduced-calorie	46	42.1	6.2	2
Rolls, hard (includes kaiser)	31	52.7	2.3	4.3
Strudel, apple	43.5	41.1	2.2	11.2
Sweet rolls, cheese	29.4	43.7	1.2	18.3
Sweet rolls, cinnamon, commercially prepared with raisins	24.8	50.9	2.4	16.4
Sweet rolls, cinnamon, refrigerated dough with frosting	28.9	51.6		12.2

Sweet rolls, cinnamon, refrigerated dough with frosting, baked	22.7	56.1		13.2
Sweet rolls, prepared from recipe with raisins and nuts	27.1	51.9		12.8
Taco shells, baked	6	62.4	7.5	22.6
Taco shells, baked, without added salt	6	62.4	7.5	22.6
Toaster pastries, brown-sugar-cinnamon	10.8	68.1	1	14.2
Toaster pastries, fruit (includes apple, blueberry, cherry, strawberry)	12.3	71.1	2.09	10.2
Tortillas, ready-to-bake or -fry, corn	44.1	46.6	5.2	2.5
Tortillas, ready-to-bake or -fry, corn, without added salt	44.1	46.6	5.2	2.5
Tortillas, ready-to-bake or -fry, flour	26.8	55.6	3.3	7.1
Tortillas, ready-to-bake or -fry, flour, without added calcium	26.8	55.6	3.1	7.1
Waffles, buttermilk, prepared from recipe	42.1	33		13.6
Waffles, plain, dry mix, prepared from complete-type	42.5	35.2	1.4	13.7
Waffles, plain, frozen, ready-to-heat (includes buttermilk)	44.9	38.6	2.2	7.8
Waffles, plain, frozen, ready-to-heat, toasted (includes buttermilk)	42.1	40.7	2.3	8.2
Waffles, plain, prepared from recipe	42	32.9		14.1
Wonton wrappers (includes egg roll wrappers)	28.8	57.9	1.84	1.5

CEREALS

	Water	Carb.	% TDF	% FAT
Cereals ready-to-eat, KELLOGG, KELLOGG'S MUESLIX Apple & Almond Crunch	4.1	74.3	8.5	9
Cereals ready-to-eat, QUAKER, QUAKER 100% Natural Cereal with Oats and Honey	2.5	68.64	7.5	16.45
Cereals ready-to-eat, 100% BRAN, (wheat bran, barley)	3	72.9	29.6	5
Cereals ready-to-eat, 100% NATURAL CEREAL, WITH APPLE AND CINNAMON, (oats, wheat)	1.9	67.1	6.6	18.8
Cereals ready-to-eat, 100% NATURAL CEREAL, WITH RAISINS AND DATES, (oats, wheat)	3.5	65.8	6.6	18.5
Cereals ready-to-eat, 40% BRAN FLAKES, RALSTON PURINA, (wheat bran)	2.5	79.8	14.1	1.4
Cereals ready-to-eat, ALPHA-BITS, (oat with other grains)	1.3	86.6	4.3	2.3
Cereals ready-to-eat, BRAN CHEX, (wheat bran, corn)	2.3	79.7	16.2	2.8
Cereals ready-to-eat, C.W. POST, PLAIN, (oats with other grains)	2.3	74.9	7.4	13.2
Cereals ready-to-eat, C.W. POST, WITH RAISINS, (oats with other grains)	3.9	71.8	13.2	14.3
Cereals ready-to-eat, COCOA PEBBLES, (rice)	2.1	85.9	1.6	5.4
Cereals ready-to-eat, COOKIE-CRISP, CHOCOLATE CHIP AND VANILLA, (corn with other grains)	1.9	87.5	1.4	3.6
Cereals ready-to-eat, CORN CHEX, (corn)	1.9	87.7	1.8	0.4

Cereals ready-to-eat, CORN FLAKES, RALSTON PURINA, (corn)	2.7	86.6	1.9	0.4
Cereals ready-to-eat, FROSTED RICE KRINKLES, (rice)	1.9	91.1	0.6	0.2
Cereals ready-to-eat, FRUITY PEBBLES, (rice)	2.9	86.1	1.3	5.2
Cereals ready-to-eat, GENERAL MILLS, WHEATIES	3.48	79.3	7	3.09
Cereals ready-to-eat, GENERAL MILLS, APPLE CINNAMON CHEERIOS	2.51	83.5	5.3	5.44
Cereals ready-to-eat, GENERAL MILLS, BASIC 4	7.14	76.3	6.1	5.16
Cereals ready-to-eat, GENERAL MILLS, BERRY BERRY KIX	2.32	87.1	0.6	3.87
Cereals ready-to-eat, GENERAL MILLS, BODY BUDDIES	2.44	86.1	3.1	3.16
Cereals ready-to-eat, GENERAL MILLS, BOO BERRY	1.69	91.1	1.3	1.77
Cereals ready-to-eat, GENERAL MILLS, CHEERIOS	3.37	76.2	8.8	5.9
Cereals ready-to-eat, GENERAL MILLS, CINNAMON TOAST CRUNCH	2.09	79.46	5	10.14
Cereals ready-to-eat, GENERAL MILLS, CLUSTERS	2.52	78.9	7.7	6.33
Cereals ready-to-eat, GENERAL MILLS, COCOA PUFFS	1.89	89.05	0.6	3.01
Cereals ready-to-eat, GENERAL MILLS, COUNT CHOCULA	1.84	88.1	1.5	2.88
Cereals ready-to-eat, GENERAL MILLS, CRISPY WHEAT 'N RAISINS	7.09	80.6	6.2	1.38
Cereals ready-to-eat, GENERAL MILLS, Country Corn Flakes	2.61	86.53	1.5	1.68
Cereals ready-to-eat, GENERAL MILLS, FIBER ONE	3.82	80.02	47.5	2.81
Cereals ready-to-eat, GENERAL MILLS, FRANKENBERRY	1.91	90.9	0.6	1.71
Cereals ready-to-eat, GENERAL MILLS, FROSTED CHEERIOS	2.22	85.12	5.2	3.32
Cereals ready-to-eat, GENERAL MILLS, GOLDEN GRAHAMS	2.64	85.63	3.1	3.6
Cereals ready-to-eat, GENERAL MILLS, HONEY FROSTED WHEATIES	2.68	88	5	0.98
Cereals ready-to-eat, GENERAL MILLS, HONEY NUT CHEERIOS	2.33	80.87	5.2	4.13
Cereals ready-to-eat, GENERAL MILLS, KABOOM	3.49	80.75	5	3.8
Cereals ready-to-eat, GENERAL MILLS, KIX	2.03	86.38	2.7	2.07
Cereals ready-to-eat, GENERAL MILLS, LUCKY CHARMS	2.36	83.9	4	3.61
Cereals ready-to-eat, GENERAL MILLS, MULTIGRAIN CHEERIOS	2.68	81.5	6.4	3.63
Cereals ready-to-eat, GENERAL MILLS, NATURE VALLEY Cinnamon & Raisins Granola	5.43	69.87	5.2	14
Cereals ready-to-eat, GENERAL MILLS, NATURE VALLEY Fruit n' Nut Granola	5.01	62.3	6.1	20.3
Cereals ready-to-eat, GENERAL MILLS, NATURE VALLEY LOW FAT FRUIT GRANOLA	4.4	79.6	6.2	5.38

Cereals ready-to-eat, GENERAL MILLS, NATURE VALLEY Toasted Oats Granola	4.29	65.88	6.4	17.62
Cereals ready-to-eat, GENERAL MILLS, OATMEAL CRISP WITH ALMONDS	2.36	76.28	7.9	8.36
Cereals ready-to-eat, GENERAL MILLS, OATMEAL CRISP WITH APPLES	2.44	84.02	8.1	3.34
Cereals ready-to-eat, GENERAL MILLS, Oatmeal Raisin Crisp	5.91	79.46	6.4	4.45
Cereals ready-to-eat, GENERAL MILLS, RAISIN NUT BRAN	4.5	75.37	9.2	8
Cereals ready-to-eat, GENERAL MILLS, REESE'S PEANUT BUTTER PUFFS	1.92	76.6	1.3	10.65
Cereals ready-to-eat, GENERAL MILLS, S'MORES GRAHAMS	2.79	85.3	2.8	4
Cereals ready-to-eat, GENERAL MILLS, SUN CRUNCHERS	2.8	79.53	4	5.74
Cereals ready-to-eat, GENERAL MILLS, TOTAL	2.82	79.6	8.8	2.32
Cereals ready-to-eat, GENERAL MILLS, TOTAL Corn Flakes	2.56	85.55	2.5	1.61
Cereals ready-to-eat, GENERAL MILLS, TOTAL Raisin Bran	9.16	77.73	9.1	1.83
Cereals ready-to-eat, GENERAL MILLS, TRIPLES	3.13	83.28	2.8	3.37
Cereals ready-to-eat, GENERAL MILLS, TRIX	2.08	86.8	2.4	5.69
Cereals ready-to-eat, GRAPE-NUTS FLAKES, (wheat, barley)	3.4	81.1	9.9	2.9
Cereals ready-to-eat, GRAPE-NUTS, (wheat, barley)	3.2	82	10	0.4
Cereals ready-to-eat, HEALTHY CHOICE from KELLOGG'S Multi-Grain Flakes	3	84.1	9.4	1.2
Cereals ready-to-eat, HEALTHY CHOICE, KELLOGG'S Almond Crunch with Raisins	3.1	85.3	8.4	1.5
Cereals ready-to-eat, HEARTLAND NATURAL CEREAL, PLAIN, (oats, wheat germ)	4.1	68.3	6.1	15.4
Cereals ready-to-eat, HEARTLAND NATURAL CEREAL, WITH COCONUT, (oats, wheat germ)	3.3	67.9	7.1	16.3
Cereals ready-to-eat, HEARTLAND NATURAL CEREAL, WITH RAISINS, (oats, wheat germ)	5	69	5.5	14.2
Cereals ready-to-eat, HONEYBRAN, (wheat)	2.5	81.8	11.1	2.1
Cereals ready-to-eat, HONEYCOMB, (corn, oats)	1.4	89.1	2.8	1.8
Cereals ready-to-eat, KELLOGG'S FROSTED MINI-WHEATS,regular and bite size	5.3	82.5	10.7	1.6
Cereals ready-to-eat, KELLOGG'S MUESLIX Raisin & Almond Crunch with Dates	10.28	73.6	6.8	5.9
Cereals ready-to-eat, KELLOGG, POP-TARTS CRUNCH Frosted Strawberry	2.3	89.2	0	2.7
Cereals ready-to-eat, KELLOGG, JUST RIGHT Fruit & Nut	6.9	80.5	5	2.9
Cereals ready-to-eat, KELLOGG, KELLOGG'S CRACKLIN' OAT BRAN	3.59	72.9	11.9	12.67
Cereals ready-to-eat, KELLOGG, KELLOGG'S RICE KRISPIES	3	86.5	1.1	1.1

Cereals ready-to-eat, KELLOGG, KELLOGG'S ALL-BRAN	3.5	73.37	32.4	3.4
Cereals ready-to-eat, KELLOGG, KELLOGG'S APPLE CINNAMON SQUARES	9.5	80.1	8.6	1.8
Cereals ready-to-eat, KELLOGG, KELLOGG'S APPLE JACKS	2.6	89.48	1.9	1.3
Cereals ready-to-eat, KELLOGG, KELLOGG'S APPLE RAISIN CRISP	5.3	84.9	8	0.9
Cereals ready-to-eat, KELLOGG, KELLOGG'S APPLE-CINNAMON RICE KRISPIES	3	89	1.5	0.5
Cereals ready-to-eat, KELLOGG, KELLOGG'S BLUEBERRY SQUARES	9.5	79.6	8.8	1.8
Cereals ready-to-eat, KELLOGG, KELLOGG'S BRAN BUDS	3	79.9	39.9	2.4
Cereals ready-to-eat, KELLOGG, KELLOGG'S CINNAMON MINI BUNS	2.3	88.7	2.2	2.1
Cereals ready-to-eat, KELLOGG, KELLOGG'S COCOA KRISPIES	2.4	87.9	1.3	2.6
Cereals ready-to-eat, KELLOGG, KELLOGG'S COMMON SENSE Oat Bran Flakes	3.3	77.4	13.2	4
Cereals ready-to-eat, KELLOGG, KELLOGG'S CORN POPS	2.89	91.7	1.4	0.58
Cereals ready-to-eat, KELLOGG, KELLOGG'S CRISPIX	3	86.2	2.2	1
Cereals ready-to-eat, KELLOGG, KELLOGG'S Complete Bran Flakes	3.64	79.86	15.9	2.2
Cereals ready-to-eat, KELLOGG, KELLOGG'S Corn Flakes	3.23	86.49	2.8	0.71
Cereals ready-to-eat, KELLOGG, KELLOGG'S DOUBLE DIP CRUNCH	3	91	1.5	0.4
Cereals ready-to-eat, KELLOGG, KELLOGG'S FROOT LOOPS	2.4	88.2	1.9	2.9
Cereals ready-to-eat, KELLOGG, KELLOGG'S FROSTED BRAN	3	84.7	11.2	1.1
Cereals ready-to-eat, KELLOGG, KELLOGG'S FROSTED FLAKES	2.7	91	1.6	0.5
Cereals ready-to-eat, KELLOGG, KELLOGG'S FROSTED KRISPIES	2.2	90.4	1.1	0.7
Cereals ready-to-eat, KELLOGG, KELLOGG'S FRUITY MARSHMALLOW KRISPIES	3	90.3	1	0.3
Cereals ready-to-eat, KELLOGG, KELLOGG'S JUST RIGHT with Crunchy Nuggets	3.2	83.7	5.1	2.7
Cereals ready-to-eat, KELLOGG, KELLOGG'S Low Fat Granola with Raisins	5.4	79.4	6	5
Cereals ready-to-eat, KELLOGG, KELLOGG'S Low Fat Granola without Raisins	3.5	80.3	5.9	5.9
Cereals ready-to-eat, KELLOGG, KELLOGG'S NUTRI-GRAIN Almond and Raisin	6.2	77.6	8	5.7
Cereals ready-to-eat, KELLOGG, KELLOGG'S NUTRI-GRAIN Wheat	3.7	80	12.6	3.3

Cereals ready-to-eat, KELLOGG, KELLOGG'S Nut & Honey Crunch	2.5	83.6	1.6	4.5
Cereals ready-to-eat, KELLOGG, KELLOGG'S PRODUCT 19	4.02	83.63	4.1	1.3
Cereals ready-to-eat, KELLOGG, KELLOGG'S RAISIN BRAN	8.67	76.59	12.8	2.34
Cereals ready-to-eat, KELLOGG, KELLOGG'S RAISIN SQUARES	9.5	78	9.4	2.8
Cereals ready-to-eat, KELLOGG, KELLOGG'S RICE KRISPIES TREATS Cereal	3.5	85.5	1	5.3
Cereals ready-to-eat, KELLOGG, KELLOGG'S SMACKS	3	87.6	3.5	2
Cereals ready-to-eat, KELLOGG, KELLOGG'S SPECIAL K	2.8	72.4	3.1	0.9
Cereals ready-to-eat, KELLOGG, KELLOGG'S STRAWBERRY SQUARES	9.1	79	9.2	3
Cereals ready-to-eat, KELLOGG, TEMPTATIONS, French Vanilla Almond	2.8	82.4	2.6	5.5
Cereals ready-to-eat, KELLOGG, TEMPTATIONS, Honey Roasted Pecan	2.8	81.4	2.3	7.5
Cereals ready-to-eat, NATURAL BRAN FLAKES, POST, (wheat bran)	3	79.3	19.5	1.6
Cereals ready-to-eat, NUTRI-GRAIN, WHEAT, see new product 08292	3	84.6	6.3	1
Cereals ready-to-eat, POST oat flakes, (oat with other grains)	3.1	75.2	3	2
Cereals ready-to-eat, QUAKER, CAP'N CRUNCH	2.3	85.35	3.2	5.06
Cereals ready-to-eat, QUAKER, CAP'N CRUNCH'S CRUNCHBERRIES	2.38	85.63	2.2	4.91
Cereals ready-to-eat, QUAKER, CAP'N CRUNCH'S PEANUT BUTTER CRUNCH	1.91	79.68	2.9	8.59
Cereals ready-to-eat, QUAKER, HONEY GRAHAM OH!S	1.7	84.24	2.6	7.07
Cereals ready-to-eat, QUAKER, KING VITAMAN	2	84.14	3.8	3.51
Cereals ready-to-eat, QUAKER, KRETSCHMER Honey Crunch Wheat Germ	3.4	58.11	10.2	7.78
Cereals ready-to-eat, QUAKER, QUAKER 100% Natural Cereal with Oats, Honey, and Raisins	4.3	70.25	7.2	14.28
Cereals ready-to-eat, QUAKER, QUAKER CINNAMON OATMEAL SQUARES	1.91	78.59	7.6	4.28
Cereals ready-to-eat, QUAKER, QUAKER CRUNCHY BRAN	2.59	84.18	17.8	3.3
Cereals ready-to-eat, QUAKER, QUAKER Low Fat 100% Natural Crispy Wholegrain Cereal with Raisins	3.87	80.68	6	5.33
Cereals ready-to-eat, QUAKER, QUAKER OAT CINNAMON LIFE	4	80.8	5.9	3.47
Cereals ready-to-eat, QUAKER, QUAKER OAT LIFE, plain	4	78.7	6.4	3.99

Cereals ready-to-eat, QUAKER, QUAKER OATMEAL SQUARES	2.39	77.35	7.6	4.62
Cereals ready-to-eat, QUAKER, QUAKER Oat Bran Cereal	4	72.62	10.5	5.17
Cereals ready-to-eat, QUAKER, QUAKER Puffed Rice	3.91	87.77	1.4	0.9
Cereals ready-to-eat, QUAKER, QUAKER Puffed Wheat	3.69	76.39	9.4	2.15
Cereals ready-to-eat, QUAKER, QUAKER Toasted Oatmeal Cereal, Honey Nut	2.5	79.5	6.8	5.53
Cereals ready-to-eat, QUAKER, SUN COUNTRY Granola with Almonds	1.37	67.2	5.2	18.02
Cereals ready-to-eat, QUAKER, SUN COUNTRY Granola, Raisin and Date	2.82	72.2	6	13.63
Cereals ready-to-eat, QUAKER, SWEET CRUNCH/ QUISP	2.51	85.08	2.5	5.51
Cereals ready-to-eat, RAISIN BRAN, POST, (wheat)	9.2	75.6	14.1	1.9
Cereals ready-to-eat, RAISIN BRAN, RALSTON PURINA, (wheat)	7.3	83	13.4	0.5
Cereals ready-to-eat, RAISINS, RICE AND RYE, (rice with other grains)	6	85.4	5.7	0.3
Cereals ready-to-eat, RICE CHEX, (rice)	2.6	89.2	1.8	0.4
Cereals ready-to-eat, SUGAR FROSTED FLAKES, RALSTON PURINA, (corn)	1.5	90.1	2.2	1.4
Cereals ready-to-eat, SUGAR SPARKLED FLAKES, (corn)	1.7	91.1	1.2	0.2
Cereals ready-to-eat, SUPER SUGAR CRISP, (wheat)	1.5	90.2	1.5	0.9
Cereals ready-to-eat, TASTEEOS, (oat with other grains)	2.1	79.1	10.6	2.8
Cereals ready-to-eat, TEAM, (rice with other grains)	3.8	85.8	1.3	1.8
Cereals ready-to-eat, TOASTIES, (corn)	3	85.8	3.4	0.2
Cereals ready-to-eat, WAFFELOS, (wheat with other grains)	2.5	86.3	4.2	
Cereals ready-to-eat, WHEAT CHEX, (wheat)	2.5	82.2	8.9	2.5
Cereals ready-to-eat, corn flakes, low sodium, (corn)	3	88.8	1.1	0.3
Cereals ready-to-eat, crisp rice, low sodium, (rice)	3	91	1.4	0.3
Cereals ready-to-eat, crispy rice, (rice)	2.5	88.6	1.2	0.4
Cereals ready-to-eat, granola, homemade, (oats, wheat germ)	5.3	53	10.5	24.6
Cereals ready-to-eat, rice, puffed, fortified, (rice)	3	89.8	1.7	0.5
Cereals ready-to-eat, wheat germ, toasted, plain, (wheat germ)	5.6	49.6	12.9	10.7
Cereals ready-to-eat, wheat, puffed, fortified, (rice)	3	79.6	4.4	1.2
Cereals ready-to-eat, wheat, shredded, large biscuit, (wheat)	3.98	81.3	9.8	1.65
Cereals ready-to-eat, wheat, shredded, small biscuit, (wheat)	5.3	80.4	9.8	1.65
Cereals ready-to-eat,HEALTHY CHOICE, KELLOGG'S Toasted Brown Sugar Squares	5	81.8	9.3	1.9
Cereals, ready-to-eat, KELLOGG, KELLOGG'S ALL-BRAN WITH EXTRA FIBER	3.7	75.6	51.1	3.1

FRUITS

	Water	Carb.	% TDF	% FAT
Acerola juice, raw	94.3	4.8	0.3	0.3
Acerola, (West Indian Cherry), raw	91.41	7.69	1.1	0.3
Apple juice, canned or bottled, unsweetened, with added ascorbic acid	87.93	11.68	0.1	0.11
Apple juice, canned or bottled, unsweetened, without added ascorbic acid	87.93	11.68	0.1	0.11
Apple juice, frozen concentrate, unsweetened, diluted with 3 volume water without added ascorbic acid	87.9	11.54	0.1	0.1
Apple juice, frozen concentrate, unsweetened, diluted with 3 volume water, with added ascorbic acid	87.9	11.54	0.1	0.1
Apple juice, frozen concentrate, unsweetened, undiluted, with added ascorbic acid	57	41	0.37	
Apple juice, frozen concentrate, unsweetened, undiluted, without added ascorbic acid	57	41	0.4	0.37
Apples, canned, sweetened, sliced, drained, heated	82.28	16.84	2	0.43
Apples, canned, sweetened, sliced, drained, unheated	82.36	16.7	1.7	0.49
Apples, dehydrated (low moisture), sulfured, stewed	79.36	19.91	2.6	0.12
Apples, dehydrated (low moisture), sulfured, uncooked	3	93.53	12.4	0.58
Apples, dried, sulfured, stewed, with added sugar	78.76	20.73	1.9	0.07
Apples, dried, sulfured, stewed, without added sugar	84.13	15.32	2	0.07
Apples, dried, sulfured, uncooked	31.76	65.89	8.7	0.32
Apples, frozen, unsweetened, heated	87.16	12	1.9	0.33
Apples, frozen, unsweetened, unheated	86.85	12.31	1.9	0.32
Apples, raw, with skin	83.93	15.25	2.7	0.36
Apples, raw, without skin	84.46	14.84	1.9	0.31
Apples, raw, without skin, cooked, boiled	85.47	13.64	2.4	0.36
Apples, raw, without skin, cooked, microwave	84.63	14.41	2.8	0.42
Applesauce, canned, sweetened, with salt	79.58	19.91	1.2	0.18
Applesauce, canned, sweetened, without salt	79.58	19.91	1.2	0.18
Applesauce, canned, unsweetened, with added ascorbic acid	88.35	11.29	1.2	0.05
Applesauce, canned, unsweetened, without added ascorbic acid	88.35	11.29	1.2	0.05
Apricot nectar, canned, with added ascorbic acid	84.87	14.39	0.6	0.09
Apricot nectar, canned, without added ascorbic acid	84.87	14.39	0.6	0.09
Apricots, canned, extra heavy syrup pack, without skin, solids and liquids	74.33	24.85	1.6	0.04
Apricots, canned, extra light syrup pack, with skin, solids and liquids	86.3	12.5	1.6	0.1
Apricots, canned, heavy syrup pack, with skin, solids and liquids	77.56	21.47	1.6	0.08
Apricots, canned, heavy syrup pack, without skin, solids and liquids	77.66	21.45	1.6	0.09
Apricots, canned, juice pack, with skin, solids and liquids	86.62	12.34	1.6	0.04
Apricots, canned, light syrup pack, with skin, solids and liquids	82.56	16.49	1.6	0.05

Apricots, canned, water pack, with skin, solids and liquids	92.36	6.39	1.6	0.16
Apricots, canned, water pack, without skin, solids and liquids	93.43	5.48	1.1	0.03
Apricots, dehydrated (low-moisture), sulfured, stewed	63.6	32.62		0.24
Apricots, dehydrated (low-moisture), sulfured, uncooked	7.5	82.89		0.62
Apricots, dried, sulfured, stewed, with added sugar	68.45	29.26	4.1	0.15
Apricots, dried, sulfured, stewed, without added sugar	75.56	21.9	3.2	0.16
Apricots, dried, sulfured, uncooked	31.09	61.75	9	0.46
Apricots, frozen, sweetened	73.3	25.1	2.2	0.1
Apricots, raw	86.35	11.12	2.4	0.39
Avocados, raw, California	72.56	6.91	4.9	17.33
Avocados, raw, Florida	79.73	8.91	5.3	8.87
Avocados, raw, all commercial varieties	74.27	7.39	5	15.32
Bananas, dehydrated, or banana powder	3	88.28	7.5	1.81
Bananas, raw	74.26	23.43	2.4	0.48
Blackberries, canned, heavy syrup, solids and liquids	75.06	23.1	3.4	0.14
Blackberries, frozen, unsweetened	82.21	15.67	5	0.43
Blackberries, raw	85.64	12.76	5.3	0.39
Blueberries, canned, heavy syrup, solids and liquids	76.78	22.06	1.5	0.33
Blueberries, frozen, sweetened	77.4	21.95	2.1	0.13
Blueberries, frozen, unsweetened	86.59	12.17	2.7	0.64
Blueberries, raw	84.61	14.13	2.7	0.38
Boysenberries, canned, heavy syrup	76.26	22.31	2.6	0.12
Boysenberries, frozen, unsweetened	85.9	12.19	3.9	0.26
Breadfruit, raw	70.65	27.12	4.9	0.23
Carambola, (starfruit), raw	90.92	7.83	2.7	0.35
Carissa, (natal-plum), raw	84.17	13.63		1.3
Cherimoya, raw	73.5	24	2.4	0.4
Cherries, sour, red, canned, extra heavy syrup pack, solids and liquids	69.73	29.23	0.8	0.09
Cherries, sour, red, canned, heavy syrup pack, solids and liquids	75.66	23.27	1.1	0.1
Cherries, sour, red, canned, light syrup pack, solids and liquids	79.62	19.3	0.8	0.1
Cherries, sour, red, canned, water pack, solids and liquids	89.93	8.94	1.1	0.1
Cherries, sour, red, frozen, unsweetened	87.2	11.02	1.6	0.44
Cherries, sour, red, raw	86.13	12.18	1.6	0.3
Cherries, sweet, canned, extra heavy syrup pack, solids and liquids	72.66	26.23	1.5	0.15
Cherries, sweet, canned, heavy syrup pack, solids and liquids	77.61	21.27	1.5	0.15
Cherries, sweet, canned, juice pack, solids and liquids	84.95	13.81	1.5	0.02
Cherries, sweet, canned, light syrup pack, solids and liquids	81.56	17.29	1.5	0.15
Cherries, sweet, canned, water pack, solids and liquids	87.05	11.76	1.5	0.13
Cherries, sweet, frozen, sweetened	75.53	22.36	2.1	0.13
Cherries, sweet, raw	80.76	16.55	2.3	0.96

Crabapples, raw	78.94	19.95		0.3
Cranberries, raw	86.54	12.68	4.2	0.2
Cranberry sauce, canned, sweetened	60.65	38.9	1	0.15
Cranberry-orange relish, canned	53.2	46.2	0	0.1
Currants, European black, raw	81.96	15.38		0.41
Currants, red and white, raw	83.95	13.8	4.3	0.2
Currants, zante, dried	19.21	74.08	6.8	0.27
Custard-apple, (bullock's-heart), raw	71.5	25.2		0.6
Dates, domestic, natural and dry	22.5	73.51	7.5	0.45
Elderberries, raw	79.8	18.4	7	0.5
Feijoa, raw	86.6	10.63		0.78
Figs, canned, extra heavy syrup pack, solids and liquids	71.39	27.86		0.1
Figs, canned, heavy syrup pack, solids and liquids	76.33	22.9	2.2	0.1
Figs, canned, light syrup pack, solids and liquids	81.26	17.95	1.8	0.1
Figs, canned, water pack, solids and liquids	85.21	13.99	2.2	0.1
Figs, dried, stewed	69.8	27.57	4.8	0.49
Figs, dried, uncooked	28.43	65.35	9.3	1.17
Figs, raw	79.11	19.18	3.3	0.3
Fruit cocktail, (peach and pineapple and pear and grape and cherry), canned, extra heavy syrup, solids and liquids	76.43	22.89	1.1	0.07
Fruit cocktail, (peach and pineapple and pear and grape and cherry), canned, extra light syrup, solids and liquids	87.7	11.63	1.1	0.07
Fruit cocktail, (peach and pineapple and pear and grape and cherry), canned, heavy syrup, solids and liquids	80.4	18.91	1	0.07
Fruit cocktail, (peach and pineapple and pear and grape and cherry), canned, juice pack, solids and liquids	87.44	11.86	1	0.01
Fruit cocktail, (peach and pineapple and pear and grape and cherry), canned, light syrup, solids and liquids	84.37	14.93	1	0.07
Fruit cocktail, (peach and pineapple and pear and grape and cherry), canned, water pack, solids and liquids	90.76	8.51	1	0.05
Fruit salad, (peach and pear and apricot and pineapple and cherry), canned, extra heavy syrup, solids and liquids	76.64	22.77	1	0.06
Fruit salad, (peach and pear and apricot and pineapple and cherry), canned, heavy syrup, solids and liquids	80.26	19.11	1	0.07
Fruit salad, (peach and pear and apricot and pineapple and cherry), canned, juice pack, solids and liquids	86.15	13.05	1	0.03
Fruit salad, (peach and pear and apricot and pineapple and cherry), canned, light syrup, solids and liquids	84.24	15.14	1	0.07
Fruit salad, (peach and pear and apricot and pineapple and cherry), canned, water pack, solids and liquids	91.5	7.87	1	0.07
Fruit salad, (pineapple and papaya and banana and guava), tropical, canned, heavy syrup, solids and liquids	76.78	22.36	1.3	0.1
Fruit, mixed, (peach and cherry-sweet and -sour and raspberry and grape and boysenberry), frozen, sweetened	73.73	24.23	1.9	0.18

Fruit, mixed, (peach and pear and pineapple), canned, heavy syrup, solids and liquids	80.56	18.76	1	0.1
Fruit, mixed, (prune and apricot and pear), dried	31.18	64.06	7.8	0.49
Gooseberries, canned, light syrup pack, solids and liquids	80.1	18.75	2.4	0.2
Gooseberries, raw	87.87	10.18	4.3	0.58
Grape juice, canned or bottled, unsweetened, without added vitamin C	84.12	14.96	0.1	0.08
Grape juice, frozen concentrate, sweetened, diluted with 3 volume water, without added vitamin C	86.9	12.75	0.1	0.09
Grape juice, frozen concentrate, sweetened, undiluted, without added vitamin C	54.4	44.37	0.3	0.31
Grapefruit juice, canned, sweetened	87.38	11.13	0.1	0.09
Grapefruit juice, canned, unsweetened	90.1	8.96	0.1	0.1
Grapefruit juice, frozen concentrate, unsweetened, diluted with 3 volume water	89.3	9.73	0.1	0.13
Grapefruit juice, frozen concentrate, unsweetened, undiluted	62	34.56	0.4	0.48
Grapefruit juice, pink, raw	90	9.2		0.1
Grapefruit juice, white, raw	90	9.2	0.1	0.1
Grapefruit, raw, pink and red and white, all areas	90.89	8.08	1.1	0.1
Grapefruit, raw, pink and red, California and Arizona	89.31	9.69		0.1
Grapefruit, raw, pink and red, Florida	91.56	7.5	1.1	0.1
Grapefruit, raw, pink and red, all areas	91.38	7.68		0.1
Grapefruit, raw, white, California	89.58	9.09		0.1
Grapefruit, raw, white, Florida	90.76	8.19		0.1
Grapefruit, raw, white, all areas	90.48	8.41	1.1	0.1
Grapefruit, sections, canned, juice pack, solids and liquids	89.67	9.21	0.4	0.09
Grapefruit, sections, canned, light syrup pack, solids and liquids	83.59	15.44	0.4	0.1
Grapefruit, sections, canned, water pack, solids and liquids	89.85	9.15	0.4	0.1
Grapes, American type (slip skin), raw	81.3	17.15	1	0.35
Grapes, canned, Thompson seedless, heavy syrup pack, solids and liquids	79.53	19.65	0.4	0.1
Grapes, canned, Thompson seedless, water pack, solids and liquids	88.84	10.3	1	0.11
Grapes, European type (adherent skin), raw	80.56	17.77	1	0.58
Groundcherries, (cape-gooseberries or poha), raw	85.4	11.2		0.7
Guava sauce, cooked	89.56	9.48	3.6	0.14
Guavas, common, raw	86.1	11.88	5.4	0.6
Guavas, strawberry, raw	80.66	17.36		0.6
Jackfruit, raw	73.23	24.01	1.6	0.3
Java-plum, (jambolan), raw	83.13	15.56		0.23
Jujube, dried	19.7	73.6		1.1
Jujube, raw	77.86	20.23		0.2
Kiwi fruit, (Chinese gooseberries), fresh, raw	83.05	14.88	3.4	0.44
Kiwifruit, (Chinese gooseberries), held in storage, raw	83.05	14.88	3.4	0.44
Kumquats, raw	81.7	16.43	6.6	0.1

Lemon juice, canned or bottled	92.46	6.48	0.4	0.29
Lemon juice, frozen, unsweetened, single strength	92.39	6.5	0.4	0.32
Lemon juice, raw	90.73	8.63	0.4	0
Lemon peel, raw	81.6	16	10.6	0.3
Lemons, raw, with peel	87.4	10.7	4.7	0.3
Lemons, raw, without peel	88.98	9.32	2.8	0.3
Lime juice, canned or bottled, unsweetened	92.52	6.69	0.4	0.23
Lime juice, raw	90.21	9.01	0.4	0.1
Limes, raw	88.26	10.54	2.8	0.2
Litchis, dried	22.3	70.7	4.6	1.2
Litchis, raw	81.76	16.53	1.3	0.44
Loganberries, frozen	84.61	13.02	4.9	0.31
Longans, dried	17.6	74		0.4
Longans, raw	82.75	15.14	1.1	0.1
Loquats, raw	86.73	12.14	1.7	0.2
Mammy-apple, (mamey), raw	86.2	12.5	3	0.5
Mangos, raw	81.71	17	1.8	0.27
Melon balls, frozen	90.26	7.94	0.7	0.25
Melons, cantaloupe, raw	89.78	8.36	0.8	0.28
Melons, casaba, raw	92	6.2	0.8	0.1
Melons, honeydew, raw	89.66	9.18	0.6	0.1
Mulberries, raw	87.68	9.8	1.7	0.39
Nectarines, raw	86.28	11.78	1.6	0.46
Oheloberries, raw	92.3	6.84		0.22
Olives, ripe, canned (jumbo-super colossal)	84.34	5.61	2.5	6.87
Olives, ripe, canned (small-extra large)	79.99	6.26	3.2	10.68
Orange juice, California, chilled, includes from concentrate	88.4	10.06		0.27
Orange juice, canned, unsweetened	89.01	9.85	0.2	0.14
Orange juice, chilled, includes from concentrate	88.4	10.06	0.2	0.27
Orange juice, frozen concentrate, unsweetened, diluted with 3 volume water	88.1	10.78	0.2	0.06
Orange juice, frozen concentrate, unsweetened, undiluted	57.85	38.17	0.8	0.21
Orange juice, raw	88.3	10.4	0.2	0.2
Orange peel, raw	72.5	25	10.6	0.2
Orange-grapefruit juice, canned, unsweetened	88.64	10.28	0.1	0.1
Oranges, raw, California, navels	86.81	11.63	2.4	0.09
Oranges, raw, California, valencias	86.34	11.89	2.5	0.3
Oranges, raw, Florida	87.14	11.54	2.4	0.21
Oranges, raw, all commercial varieties	86.75	11.75	2.4	0.12
Oranges, raw, with peel	82.3	15.5	4.5	0.3
Papaya nectar, canned	85.02	14.51	0.6	0.15
Papayas, raw	88.83	9.81	1.8	0.14
Passion-fruit juice, purple, raw	85.62	13.6	0.2	0.05
Passion-fruit juice, yellow, raw	84.21	14.45	0.2	0.18
Passion-fruit, (granadilla), purple, raw	72.93	23.38	10.4	0.7
Peach nectar, canned, with added ascorbic acid	85.64	13.92	0.6	0.02
Peach nectar, canned, without added ascorbic acid	85.64	13.92	0.6	0.02

Peaches, canned, extra heavy syrup pack, solids and liquids	73.19	26.06	1	0.03
Peaches, canned, extra light syrup, solids and liquids	88.2	11.1	1	0.1
Peaches, canned, heavy syrup pack, solids and liquids	79.28	19.94	1.3	0.1
Peaches, canned, juice pack, solids and liquids	87.49	11.57	1.3	0.03
Peaches, canned, light syrup pack, solids and liquids	84.72	14.55	1.3	0.03
Peaches, canned, water pack, solids and liquids	93.13	6.11	1.3	0.06
Peaches, dehydrated (low-moisture), sulfured, stewed	62.04	34.14		0.42
Peaches, dehydrated (low-moisture), sulfured, uncooked	7.5	83.18		1.03
Peaches, dried, sulfured, stewed, with added sugar	71.38	26.6	2.4	0.22
Peaches, dried, sulfured, stewed, without added sugar	78.1	19.69	2.7	0.25
Peaches, dried, sulfured, uncooked	31.8	61.33	8.2	0.76
Peaches, frozen, sliced, sweetened	74.73	23.98	1.8	0.13
Peaches, raw	87.66	11.1	2	0.09
Peaches, spiced, canned, heavy syrup pack, solids and liquids	79.2	20.08	1.3	0.1
Pear nectar, canned, with added ascorbic acid	84.01	15.76	0.6	0.01
Pear nectar, canned, without added ascorbic acid	84.01	15.76	0.6	0.01
Pears, Asian, raw	88.25	10.65	3.6	0.23
Pears, canned, extra heavy syrup pack, solids and liquids	74.28	25.25	1.6	0.13
Pears, canned, extra light syrup pack, solids and liquids	87.3	12.2	1.6	0.1
Pears, canned, heavy syrup pack, solids and liquids	80.35	19.17	1.6	0.13
Pears, canned, juice pack, solids and liquids	86.47	12.94	1.6	0.07
Pears, canned, light syrup pack, solids and liquids	84.46	15.17	1.6	0.03
Pears, canned, water pack, solids and liquids	91.81	7.81	1.6	0.03
Pears, dried, sulfured, stewed, with added sugar	61.2	37.14	5.8	0.29
Pears, dried, sulfured, stewed, without added sugar	64.44	33.81	6.4	0.31
Pears, dried, sulfured, uncooked	26.69	69.7	7.5	0.63
Pears, raw	83.81	15.11	2.4	0.4
Persimmons, Japanese, dried	23.01	73.43	14.5	0.59
Persimmons, Japanese, raw	80.32	18.59	3.6	0.19
Persimmons, native, raw	64.4	33.5		0.4
Pineapple juice, canned, unsweetened, without added ascorbic acid	85.53	13.78	0.2	0.08
Pineapple juice, canned, with added ascorbic acid, unsweetened	85.53	13.78	0.2	0.08
Pineapple juice, frozen concentrate, unsweetened, diluted with 3 volume water	86.5	12.77	0.2	0.03
Pineapple juice, frozen concentrate, unsweetened, undiluted	53.1	44.3	0.7	0.1
Pineapple, canned, extra heavy syrup pack, solids and liquids	77.71	21.5	0.8	0.11
Pineapple, canned, heavy syrup pack, solids and liquids	78.99	20.2	0.8	0.11
Pineapple, canned, juice pack, solids and liquids	83.51	15.7	0.8	0.08
Pineapple, canned, light syrup pack, solids and liquids	85.73	13.45	0.8	0.12
Pineapple, canned, water pack, solids and liquids	90.82	8.3	0.8	0.09
Pineapple, frozen, chunks, sweetened	77.1	22.2	1.1	0.1
Pineapple, raw	86.5	12.39	1.2	0.43
Pitanga, (Surinam-cherry), raw	90.81	7.49		0.4

Plantains, cooked	67.3	31.15	2.3	0.18
Plantains, raw	65.28	31.89	2.3	0.37
Plums, canned, purple, extra heavy syrup pack, solids and liquids	73	26.31	1	0.1
Plums, canned, purple, heavy syrup pack, solids and liquids	76.06	23.24	1	0.1
Plums, canned, purple, juice pack, solids and liquids	84.02	15.15	1	0.02
Plums, canned, purple, light syrup pack, solids and liquids	83	16.28	1	0.1
Plums, canned, purple, water pack, solids and liquids	88.35	11.03	1	0.01
Plums, raw	85.2	13.01	1.5	0.62
Pomegranates, raw	80.97	17.17	0.6	0.3
Prickly pears, raw	87.55	9.57	3.6	0.51
Prune juice, canned	81.24	17.45	1	0.03
Prunes, canned, heavy syrup pack, solids and liquids	70.67	27.8	3.8	0.2
Prunes, dehydrated (low-moisture), stewed	67.99	29.7		0.24
Prunes, dehydrated (low-moisture), uncooked	4	89.07		0.73
Prunes, dried, stewed, with added sugar	65.08	32.88	3.8	0.22
Prunes, dried, stewed, without added sugar	69.73	28.08	6.6	0.23
Prunes, dried, uncooked	32.39	62.73	7.1	0.52
Pummelo, raw	89.1	9.62	1	0.04
Quinces, raw	83.8	15.3	1.9	0.1
Raisins, golden seedless	14.97	79.52	4	0.46
Raisins, seeded	16.57	78.47	6.8	0.54
Raisins, seedless	15.42	79.13	4	0.46
Raspberries, canned, red, heavy syrup pack, solids and liquids	75.33	23.36	3.3	0.12
Raspberries, frozen, red, sweetened	72.75	26.16	4.4	0.16
Raspberries, raw	86.57	11.57	6.8	0.55
Rhubarb, frozen, cooked, with sugar	67.79	31.2	2	0.05
Rhubarb, frozen, uncooked	93.51	5.1	1.8	0.11
Rhubarb, raw	93.61	4.54	1.8	0.2
Rose-apples, raw	93	5.7	0.3	
Roselle, raw	86.58	11.31		0.64
Sapodilla, raw	78	19.96	5.3	1.1
Sapotes, (marmalade plum), raw	62.43	33.76	2.6	0.6
Soursop, raw	81.16	16.84	3.3	0.3
Strawberries, canned, heavy syrup pack, solids and liquids	75.35	23.53	1.7	0.26
Strawberries, frozen, sweetened, sliced	73.18	25.92	1.9	0.13
Strawberries, frozen, sweetened, whole	78.05	21	1.9	0.14
Strawberries, frozen, unsweetened	89.97	9.13	2.1	0.11
Strawberries, raw	91.57	7.02	2.3	0.37
Sugar-apples, (sweetsop), raw	73.23	23.64	4.4	0.29
Tamarinds, raw	31.4	62.5	5.1	0.6
Tangerine juice, canned, sweetened	87	12	0.2	0.2
Tangerine juice, frozen concentrate, sweetened, diluted with 3 volume water	88.1	11.06		0.11

Tangerine juice, frozen concentrate, sweetened, undiluted	58.2	38.85	0.6	0.39
Tangerine juice, raw	88.9	10.1	0.2	0.2
Tangerines, (mandarin oranges), canned, juice pack	89.51	9.57	0.7	0.03
Tangerines, (mandarin oranges), canned, light syrup pack	83.06	16.19	0.7	0.1
Tangerines, (mandarin oranges), raw	87.6	11.19	2.3	0.19
Watermelon, raw	91.51	7.18	0.5	0.43

LEGUMES

	Water	Carb.	% TDF	% FAT
Bacon, meatless	48.98	6.33	2.6	29.52
Beans, adzuki, mature seed, cooked, boiled, with salt	66.29	24.77		0.1
Beans, adzuki, mature seeds, canned, sweetened	40.58	55.01		0.03
Beans, adzuki, mature seeds, cooked, boiled, without salt	66.29	24.77		0.1
Beans, adzuki, mature seeds, raw	13.44	62.9	12.7	0.53
Beans, adzuki, yokan, mature seeds	35.45	60.72		0.12
Beans, baked, canned, plain or vegetarian	72.65	20.51	5	0.45
Beans, baked, canned, with beef	71.33	16.91		3.45
Beans, baked, canned, with franks	69.34	15.39	6.9	6.57
Beans, baked, canned, with pork	71.46	19.98	5.5	1.55
Beans, baked, canned, with pork and sweet sauce	70.71	20.99	5.2	1.46
Beans, baked, canned, with pork and tomato sauce	72.69	19.39	4.8	1.03
Beans, baked, home prepared	65.17	21.39	5.5	5.15
Beans, black turtle soup, mature seeds, canned	75.64	16.56	6.9	0.29
Beans, black turtle soup, mature seeds, cooked, boiled, with salt	65.74	24.35	5.3	0.35
Beans, black turtle soup, mature seeds, cooked, boiled, without salt	65.74	24.35	5.3	0.35
Beans, black turtle soup, mature seeds, raw	11	63.25	24.9	0.9
Beans, black, mature seeds, cooked, boiled, with salt	65.74	23.71	8.7	0.54
Beans, black, mature seeds, cooked, boiled, without salt	65.74	23.71	8.7	0.54
Beans, black, mature seeds, raw	11.02	62.37	15.2	1.42
Beans, cranberry (roman), mature seeds, canned	77.56	15.12	6.3	0.28
Beans, cranberry (roman), mature seeds, cooked, boiled, with salt	64.65	24.46	10	0.46
Beans, cranberry (roman), mature seeds, cooked, boiled, without salt	64.65	24.46	10	0.46
Beans, cranberry (roman), mature seeds, raw	12.39	60.05	24.7	1.23
Beans, French, mature seeds, cooked, boiled, with salt	66.57	24.02	9.4	0.76
Beans, French, mature seeds, cooked, boiled, without salt	66.57	24.02	9.4	0.76
Beans, French, mature seeds, raw	10.77	64.11	25.2	2.02
Beans, great northern, mature seeds, canned	69.89	21.03	4.9	0.39
Beans, great northern, mature seeds, cooked, boiled, with salt	69	21.09	7	0.45
Beans, great northern, mature seeds, cooked, boiled, without salt	69	21.09	7	0.45

Beans, great northern, mature seeds, raw	10.7	62.37	20.2	1.14
Beans, kidney, all types, mature seeds, canned	77.95	14.88	3.5	0.31
Beans, kidney, all types, mature seeds, cooked, boiled, with salt	66.94	22.81	6.4	0.5
Beans, kidney, all types, mature seeds, cooked, boiled, without salt	66.94	22.81	6.4	0.5
Beans, kidney, all types, mature seeds, raw	11.75	60.01	24.9	0.83
Beans, kidney, california red, mature seeds, cooked, boiled, with salt	66.93	22.41	9.3	0.09
Beans, kidney, california red, mature seeds, cooked, boiled, without salt	66.93	22.41	9.3	0.09
Beans, kidney, california red, mature seeds, raw	11.75	59.8	24.9	0.25
Beans, kidney, red, mature seeds, canned	77.36	15.6	6.4	0.34
Beans, kidney, red, mature seeds, cooked, boiled, with salt	66.94	22.81	7.4	0.5
Beans, kidney, red, mature seeds, cooked, boiled, without salt	66.94	22.81	7.4	0.5
Beans, kidney, red, mature seeds, raw	11.75	61.3	15.2	1.06
Beans, kidney, royal red, mature seeds, cooked, boiled with salt	66.99	21.85	9.3	0.17
Beans, kidney, royal red, mature seeds, cooked, boiled, without salt	66.99	21.85	9.3	0.17
Beans, kidney, royal red, mature seeds, raw	11.9	58.33	24.9	0.45
Beans, navy, mature seeds, canned	70.45	20.45	5.1	0.43
Beans, navy, mature seeds, cooked, boiled, with salt	63.18	26.31	15.9	0.57
Beans, navy, mature seeds, cooked, boiled, without salt	63.18	26.31	6.4	0.57
Beans, navy, mature seeds, raw	12.36	60.65	24.4	1.28
Beans, pink, mature seeds, cooked, boiled, with salt	61.2	27.91	5.3	0.49
Beans, pink, mature seeds, cooked, boiled, without salt	61.2	27.91	5.3	0.49
Beans, pink, mature seeds, raw	10.06	64.19	12.7	1.13
Beans, pinto, mature seeds, canned	77.54	15.25	4.6	0.81
Beans, pinto, mature seeds, cooked, boiled, with salt	64.27	25.65	8.6	0.52
Beans, pinto, mature seeds, cooked, boiled, without salt	64.27	25.65	8.6	0.52
Beans, pinto, mature seeds, raw	10.95	63.41	24.4	1.13
Beans, small white, mature seeds, cooked, boiled, with salt	63.24	25.81	10.4	0.64
Beans, small white, mature seeds, cooked, boiled, without salt	63.24	25.81	10.4	0.64
Beans, small white, mature seeds, raw	11.71	62.25	24.9	1.18
Beans, white, mature seeds, canned	70.1	21.94	4.8	0.29
Beans, white, mature seeds, cooked, boiled, with salt	63.08	25.1	6.3	0.35
Beans, white, mature seeds, cooked, boiled, without salt	63.08	25.1	6.3	0.35
Beans, white, mature seeds, raw	11.32	60.27	15.2	0.85
Beans, winged, mature seeds, cooked, boiled, without salt	67.19	14.94		5.84
Beans, yellow, mature seeds, cooked, boiled, with salt	62.98	25.27	10.4	1.08
Beans, yellow, mature seeds, cooked, boiled, without salt	62.98	25.27	10.4	1.08
Beans, yellow, mature seeds, raw	11.1	60.7	25.1	2.6

Broadbeans (fava beans), mature seeds, canned	80.32	12.41	3.7	0.22
Broadbeans (fava beans), mature seeds, cooked, boiled, with salt	71.54	19.65	5.4	0.4
Broadbeans (fava beans), mature seeds, cooked, boiled, without salt	71.54	19.65	5.4	0.4
Broadbeans (fava beans), mature seeds, raw	10.98	58.3	25	1.53
Carob flour	3.58	88.88	39.8	0.65
Chickpeas (garbanzo beans, bengal gram), mature seeds, canned	69.69	22.62	4.4	1.14
Chickpeas (garbanzo beans, bengal gram), mature seeds, cooked, boiled, with salt	60.21	27.41	7.6	2.59
Chickpeas (garbanzo beans, bengal gram), mature seeds, cooked, boiled, without salt	60.21	27.41	7.6	2.59
Chickpeas (garbanzo beans, bengal gram), mature seeds, raw	11.53	60.66	17.4	6.04
Chili with beans, canned	75.51	11.91	4.4	5.49
Cowpeas, catjang, mature seeds, cooked, boiled, with salt	69.7	20.32	3.6	0.71
Cowpeas, catjang, mature seeds, cooked, boiled, without salt	69.7	20.32	3.6	0.71
Cowpeas, catjang, mature seeds, raw	11.05	59.64	10.7	2.07
Cowpeas, common (black-eyed, crowder, southern), mature seeds, canned with pork	77.59	16.53	3.3	1.6
Cowpeas, common (black-eyed, crowder, southern), mature seeds, canned, plain	79.63	13.63	3.3	0.55
Cowpeas, common (black-eyed, crowder, southern), mature seeds, cooked, boiled, with salt	70.04	20.77	6.5	0.53
Cowpeas, common (black-eyed, crowder, southern), mature seeds, cooked, boiled, without salt	70.04	20.77	6.5	0.53
Cowpeas, common (black-eyed, crowder, southern), mature seeds, raw	11.95	60.03	10.6	1.26
Falafel	34.62	31.84		17.8
Humus, raw	64.91	20.17	5.1	8.45
Hyacinth beans, mature seeds, cooked, boiled, with salt	69.13	20.7		0.58
Hyacinth beans, mature seeds, cooked, boiled, without salt	69.13	20.7		0.58
Hyacinth beans, mature seeds, raw	9.38	60.76		1.69
Lentils, mature seeds, cooked, boiled, with salt	69.64	20.14	7.9	0.38
Lentils, mature seeds, cooked, boiled, without salt	69.64	20.14	7.9	0.38
Lentils, mature seeds, raw	11.19	57.09	30.5	0.96
Lima beans, large, mature seeds, canned	77.08	14.91	4.8	0.17
Lima beans, large, mature seeds, cooked, boiled, with salt	69.79	20.89	7	0.38
Lima beans, large, mature seeds, cooked, boiled, without salt	69.79	20.89	7	0.38
Lima beans, large, mature seeds, raw	10.17	63.38	19	0.69
Lima beans, thin seeded (baby), mature seeds, cooked, boiled, with salt	67.15	23.31	7.7	0.38
Lima beans, thin seeded (baby), mature seeds, cooked, boiled, without salt	67.15	23.31	7.7	0.38

Lima beans, thin seeded (baby), mature seeds, raw	12.07	62.83	20.6	0.93
Lupins, mature seeds, cooked, boiled, with salt	71.08	9.88	2.8	2.92
Lupins, mature seeds, cooked, boiled, without salt	71.08	9.88	2.8	2.92
Lupins, mature seeds, raw	10.44	40.38		9.74
Meat extender	7.48	38.32	17.5	2.97
Miso	41.45	27.96	5.4	6.07
Mothbeans, mature seeds, cooked, boiled, with salt	69.23	20.96		0.55
Mothbeans, mature seeds, cooked, boiled, without salt	69.23	20.96		0.55
Mothbeans, mature seeds, raw	9.68	61.52		1.61
Mung beans, mature seeds, cooked, boiled, with salt	72.66	19.14	7.6	0.38
Mung beans, mature seeds, cooked, boiled, without salt	72.66	19.14	7.6	0.38
Mung beans, mature seeds, raw	9.05	62.62	16.3	1.15
Mungo beans, mature seeds, cooked, boiled, with salt	72.51	18.34	6.4	0.55
Mungo beans, mature seeds, cooked, boiled, without salt	72.51	18.34	6.4	0.55
Mungo beans, mature seeds, raw	8.58	61.01	16.4	1.83
Natto	55.02	14.35	5.4	11
Noodles, chinese, cellophane or long rice (mung beans), dehydrated	13.42	86.1	0.5	0.06
Peanut butter, chunk style, with salt	1.13	21.59	6.6	49.94
Peanut butter, chunk style, without salt	1.13	21.59	6.6	49.94
Peanut butter, smooth style, with salt	1.22	19.28	5.9	51.03
Peanut butter, smooth style, without salt	1.22	19.28	5.9	51.03
Peanut flour, defatted	7.8	34.7	15.8	0.55
Peanut flour, low fat	7.8	31.27	15.8	21.9
Peanuts, all types, cooked, boiled, with salt	41.78	21.26	8.8	22.01
Peanuts, all types, dry-roasted, with salt	1.55	21.51	8	49.66
Peanuts, all types, dry-roasted, without salt	1.55	21.51	8	49.66
Peanuts, all types, oil-roasted, with salt	1.95	18.93	9.2	49.3
Peanuts, all types, oil-roasted, without salt	1.95	18.93	6.9	49.3
Peanuts, all types, raw	6.5	16.14	8.5	49.24
Peanuts, Spanish, oil-roasted, with salt	1.78	17.45	8.9	49.04
Peanuts, Spanish, oil-roasted, without salt	1.78	17.45	8.9	49.04
Peanuts, Spanish, raw	6.39	15.82	9.5	49.6
Peanuts, Valencia, oil-roasted, with salt	2.12	16.3	8.9	51.24
Peanuts, Valencia, oil-roasted, without salt	2.12	16.3	8.9	51.24
Peanuts, Valencia, raw	4.26	20.91	8.7	47.58
Peanuts, Virginia, oil-roasted, with salt	2.17	19.86	8.9	48.62
Peanuts, Virginia, oil-roasted, without salt	2.17	19.86	8.9	48.62
Peanuts, Virginia, raw	6.91	16.54	8.5	48.75
Peas, split, mature seeds, cooked, boiled, with salt	69.49	21.11	8.3	0.39
Peas, split, mature seeds, cooked, boiled, without salt	69.49	21.11	8.3	0.39
Peas, split, mature seeds, raw	11.27	60.38	25.5	1.16
Pigeon peas (red gram), mature seeds, cooked, boiled, with salt	68.55	23.25	6.7	0.38
Pigeon peas (red gram), mature seeds, cooked, boiled, without salt	68.55	23.25	6.7	0.38
Pigeon peas (red gram), mature seeds, raw	10.59	62.78	15	1.49
Refried beans, canned	75.97	15.53	5.3	1.26
Sausage, meatless	50.4	9.85	2.8	18.16

Soy flour, defatted	7.25	38.37	17.5	1.22
Soy flour, defatted, crude protein basis (N x 6.25)	7.25	33.93	17.5	1.22
Soy flour, full-fat, raw	5.16	35.2	9.6	20.65
Soy flour, full-fat, raw, crude protein basis (N x 6.25)	5.16	31.93	9.6	20.65
Soy flour, full-fat, roasted	3.81	33.67	9.7	21.86
Soy flour, full-fat, roasted, crude protein basis (N x 6.25)	3.81	30.38		21.86
Soy flour, low-fat	2.7	37.98	10.2	6.7
Soy flour, low-fat, crude protein basis (N x 6.25)	2.7	33.58	10.2	6.7
Soy meal, defatted, raw	6.94	40.14		2.39
Soy meal, defatted, raw, crude protein basis (N x 6.25)	6.94	35.89		2.39
Soy milk, fluid	93.27	1.81	1.3	1.91
Soy protein concentrate, crude protein basis (N x 6.25), produced by acid wash	5.8	25.41	5.5	0.46
Soy protein concentrate, produced by acid wash	5.8	31.21	5.5	0.46
Soy protein concentrate, produced by alcohol extraction	5.8	31.21	5.5	0.46
Soy protein isolate	4.98	7.36	5.6	3.39
Soy protein isolate, potassium type	4.98	10.23	5.6	0.53
Soy protein isolate, potassium type, crude protein basis	4.98	2.59	2	0.53
Soy sauce made from hydrolyzed vegetable protein	75.66	7.73	0.5	0.08
Soy sauce made from soy (tamari)	66	5.57	0.8	0.1
Soy sauce made from soy and wheat (shoyu)	71.09	8.51	0.8	0.08
Soy sauce made from soy and wheat (shoyu), low sodium	71.09	8.51	0.8	0.08
Soybeans, mature cooked, boiled, without salt	62.55	9.92	6	8.97
Soybeans, mature seeds, cooked, boiled, with salt	62.55	9.92	6	8.97
Soybeans, mature seeds, dry roasted	0.8	32.72	8.1	21.62
Soybeans, mature seeds, raw	8.54	30.16	9.3	19.94
Soybeans, mature seeds, roasted, no salt added	1.95	33.56	17.7	25.4
Soybeans, mature seeds, roasted, salted	1.95	33.56	17.7	25.4
Tempeh	54.95	17.03		7.68
Tofu, dried-frozen (koyadofu)	5.78	14.56	7.2	30.34
Tofu, dried-frozen (koyadofu), prepared with calcium sulfate	5.78	14.56	1.2	30.34
Tofu, fried	50.52	10.5	3.9	20.18
Tofu, fried, prepared with calcium sulfate	50.52	10.5	3.9	20.18
Tofu, okara	81.64	12.54		1.73
Tofu, raw, firm	69.83	4.28	2.3	8.72
Tofu, raw, firm, prepared with calcium sulfate	69.83	4.28	2.3	8.72
Tofu, raw, regular	84.55	1.88	1.2	4.78
Tofu, raw, regular, prepared with calcium sulfate	84.55	1.88	0.3	4.78
Tofu, salted and fermented (fuyu)	70.01	5.15		8
Tofu, salted and fermented (fuyu), prepared with calcium sulfate	70.01	5.15		8
Winged beans, mature seeds, cooked, boiled, with salt	67.19	14.94		5.84
Winged beans, mature seeds, raw	8.34	41.71		16.32
Yardlong beans, mature seeds, cooked, boiled, without salt	68.8	21.09	3.8	0.45
Yardlong beans, mature seeds, raw	8.43	61.91	11	1.31

Yardlong beans, yardlong, mature seeds, cooked, boiled, with salt	68.8	21.09	3.8	0.45

GRAINS

	Water	Carb.	% TDF	% FAT
Amaranth	9.84	66.17	15.2	6.51
Arrowroot flour	11.37	88.15	3.4	0.1
Barley	9.44	73.48	17.3	2.3
Barley, pearled, cooked	68.8	28.22	3.8	0.44
Barley, pearled, raw	10.09	77.72	15.6	1.16
Buckwheat	9.75	71.5	10	3.4
Buckwheat flour, whole-groat	11.15	70.59	10	3.1
Buckwheat groats, roasted, cooked	75.63	19.94	2.7	0.62
Buckwheat groats, roasted, dry	8.41	74.95	10.3	2.71
Bulgur, cooked	77.76	18.58	4.5	0.24
Bulgur, dry	9	75.87	18.3	1.33
Corn bran, crude	4.71	85.64	85.5	0.92
Corn flour, masa, enriched	9.03	76.27	9.6	3.78
Corn flour, masa, enriched, yellow	9.03	76.27		3.78
Corn flour, whole-grain, white	10.91	76.85	9.6	3.86
Corn flour, whole-grain, yellow	10.91	76.85	13.4	3.86
Corn, white	10.37	74.26		4.74
Corn, yellow	10.37	74.26		4.74
Cornmeal, degermed, enriched, white	11.59	77.68	7.4	1.65
Cornmeal, degermed, enriched, yellow	11.59	77.68	7.4	1.65
Cornmeal, degermed, unenriched, white	11.59	77.68	7.4	1.65
Cornmeal, degermed, unenriched, yellow	11.59	77.68	7.4	1.65
Cornmeal, self-rising, bolted, plain, enriched, white	12.59	70.28	6.7	3.4
Cornmeal, self-rising, bolted, plain, enriched, yellow	12.59	70.28	6.7	3.4
Cornmeal, self-rising, bolted, with wheat flour added, enriched, white	10.33	73.43	6.3	2.85
Cornmeal, self-rising, bolted, with wheat flour added, enriched, yellow	10.33	73.43	6.3	2.85
Cornmeal, self-rising, degermed, enriched, white	10.17	74.79	7.1	1.72
Cornmeal, self-rising, degermed, enriched, yellow	10.17	74.79	7.1	1.72
Cornmeal, whole-grain, white	10.26	76.89	7.3	3.59
Cornmeal, whole-grain, yellow	10.26	76.89	7.3	3.59
Cornstarch	8.32	91.27	0.9	0.05
Couscous, cooked	72.57	23.22	1.4	0.16
Couscous, dry	8.56	77.43	5	0.64
Hominy, canned, white	82.53	14.26	2.5	0.88
Hominy, canned, yellow	82.53	14.26	2.5	0.88
Macaroni, cooked, enriched	65.99	28.34	1.3	0.67
Macaroni, cooked, unenriched	65.99	28.34	1.3	0.67
Macaroni, dry, enriched	10.25	74.69	2.4	1.58
Macaroni, dry, unenriched	10.25	74.69	2.4	1.58
Macaroni, protein-fortified, cooked, enriched, (n x 5.70)	59.73	31.66		0.21
Macaroni, protein-fortified, cooked, enriched, (n x 6.25)	59.73	30.88	1.5	0.21
Macaroni, protein-fortified, dry, enriched, (n x 5.70)	9.23	67.56	2.4	2.23

Macaroni, protein-fortified, dry, enriched, (n x 6.25)	9.23	65.65	2.4	2.23
Macaroni, vegetable, cooked, enriched	68.37	26.61	4.3	0.11
Macaroni, vegetable, dry, enriched	9.89	74.88	4.3	1.04
Macaroni, whole-wheat, cooked	67.15	26.54	2.8	0.54
Macaroni, whole-wheat, dry	7.34	75.03	8.3	1.4
Millet, cooked	71.41	23.67	1.3	1
Millet, raw	8.67	72.85	8.5	4.22
Noodles, Chinese, chow mein	0.73	57.54	3.9	30.76
Noodles, egg, cooked, enriched	68.7	24.84	1.1	1.47
Noodles, egg, cooked, enriched, with added salt	68.7	24.84	1.1	1.47
Noodles, egg, cooked, unenriched, with added salt	68.7	24.84		1.47
Noodles, egg, cooked, unenriched, without added salt	68.7	24.84	1.1	1.47
Noodles, egg, dry, enriched	9.67	71.13	2.7	4.21
Noodles, egg, dry, unenriched	9.67	71.13	2.7	4.21
Noodles, egg, spinach, cooked, enriched	68.52	24.25	2.3	1.57
Noodles, egg, spinach, dry, enriched	8.72	70.32	6.8	4.55
Noodles, Japanese, soba, cooked	73.01	21.44		0.1
Noodles, Japanese, soba, dry	6.88	74.62		0.71
Noodles, Japanese, somen, cooked	67.91	27.54		0.18
Noodles, Japanese, somen, dry	9.21	74.1	4.3	0.81
Oat bran, cooked	84	11.44	2.6	0.86
Oat bran, raw	6.55	66.22	15.4	7.03
Oats	8.22	66.27	10.6	6.9
Pasta, corn, cooked	68.31	27.91	4.8	0.73
Pasta, corn, dry	10	79.26	11	2.08
Pasta, fresh-refrigerated, plain, as purchased	31	54.73		2.3
Pasta, fresh-refrigerated, plain, cooked	68.56	24.93		1.05
Pasta, fresh-refrigerated, spinach, as purchased	30.1	55.72	2.1	
Pasta, fresh-refrigerated, spinach, cooked	68.58	25.04		0.94
Pasta, homemade, made with egg, cooked	68.71	23.54		1.74
Pasta, homemade, made without egg, cooked	68.86	25.12		0.98
Quinoa	9.3	68.9	5.9	5.8
Rice bran, crude	6.13	49.69	21	20.85
Rice flour, brown	11.97	76.48	4.6	2.78
Rice flour, white	11.89	80.13	2.4	1.42
Rice, brown, long-grain, cooked	73.09	22.96	1.8	0.9
Rice, brown, long-grain, raw	10.37	77.24	3.5	2.92
Rice, brown, medium-grain, cooked	72.96	23.51	1.8	0.83
Rice, brown, medium-grain, raw	12.37	76.17	3.4	2.68
Rice, white, glutinous, cooked	76.63	21.09		10.19
Rice, white, glutinous, raw	10.46	81.68	2.8	0.55
Rice, white, long-grain, parboiled, cooked, enriched	72.49	24.73	0.4	0.27
Rice, white, long-grain, parboiled, cooked, unenriched	72.49	24.73	0.4	0.27
Rice, white, long-grain, parboiled, dry	10.16	81.72	1.7	0.56
Rice, white, long-grain, parboiled, dry, unenriched	10.16	81.72	1.7	0.56
Rice, white, long-grain, precooked or instant, enriched, dry	8.14	83.59	1.6	0.29
Rice, white, long-grain, precooked or instant, enriched, prepared	76.44	21.27	0.6	0.16
Rice, white, long-grain, regular, cooked	68.44	28.17	0.4	0.28

Rice, white, long-grain, regular, cooked, enriched, with salt	68.44	28.17	0.4	0.28
Rice, white, long-grain, regular, cooked, unenriched, with salt	68.44	28.17	0.4	0.28
Rice, white, long-grain, regular, cooked, unenriched, without salt	68.44	28.17	0.4	0.28
Rice, white, long-grain, regular, raw, enriched	11.62	79.95	1.3	0.66
Rice, white, long-grain, regular, raw, unenriched	11.62	79.95	1.3	0.66
Rice, white, medium-grain, cooked	68.61	28.59	0.3	0.21
Rice, white, medium-grain, cooked, unenriched	68.61	28.59		0.21
Rice, white, medium-grain, raw, enriched	12.89	79.34	1.4	0.58
Rice, white, medium-grain, raw, unenriched	12.89	79.34		0.58
Rice, white, short-grain, cooked	68.53	28.73		0.19
Rice, white, short-grain, cooked, unenriched	68.53	28.73		0.19
Rice, white, short-grain, raw	13.29	79.15	2.8	0.52
Rice, white, short-grain, raw, unenriched	13.29	79.15		0.52
Rice, white, with pasta, cooked	71.74	21.43	2.5	2.82
Rice, white, with pasta, dry	7.13	75.32		2.44
Rye	10.95	69.76	14.6	2.5
Rye flour, dark	11.07	68.74	22.6	2.69
Rye flour, light	8.78	80.23	14.6	1.36
Rye flour, medium	9.85	77.49	14.6	1.77
Semolina, enriched	12.67	72.83	3.9	1.05
Semolina, unenriched	12.67	72.83	3.9	1.05
Sorghum	9.2	74.63		3.3
Spaghetti, cooked, enriched, with added salt	65.99	28.34	1.7	0.67
Spaghetti, cooked, enriched, without added salt	65.99	28.34	1.7	0.67
Spaghetti, cooked, unenriched, with added salt	65.99	28.34		0.67
Spaghetti, cooked, unenriched, without added salt	65.99	28.34	1.7	0.67
Spaghetti, dry, enriched	10.25	74.69	2.4	1.58
Spaghetti, dry, unenriched	10.25	74.69	2.4	1.58
Spaghetti, protein-fortified, cooked, enriched (n x 5.70)	59.73	31.66	1.7	0.21
Spaghetti, protein-fortified, cooked, enriched (n x 6.25)	59.73	30.88	2	0.21
Spaghetti, protein-fortified, dry, enriched (n x 5.70)	9.23	67.56		2.23
Spaghetti, protein-fortified, dry, enriched (n x 6.25)	9.23	65.65	2.4	2.23
Spaghetti, spinach, cooked	68.14	26.15		0.63
Spaghetti, spinach, dry	8.34	74.81	10.6	1.57
Spaghetti, whole-wheat, cooked	67.15	26.54	4.5	0.54
Spaghetti, whole-wheat, dry	7.34	75.03		1.4
Tapioca, pearl, dry	10.99	88.69	0.9	0.02
Triticale	10.51	72.13		2.09
Triticale flour, whole-grain	10.01	73.14	14.6	1.81
Wheat bran, crude	9.89	64.51	42.8	4.25
Wheat flour, white, all-purpose, enriched, bleached	11.92	76.31	2.7	0.98
Wheat flour, white, all-purpose, enriched, calcium-fortified	11.92	76.31	2.7	0.98
Wheat flour, white, all-purpose, enriched, unbleached	11.92	76.31	2.7	0.98
Wheat flour, white, all-purpose, self-rising, enriched	10.59	74.22	2.7	0.97
Wheat flour, white, all-purpose, unenriched	11.92	76.31	2.7	0.98

Wheat flour, white, bread, enriched	13.36	72.53	2.4	1.66
Wheat flour, white, cake, enriched	12.51	78.03	1.7	0.86
Wheat flour, white, tortilla mix, enriched	10.08	67.14		10.63
Wheat flour, whole-grain	10.27	72.57	12.2	1.87
Wheat germ, crude	11.12	51.8	13.2	9.72
Wheat, durum	10.94	71.13		2.47
Wheat, hard red spring	12.76	68.03	12.2	1.92
Wheat, hard red winter	13.1	71.18	12.2	1.54
Wheat, hard white	9.57	75.9		1.71
Wheat, soft red winter	12.17	74.24	12.5	1.56
Wheat, soft white	10.42	75.36	12.7	1.99
Wheat, sprouted	47.75	42.53	1.1	1.27
Wild rice, cooked	73.93	21.34	1.8	0.34
Wild rice, raw	7.76	74.9	6.2	1.08

VEGETABLES

	Water	Carb.	% TDF	% FAT
Alfalfa seeds, sprouted, raw	91.14	3.78	2.5	0.69
Amaranth leaves, cooked, boiled, drained, with salt	91.49	4.11		0.18
Amaranth leaves, cooked, boiled, drained, without salt	91.49	4.11		0.18
Amaranth leaves, raw	91.69	4.03		0.33
Arrowhead, cooked, boiled, drained, with salt	77.08	16.14		0.1
Arrowhead, cooked, boiled, drained, without salt	77.08	16.14		0.1
Arrowhead, raw	72.48	20.23		0.29
Artichokes, (globe or French), cooked, boiled, drained, with salt	83.97	11.18	5.4	0.16
Artichokes, (globe or French), cooked, boiled, drained, without salt	83.97	11.18	5.4	0.16
Artichokes, (globe or French), frozen, cooked, boiled, drained, with salt	86.5	9.18	4.6	0.5
Artichokes, (globe or French), frozen, cooked, boiled, drained, without salt	86.5	9.18	4.6	0.5
Artichokes, (globe or French), frozen, unprepared	88.59	7.76	3.9	0.43
Artichokes, (globe or French), raw	84.94	10.51	5.4	0.15
Arugula, raw	91.71	3.65	1.6	0.66
Asparagus, canned, drained solids	93.98	2.48	1.6	0.65
Asparagus, canned, no salt added, solids and liquids	94.32	2.47	1	0.18
Asparagus, canned, regular pack, solids and liquids	94.32	2.47	1	0.18
Asparagus, cooked, boiled, drained	92.2	4.23	1.6	0.31
Asparagus, cooked, boiled, drained, with salt	92.2	4.23	2.1	0.31
Asparagus, frozen, cooked, boiled, drained, with salt	91.15	4.87	1.6	0.42
Asparagus, frozen, cooked, boiled, drained, without salt	91.15	4.87	1.6	0.42
Asparagus, frozen, unprepared	91.82	4.1	1.9	0.23
Asparagus, raw	92.4	4.54	2.1	0.2
Balsam-pear, leafy tips, cooked, boiled, drained, with salt	88.69	6.78	1.9	0.2
Balsam-pear, leafy tips, cooked, boiled, drained, without salt	88.69	6.78	1.9	0.2
Balsam-pear, leafy tips, raw	89.25	3.29		0.69

Balsam-pear, pods, cooked, boiled, drained, with salt	93.95	4.32	2	0.18
Balsam-pear, pods, cooked, boiled, drained, without salt	93.95	4.32	2	0.18
Balsam-pear, pods, raw	94.03	3.7	2.8	0.17
Bamboo shoots, canned, drained solids	94.32	3.22	1.4	0.4
Bamboo shoots, cooked, boiled, drained, with salt	95.92	1.92	1	0.22
Bamboo shoots, cooked, boiled, drained, without salt	95.92	1.92	1	0.22
Bamboo shoots, raw	91	5.2	2.2	0.3
Beans, kidney, mature seeds, sprouted, cooked, boiled, drained, with salt	89.3	4.72		0.58
Beans, kidney, mature seeds, sprouted, cooked, boiled, drained, without salt	89.3	4.72		0.58
Beans, kidney, mature seeds, sprouted, raw	90.7	4.1		0.5
Beans, lima, immature seeds, canned, regular pack, solids and liquids	81.17	13.33	3.6	0.29
Beans, mung, mature seeds, sprouted, canned, drained solids	96.1	2.15	0.8	0.06
Beans, navy, mature seeds, sprouted, cooked, boiled, drained, with salt	76.02	15.01		0.81
Beans, navy, mature seeds, sprouted, cooked, boiled, drained, without salt	76.02	15.01		0.81
Beans, navy, mature seeds, sprouted, raw	79.15	13.05		0.7
Beans, pinto, immature seeds, frozen, cooked, boiled, drained, with salt	58.01	30.88	8.6	0.48
Beans, pinto, immature seeds, frozen, cooked, boiled, drained, without salt	58.01	30.88	8.6	0.48
Beans, pinto, immature seeds, frozen, unprepared	55.8	32.5	5.7	0.5
Beans, pinto, mature seeds, sprouted, cooked, boiled, drained, with salt	93.39	4.1		0.32
Beans, pinto, mature seeds, sprouted, cooked, boiled, drained, without salt	93.39	4.1		0.32
Beans, pinto, mature seeds, sprouted, raw	81.3	11.6		0.9
Beans, shell, canned, solids and liquids	90.69	6.19	3.4	0.19
Beans, snap, canned, all styles, seasoned, solids and liquids	94.3	3.49	1.5	0.2
Beans, snap, green variety, canned, regular pack, solids and liquids	94.68	3.5	1.5	0.1
Beans, snap, green, canned, no salt added, solids and liquids	94.68	3.5	1.5	0.1
Beans, snap, green, canned, regular pack, drained solids	93.3	4.5	1.9	0.1
Beans, snap, green, canned, special dietary pack, drained solids	93.3	4.5	1.9	0.1
Beans, snap, green, cooked, boiled, drained, with salt	89.22	7.89	3.2	0.28
Beans, snap, green, cooked, boiled, drained, without salt	89.22	7.89	3.2	0.28
Beans, snap, green, frozen, all styles, unprepared	89.88	7.57	2.8	0.21
Beans, snap, green, frozen, cooked, boiled, drained without salt	91.42	6.45	3	0.17
Beans, snap, green, frozen, cooked, boiled, drained, with salt	91.42	6.45	3	0.17

Beans, snap, green, raw	90.27	7.14	3.4	0.12
Beans, snap, yellow, canned, no salt added, drained solids	93.3	4.5	1.3	0.1
Beans, snap, yellow, canned, no salt added, solids and liquids	94.68	3.5	1.5	0.1
Beans, snap, yellow, canned, regular pack, drained solids	93.3	4.5	1.3	0.1
Beans, snap, yellow, canned, regular pack, solids and liquids	94.68	3.5	1.5	0.1
Beans, snap, yellow, cooked, boiled, drained, with salt	89.22	7.89	3.3	0.28
Beans, snap, yellow, cooked, boiled, drained, without salt	89.22	7.89	3.3	0.28
Beans, snap, yellow, frozen, all styles, unprepared	89.88	7.57	2.8	0.21
Beans, snap, yellow, frozen, cooked, boiled, drained, with salt	91.42	6.45	3	0.17
Beans, snap, yellow, frozen, cooked, boiled, drained, without salt	91.42	6.45	3	0.17
Beans, snap, yellow, raw	90.27	7.14	3.4	0.12
Beet greens, cooked, boiled, drained, with salt	89.13	5.46	2.9	0.2
Beet greens, cooked, boiled, drained, without salt	89.13	5.46	2.9	0.2
Beet greens, raw	92.15	3.97	3.7	0.06
Beets, canned, drained solids	90.96	7.2	1.7	0.14
Beets, canned, no salt added, solids and liquids	91.62	6.58	1.2	0.07
Beets, canned, regular pack, solids and liquids	91.62	6.58	1.2	0.07
Beets, cooked, boiled, drained	87.06	9.96	2	0.18
Beets, cooked, boiled. drained, with salt	87.06	9.96	2	0.18
Beets, harvard, canned, solids and liquids	80.16	18.18	2.5	0.06
Beets, pickled, canned, solids and liquids	81.88	16.28		0.08
Beets, raw	87.58	9.56	2.8	0.17
Borage, cooked, boiled, drained, with salt	91.88	3.55		0.81
Borage, cooked, boiled, drained, without salt	91.88	3.55		0.81
Borage, raw	93	3.06		0.7
Broadbeans, immature seeds, cooked, boiled, drained, with salt	83.7	10.1		0.5
Broadbeans, immature seeds, cooked, boiled, drained, without salt	83.7	10.1	3.6	0.5
Broadbeans, immature seeds, raw	81	11.7	4.2	0.6
Broccoli, cooked, boiled, drained, with salt	90.69	5.06	2.9	0.35
Broccoli, cooked, boiled, drained, without salt	90.69	5.06	2.9	0.35
Broccoli, flower clusters, raw	90.69	5.24		0.35
Broccoli, frozen, chopped, cooked, boiled, drained, with salt	90.72	5.35	3	0.12
Broccoli, frozen, chopped, cooked, boiled, drained, without salt	90.72	5.35	3	0.12
Broccoli, frozen, chopped, unprepared	91.46	4.79	3	0.29
Broccoli, frozen, spears, cooked, boiled, drained, with salt	90.72	5.35	3	0.11
Broccoli, frozen, spears, cooked, boiled, drained, without salt	90.72	5.35	3	0.11
Broccoli, frozen, spears, unprepared	90.55	5.35	3	0.34

Broccoli, leaves, raw	90.69	5.24		0.35
Broccoli, raw	90.69	5.24	3	0.35
Broccoli, stalks, raw	90.69	5.24		0.35
Brussels sprouts, cooked, boiled, drained, with salt	87.32	8.67	2.6	0.51
Brussels sprouts, cooked, boiled, drained, without salt	87.32	8.67	2.6	0.51
Brussels sprouts, frozen, cooked, boiled, drained, with salt	86.74	8.32	4.1	0.39
Brussels sprouts, frozen, cooked, boiled, drained, without salt	86.74	8.32	4.1	0.39
Brussels sprouts, frozen, unprepared	87.07	7.87	3.8	0.41
Brussels sprouts, raw	86	8.96	3.8	0.3
Burdock root, cooked, boiled, drained, with salt	75.64	21.15	1.8	0.14
Burdock root, cooked, boiled, drained, without salt	75.64	21.15	1.8	0.14
Burdock root, raw	80.09	17.35	3.3	0.15
Butterbur, (fuki), raw	94.5	3.61		0.04
Butterbur, canned	97.92	0.38		0.13
Butterbur, cooked, boiled, drained, with salt	96.7	2.16		0.02
Butterbur, cooked, boiled, drained, without salt	96.7	2.16		0.02
Cabbage, Chinese (pak-choi), cooked, boiled, drained, with salt	95.55	1.78	1.6	0.16
Cabbage, Chinese (pak-choi), cooked, boiled, drained, without salt	95.55	1.78	1.6	0.16
Cabbage, Chinese (pak-choi), raw	95.32	2.18	1	0.2
Cabbage, Chinese (pe-tsai), cooked, boiled, drained, with salt	95.24	2.41	2.7	0.17
Cabbage, Chinese (pe-tsai), cooked, boiled, drained, without salt	95.24	2.41	2.7	0.17
Cabbage, Chinese (pe-tsai), raw	94.39	3.23	3.1	0.2
Cabbage, common (Danish, domestic, and pointed types), freshly harvest, raw	92.52	5.37	2.3	0.18
Cabbage, common (Danish, domestic, and pointed types), stored, raw	92.52	5.37	2.3	0.18
Cabbage, common, cooked, boiled, drained, with salt	93.6	4.46	2.8	0.43
Cabbage, cooked, boiled, drained, without salt	93.6	4.46	2.3	0.43
Cabbage, raw	92.15	5.43	2.3	0.27
Cabbage, red, cooked, boiled, drained, with salt	93.6	4.64	2	0.2
Cabbage, red, cooked, boiled, drained, without salt	93.6	4.64	2	0.2
Cabbage, red, raw	91.55	6.12	2	0.26
Cabbage, savoy, cooked, boiled, drained, with salt	92	5.41	2.8	0.09
Cabbage, savoy, cooked, boiled, drained, without salt	92	5.41	2.8	0.09
Cabbage, savoy, raw	91	6.1	3.1	0.1
Cardoon, cooked, boiled, drained, with salt	93.46	5.33	1.7	0.11
Cardoon, cooked, boiled, drained, without salt	93.46	5.33	1.7	0.11
Cardoon, raw	94	4.89	1.6	0.1
Carrot juice, canned	88.87	9.29	0.8	0.15
Carrots, baby, raw	89.81	8.16	1.8	0.53
Carrots, canned, no salt added, solids and liquids	92.99	5.37	1.8	0.14
Carrots, canned, regular pack, drained solids	92.95	5.54	1.5	0.19
Carrots, canned, regular pack, solids and liquids	92.99	5.37	1.8	0.14
Carrots, canned, special dietary pack, drained solids	92.95	5.54	1.5	0.19

Carrots, cooked, boiled, drained, with salt	87.38	10.48	3.3	0.18
Carrots, cooked, boiled, drained, without salt	87.38	10.48	3.3	0.18
Carrots, frozen, cooked, boiled, drained, with salt	89.88	8.25	3.5	0.11
Carrots, frozen, cooked, boiled, drained, without salt	89.88	8.25	3.5	0.11
Carrots, frozen, unprepared	89.05	8.99	3.2	0.21
Carrots, raw	87.79	10.14	3	0.19
Cassava, raw	68.51	26.92	1.6	0.39
Catsup	66.58	27.29	1.3	0.36
Catsup, low sodium	66.58	27.29	1.3	0.36
Cauliflower, cooked, boiled, drained, with salt	93	4.11	2.7	0.45
Cauliflower, cooked, boiled, drained, without salt	93	4.11	2.7	0.45
Cauliflower, frozen, cooked, boiled, drained, with salt	94	3.75	2.7	0.22
Cauliflower, frozen, cooked, boiled, drained, without salt	94	3.75	2.7	0.22
Cauliflower, frozen, unprepared	92.51	4.68	2.3	0.27
Cauliflower, green, cooked, no salt	89.47	6.28	3.3	0.31
Cauliflower, green, cooked, salt	89.47	6.28	3.3	0.31
Cauliflower, green, raw	89.79	6.09	3.2	0.3
Cauliflower, raw	91.91	5.2	2.5	0.21
Celeriac, cooked, boiled, drained, with salt	92.3	5.9		0.19
Celeriac, cooked, boiled, drained, without salt	92.3	5.9	1.2	0.19
Celeriac, raw	88	9.2	1.8	0.3
Celery, cooked, boiled, drained, with salt	94.11	4.01	1.6	0.16
Celery, cooked, boiled, drained, without salt	94.11	4.01	1.6	0.16
Celery, raw	94.64	3.65	1.7	0.14
Celtuce, raw	94.5	3.65	1.7	0.3
Chard, Swiss, cooked, boiled, drained, with salt	92.65	4.14	2.1	0.08
Chard, Swiss, cooked, boiled, drained, without salt	92.65	4.14	2.1	0.08
Chard, Swiss, raw	92.66	3.74	1.6	0.2
Chayote, fruit, cooked, boiled, drained, with salt	93.43	5.09		0.48
Chayote, fruit, cooked, boiled, drained, without salt	93.43	5.09	2.8	0.48
Chayote, fruit, raw	93	5.4	3	0.3
Chicory greens, raw	92	4.7	4	0.3
Chicory roots, raw	80	17.51		0.2
Chicory, witloof, raw	94.52	4	3.1	0.1
Chives, freeze-dried	2	64.29	26.2	3.5
Chives, raw	90.65	4.35	2.5	0.73
Chrysanthemum, garland, cooked, boiled, drained, with salt	92.49	4.31	2.3	0.09
Chrysanthemum, garland, cooked, boiled, drained, without salt	92.49	4.31	2.3	0.09
Chrysanthemum, garland, raw	92.56	4.37	2.9	0.17
Coleslaw	81.5	12.41	1.5	2.61
Collards, cooked, boiled, drained, with salt	91.86	6.13	2.8	0.19
Collards, cooked, boiled, drained, without salt	91.86	6.13	2.8	0.19
Collards, frozen, chopped, cooked, boiled, drained, with salt	88.47	7.11	2.8	0.41
Collards, frozen, chopped, cooked, boiled, drained, without salt	88.47	7.11	2.8	0.41
Collards, frozen, chopped, unprepared	89.53	6.45	3.6	0.37

Collards, raw	90.55	7.11	3.6	0.22
Coriander, raw	92.8	2.59	2.3	0.588
Corn pudding	76.32	12.76		5.32
Corn with red and green peppers, canned, solids and liquids	77.5	18.17		0.55
Corn, sweet, white, canned, cream style, no salt added	78.73	18.13	1.2	0.42
Corn, sweet, white, canned, cream style, regular pack	78.73	18.13	1.2	0.42
Corn, sweet, white, canned, vacuum pack, no salt added	76.58	19.44	2	0.5
Corn, sweet, white, canned, vacuum pack, regular pack	76.58	19.44	2	0.5
Corn, sweet, white, canned, whole kernel, drained solids	76.92	18.59	2	1
Corn, sweet, white, canned, whole kernel, no salt added, solids and liquids	81.34	15.4	0.7	0.5
Corn, sweet, white, canned, whole kernel, regular pack, solids and liquids	81.34	15.4	1.7	0.5
Corn, sweet, white, cooked, boiled, drained, with salt	69.57	25.11	2.7	1.28
Corn, sweet, white, cooked, boiled, drained, without salt	69.57	25.11	2.7	1.28
Corn, sweet, white, frozen, kernels cut off cob, boiled, drained, with salt	76.73	19.56	2.4	0.43
Corn, sweet, white, frozen, kernels cut off cob, boiled, drained, without salt	76.73	19.56	2.4	0.43
Corn, sweet, white, frozen, kernels cut off cob, unprepared	74.92	20.8	2.4	0.77
Corn, sweet, white, frozen, kernels on cob, cooked, boiled, drained, with salt	73.2	22.33	2.8	0.74
Corn, sweet, white, frozen, kernels on cob, cooked, boiled, drained, without salt	73.2	22.33	2.1	0.74
Corn, sweet, white, frozen, kernels on cob, unprepared	71.79	23.5	2.8	0.78
Corn, sweet, white, raw	75.96	19.02	2.7	1.18
Corn, sweet, yellow, canned, brine pack, regular pack, solids and liquids	81.34	15.4	1.7	0.5
Corn, sweet, yellow, canned, cream style, regular pack	78.73	18.13	1.2	0.42
Corn, sweet, yellow, canned, cream style, special dietary pack	78.73	18.13	1.2	0.42
Corn, sweet, yellow, canned, no salt added, solids and liquids	81.34	15.4	1.7	0.5
Corn, sweet, yellow, canned, vacuum pack, no salt added	76.58	19.44	2	0.5
Corn, sweet, yellow, canned, vacuum pack, regular pack	76.58	19.44	2	0.5
Corn, sweet, yellow, canned, whole kernel, drained solids	76.92	18.59	2	1
Corn, sweet, yellow, cooked, boiled, drained, with salt	69.57	25.11	2.8	1.28
Corn, sweet, yellow, cooked, boiled, drained, without salt	69.57	25.11	2.8	1.28
Corn, sweet, yellow, frozen, kernels cut off cob, boiled, drained, without salt	76.73	19.56	2.4	0.43

Corn, sweet, yellow, frozen, kernels cut off cob, unprepared	74.92	20.8	2.4	0.77
Corn, sweet, yellow, frozen, kernels on cob, cooked, boiled, drained, with salt	73.2	22.33	2.8	0.74
Corn, sweet, yellow, frozen, kernels on cob, cooked, boiled, drained, without salt	73.2	22.33	2.8	0.74
Corn, sweet, yellow, frozen, kernels on cob, unprepared	71.79	23.5	2.8	0.78
Corn, sweet, yellow, frozen, kernels, cut off cob, boiled, drained, with salt	76.73	19.56	2.4	0.43
Corn, sweet, yellow, raw	75.96	19.02	2.7	1.18
Cornsalad, raw	92.8	3.6		0.4
Cowpeas, immature seeds, cooked, boiled, drained, with salt	75.48	20.33	5	0.38
Cowpeas, immature seeds, cooked, boiled, drained, without salt	75.48	20.33	5	0.38
Cowpeas, immature seeds, frozen, cooked, boiled, drained, with salt	66.1	23.76	6.4	0.66
Cowpeas, immature seeds, frozen, cooked, boiled, drained, without salt	66.1	23.76	6.4	0.66
Cowpeas, immature seeds, frozen, unprepared	64.15	25.13	5	0.7
Cowpeas, immature seeds, raw	77.2	18.9	5	0.35
Cowpeas, leafy tips, cooked, boiled, drained, with salt	91.3	2.8		0.1
Cowpeas, leafy tips, cooked, boiled, drained, without salt	91.3	2.8		0.1
Cowpeas, leafy tips, raw	89.78	4.82		0.25
Cowpeas, young pods with seeds, cooked, boiled, drained, with salt	89.5	7		0.3
Cowpeas, young pods with seeds, cooked, boiled, drained, without salt	89.5	7		0.3
Cowpeas, young pods with seeds, raw	86	9.5		0.3
Cress, garden, cooked, boiled, drained, with salt	92.5	3.8	0.7	0.6
Cress, garden, cooked, boiled, drained, without salt	92.5	3.8	0.7	0.6
Cress, garden, raw	89.4	5.5	1.1	0.7
Cucumber, with peel, raw	96.01	2.76	0.8	0.13
Dandelion greens, cooked, boiled, drained, with salt	89.8	6.4	2.9	0.6
Dandelion greens, cooked, boiled, drained, without salt	89.8	6.4	2.9	0.6
Dandelion greens, raw	85.6	9.2	3.5	0.7
Dock, cooked, boiled, drained, with salt	93.6	2.93		0.64
Dock, cooked, boiled, drained, without salt	93.6	2.93	2.6	0.64
Dock, raw	93	3.2	2.9	0.7
Eggplant, cooked, boiled, drained, with salt	91.77	6.64	2.5	0.23
Eggplant, cooked, boiled, drained, without salt	91.77	6.64	2.5	0.23
Eggplant, raw	92.03	6.07	2.5	0.18
Endive, raw	93.79	3.35	3.1	0.2
Eppaw, raw	60	31.68		1.8
Fennel, bulb, raw	90.21	7.29	3.1	0.2
Garlic, raw	58.58	33.07	2.1	0.5
Ginger root, raw	81.67	15.09	2	0.73
Gourd, dishcloth (towelgourd), cooked, boiled, drained, with salt	84.29	14.34		0.34

Gourd, dishcloth (towelgourd), cooked, boiled, drained, without salt	84.29	14.34		0.34
Gourd, dishcloth (towelgourd), raw	93.85	4.36		0.2
Gourd, white-flowered (calabash), cooked, boiled, drained, with salt	95.32	3.69		0.02
Gourd, white-flowered (calabash), cooked, boiled, drained, without salt	95.32	3.69		0.02
Gourd, white-flowered (calabash), raw	95.54	3.39		0.02
Hearts of palm, canned	90.2	4.62	2.4	0.62
Horseradish-tree leafy tips, raw	78.66	8.28	2	1.4
Horseradish-tree, leafy tips, cooked, boiled, drained, with salt	81.65	11.15	2	0.93
Horseradish-tree, leafy tips, cooked, boiled, drained, without salt	81.65	11.15	2	0.93
Horseradish-tree, pods, cooked, boiled, drained, with salt	88.42	8.18	4.2	0.19
Horseradish-tree, pods, cooked, boiled, drained, without salt	88.42	8.18	4.2	0.19
Horseradish-tree, pods, raw	88.2	8.53	3.2	0.2
Hyacinth-beans, immature seeds, cooked, boiled, drained, with salt	86.9	9.2		0.27
Hyacinth-beans, immature seeds, cooked, boiled, drained, without salt	86.9	9.2		0.27
Hyacinth-beans, immature seeds, raw	87.87	9.19		0.2
Jerusalem-artichokes, raw	78.01	17.44	1.6	0.01
Jew's ear, (pepeao), dried	11.14	81.04		0.44
Jew's ear, (pepeao), raw	92.59	6.75		0.04
Jute, potherb, cooked, boiled, drained, with salt	87.15	7.3	2	0.2
Jute, potherb, cooked, boiled, drained, without salt	87.15	7.3	2	0.2
Jute, potherb, raw	87.72	5.8		0.25
Kale, cooked, boiled, drained, with salt	91.2	5.63	2	0.4
Kale, cooked, boiled, drained, without salt	91.2	5.63	2	0.4
Kale, frozen, cooked, boiled, drained, with salt	90.5	5.24	2	0.49
Kale, frozen, cooked, boiled, drained, without salt	90.5	5.24	2	0.49
Kale, frozen, unprepared	91.12	4.9	2	0.46
Kale, raw	84.46	10.01	2	0.7
Kale, scotch, cooked, boiled, drained, with salt	91.2	5.63		0.41
Kale, scotch, cooked, boiled, drained, without salt	91.2	5.63	1.2	0.41
Kale, scotch, raw	87	8.32	1.7	0.6
Kanpyo, (dried gourd strips)	19.97	65.04		0.56
Kohlrabi, cooked, boiled, drained, with salt	90.3	6.69	1.1	0.11
Kohlrabi, cooked, boiled, drained, without salt	90.3	6.69	1.1	0.11
Kohlrabi, raw	91	6.2	3.6	0.1
Lambs quarters, cooked, boiled, drained, with salt	88.9	5	2.1	0.7
Lambsquarters, cooked, boiled, drained, without salt	88.9	5	2.1	0.7
Lambsquarters, raw	84.3	7.3	4	0.8
Leeks, (bulb and lower leaf-portion), cooked, boiled, drained, with salt	90.8	7.62	1	0.2
Leeks, (bulb and lower leaf-portion), cooked, boiled, drained, without salt	90.8	7.62	1	0.2

Leeks, (bulb and lower leaf-portion), raw	83	14.15	1.8	0.3
Leeks, (bulb and lower-leaf portion), freeze-dried	2	74.65	10.4	2.1
Lentils, sprouted, cooked, stir-fried, with salt	68.7	21.25		0.45
Lentils, sprouted, cooked, stir-fried, without salt	68.7	21.25		0.45
Lentils, sprouted, raw	67.34	22.14		0.55
Lettuce, butterhead (includes Boston and bibb types), raw	95.58	2.32	1	0.22
Lettuce, cos or romaine, raw	94.91	2.37	1.7	0.2
Lettuce, iceberg (includes crisphead types), raw	95.89	2.09	1.4	0.19
Lettuce, looseleaf, raw	94	3.5	1.9	0.3
Lima beans, immature seeds, canned, no salt added, solids and liquids	81.17	13.33	3.6	0.29
Lima beans, immature seeds, cooked, boiled, drained, with salt	67.17	23.64	5.3	0.32
Lima beans, immature seeds, cooked, boiled, drained, without salt	67.17	23.64	5.3	0.32
Lima beans, immature seeds, frozen, baby, cooked, boiled, drained, with salt	72.35	19.45	6	0.3
Lima beans, immature seeds, frozen, baby, cooked, boiled, drained, without salt	72.35	19.45	6	0.3
Lima beans, immature seeds, frozen, baby, unprepared	65.46	25.13	6	0.44
Lima beans, immature seeds, frozen, fordhook, cooked, boiled, drained, with salt	73.5	18.8	5.8	0.34
Lima beans, immature seeds, frozen, fordhook, cooked, boiled, drained, without salt	73.5	18.8	5.8	0.34
Lima beans, immature seeds, frozen, fordhook, unprepared	72.05	19.83	5.5	0.35
Lima beans, immature seeds, raw	70.24	20.16	4.9	0.86
Lotus root, cooked, boiled, drained, with salt	81.42	16.03	3.1	0.07
Lotus root, cooked, boiled, drained, without salt	81.42	16.03	3.1	0.07
Lotus root, raw	79.1	17.24	4.9	0.1
Mountain yam, Hawaii, cooked, steamed, with salt	77.14	20		0.08
Mountain yam, Hawaii, cooked, steamed, without salt	77.14	20		0.08
Mountain yam, Hawaii, raw	81.44	16.31		0.1
Mung beans, mature seeds, sprouted, cooked, boiled, drained, with salt	93.39	4.19	0.8	0.09
Mung beans, mature seeds, sprouted, cooked, boiled, drained, without salt	93.39	4.19	0.8	0.09
Mung beans, mature seeds, sprouted, cooked, stir-fried	84.3	10.59	1.9	0.21
Mung beans, mature seeds, sprouted, raw	90.4	5.93	1.8	0.18
Mushrooms, canned, drained solids	91.08	4.96	2.4	0.29
Mushrooms, cooked, boiled, drained, with salt	91.08	5.14	2.2	0.47
Mushrooms, cooked, boiled, drained, without salt	91.08	5.14	2.2	0.47
Mushrooms, enoki, raw	89.36	7.02	2.6	0.39
Mushrooms, raw	91.81	4.65	1.2	0.42
Mushrooms, shiitake, cooked, with salt	83.48	14.28	2.1	0.22
Mushrooms, shiitake, cooked, without salt	83.48	14.28	2.1	0.22
Mushrooms, shiitake, dried	9.5	75.37	11.5	0.99
Mustard greens, cooked, boiled, drained, with salt	94.46	2.1	2	0.24
Mustard greens, cooked, boiled, drained, without salt	94.46	2.1	2	0.24

Mustard greens, frozen, cooked, boiled, drained, with salt	93.8	3.12	2.8	0.25
Mustard greens, frozen, cooked, boiled, drained, without salt	93.8	3.12	2.8	0.25
Mustard greens, frozen, unprepared	93.21	3.41	3.3	0.27
Mustard greens, raw	90.8	4.9	3.3	0.2
Mustard spinach, (tendergreen), cooked, boiled, drained, with salt	94.5	2.8	2	0.2
Mustard spinach, (tendergreen), cooked, boiled, drained, without salt	94.5	2.8	2	0.2
Mustard spinach, (tendergreen), raw	92.2	3.9	2.8	0.3
New Zealand spinach, cooked, boiled, drained, without salt	94.8	2.2		0.17
New Zealand spinach, raw	94	2.5		0.2
New zealand spinach, cooked, boiled, drained, with salt	94.8	2.2		0.17
Nopales, cooked, without salt	94.31	3.27	2	0.05
Nopales, raw	93.93	3.39	2.3	0.12
Okra, cooked, boiled, drained, with salt	89.91	7.21	2.5	0.17
Okra, cooked, boiled, drained, without salt	89.91	7.21	2.5	0.17
Okra, frozen, cooked, boiled, drained, with salt	91.12	5.75	2.8	0.3
Okra, frozen, cooked, boiled, drained, without salt	91.12	5.75	2.8	0.3
Okra, frozen, unprepared	90.82	6.64	2.2	0.25
Okra, raw	89.58	7.63	3.2	0.1
Onion rings, breaded, par fried, frozen, prepared, heated in oven	28.5	38.16	1.3	26.7
Onion rings, breaded, par fried, frozen, unprepared	51.22	30.53	1.8	14.1
Onions, canned, solids and liquids	94.1	4.01	1.2	0.09
Onions, cooked, boiled, drained, with salt	87.86	10.15	1.4	0.19
Onions, cooked, boiled, drained, without salt	87.86	10.15	1.4	0.19
Onions, dehydrated flakes	3.93	83.28	9.2	0.46
Onions, frozen, chopped, cooked, boiled, drained, with salt	92.24	6.6	1.7	0.1
Onions, frozen, chopped, cooked, boiled, drained, without salt	92.24	6.6	1.8	0.1
Onions, frozen, chopped, unprepared	91.99	6.81	1.8	0.1
Onions, frozen, whole, cooked, boiled, drained, with salt	92.24	6.7	1.4	0.05
Onions, frozen, whole, cooked, boiled, drained, without salt	92.24	6.7	1.4	0.05
Onions, frozen, whole, unprepared	90.22	8.44	1.7	0.06
Onions, raw	89.68	8.63	1.8	0.16
Onions, spring (includes tops and bulb), raw	89.83	7.34	2.6	0.19
Onions, welsh, raw	90.5	6.5		0.4
Parsley, freeze-dried	2	42.38	32.7	5.2
Parsley, raw	87.71	6.33	3.3	0.79
Parsnips, cooked, boiled, drained, with salt	77.72	19.53	4	0.3
Parsnips, cooked, boiled, drained, without salt	77.72	19.53	4	0.3
Parsnips, raw	79.53	17.99	4.9	0.3
Peas and carrots, canned, no salt added, solids and liquids	88.15	8.48	3.3	0.27

Peas and carrots, canned, regular pack, solids and liquids	88.15	8.48	2	0.27
Peas and carrots, frozen, cooked, boiled, drained, with salt	85.8	10.12	3.1	0.42
Peas and carrots, frozen, cooked, boiled, drained, without salt	85.8	10.12	3.1	0.42
Peas and carrots, frozen, unprepared	84.36	11.15	3.4	0.47
Peas and onions, canned, solids and liquids	86.4	8.57	2.3	0.38
Peas and onions, frozen, cooked, boiled, drained, with salt	88.18	8.63	2.2	0.2
Peas and onions, frozen, cooked, boiled, drained, without salt	88.18	8.63	2.2	0.2
Peas and onions, frozen, unprepared	81.5	13.51	3.5	0.32
Peas, edible-podded, cooked, boiled, drained, with salt	88.91	7.05	2.8	0.23
Peas, edible-podded, cooked, boiled, drained, without salt	88.91	7.05	2.8	0.23
Peas, edible-podded, frozen, cooked, boiled, drained, with salt	86.6	9.02	3.1	0.38
Peas, edible-podded, frozen, cooked, boiled, drained, without salt	86.6	9.02	3.1	0.38
Peas, edible-podded, frozen, unprepared	89.3	7.2	3.1	0.3
Peas, edible-podded, raw	88.89	7.56	2.6	0.2
Peas, green, canned, dietary pack, drained solids	81.7	12.58	4.1	0.35
Peas, green, canned, no salt added, solids and liquids	85.92	9.75	3.2	0.3
Peas, green, canned, regular pack, drained solids	81.7	12.58	4.1	0.35
Peas, green, canned, regular pack, solids and liquids	85.92	9.75	3.2	0.3
Peas, green, canned, seasoned, solids and liquids	86.51	9.25	2	0.27
Peas, green, cooked, boiled, drained, with salt	77.87	15.64	5.5	0.22
Peas, green, cooked, boiled, drained, without salt	77.87	15.64	5.5	0.22
Peas, green, frozen, cooked, boiled, drained, with salt	79.52	14.26	5.5	0.27
Peas, green, frozen, cooked, boiled, drained, without salt	79.52	14.26	5.5	0.27
Peas, green, frozen, unprepared	79.93	13.7	4.7	0.37
Peas, green, raw	78.86	14.46	5.1	0.4
Peas, mature seeds, sprouted, cooked, boiled, drained, with salt	74.37	21.86		0.51
Peas, mature seeds, sprouted, cooked, boiled, drained, without salt	74.37	21.86		0.51
Peas, mature seeds, sprouted, raw	62.27	28.26		0.68
Peppers, hot chile, sun-dried	7.15	69.86	28.7	5.81
Peppers, hot chili, green, canned, pods, excluding seeds, solids and liquids	92.5	5.1	1.3	0.1
Peppers, hot chili, green, raw	87.74	9.46	1.5	0.2
Peppers, hot chili, red, canned, excluding seeds, solids and liquids	92.5	5.1	1.3	0.1
Peppers, hot chili, red, raw	87.74	9.46	1.5	0.2
Peppers, jalapeno, canned, solids and liquids	89.9	4.9	1.9	0.6
Peppers, sweet, green, canned, solids and liquids	91.25	3.9	1.2	0.3
Peppers, sweet, green, cooked, boiled, drained, with salt	91.87	6.7	1.2	0.2

Peppers, sweet, green, cooked, boiled, drained, without salt	91.87	6.7	1.2	0.2
Peppers, sweet, green, freeze-dried	2	68.7	21.3	3
Peppers, sweet, green, frozen, chopped, boiled, drained, without salt	94.7	3.9	0.9	0.18
Peppers, sweet, green, frozen, chopped, cooked, boiled, drained, with salt	94.7	3.9		0.18
Peppers, sweet, green, frozen, chopped, unprepared	93.96	4.45	1.6	0.21
Peppers, sweet, green, raw	92.19	6.43	1.8	0.19
Peppers, sweet, red, canned, solids and liquids	91.25	3.9	1.2	0.3
Peppers, sweet, red, cooked, boiled, drained, with salt	91.87	6.7	1.2	0.2
Peppers, sweet, red, cooked, boiled, drained, without salt	91.87	6.7	1.2	0.2
Peppers, sweet, red, freeze-dried	2	68.7	21.3	3
Peppers, sweet, red, frozen, chopped, cooked, boiled, drained, with salt	94.7	3.9		0.18
Peppers, sweet, red, frozen, chopped, cooked, boiled, drained, without salt	94.7	3.9		0.18
Peppers, sweet, red, frozen, chopped, unprepared	93.96	4.45	1.6	0.21
Peppers, sweet, red, raw	92.19	6.43	2	0.19
Peppers, sweet, yellow, raw	92.02	6.32	0.9	0.21
Pickle relish, hamburger	61.12	34.48	3.2	0.54
Pickle relish, hot dog	71.65	23.35	1.5	0.46
Pickle relish, sweet	62.07	35.05	1.1	0.47
Pickle, cucumber, sour	94.08	2.25	1.2	0.2
Pickle, cucumber, sour, low sodium	94.08	2.25	1.2	0.2
Pickle, cucumber, sweet	65.26	31.81	1.1	0.26
Pickle, cucumber, sweet, low sodium	65.26	31.81	1.1	0.26
Pickles, cucumber, dill	91.67	4.13	1.2	0.19
Pickles, cucumber, dill, low sodium	91.67	4.13	1.2	0.19
Pigeonpeas, immature seeds, cooked, boiled, drained, with salt	71.8	19.49	6.2	1.36
Pigeonpeas, immature seeds, cooked, boiled, drained, without salt	71.8	19.49	6.2	1.36
Pigeonpeas, immature seeds, raw	65.88	23.88	5.1	1.64
Pimento, canned	93.1	5.1	1.9	0.3
Poi	71.64	27.23	0.4	0.14
Pokeberry shoots, (poke), cooked, boiled, drained, with salt	92.9	3.1	1.5	0.4
Pokeberry shoots, (poke), cooked, boiled, drained, without salt	92.9	3.1	1.5	0.4
Pokeberry shoots, (poke), raw	91.6	3.7	1.7	0.4
Potato flour	7.6	79.9	6.1	0.8
Potato pancakes, home-prepared	47.26	28.64	2	15.24
Potato puffs, frozen, prepared	52.9	30.48	3.2	10.73
Potato puffs, frozen, unprepared	62.44	24.31	2.3	8.55
Potato salad	76	11.17	1.3	8.2
Potatoes, au gratin, dry mix, prepared with water, whole milk and butter	78.98	12.84	0.9	4.12

Potatoes, au gratin, dry mix, unprepared	4.97	74.31	4.1	3.7
Potatoes, au gratin, home-prepared from recipe using butter	74	11.27	1.8	7.59
Potatoes, au gratin, home-prepared from recipe using margarine	74	11.27	1.8	7.59
Potatoes, baked, flesh and skin, with salt	71.2	25.23	2.4	0.1
Potatoes, baked, flesh and skin, without salt	71.2	25.23	2.4	0.1
Potatoes, baked, flesh, with salt	75.42	21.56	1.5	0.1
Potatoes, baked, flesh, without salt	75.42	21.56	1.5	0.1
Potatoes, baked, skin, with salt	47.31	46.07	7.9	0.1
Potatoes, baked, skin, without salt	47.31	46.07	7.9	0.1
Potatoes, boiled, cooked in skin, flesh, with salt	76.98	20.13	2	0.1
Potatoes, boiled, cooked in skin, flesh, without salt	76.98	20.13	1.8	0.1
Potatoes, boiled, cooked in skin, skin, with salt	77.8	17.21	3.3	0.1
Potatoes, boiled, cooked in skin, skin, without salt	77.8	17.21	3.3	0.1
Potatoes, boiled, cooked without skin, flesh, with salt	77.46	20.01	2	0.1
Potatoes, boiled, cooked without skin, flesh, without salt	77.46	20.01	1.8	0.1
Potatoes, canned, drained solids	84.28	13.61	2.3	0.21
Potatoes, canned, solids and liquids	87.83	9.89	1.4	0.11
Potatoes, French fried, frozen, home-prepared, heated in oven, with salt	57.15	31.19	3.2	7.56
Potatoes, French fried, frozen, home-prepared, heated in oven, without salt	57.15	31.19	3.2	7.56
Potatoes, French fried, frozen, unprepared	66.58	24.33	3	5.9
Potatoes, frozen, French fried, par fried, cottage-cut, prepared, heated in oven, with salt	52.9	34.04	3.2	8.2
Potatoes, frozen, French fried, par fried, cottage-cut, prepared, heated in oven, without salt	52.9	34.04	3.2	8.2
Potatoes, frozen, French fried, par fried, cottage-cut, unprepared	66.82	23.98	3	5.78
Potatoes, frozen, French fried, par fried, extruded, prepared, heated in oven, without salt	35.4	39.68	3.2	18.71
Potatoes, frozen, French fried, par fried, extruded, unprepared	49.94	30.15	4.5	14.95
Potatoes, frozen, whole, cooked, boiled, drained, with salt	82.8	14.52	1.4	0.13
Potatoes, frozen, whole, cooked, boiled, drained, without salt	82.8	14.52	1.4	0.13
Potatoes, frozen, whole, unprepared	79.3	17.48	1.2	0.16
Potatoes, hashed brown, frozen, plain, prepared	56.1	28.1	2	11.5
Potatoes, hashed brown, frozen, plain, unprepared	78.85	17.72	1.4	0.62
Potatoes, hashed brown, frozen, with butter sauce, prepared	63.71	24.13	3.8	8.79
Potatoes, hashed brown, frozen, with butter sauce, unprepared	72.51	18.28	2.9	6.66
Potatoes, hashed brown, home-prepared	61.55	21.32	2	13.91
Potatoes, mashed, dehydrated, flakes without milk, dry form	6.51	81.21	6.9	0.39

Potatoes, mashed, dehydrated, granules with milk, dry form	6.3	77.7		1.1
Potatoes, mashed, dehydrated, granules without milk, dry form	3.63	85.51	7.1	0.54
Potatoes, mashed, dehydrated, prepared from flakes without milk, whole milk and butter add	76.3	15.02	2.3	5.6
Potatoes, mashed, dehydrated, prepared from granules with milk, water and margarine added	81.4	13.1	1.8	2.2
Potatoes, mashed, dehydrated, prepared from granules without milk, whole milk and butter added	77.49	14.36	2.2	4.96
Potatoes, mashed, home-prepared, whole milk added	78.46	17.55	2	0.59
Potatoes, mashed, home-prepared, whole milk and butter added	76.26	16.71	2	4.23
Potatoes, mashed, home-prepared, whole milk and margarine added	76.26	16.71	2	4.23
Potatoes, mashed, prepared from flakes, without milk, whole milk and margarine	76.3	15.02	2.3	5.6
Potatoes, mashed, prepared from granules, without milk, whole milk and margarine	77.48	14.4	2.2	4.93
Potatoes, microwaved, cooked in skin, flesh and skin, without salt	72.04	24.13	2.3	0.1
Potatoes, microwaved, cooked in skin, flesh, with salt	73.55	23.28	1.6	0.1
Potatoes, microwaved, cooked in skin, flesh, without salt	73.55	23.28	1.6	0.1
Potatoes, microwaved, cooked in skin, skin, without salt	63.5	29.63	5.5	0.1
Potatoes, microwaved, cooked, in skin, flesh and skin, with salt	72.04	24.13	2.3	0.1
Potatoes, microwaved, cooked, in skin, skin with salt	63.5	29.63	5.5	0.1
Potatoes, O'brien, frozen, prepared	61.96	21.86	1.7	13.21
Potatoes, O'brien, frozen, unprepared	79.97	17.47	1.9	0.14
Potatoes, O'brien, home-prepared	79.6	15.47		1.28
Potatoes, raw, flesh and skin	78.96	17.98	1.6	0.1
Potatoes, raw, skin	83.29	12.44	2.5	0.1
Potatoes, scalloped, dry mix, prepared with water, whole milk and butter	79.17	12.77	1.1	4.3
Potatoes, scalloped, dry mix, unprepared	6.22	73.93	8.6	4.59
Potatoes, scalloped, home-prepared with butter	80.94	10.78	1.9	3.68
Potatoes, scalloped, home-prepared with margarine	80.94	10.78	1.9	3.68
Pumpkin flowers, cooked, boiled, drained, without salt	95.2	3.3	0.9	0.08
Pumpkin flowers, raw	95.15	3.28	0.07	
Pumpkin leaves, cooked, boiled, drained, without salt	92.51	3.39	2.7	0.22
Pumpkin leaves, raw	92.88	2.33		0.4
Pumpkin pie mix, canned	71.49	26.39	8.3	0.13
Pumpkin, canned, with salt	89.97	8.08	2.9	0.28
Pumpkin, canned, without salt	89.97	8.08	2.9	0.28
Pumpkin, cooked, boiled, drained, with salt	93.69	4.89	1.1	0.07
Pumpkin, cooked, boiled, drained, without salt	93.69	4.89	1.1	0.07
Pumpkin, flowers, cooked, boiled, drained, with salt	95.2	3.3	0.9	0.08
Pumpkin, leaves, cooked, boiled, drained, with salt	92.51	3.39	2.7	0.22

Pumpkin, raw	91.6	6.5	0.5	0.1
Purslane, cooked, boiled, drained, with salt	93.52	3.55		0.19
Purslane, cooked, boiled, drained, without salt	93.52	3.55		0.19
Purslane, raw	93.92	3.43		0.1
Radicchio, raw	93.14	4.48	0.9	0.25
Radish seeds, sprouted, raw	90.07	3.6		2.53
Radishes, oriental, cooked, boiled, drained, with salt	95.04	3.43	1.6	0.24
Radishes, oriental, cooked, boiled, drained, without salt	95.04	3.43	1.6	0.24
Radishes, oriental, dried	19.68	63.37		0.72
Radishes, oriental, raw	94.62	4.11	1.6	0.1
Radishes, raw	94.84	3.59	1.6	0.54
Radishes, white icicle, raw	95.37	2.63	1.4	0.1
Rutabagas, cooked, boiled, drained, with salt	88.88	8.74	1.8	0.22
Rutabagas, cooked, boiled, drained, without salt	88.88	8.74	1.8	0.22
Rutabagas, raw	89.66	8.13	2.5	0.2
Salsify, (vegetable oyster), raw	77	18.6	3.3	0.2
Salsify, cooked, boiled, drained, with salt	81	15.37	3.1	0.17
Salsify, cooked, boiled, drained, without salt	81	15.37	3.1	0.17
Sauerkraut, canned, solids and liquids	92.52	4.28	2.5	0.14
Seaweed, agar, dried	8.68	80.89	7.7	0.3
Seaweed, agar, raw	91.32	6.75	0.5	0.03
Seaweed, irishmoss, raw	81.34	12.29	1.3	0.16
Seaweed, kelp, raw	81.58	9.57	1.3	0.56
Seaweed, laver, raw	85.03	5.11	0.3	0.28
Seaweed, spirulina, dried	4.68	23.9	3.6	7.72
Seaweed, spirulina, raw	90.67	2.42		0.39
Seaweed, wakame, raw	79.99	9.14	0.5	0.64
Sesbania flower, cooked, steamed, with salt	93.3	5.23		0.05
Sesbania flower, cooked, steamed, without salt	93.3	5.23		0.05
Sesbania flower, raw	91.58	6.73		0.04
Shallots, freeze-dried	2	80.7		0.5
Shallots, raw	79.8	16.8		0.1
Soybeans, green, cooked, boiled, drained, with salt	68.6	11.05	4.2	6.4
Soybeans, green, cooked, boiled, drained, without salt	68.6	11.05	4.2	6.4
Soybeans, green, raw	67.5	11.05	4.2	6.8
Soybeans, mature seeds, sprouted, cooked, steamed	79.45	6.53	0.8	4.45
Soybeans, mature seeds, sprouted, cooked, steamed, with salt	79.45	6.53	0.8	4.45
Soybeans, mature seeds, sprouted, cooked, stir-fried	67.2	9.4	0.8	7.1
Soybeans, mature seeds, sprouted, cooked, stir-fried, with salt	67.2	9.4	0.8	7.1
Soybeans, mature seeds, sprouted, raw	69.05	9.57	1.1	6.7
Spinach souffle	73.94	2.08		13.5
Spinach, canned, drained solids	91.78	3.4	2.4	0.5
Spinach, canned, no salt added, solids and liquids	93.22	2.92	2.2	0.37
Spinach, canned, regular pack, solids and liquids	93.22	2.92	1.6	0.37
Spinach, cooked, boiled, drained, with salt	91.21	3.75	2.4	0.26
Spinach, cooked, boiled, drained, without salt	91.21	3.75	2.4	0.26
Spinach, frozen, chopped or leaf, cooked, boiled, drained, with salt	89.98	5.34	3	0.21

Spinach, frozen, chopped or leaf, cooked, boiled, drained, without salt	89.98	5.34	3	0.21
Spinach, frozen, chopped or leaf, unprepared	91.64	4	3	0.31
Spinach, raw	91.58	3.5	2.7	0.35
Squash, summer, all varieties, cooked, boiled, drained, with salt	93.7	4.31	1.4	0.31
Squash, summer, all varieties, cooked, boiled, drained, without salt	93.7	4.31	1.4	0.31
Squash, summer, all varieties, raw	93.68	4.35	1.9	0.21
Squash, summer, crookneck and straightneck, canned, drained, solid, without salt	96.04	2.96	1.4	0.07
Squash, summer, crookneck and straightneck, cooked, boiled, drained, with salt	93.7	4.31	1.4	0.31
Squash, summer, crookneck and straightneck, cooked, boiled, drained, without salt	93.7	4.31	1.4	0.31
Squash, summer, crookneck and straightneck, frozen, cooked, boiled, drained, with salt	92.24	5.54	1.4	0.2
Squash, summer, crookneck and straightneck, frozen, cooked, boiled, drained, without salt	92.24	5.54	1.4	0.2
Squash, summer, crookneck and straightneck, frozen, unprepared	93.66	4.8	1.2	0.14
Squash, summer, crookneck and straightneck, raw	94.2	4.04	1.9	0.24
Squash, summer, scallop, cooked, boiled, drained, with salt	95	3.3	1.9	0.17
Squash, summer, scallop, cooked, boiled, drained, without salt	95	3.3	1.9	0.17
Squash, summer, scallop, raw	94.18	3.84		0.2
Squash, summer, zucchini, includes skin, cooked, boiled, drained, with salt	94.74	3.93	1.4	0.05
Squash, summer, zucchini, includes skin, cooked, boiled, drained, without salt	94.74	3.93	1.4	0.05
Squash, summer, zucchini, includes skin, frozen, cooked, boiled, drained, with salt	94.74	3.56	1.3	0.13
Squash, summer, zucchini, includes skin, frozen, cooked, boiled, drained, without salt	94.74	3.56	1.3	0.13
Squash, summer, zucchini, includes skin, frozen, unprepared	94.7	3.59	1.3	0.13
Squash, summer, zucchini, includes skin, raw	95.28	2.9	1.2	0.14
Squash, summer, zucchini, italian style, canned	90.61	6.85	0.11	
Squash, winter, acorn, cooked, baked, with salt	82.9	14.58	4.4	0.14
Squash, winter, acorn, cooked, baked, without salt	82.9	14.58	4.4	0.14
Squash, winter, acorn, cooked, boiled, mashed, with salt	89.7	8.78	2.6	0.08
Squash, winter, acorn, cooked, boiled, mashed, without salt	89.7	8.78	2.6	0.08
Squash, winter, acorn, raw	87.78	10.42	1.5	0.1
Squash, winter, all varieties, cooked, baked, with salt	89.02	8.75	2.8	0.63
Squash, winter, all varieties, cooked, baked, without salt	89.02	8.75	2.8	0.63
Squash, winter, all varieties, raw	88.72	8.8	1.5	0.23
Squash, winter, butternut, cooked, baked, with salt	87.8	10.49		0.09

Squash, winter, butternut, cooked, baked, without salt	87.8	10.49		0.09
Squash, winter, butternut, frozen, cooked, boiled, with salt	87.8	10.05		0.07
Squash, winter, butternut, frozen, cooked, boiled, without salt	87.8	10.05		0.07
Squash, winter, butternut, frozen, unprepared	82.5	14.41	1.3	0.1
Squash, winter, butternut, raw	86.41	11.69		0.1
Squash, winter, hubbard, cooked, baked, with salt	85.1	10.81		0.62
Squash, winter, hubbard, cooked, baked, without salt	85.1	10.81		0.62
Squash, winter, hubbard, cooked, boiled, mashed, with salt	91.1	6.45	2.9	0.37
Squash, winter, hubbard, cooked, boiled, mashed, without salt	91.1	6.45	2.9	0.37
Squash, winter, hubbard, raw	88	8.7	0.5	
Squash, winter, spaghetti, cooked, boiled, drained, or baked, with salt	92.3	6.46	1.4	0.26
Squash, winter, spaghetti, cooked, boiled, drained, or baked, without salt	92.3	6.46	1.4	0.26
Squash, winter, spaghetti, raw	91.6	6.91		0.57
Squash, zucchini, baby, raw	92.73	3.1	1.1	0.4
Succotash, (corn and limas), canned, with cream style corn	78.17	17.61	3	0.54
Succotash, (corn and limas), canned, with whole kernel corn, solids and liquids	81.96	13.98	2.6	0.49
Succotash, (corn and limas), cooked, boiled, drained, with salt	68.37	24.38		0.8
Succotash, (corn and limas), cooked, boiled, drained, without salt	68.37	24.38	4.5	0.8
Succotash, (corn and limas), frozen, cooked, boiled, drained, with salt	74.1	19.95	4.1	0.89
Succotash, (corn and limas), frozen, cooked, boiled, drained, without salt	74.1	19.95	4.1	0.89
Succotash, (corn and limas), frozen, unprepared	74.11	19.94	4	0.89
Succotash, (corn and limas), raw	73.1	19.59	3.8	1.02
Swamp cabbage, (skunk cabbage), raw	92.47	3.14	2.1	0.2
Swamp cabbage, cooked, boiled, drained, with salt	92.93	3.71	1.9	0.24
Swamp cabbage, cooked, boiled, drained, without salt	92.93	3.71	1.9	0.24
Sweetpotato leaves, cooked, steamed, with salt	88.71	7.32	1.9	0.3
Sweetpotato leaves, cooked, steamed, without salt	88.71	7.32	1.9	0.3
Sweetpotato leaves, raw	87.96	6.38	2	0.3
Sweetpotato, canned, mashed	73.88	23.2	1.7	0.2
Sweetpotato, canned, syrup pack, drained solids	72.47	25.36	3	0.32
Sweetpotato, canned, syrup pack, solids and liquids	77.39	20.93	2.5	0.2
Sweetpotato, canned, vacuum pack	76.03	21.13	1.8	0.2
Sweetpotato, cooked, baked in skin, with salt	72.85	24.27	3	0.11
Sweetpotato, cooked, baked in skin, without salt	72.85	24.27	3	0.11
Sweetpotato, cooked, boiled, without skin, with salt	72.84	24.28	1.8	0.3
Sweetpotato, cooked, boiled, without skin, without salt	72.84	24.28	1.8	0.3
Sweetpotato, cooked, candied	66.94	27.86	2.4	3.25
Sweetpotato, frozen, cooked, baked, with salt	73.7	23.4	1.8	0.12

Sweetpotato, frozen, cooked, baked, without salt	73.7	23.4	1.8	0.12
Sweetpotato, frozen, unprepared	74.89	22.22	1.7	0.18
Sweetpotato, raw	72.84	24.28	3	0.3
Taro leaves, cooked, steamed, without salt	92.15	4.02	2	0.41
Taro leaves, raw	85.66	6.71	3.7	0.74
Taro shoots, cooked, without salt	95.3	3.2		0.08
Taro shoots, raw	95.82	2.32		0.09
Taro, cooked, with salt	63.8	34.6	5.1	0.11
Taro, cooked, without salt	63.8	34.6	5.1	0.11
Taro, leaves, cooked, steamed, with salt	92.15	4.02	2	0.41
Taro, raw	70.64	26.46	4.1	0.2
Taro, shoots, cooked, with salt	95.3	3.2		0.08
Taro, tahitian, cooked, with salt	86.46	6.85		0.68
Taro, tahitian, cooked, without salt	86.46	6.85	0.68	
Taro, tahitian, raw	87.96	6.91		0.97
Tomatillos, raw	91.63	5.83	1.9	1.02
Tomato juice, canned, with salt added	93.9	4.23	0.4	0.06
Tomato juice, canned, without salt added	93.9	4.23	0.8	0.06
Tomato powder	3.06	74.68	16.5	0.44
Tomato products, canned, paste, with salt added	73.8	19.3	4.1	0.55
Tomato products, canned, paste, without salt added	73.8	19.3	4.1	0.55
Tomato products, canned, puree, with salt added	87.46	9.56	2	0.16
Tomato products, canned, puree, without salt added	87.46	9.56	2	0.16
Tomato products, canned, sauce	89.07	7.18	1.4	0.17
Tomato products, canned, sauce, spanish style	89.08	7.24	1.4	0.27
Tomato products, canned, sauce, with herbs and cheese	83.43	10.24	2.2	1.93
Tomato products, canned, sauce, with mushrooms	87.97	8.43	1.5	0.13
Tomato products, canned, sauce, with onions	86.09	9.94	1.8	0.19
Tomato products, canned, sauce, with onions, green peppers, and celery	88.28	8.76	1.4	0.74
Tomato products, canned, sauce, with tomato tidbits	89.09	7.09	1.4	0.39
Tomatoes, crushed, canned	89.44	7.29	1.9	0.28
Tomatoes, green, raw	93	5.1	1.1	0.2
Tomatoes, red, ripe, canned, stewed	91.01	6.78	1	0.13
Tomatoes, red, ripe, canned, wedges in tomato juice	91.78	6.31		0.16
Tomatoes, red, ripe, canned, whole, no salt added	93.65	4.37	1	0.13
Tomatoes, red, ripe, canned, whole, regular pack	93.65	4.37	1	0.13
Tomatoes, red, ripe, canned, with green chilies	94.23	3.62		0.08
Tomatoes, red, ripe, cooked, boiled, with salt	92.16	5.83	1.1	0.41
Tomatoes, red, ripe, cooked, boiled, without salt	92.16	5.83	1	0.41
Tomatoes, red, ripe, cooked, stewed	80.63	13.05	1.7	2.68
Tomatoes, red, ripe, raw, June thru October average	93.76	4.64	1.1	0.33
Tomatoes, red, ripe, raw, November thru May average	93.76	4.64	1.1	0.33
Tomatoes, red, ripe, raw, year round average	93.76	4.64	1.1	0.33
Tomatoes, sun-dried	14.56	55.76	12.3	2.97
Tomatoes, sun-dried, packed in oil, drained	53.83	23.33	5.8	14.08
Tree fern, cooked, with salt	88.6	10.98	3.7	0.07
Tree fern, cooked, without salt	88.6	10.98	3.7	0.07
Turnip greens and turnips, frozen, cooked, boiled, drained, with salt	94.19	2.88	2.4	0.16

Turnip greens and turnips, frozen, cooked, boiled, drained, without salt	94.19	2.88	1.8	0.16
Turnip greens and turnips, frozen, unprepared	93.13	3.4	2.4	0.19
Turnip greens, canned, solids and liquids	94.69	2.42	1.7	0.3
Turnip greens, cooked, boiled, drained, with salt	93.2	4.36	3.5	0.23
Turnip greens, cooked, boiled, drained, without salt	93.2	4.36	3.5	0.23
Turnip greens, frozen, cooked, boiled, drained, with salt	90.4	4.98	3.4	0.42
Turnip greens, frozen, cooked, boiled, drained, without salt	90.4	4.98	3.4	0.42
Turnip greens, frozen, unprepared	92.93	3.67	2.5	0.31
Turnip greens, raw	91.07	5.73	3.2	0.3
Turnips, cooked, boiled, drained, with salt	93.6	4.9	2	0.08
Turnips, cooked, boiled, drained, without salt	93.6	4.9	2	0.08
Turnips, frozen, cooked, boiled, drained, with salt	93.6	4.35	2	0.24
Turnips, frozen, cooked, boiled, drained, without salt	93.6	4.35	2	0.24
Turnips, frozen, unprepared	95.67	2.94	1.8	0.16
Turnips, raw	91.87	6.23	1.8	0.1
Vegetable juice cocktail, canned	93.52	4.55	0.8	0.09
Vegetables, mixed, canned, drained solids	87.01	9.26	3	0.25
Vegetables, mixed, canned, solids and liquids	90.24	7.12	3.8	0.25
Vegetables, mixed, frozen, cooked, boiled, drained, with salt	83.23	13.09	4.4	0.15
Vegetables, mixed, frozen, cooked, boiled, drained, without salt	83.23	13.09	4.4	0.15
Vegetables, mixed, frozen, unprepared	82.08	13.46	4	0.52
Vinespinach, (basella), raw	93.1	3.4		0.3
Waterchestnuts, Chinese, (matai), raw	73.46	23.94	3	0.1
Waterchestnuts, Chinese, canned, solids and liquids	86.42	12.43	2.5	0.06
Watercress, raw	95.11	1.29	1.5	0.1
Waxgourd, (Chinese preserving melon), cooked, boiled, drained, with salt	96.06	3.03	1	0.2
Waxgourd, (Chinese preserving melon), cooked, boiled, drained, without salt	96.06	3.03	1	0.2
Waxgourd, (Chinese preserving melon), raw	96.1	3	2.9	0.2
Winged bean leaves, raw	76.85	14.1		1.1
Winged bean tuber, raw	57.4	28.1		0.9
Winged bean, immature seeds, cooked, boiled, drained, with salt	90.11	3.21		0.66
Winged beans, immature seeds, cooked, boiled, drained, without salt	90.11	3.21		0.66
Winged beans, immature seeds, raw	87.04	4.31		0.87
Yam, cooked, boiled, drained, or baked, with salt	70.13	27.6	3.9	0.14
Yam, cooked, boiled, drained, or baked, without salt	70.13	27.6	3.9	0.14
Yam, raw	69.6	27.89	4.1	0.17
Yambean, cooked, boiled, drained, with salt	90.07	8.82		0.09
Yambean, cooked, boiled, drained, without salt	90.07	8.82		0.09
Yambean, raw	90.07	8.82	4.9	0.09
Yardlong bean, cooked, boiled, drained, with salt	87.47	9.18		0.1
Yardlong bean, cooked, boiled, drained, without salt	87.47	9.18		0.1
Yardlong bean, raw	87.85	8.35		0.4

Index

Advance Notice of Proposed Rule Making (ANPRM) of the FDA, 17
Alcohol, dietary guidelines for, 9
Alginates, 343
Alkaline hydrogen peroxide (AMP) treatment, 363–364
Allium compounds, 67
American Dietetic Association (ADA):
  DF guidelines, 10
  functional food development and, 595
Amylopectin, 117–119
  HPAE-PAD in structural studies of, 279
Amylose, 117–119
Anaerobic colonic bacteria, fermentation of, 28
Analysis of dietary fiber, 74, 305–316
  component analysis procedures, 76–77
    DNS reduction method for soluble and insoluble NSP, 77
    unavailable carbohydrate method, 76
    Uppsalla GLC methods, 76–77
  gravimetric procedures, 74–76
    crude fiber determination, 74–75
    detergent methods of fiber analysis, 75
    Hellendoorn method, 75–76
Analytical method to measure complex carbohydrates, 137–141
  analytical results, 139–141
  sample, 138
Antioxidants, dietary fiber and, 60
Antioxidant vitamins, 67
Asia-Pacific region:
  actual DF intake levels in, 102–103
  DF intake recommendations in, 85–89, 90
Association of Official Analytical Chemists (AOAC), 2, 3
  analytical measurement of polydextrose, 238
  defining and labeling of complex carbohydrates, 21, 41–42, 47–48
  modified AOAC method for recovery of inulin and oligofructose, 208–209
    combined with inulinase method, 211
    in determination of occurrence in food products, 213–227
AOAC International Workshop (1995):
  defining complex carbohydrates, 137
  Task Force on Nutrient Labeling Analysis, 47–48

Australia:
DF recommendations for, 90
daily intake, 79
estimate of DF intake in, 93
Autoclaving, 378

Bacterial cellulose, 419
Bakery products:
DF applications in, 350–351
DF-based fat substitutes for, 501–502
DF content of, 330–332
hydrocolloids/gums in low-calorie product development, 517–518
recovery of FOS contained in, 199, 200
starch-based fat substitutes for, 481–486
total carbohydrates and total DF in, 609–621
total sugar, starches and total DF in, 150
Baking, effect on dietary fiber composition, 379
Barley bran, 361–362
Belgium:
DF daily intake rcommendations for, 79
estimate of DF intake in, 93
Beta-glutan, 356–357
Beverages:
DF-based fat substitutes for, 501
DF supplements in, 349–350
hydrocolloids/gums for low-calorie product development, 518–519
starch-based fat substitutes for, 486–487
Bile acids, interaction between dietary fiber and, 66
Bleaching, effect on dietary fiber composition, 377
Blood cholesterol, dietary fiber in lowering of, 58–60, 595
Blood sugar, control of, 595
Boiling, effect on dietary fiber composition, 378
Botanical structure of dietary fiber, 307–310
Bowel cancer, 65–66
Breads:
DF in, 402
bread staling, 351
as a structure enhancer, 350–351
guidelines for complex carbohydrates from, 11
resistant starch in, 387
Breakfast cereals:
DF in, 332
resistant starch in, 387
British Nutrition Foundation Report, 8
defining complex carbohydrates, 43
dietary guidelines for complex carbohydrates, 11
Bulgaria, estimate of DF intake in, 93

Canada:
DF recommendations for, 84–85
daily intake, 79
estimate of DF intake in, 93
Canadian Nutrition Recommendations (1990), 35
Calibration of the NIRS, 293–295
Cancer, 71, 594, 595
bowel, 65–66
colon, 66, 595
Canning, effect on dietary fiber composition, 378
Carbohydrate-based fat replacers, 414–418
in low-fat products, 425–426
maltodextrins, 417–418
polydextrose, 415–417
Carbohydrate-rich foods, 44–45
Carbohydrates:
dietary guidelines for, 9–10
HPAE chromatography of, 273–274
total carbohydrates in grain based food, 609–660
bakery products, 609–621
cereals, 621–626
fruits, 627–634
grains, 639–642
legumes, 634–639
vegetables, 642–660

Carboxymethyl cellulose (CMC), 431
Carrageenans, 343–344, 425, 431
Cartenoids, 67
Cellulose, 119, 351–363
  hemicellulose, 355–363
  microcrystalline cellulose, 353–355
  powdered cellulose, 351–353
Cellulose derivatives, 418–420
  bacterial cellulose, 419
  methylcellose gums, 419
  microcrystalline cellulose, 418–419
  pectin, 420
Cellulose gel, 425
Cellulose gums, 348–349
Central America, DF recommendations for, 91
  daily intake, 79
Cereal brans, 358
Cereals:
  DF content of cereal grains, 332–333
  guidelines for complex carbohyrates from, 11
  total carbohydrates and total DF in, 621–626
  total sugar, starches and total DF in, 151
  See also Breakfast cereals; Whole-grain cereals
Certification of five new food reference materials. *See* New food reference materials, certification of
Chemical treatment of dietary fiber, 377–381
  chemical modifications, 377–378
    bleaching, 377
    enzymes, 377–378
    food processing, 378
  dry heat treatment, 379–381
  non-thermal treament, 381
  wet heat treatment, 378–379
Chemistry of complex carbohydrates, 115–129
  cellulose, 119
  hemicellulose, 119–122
  hydrocolloids (gums, mucilages), 122–123
[Chemistry of complex carbohydrates]
  modified starches, 123–125
  pectic substances, 122
  resistant starch, 125–127
  starch, 117–119
Chicory fructooligosaccharides, 26
  behavior and effects in the gastrointestinal tract, 28–29
    bulking effect, 28–29
    fermentation by anaerobic colonic bacteria, 28
    non-digestibility, 28
    as prebiotics, 29
  systemic effects of, 30–31
    caloric value, 30–31
    effects on lipid metabolism, 30
    mineral bioavailability, 31
Chile:
  DF recommendations for, 91
  estimate of DF intake in, 93
China:
  DF recommendations for, 90
  estimate of DF intake in, 93
Cholesterol:
  coronary heart disease and, 412
  lowering, 58–60, 595
Colombia, DF recommendations for, 91
  daily intake, 79
Colon cancer, 66, 595
Colonic function, effect of dietary fiber on, 307–309
Column packing for high pH anion exchange chromatography, 275–276
Committee on Medical Aspects of Food Policy (COMA), 413
Complex carbohydrate fractions in foods, determination of, 145–153
  method, 146
  results and discussion, 146–153
Complex carbohydrates:
  definitions, 1–4, 131–137, 234
    the FDA and, 1–2, 3, 15, 20–22, 45–46
  international survey on definition and results, 133–137

Complex Carbohydrates: The Science and the Label (ILSI workshop), 39–52
Composition of dietary fiber 329–340
Constipation, 71
Corn bran, 360
Coronary heart disease (CHD), 71, 412, 594, 595
  DF and, 64–65
  prevention of, 54–55
Coumarins, 67
Crude fiber (CF) determination, 74–75
Cuba, estimate of DF intake in, 93
Czechoslovakia, estimate of DF intake in, 93

Daily intake of dietary fiber, recommendations for (worldwide), 67, 78–80
Dairy products:
  hydrocolloids/gums in low-calorie product development, 519–528
  recovery of FOS contained in, 199, 200
  starch-based fat substitutes for, 488–490
Deep fat frying, 406–407
Definitions:
  AOAC International Workshop results (1995), 137
  of complex carbohydrates, 1–4, 131–137, 234
    the FDA and, 1–2, 3, 15, 20–22, 45–46
    international survey on, 133–137
  of DF, 72–74, 232–234, 310–311
    international survey on, 135–136
    methods for determination, 605–608
Denmark:
  DF daily intake recommendations for, 79
  estimate of DF intake in, 93
Dessert:
  hydrocolloids/gums in low-calorie product development, 528–531
[Dessert]
  starch-based fat substitutes for, 496–498
Detergent method of fiber analysis, 75
Diabetes, 71, 594, 595
Dietary fiber (DF), 2, 3, 4, 46, 329
  antioxidants and, 60
  bakery product applications, 350–351
    bread staling, 351
    as a structure enhancer, 350–351
  bulking effect of chicory fructooligosaccharides compared to, 29
  calculation of, 46
  cellulose and, 351–363
    hemicellulose, 355–363
    microcrystalline cellulose, 353–355
    powdered cellulose, 351–353
  chemical and physical modifications of, 373–384
  common components and sources of, 351
  definition and analysis of, 72–74, 232–234, 310–311
    botanical structure and physiological effects, 307–310
    international survey, 135–136
    methods, 311–313, 605–608
  dietary guidelines for, 10–11
  food sources of, 328–329
    insoluble fiber, 329
    soluble fiber, 329
    soluble and insoluble fibers, 329
    specific food sources, 329, 330–339
  HPAE-PAD for determination of, 268–269, 286
  hydrocolloids as, 342–343
  hydrolipidemic effects of chicory fructooligosaccharides compared to, 30
  identification of, 37
  measurement by NIRS, 296–301
  microbial gums and, 347–348
    gellan gum, 348
    xanthan gum, 347–348

[Dietary fiber (DF)]
modified cellulose, pectin and, 348–349
NDOs as, 31–32
plant exudates and, 346–347
gum arabic, 346
gum karayu, 346–347
gum tragacanth, 347
in prevention of lipid metabolism disorders, 53–62
animal studies, 55–56
clinical and metabolic studies, 56–58
epidemiologic studies, 54–55
mechanisms of action, 58–60
root flour and, 345–346
seaweed extracts and, 343–344
alginates, 343
carrageenan, 343–344
seed extracts and, 344–345
guar gum, 345
locust bean gum, 344
selected hydrocolloid properties, 349–350
DF supplements in beverages, 349–350
reduced fat foods, 350
sources and properties of, 66–67, 329–342
component classification, 341–342
composition of DF, 329–340
industry availability, 340–341
variation in source composition, 341
total DF content in grain-based foods, 609–660
bakery products, 609–621
cereals, 621–626
fruits, 627–634
grains, 639–642
legumes, 634–639
vegetables, 642–660
treatment to improve fiber functionality and unique fiber sources, 363–365
[Dietary fiber (DF)]
alkaline hydrogen peroxide treatment, 363–364
encapsulation, 365
enzymatic modification, 365
extrusion modification, 364–365
See also New food reference materials, certification of; Polydextrose
Dietary fiber-based fat substitutes (patent literature review), 498–505
bakery, 501–502
beverage, 501
fruit paste, 503–504
general, 498–500
low-calorie foods, 504–505
meat product, 502–503
Dietary fiber intake, 71–111
analytical methods for DF, 74
component analysis procedures, 76–77
DNS reduction method for soluble and insoluble NSF, 77
unavailable carbohydrate method, 76
Uppsalla GLC method, 76–77
gravimetric procedures, 74–76
crude fiber determination, 74–75
detergent method of fiber analysis, 75
Hellendoorn method, 75–76
intake levels around the world, 94–106
Asia-Pacific region, 102–103
Europe, 98–100, 102
North American and Latin America, 95–97
problems in assessing intake, 92–94
recommendations for intake levels, 77–92
Asia-Pacific region, 85–89, 90
Europe, 79, 81–85, 86–88
Latin America, 89, 91
North America, 80–81, 82–85
South Africa, 89–92
worldwide intake recommendations, 78–80

Dietary Goals for the United States (1977), 8, 41
Dietary guidelines, 7–14
  for carbohydrates, 9–10
  for complex carbohydrates, 11–12
  for DF, 10–11
  dietary guidance, 8–9
Dietary Guidelines for Americans, 8–9, 15, 16, 17
Dionex Ion Chromatograph, 195–196
Directive on Nutrition Labeling of Foodstuffs (issued by EU), 252
Disaccharides, 10
Disease status, role of dietary fiber in prevention and management of, 235
Dithiolthiones, 67
Diverticular disease, 65
Dry heat treatment of dietary fiber, 379–381
  baking, 379
  extrusion, 380–381
  roasting, 379–380

Energy metabolism, effect of carbohyrates on, 12
Enzymes, 377–378
  enzymatic modification of DF, 365
Europe:
  actual df intake levels in, 98–100, 102
  benefits of oligosaccharides in, 597–598
  DF intake recommendations for, 79, 81–85, 86–88
European Commission/Scientific Committee for Foods (EC/SCF), 232
European Union (EU):
  Directive on Nutrition Labeling of Foodstuffs issued by, 252
  functional food development in, 600–601
Extrusion cooking, 380–381, 407

Fat intake:
  dietary guidelines for, 9
  disease and, 411–413
  effect of DF on fat absorption, 310
Fat mimetics, complex carbohydrates as, 411–429
  applicability of carbohydrate-based fat mimetics, 425–426
  carbohydrate-based fat replacers, 414–418
    maltodextrins, 417–418
    polydextrose, 415–417
  cellulose derivatives, 418–420
    bacterial cellulose, 419
    methylcellulose gums, 419
    microcrystalline cellulose, 418–419
    pectin, 420
  development of fat replacer market, 413–414
  fat intake and disease, 411–413
  gums, 420–425
    fibers, 423
    gelactomannan gums, 420–421
    hydrocolloid gum blends, 422–423
    inulin, 424–425
    oatrim, 423–424
    other gums, 421–422
    Vitacel, 424
    xanthan gum, 421
    Z-trim, 424
  See also Patent literature review
Federal Trade Commission (FTC), food label reform and, 17–19
Fermentation, 28, 381
Fibers as fat mimetics, 423
Finland:
  DF recommendations for, 88
    daily intake, 79
  estimate of DF intake in, 93
Flavinoids, 67
Food additives, HPAE-PAD in analysis of, 281–282
Food and Drug Administration (FDA):
  defining complex carbohydrates, 1–2, 3, 15, 20–22, 45–46
  food labeling regulations and, 17–19, 132, 605
    complex carbohydrates, 41–42, 46–47
  functional food development and, 601–602

Food Guide Pyramid of the USDA, 7, 9, 16, 40, 41
Food guides. *See* Dietary guidelines
Food labels. *See* Labeling (food labels)
Food reference materials for dietary fiber analysis. *See* New food reference materials, confirmation of
Foods for Specified Health Use (FOSHU) in Japan, 232, 599–600
France:
  DF recommendations for, 86
    daily intake, 79
  estimate of DF intake in, 93
Freezing, 381
Fructans, 126–127
Fructooligosaccharides (FOS), 27, 126–127
  measuring FOS in food products, 191–201
    materials and methods, 193–196
    results and discussion, 196–200
  See also Chicory fructooligosaccharides
Fructose determination methods, 209–210
Fruit paste, 503–504
Fruits:
  DF content of fruit and fruit products, 334–335
  DF intake from, 10
  guidelines for complex carbohydrates from, 9–10, 11
  hydrocolloids/gums in low-calorie product development, 533–535
  starch-based fat substitutes for, 480–481
  total carbohydrates and total DF in, 627–634
Functional food development, 593–604
  definition of functional foods, 593
  food production development perspectives, 595–599
  regulations, opportunities, and constraints, 599–602
    European Union, 600–601
    Japan, 599–600
    the U.S., 601–602
  three categories of functional foods, 594
Galactomannan gums, 420–421
Gas chromatography (GC), 209
Gas-liquid chromatography (GLC), 76–77, 145–146, 209
Gastrointestinal (GI) tract:
  behavior and effects of chicory fructooligosaccharides in, 28–29
  DF and disorders of, 65
  polydextrose effect on, 237
Gellan gum, 348, 422
Generally recognized as safe (GRAS), inulin and oligofructose as, 206
Germany:
  DF recommendations for, 86
    daily intake, 79
  estimate of DF intake in, 93
Glucosinolates, 67
Glycemic index, polydextrose effect on, 237
Grain-based foods:
  carbohydrates in RDA from, 9
  hydrocolloids/gums in low-calorie product development, 517–518
  starch-based fat substitutes for, 481–486
  total carbohydrates and total DF content in, 609–660
Grains, total carbohydrates and total DF content in, 639–642
Gravimetric procedures for dietary fiber analysis, 74–76
  crude fiber determination, 74–75
  detergent methods of fiber analysis, 75
  Hellendoorn method, 75–76
Greece, estimate of DF intake in, 93
Guam gum, 345, 425
Gum arabic, 346
Gum karaya, 346–347
Gums, 420–425
  fibers, 423
  gelactomannan gums, 420–421
  hydrocolloid gum blends, 422–423
  inulin, 424–425
  oatrim, 423–424
  other gums, 421–422

[Gums]
Vitacel, 424
xanthan gum, 421
Z-trim, 424
Gum tragacanth, 347

Health benefits of complex carbohydrates, 63–69
Hellendoorn method of dietary fiber analysis, 75–76
Hemicelluloses, 119–122, 355–363
barley bran, 361–362
beta-glucan, 356–357
cereal bran, 358
corn bran, 360
lignin, 357
oat bran, 362–363
resistant starch, 357–358
rice bran, 360–361
wheat bran, 358–360
High-density lipoproteins (HDLs), 412–413
High performance anion exchange chromatography with pulsed amperometric detection (HPAE-PAD), 267–289
for analysis of inulin and oligofructose, 209, 221–223
for analysis of physiologically functional food additives, 281–282
for analysis of starch and non-starch polysaccharides, 277–278, 279, 282–284
application in pectin research, 286–287
column packings for high pH anion exchange chromatography, 275–276
for determination of complex carbohydrates and DF, 268–279
for determination of sugars and oligosaccharides, 276, 277
principle of PAD, 269–273
for quantitation of polysaccharides, 279–281
for structural studies on amylopectins, 279
High pH, anion exchange chromatography at, 275–276
High pressure liquid chromatography (HPLC):
for analysis of oligofructose, 209
for analysis of polydextrose, 240–244, 245
for determination of inulin in food products, 215–221
for measuring complex carbohydrates in food products, 138–141
HIST (high-temperature, short-time) extrusion cooking, 407
Hungary, estimate of DF intake in, 93
Hydrocolloids, 122–123, 422–423
as fat mimetics (patent literature review), 505–591
bakery and grain, 517–518
beverage, 518–519
dairy, 519–528
dessert, 528–531
emulsifier, stabilizer, and suspending agent, 531–533
fruits and vegetables, 533–535
general, 505–517
low-calorie foods: laxative, 559–560
low-calorie foods: satiety and weight control, 554–559
miscellaneous low-calorie foods, 560–591
snacks, 536
spread and salad dressing, 536–554
as functional soluble DF, 342–343
selected applications, 349–350
H_2 breath test to estimate resistant starch in humans, 160–165
Hydroxypropyl methylcellulose (HPMC), 419

Iceland, estimate of DF intake in, 93
Identification of carbohydrates, 36
Ileostomy model to estimate resistant starch in humans, 163, 165
India, DF recommendations for, 90
daily intake, 79

Indoles, 67
Industrial process of dietary fiber, 374–381
  chemical treatments, 377–381
    chemical modifications, 377–378
    dry heat treatments, 379–381
    non-thermal treatments, 381
    wet heat treatments, 378–379
  fiber separation techniques, 374–376
  particle size reduction, 376–377
Inositol hexaphosphate, 67
Insoluble dietary fiber, 329
International Life Science Institute (ILSI), 21, 40
International survey on complex carbohydrate definition, 133–134
International survey on dietary fiber definition, 135–136
Intubation technique to estimate resistant starch in humans, 163, 165–166
Inulin, 27, 203–212, 424–425, 432
  analytical methods, 209–212
    direct GC, 209
    direct HPLC, 209
    fructose determination method, 209–210
    HPAE-PAD methods, 209, 221–223
    inulinase method, 209–211
  as DF, 205–206
  elimination of pectolytic activities of Novozym SP 230 by thermic treatment, 224–226
  in food products, determination of (modified AOAC dietary fiber method), 213–227
    HPLC method for, 215–221
    quantitative analysis for, 214–215
  legal status, 206–207
  natural occurrence of, 204–205
  recovery by DF methods, 207–208
Inulinase method for determination of total fructan content in foods, 210, 211
In vivo techniques to quantify resistant starch, 157–168
  comparison of in vivo models, 166
  quantification of RS in animal models, 159–160, 161, 162
    pig model, 159–160
    rat model, 160, 161, 162
  quantification of RS in humans, 160–166
    H_2 breath test, 160–165
    ileostomy model, 163, 165
    intubation technique, 163, 165–166
    sample test, 162–163
  starch digestion in humans, 158–159
Ireland:
  DF recommendations for, 88
    daily intake, 79
  estimate of DF intake in, 93
Irritable bowel syndrome, 65
Isomaltooligosaccharides (IMO), 26
Isothiocyanates, 67
Italy:
  DF recommendations for, 88
    daily intake, 79
  estimate of DF intake in, 93

Japan:
  benefits of oligosaccharides in, 597
  DF recommendations for, 90
    daily intake, 79
  estimate of DF intake in, 93
  functional food development in, 593, 594, 595–597
    regulations, opportunities and constraints, 599–600
Japanese Foods for Specified Health Use (FOSHU), 599–600
  status of polydextrose and, 232
Joint FAO/WHO Expert Committee on Food Additives (JECFA), 232

Konjac flour gel, 422
Konjac powder, 345–346
Korea, DF recommendations for, 90

Labeling (food labels), 15–23, 37, 46–47, 605
  dietary guidelines and, 16
  educating consumers on the term "complex carbohydrates," 40
  FDA regulations for, 17–19, 132, 605
  FTC and food label reform, 17–19
  post-NLEA, 19–21
  pre-NLEA, 17–19
  See also Science and the label
Latin America:
  actual DF intake levels in, 95–97
  DF intake recommendations for, 89, 91
Legumes:
  DF content of, 335
  total carbohydrates and total DF in, 634–639
  total sugar, starches, and total DF in, 151
Lignin, 2, 72, 73, 357, 606
  defining complex carbohydrates and, 134
Lipid metabolism:
  DF in prevention of disorders of, 53–62
    animal studies, 55–56
    clinical and metabolic studies 56–58
    epidemiologic studies, 54–55
    mechanisms of action, 58–60
  systemic effects of chicory fructo-oligosaccharides on, 30
Lipogenesis, carbohydrate intake effect on, 12
Locust bean gum, 344
Low-calorie foods:
  DF-based fat substitutes for, 504–505
  hydrocolloids/gums in product development, 554–591
Low-density lipoproteins (LDLs), 412–413
LDL cholesterol levels, 55
Luxembourg, estimate of DF intake in, 93

McGovern Commission, 45–46
Malting, 381
Maltodextrins, 417–418, 431
Measurements and Testing (M&T) Programme, 251, 252–253
  requirements for homogeneity, 255–256
Measuring fructooligosaccharides (FOS) in food products, 191–201
  materials and methods, 193–196
  results and discussion, 196–200
    recovery of FOS, 199, 200
    sensitivity of method for determining FOS in cakes and dairy products, 200
    validity of method and determination of the recovery, 196–199
Meat products:
  DF-based fat substitutes for, 502–503
  starch-based fat substitutes for, 454–463
Metabolic effects:
  of carbohydrate intake, 12
  of DF, 235
Methylcellulose gums, 419
Mexico:
  DF recommendations for, 91
    daily intake, 79
  estimate of DF intake in, 93
Microbial gums, 347–348
Microcrystalline cellulose, 353–355, 418–419
Microwaving, 379
Modifications of dietary fiber, 373–384
  industrial processing, 374–381
    chemical treatments, 377–381
    fiber separation techniques, 374–376
    particle size reduction, 376–377
Modified starches, 123–125
Monosaccharides, 10

National Advisory Committee on Nutrition Education (NACNE), 413

National Cancer Institute (NCI), functional food development and, 593–594
National Labeling and Education Act of 1990 (NLEA), 2, 40, 132, 601
  food label reform and, 19–21
  labeling for complex carbohydrates, 47
National Health and Nutrition Examination Survey (NHNES III), 413
National Research Council dietary guidelines for complex carbohydrates, 12
Near-infrared spectroscopy (NIRS), 291–303
  application of NIRS to foods, 296
  chemometrics, 293–295
  instrumentation, 292–293
  measurement of DF by NIRS, 296–301
Neosugar, 27
Netherlands:
  DF daily intake recommendations for, 79
  estimate of DF intake in, 93
Neutral detergent fiber (NDF) method of analysis, 75
Neutral sugars, determination in foods of, 146, 150
New food reference materials, 251–260
  cell wall study, 253–254
  certification study, 259–263
    control materials, 260
    enzyme testing, 261
    structure, 259–260
  intercomparison study, 256–259
  main study, 254–256
    M&T Programme requirements for homogeneity, 255–256
    preparation, packing, homogeneity and stability check, 254–255
  supplementary study, 263–264
New Zealand, estimate of DF intake in, 93
Non-digestible oligosaccharides (NDOs), 25–33
  behavior and effects of chicory fructooligosaccharides in the GI tract, 28–29
    bulking effect, 28–29
    fermentation by anaerobic colonic bacteria, 28
    non-digestibility, 28
    as prebiotics, 29
  as DF, 31–32
  systemic effects of chicory fructo-oligosaccharides, 30–31
    caloric value, 30–31
    effects on lipid metabolism, 30
    mineral bioavailability, 31
Non-starch polysaccharides (NSP):
  defining complex carbohydrates and, 134
  DNS reduction method for soluble and insoluble NSP, 77
  HPAE-PAD in analysis of, 277–278, 279, 282–284
Non-starch saccharides, 3
Non-thermal treatments for dietary fiber, 381
North America:
  actual DF intake levels in, 95–97
  DF intake recommendations for, 80–81, 82–85
Norway:
  DF recommendations for, 88
    daily intake, 79
  estimate DF intake in, 93
Novozym SP 230 (commercial inulinase), 224–226
Nutraceuticals, 593, 594–595
Nutrient absorption, polydextrose effect on, 237–238
Nutrition and Your Health: Dietary Guidelines for Americans, 8–9, 15, 16, 17
Nuts and seeds, DF content of, 335–336

Oat bran, 362–363
  influence on lipoprotein cholestrol levels, 57

Oatrim, 423–424, 431
Obesity, dietary fiber in treatment of, 65
Oligofructose, 27, 203–212
  analytical methods, 209–212
    direct GC, 209
    direct HPLC, 209
    fructose determination method, 209–210
    HPAE-PAD methods, 209, 221–223
    inulinase method, 209–211
  in food products, determination of (modified AOAC dietary fiber method), 213–227
    HPLC method for, 215–221
    quantitative analysis for, 214–215
  legal status, 206–207
  natural occurrence of, 204–205
Oligosaccharides, 2–3, 595
  benefits of, 596–599
  in definition of complex carbohydrates, 134
  in definition of DF, 606
  HPAE-PAD in determination of, 276, 277
  See also Non-digestible oligosaccharides (NDOs); Resistant oligosaccharides (ROs)
"Other carbohydrates," 20–21, 46–47

Palatinose condensates (PC), 27
Pasta:
  DF content of, 336–337
  guidelines for complex carbohydrates from, 11
  resistant starch in, 387, 399
  total sugar, starches, and total DF content in, 151
Patent literature review (complex carbohydrates as fat mimetics), 431–591
  DF-based fat substitutes, 498–505
    bakery, 501–502
[Patent literature review]
    beverage, 501
    fruit paste, 503–504
    general, 498–500
    low-calorie foods, 504–505
    meat product, 502–503
  hydrocolloids/gums for low-fat and low-calorie food product development, 505–591
    bakery and grain, 517–518
    beverage, 518–519
    dairy, 519–528
    dessert, 528–531
    emulsifier, stabilizer, and suspending agent, 531–533
    fruits and vegetables, 533–535
    general, 505–517
    low-calorie foods: laxative, 559–560
    low-calorie foods: satiety and weight control, 554–559
    miscellaneous low-calorie foods, 560–591
    snacks, 536
    spread and salad dressing, 536–554
  starch-based fat substitutes, 432–498
    bakery and grain, 481–486
    beverages, 486–487
    dairy, 488–490
    dessert, 496–498
    emulsifier, stabilizer, and suspending agent, 490–496
    flavor, 479
    fruits and vegetables, 480–481
    general, 432–454
    meat products, 454–463
    method, 477–479
    snacks, 463
    spread and salad dressing, 463–477
Pectic substances, 122
Pectin, 349, 420
  HPAE-PAD in pectin research, 286–287
pH, high, anion exchange chromatography in, 275–276
Phenols, 67

Physically trapped starch (RS1), 125
Physiological effects of dietary fiber, 37, 43–44, 307–310
colonic function, 307–309
fat absorption, 310
polydextrose as soluble fiber, 234–238
disease prevention/intervention, 234–236
fermentation to short chain fatty acids, 236
gastrointestinal function, 237
glycemic index, 237
nutrient interference, 237–238
postprandial glucose response, 309
Plant exudates, 346–347
Poland, estimate of DF intake in, 93
Polydextrose, 27, 229–247, 415–417, 432
analytical measurement of DF, 238–244
AOAC method, 238–240
HPLC methods, 240–244, 245
complex carbohydrate definition and, 234
DF definition and, 232–234
physiological effects of DF, 234–238
disease prevention/intervention, 234–236
fermentation to short chain fatty acids, 236
gastrointestinal function, 237
glycemic index, 237
nutrient interference, 237–238
regulatory status around the world, 232
structure of, 230–232
Polysaccharides, 2, 72, 73, 606
PAD in quantitation of, 279–281
starch and non-starch, HPAE-PAD in analysis of, 277–278, 279, 282–284
Portugal, estimate of DF intake in, 93
Postprandial glucose response, effect of DF on, 309
Potato(es):
effect of cooking on DF in, 400
resistant starch in, 387, 399
Powdered cellulose, 351–353
Prebiotics, chicory fructooligosaccharides as, 29
Processing effect on dietary fiber in foods, 395–409
effects of different processes, 405–408
effects of processing on different foods, 399–405
possible changes in processing, 396–399
Psyllium content in ready-to-eat cereals, 317–325
materials and methods, 319–322
apparatus, 319
psyllium determination, 321–322
reagents, 319–320
sample preparation, 320–321
results and discussion, 322–324
Puerto Rico, DF recommendations for, 91
daily intake, 79
Pulsed amperometric detection (PAD), principle of, 269–273
Pulses:
DF content in, 335
resistant starch in, 387

Ready-to-eat (RTE) cereals, psyllium content in. *See* Psyllium content in ready-to-eat cereals
Recommended Dietary Allowances (RDAs), 8–9
carbohydrates in diet, 9–10
DF in diet, 10
Resistant oligosaccharides (ROs), 2–3, 25, 126–127, 229–230, 595
defining complex carbohydrates and, 134
defining DF and, 606–607

Resistant starch (RS), 125–127, 171–189, 357–358, 385–394, 397
analysis of total starch, 173–174
analytical methods for, 174–186
Champ method, 181–182
comparison of main methods, 182–185
method of Bjôrck et al., 175–176
method of Englyst et al., 176
method of Muir and O'Dea, 179, 180
classification of, 172
defining complex carbohydrates and, 134
effects of processing on, 397–399
in foods, 377
production of, 388–392
See also In vivo techniques to quantify resistant starch
Resistant starch granules (RS2), 125–126
Retrograded starch (RS3), 126–127
Rice:
guidelines for complex carbohydrates from, 11
resistant starch formation in reheated food, 399
Rice bran, 360–361
Roasting, 379–380
Romania, estimate of DF intake in 93
Root flour, 345–346

Salad dressing:
hydrocolloids/gums in low-calorie product development, 536–554
starch-based fat substitutes for, 463–477
Salt intake, dietary guidelines for, 9
Saponins, 67
Saturated fat, dietary guidelines for, 9
Science and the label, 39–52
AOAC survey on complex carbohydrates, 47–48
defining simple and complex carbohydrates, 44–45
dietary guidance issues, 42–43
[Science and the label]
methodology development, 45–46
overview, 40
panel discussion, 48–50
perspective on labeling, 46–47
physiologic effects, 43–44
Scientific Committee for Foods of the European Commission, 206–207
Seaweed extracts, 343–344
Seed extracts, 344–345
Seeds and nuts, DF content of, 335–336
Selenium, 67
Serum cholesterol, coronary heart disease and, 412
Short chain carboxylic acid (SCCA), 26
Short chain fatty acids (SCFA), 597
polydextrose fermented to (in large intestine), 236
Simple carbohydrates, 44–45
Singapore, estimate of DF intake in, 93
Snacks:
hydrocolloids/gums in low-calorie product development, 536
starch-based fat substitutes for, 463
Soluble dietary fiber, 329
hydrocolloids as, 342–343
South Africa, DF intake recommendations for, 89–92
daily intake, 79
Soybean oligosaccharides (SOS), 26, 27
Spain:
DF daily recommendations for, 79
estimate of DF intake in, 93
Sprouting, 381
Starch (starches), 36, 117–119
defining complex carbohydrates and, 134
definition and identification of, 36
determination of starch content in foods, 146, 148
digestion in humans of, 158–159
modified starch, 123–125
total starches, sugar, and total DF content in cereal grains, legumes, pasta and vegetables, 151
See also Resistant starch (RS)

Starch-based fat substitutes (patent literature review), 432–498
bakery and grain, 481–486
beverages, 486–487
dairy, 488–490
dessert, 496–498
emulsifier, stabilizer, and suspending agent, 490–496
flavor, 479
fruits and vegetables, 480–481
general, 432–454
meat products, 454–463
method, 477–479
snacks, 463
spread and salad dressing, 463–477
Starch polysaccharides, HPAE-PAD in analysis of, 277–278, 279
Steaming, 379
Sterols, 67
Sugars:
HPAE-PAD in analysis of, 276, 277
total sugar, starches, and total DF content in cereal grains, legumes, pasta and vegetables, 151
Suggested alternatives to the ''complex carbohydrates'' term, 35–38
Surgeon Generals's Report on Nutrition and Health, 10, 11–12
Sweden:
DF recommendations for, 88
daily intake, 79
estimate of DF intake in, 93
Switzerland, estimate of DF intake in, 93

Taiwan, DF recommendations for, 90
Task Force on Nutrient Labeling Analysis of the AOAC Internatinoal, 47–48
Technical Committee on Carbohydrates, 40
Thiocyanates, 67
Total dietary fiber (TDF). *See* Dietary fiber (DF)
Trans-galacto-oligosaccharides (TOS or GOS), 26, 27

Unavailable carbohydrate method of DF analysis, 76
United Kingdom (U.K.):
DF guidelines in, 10
DF recommendations for, 87
daily intake, 80
estimate of DF intake in, 93
United States (U.S.):
DF recommendations for, 82–84
daily intake, 80
estimate of DF intake in, 93
functional food development in, 598, 601–602
United States Department of Agriculture (USDA):
food guide published by, 8–9
Food Guide Pyramid of, 7, 9, 16, 40, 41
food label reform and, 17–19, 605
U.S. Senate Select Committee on Nutrition and Human Needs (1977), 8, 41
Uppsalla gas-liquid chromatography method for DF analysis, 76–77
Uronic acid, 146, 150
Uruguay, estimate of DF intake in, 93

Vegetables:
DF content of, 10, 337–339
guidelines for complex carbohydrates from, 11
hydrocolloids/gums in low-fat calorie product development, 533–535
starch-based fat substitutes for, 480–481
total carbohydrates and total DF in, 642–660
total sugar, starches and total DF in, 151
Venezuela, DF recommendations for, 91
daily intake, 80
Very low-density lipoprotein (VLDL) cholesterol levels, 55
Vitacel, 424, 431

Water binding capacity (WBC) of powdered cellulose, 352
Weight control:
DF in treatment of obesity, 65
dietary guidelines for, 9
relationship between fat intake and, 412–413
Wet heat treatment of dietary fiber, 378–379
autoclaving, 378
boiling, 378
canning, 378
microwaving, 379
steaming, 379
Wheat brans, 358–360
thermal treatment of, 399–400
Wholegrain cereals, resistant starch in, 387
World Health Organization (WHO), recommendations for dietary fiber intake by, 78–80
Worldwide dietary fiber intake. *See* Dietary fiber intake

Xanthan gum, 347–348, 421, 425, 431
Xylooligosaccharides (XOS), 26

Yogurt (yoghurt), 594
determination of recovery of FOS contained in, 194
Yugoslavia, estimate of DF intake in, 93

Z-trim, 424, 431